# Diseases of the Knee Joint

# Diseases of the Knee Joint

**I. S. Smillie**

*O.B.E.,* Ch.M., F.R.C.S.(Ed.), F.R.C.S.(Glas.)

Sometime Professor of Orthopaedic Surgery, University of St. Andrews
Emeritus Professor of Orthopaedic Surgery, University of Dundee
Honorary Research Fellow in Orthopaedic Surgery, University of Dundee
Honorary Consultant in Orthopaedic Surgery, Tayside Health Board
First Vice President of the International Society of the Knee

SECOND EDITION

CHURCHILL LIVINGSTONE  EDINBURGH LONDON AND NEW YORK  1980

CHURCHILL LIVINGSTONE
Medical Division of Longman Group Limited

Distributed in the United States of America by
Churchill Livingstone Inc., 19 West 44th Street,
New York, N.Y. 10036 and by associated companies,
branches and representatives throughout the world.

First published 1974
Second Edition 1980

ISBN 0 443 01382 9

**British Library Cataloguing in Publication Data**
Smillie, Ian Scott
    Diseases of the knee joint.—2nd ed.
    1. Knee—Diseases
    I. Title
    616.7′2     RC932     79-40943

Printed in Great Britain by T. & A. Constable, Edinburgh.

# Preface to the Second Edition

In this second edition I have completed, in so far as is possible, the separation of 'Injuries' from 'Diseases'. I have, for example, retained osteochondral fractures in *Injuries of the Knee Joint* whereas osteochondritis dissecans in considerably expanded form has, rightly or wrongly, been placed in *Diseases of the Knee Joint*. Developments in total joint replacement proceed apace. I have brought this section up to date in so far as my personal experience is concerned and in relation to the apprehension engendered by having witnessed over thirty different operations performed in a variety of countries in Europe and in the Americas. In the present state of our knowledge this procedure remains one to be approached with caution. If positive recommendations have to be made it is in the knowledge that problems of pain and loss of function in the age range concerned demand urgent topical solution. There are numerous other changes and additions to the extent of 40 000 words of new writing, 172 new illustrations and 110 new references.

I acknowledge the willing help and co-operation of my colleagues in the Department of Ortho-paedic and Traumatic Surgery of the University of Dundee, and in the Department of Orthopaedic and Traumatic Surgery of the Tayside Health Board: Mr J. Hutchison, Mr I. D. Sutherland, Professor G. Murdoch, Mr R. D. Muckart, Mr G. L. Clark, Mr C. S. Campbell, Mr W. Waldie, Mr B. C. Colvin, Mr T. Thulbourne, Mr J. W. Innes, Mr M. S. Turner, Mr K. C. Rankin and Mr H. Cuthbert.

There are many others who have assisted me and to whom I am grateful. In particular, Mrs A. M. McGregor, my secretary, who not only typed and re-typed the script but corrected the proofs; Miss J. B. Mudie, secretary in the Department of Orthopaedic and Traumatic Surgery in the Royal Infirmary, Dundee, and Miss M. Russell, secretary in the department in Bridge of Earn Hospital, Perthshire, have helped me with statistics. Miss A. Morrison, sister in charge of the operating theatres has helped me with the development of techniques and patiently preserved the aseptic regime on innumerable occasions while photographs were taken. Miss M. Benstead, lately medical artist in the University of Dundee, has been responsible for the line drawings. The other new half-tone illustrations are the work of Mr B. S. Mireylees, senior medical photographer, Bridge of Earn Hospital, Perthshire.

I wish to acknowledge the facilities made available to me by the University of Dundee and the Tayside Health Board.

My special thanks are due for the assistance I have received from Churchill Livingstone.

Milton of Drimmie,
Bridge of Cally,
Blairgowrie, PH10 7JR,
Perthshire, Scotland.
Telephone 025-086-245.
1980

I. S. Smillie

# Contents

# 1. Examination and Investigation

## Introduction

The knee is the largest of human joints in area of articular cartilage and of synovial membrane. It is the most complicated in terms of internal components. It is the most complicated in terms of mechanics: flexion is successively a combination of rotation, rocking and gliding movements far removed from the concept of a simple hinge. It occupies an exposed position at the junction of the longest and strongest levers in the body. It is, of the weight-bearing joints, the most vulnerable to trauma, incidental or repetitive in the form of wear and tear. There are few disease processes affecting joints to which it is not the most susceptible. It is thought appropriate that the introduction to a subject of such proportions and diversity should be devoted to examination and investigation. There are complexities which apply to no other joint.

The problems of diagnosis in disease, as opposed to injury, are different. If there is a dividing line between the two, which, in many instances is difficult to define, it is that disease involves the joint as a whole while injury involves individual components. In disease, the subtleties of clinical examination are few. In any event the ultimate diagnosis may be determined by the outcome of laboratory tests. In injury, the diagnosis depends on the interpretation of the detailed findings of clinical examination and, with the possible exception of radiography, seldom rests on ancillary investigations. It is a matter of difference of approach, adopted subconsciously by the experienced but to be learnt at considerable cost in other circumstances. Nevertheless, it is important that clinicians undertaking the treatment of diseases of the joint are familiar with every aspect of history-taking and clinical examination and of the possible interpretation of the findings.

In this first chapter it is proposed to suggest a sequence of events in order of importance which may lead to ,the establishment of a diagnosis.

## History

The importance of the history in any derangement based on a mechanical or disease process cannot be overstressed. The secret of success is thoroughness, and this applies to the history in particular because, in many cases of internal derangement, physical examination reveals no sign upon which a diagnosis can be based. It is hardly an exaggeration to cite the hypothetical situation in which it is required to establish the diagnosis, either from the history or from physical examination; but not on both. There is no orthopaedic surgeon of experience who would not choose to make his diagnosis from the history.

But listening to a patient's description of his complaints is time consuming. It is one reason why this aspect of investigation tends to be neglected. An experienced clinician will recognise the unintelligent and those garrulous with irrelevancies. The former must be questioned following a plan; the latter cut short without offence, with the explanation of the necessity to obtain the history in an orderly manner.

Time spent on purposeful history-taking is seldom wasted. A point, picked up in the course of a detailed history, can direct the way to a particular aspect of clinical examination which can confirm a provisional diagnosis. In routine examination, the sign, or the significance of it, can pass unnoticed.

**Method.** Time, it is repeated, is valuable in the contemporary scene. It can be expended in limitless quantities on the examination of a knee. If the examination must not be so slow and meticulous as to bore the clinician it is even more important that it is not so slow and meticulous as to bore the patient.

To take a history of maximum assistance in diagnosis the questioner must know his subject and thus know what he is looking for; and without, initially at least, leading questions. The history, unfortunately, cannot be taken by a secretary no matter how experienced; not even by another doctor. There is no short-cut. The proforma has uses in the field of medical records and in the assessment of the results of treatment in disease processes; but not in diagnosis. The history you must take yourself; and moreover, know how to do it.

What follows is a general guide in the approach to diagnosis. It is not intended to be comprehensive. The detail as it concerns systems or diseases will be found in the related sections.

### Name, Age and Sex

The first action in the approach to a knee joint problem is to read the letter of referral, if such exists. The history, taken by somebody else, is of limited value; but it may contain vital background information of which the consultant might otherwise be unaware. Note will have been taken of the age and sex, and whether the condition is the result of trauma, or of a disease process of acute or of insidious origin. These few details will permit a reduction of the probabilities to a minimum; but not the possibilities.

It is not intended and it would be tedious to attempt to cover every eventuality. The list reflects the approach of an experienced clinician to a problem of diagnosis armed with no more information than the age and sex of the patient and the bare facts of background such as might be contained in a letter of referral:

1. IN EARLY CHILDHOOD. The probability is so-called physiological genu valgum and the possibility, one of the rarer forms (Ch. 8).

2. IN ADOLESCENT MALE. With pain at the tibial tubercle, traction epiphysitis (Schlatter's disease) (Ch. 2), in other and more vague circumstances, osteochondritis dissecans.

3. IN ADOLESCENT FEMALE. With giving-way incidents, recurrent subluxation of the patella (Ch. 2) or a congenital discoid lateral meniscus (Ch. 12). If with bilateral intermittent pain and mid-line swelling, the possibility of a fat pad lesion (Ch. 4).

4. IN YOUNG ADULT MALE ATHLETE. With a history of an injury involving rotation, a meniscus tear; with injury involving considerable contact violence, a ligamentous tear.

5. IN YOUNG ADULT FEMALE. Recurrent subluxation of the patella or congenital discoid lateral meniscus are probabilities; the rarity of

meniscus lesions on the medial side is a point to be remembered. In the circumstances of persistent synovial swelling the wish to eliminate the possibility of rheumatoid arthritis will be paramount.

6. IN MALE OF MIDDLE AGE. With pain on the medial side of the joint in the absence of trauma will be recognised the probability of a horizontal cleavage lesion of the posterior segment of the meniscus.

7. IN FEMALE OF MIDDLE AGE. An attitude of caution with the probability of patello-femoral osteoarthrosis to be considered and the possibility of rheumatoid arthritis to be eliminated.

8. IN OLDER AGE. Osteoarthrosis in local or general form is the probability.

In general, it is a matter of knowing what to expect but not to be surprised by the unexpected.

It is at this point that particular questions arise:

WHICH KNEE? BOTH KNEES? OTHER JOINTS ALSO? That both knees are affected in relation to age and sex reduces the possibilities. That other joints are affected reduces the probabilities to a minimum.

DURATION OF COMPLAINT? The time the condition has existed distinguishes the acute from the chronic and is thus important both in diagnosis and prognosis.

INITIAL INJURY? The tendency to attribute human ills to an incident of trauma is well-known. It is important, therefore, that the nature and particularly the degree of the violence be assessed, i. e. *non-contact* in the form of rotation or *contact* in the form of a direct injury or blow. On the other hand, horizontal cleavage of the posterior segment of the medial meniscus can be initiated by a simple twist or, indeed, occur with no injury at all.

INSIDIOUS ORIGIN? If so, what was the presenting symptom, pain, swelling or loss of function in form of stiffness, block or obstruction to movement, or what?

## INTERPRETATION OF PRESENTING SYMPTOM OR COMBINATION OF SYMPTOMS

### Pain

The principal reasons for seeking advice are *pain*

and *loss of function*. It is well-known that of the two, pain, the most variable, unreliable and unassessable of symptoms, is yet the most common and most important single cause for seeking advice. It is a phenomenon that it has not been possible to quantify. 'What is one woman's ache is another woman's agony.'

**Sources of pain.** The most important single source of pain is the synovial membrane. The major example is that produced by the aggressive vascular hypertrophic tissue characteristic of rheumatoid arthritis; or of infective arthritis; or of the condition which simulates infective arthritis, calcium pyrophosphate deposition disease or pseudo-gout.

The other source is any *tension-situation* within the synovial cavity or other soft tissue stimulating nerve endings. The obvious example is haematoma in a situation such as partial, as opposed to total, rupture of the medial ligament.

**Nature and site.** If it is the presenting symptom the nature and site must be determined. Was it acute, as in an incident of locking, or a constant ache? Is it general throughout the joint or can it be located? The patient's opinion on the site of the pain is of diagnostic importance as, for example, medial joint line posteriorly, infrapatellar fat pad, patello-femoral joint, etc. Is it constant, related to movement after rest, or at a particular time, for example, in bed at night? A positive answer to any of these questions would point to a possible diagnosis to be confirmed or refuted by clinical examination. Pain in bed at night, for example, in a male of middle age, located to the joint line posterior to the medial ligament, would indicate a degenerative lesion of the meniscus.

A classical trap for the unwary, recorded in every text-book and taught to generations of students, whereby pain complained of in a knee originates in the hip joint, still accounts for misdiagnosis. The error occurs in the earliest degree of tuberculosis in childhood or of osteoarthrosis in later life at a stage revealed only by careful clinical examination; not when the diagnosis is obvious. The patient indicates the anterior aspect of the thigh and the inner side of the knee as the site of the pain. The exact mechanism is debatable. But the knee and hip joints share a common nerve supply through the obturator nerve, the anterior branch of which supplies the hip joint; the posterior branch terminates in the knee.

## Loss of Function

This description of disability, from the patient's viewpoint, covers a variety of complaints.

**Stiffness.** Stiffness may be defined as resistance to mobility. There are normal physiological variations in the sensation. It is greatest at the beginning and at the end of the day. In addition the phenomenon is closely related to atmospheric conditions increasing as the temperature decreases. In general this symptom, the inability to move freely after rest, is indicative of ageing articular cartilage and the breakdown of the lubrication system. It covers a multiplicity of circumstances, the most common of which are the various forms of arthritis and arthrosis. It is a symptom, but not the major complaint, in the commonest of all internal derangements of degenerative origin, horizontal cleavage of the posterior segment of the medial meniscus. In such circumstances it is explained by contact between the rough surface of the meniscus with the damaged opposing articular cartilage. In other circumstances the underlying gross pathology will be recognised as the source of the symptom. On the other hand it is unlikely in the early stages of a disease process, in view of what is known of the low coefficient of friction between articular surfaces, that stiffness is so related. It is probably located within the soft tissue elements from stretching of abnormal synovial membrane and/or friction between opposing synovial layers.

**Insecurity: giving-way.** This common symptom arises as a result of the interposition of some small object (as opposed to a large one as in locking, see below) in the form of a fragment of meniscus, articular cartilage or loose body between opposing articular surfaces under circumstances of stress. It can thus relate to a wide variety of pathological processes. Interposed in the hinge action of tibia on femur, or rotatory action of the screw-home movement, the most common underlying lesion is a tear of degenerative or traumatic origin of the posterior segment of the medial meniscus. In the patello-femoral joint, particularly in the presence of a flexion deformity, a tag of articular cartilage from chondromalacia is the most likely obstructive object. In gross osteoarthrosis the sensation can be produced by contact between irregular surfaces in some unguarded action. There is finally to be considered, in the absence of obvious explanation, the possibility that the symptom is related to no more than the existence of a minor flexion deformity and the related quadriceps wasting.

**Locking.** This is a symptom associated with the young male athlete rather than the patient suffering from a disease process. It is defined as a sudden and complete painful block to extension sustained by the mechanism of rotation in flexion usually in some contact game, commonly football. In such circumstances the block to extension, and to the screw-home movement, is due to the classical internal derangement, the displaced complete longitudinal or bucket-handle tear of the medial meniscus. In the realm of disease process, as opposed to trauma, locking occurs totally unexpectedly, out of the blue as it were, in the course of some simple domestic action from the interposition of a loose body between femur and tibia.

If these are the classical situations in which locking occurs exceptions are almost the rule: A displaced longitudinal tear may lock the joint at the age of 70; and a loose body separate from an osteochondritis dissecans lesion without previous warning in an adolescent.

In taking the history the statement that the knee 'locked' should not be accepted in terms of the definition and implications outlined above. The patient must be asked to explain what he means by 'locking' and demonstrate the angle at which the block to extension occurred. The sensation experienced at unlocking, if such occurred, is also important. In general, knees lock at 45° to 10° short of extension; and unlock dramatically. The description of 'locking' in full flexion, or full extension, or with a gradual return of movement should be accepted with reserve.

**Limitation of movement.** The complaint of loss of range of movement as such is unusual. But it depends on the circumstances of the case; and this varies widely. It is seldom, for example, that loss of those important last few degrees of extension which constitute the screw-home movement is recognised other than by the young

athlete seeking perfection of function. In circumstances of the ageing knee a flexion deformity of considerable degree may pass unnoticed. It will be recognised, in circumstances of gross pathology, that right-angled flexion is an acceptable range of motion for most social and domestic purposes; but anything less constitutes a disability.

## Swelling

Is it general or local? Was it of sudden or of insidious origin? Does the swelling involve the entire joint? Is it fluid, filling the synovial cavity, or is it the membrane lining the cavity?

A sudden swelling of the entire joint, within, say, half an hour, is a haemarthrosis. If it is superficial and located in the mid-line anteriorly, it is a haemobursitis; elsewhere it is probably a haematoma.

The insidious swellings of the entire joint are likely to have a more serious pathological background and often provide considerable problems of diagnosis. The most common local swelling of insidious origin is located on the lateral joint line in the form of cystic degeneration of the meniscus. In spite of the small size, its existence is likely to be known to the patient on account of pain associated with physical activity with the creation of a temporary tension situation.

## PHYSICAL EXAMINATION

### Prerequisites

If the history can be taken anywhere certain prerequisites are necessary for physical examination.

**Lighting.** It will be shown that observation is the most important act of physical examination. It is important that the lighting of the room is even and the same on one side as on the other. In this respect the walls of a room used for such examinations must be white; never one of one colour and one of another. Inspection is useless carried out on a couch against a wall from which there is no reflected light.

**Examination couch.** To examine the knee the couch must be free-standing and of suitable height so that the clinician can stand not only at the foot-end to observe both joints at once but at either side to undertake the necessary observations and manipulations. Furthermore, it is desirable that sufficient space exist on either side so that the profile of the joints can be observed from a distance in flexion (Fig. 1,4).

**Adequate exposure.** Patients are normally resistant to removing clothes. They are prepared for limited exposure of the affected knee; but not the other one. When the normal is examined first, as it should be, how often is it exclaimed: 'But it's the other knee, Doctor'.

It is essential to have the other knee visible for comparison, even if it too is abnormal. To pull up the trouser leg above the knee, if such is possible, is not enough. Both knees and both thighs must be exposed if embarrassing mistakes are to be avoided.

**Relaxation.** A patient, required to lie on his back while his knee is examined, will almost invariably raise his head to see what is going on in what for him is a new experience. It is understandable; after all, it is his knee. In such circumstances it should be explained why relaxation is important and why the head should remain on the pillow.

**Induction of pain.** In this respect also, and with the purpose of achieving and maintaining confidence, pain should never be induced without warning. If it is essential to invoke such reaction, the provocative movement should be purposefully relegated to the termination of the examination; and the possibility indicated. To induce pain precipitatively and unnecessarily at an early stage is to create a situation in which co-operation is lost in the atmosphere of apprehension. In such circumstances an erroneous conclusion may be achieved.

**Privacy.** When confronted with 'a difficult patient' with 'a difficult knee' it may be important to take the history and examine the patient alone; not in the presence of nurse, secretary, students or other patients as in an open hospital ward. The assessment of such patients is easier when they are deprived of an audience. In this regard too, and in circumstances in which exaggeration is evident, a second examination a week or so later may be conducted in a calmer atmosphere in which a more accurate evaluation of symptoms is possible.

## Approach

It is unrealistic to pretend that a complete examination is undertaken in every case. Examination of the joint, no matter how complete, leads in no particular direction without background knowledge. In any age group of either sex, there is a minimum of possibilities; and these are known to the experienced. In other words, the clinician, having heard the history, and confined the patient to the relevant details, examines the knee only in regard to the possible diagnoses to which his experience directs him: complete examination is irrelevant.

He looks at the patient's quadriceps 'perfect quadriceps seldom control imperfect knees'. If there is wasting, it is observed but not measured (Ch. 2). He looks then for points to which he has been directed by the history, the common degenerative lesion of the medial meniscus, patello-femoral osteoarthrosis, etc. In short, he confirms or refutes the diagnosis to which he has been directed; **or he begins again.**

The ability to diagnose internal derangements of the knee, and the massive related pathology, cannot be acquired from a book; not even this one. If the art of clinical diagnosis is to be mastered there is no alternative to acquaintance with the attitude and techniques of the expert: More can be learnt in minutes than in hours of reading.

## Inspection

The human eye is the most sensitive of the instruments of clinical examination. It can detect what cannot be palpated, measured or otherwise recorded. It is the facility to be exploited. It is important at all stages of the investigation of a knee complaint.

The patient should give his history in answer to relevant questions; and not otherwise. While doing so the clinician should be observing the uncovered knees in general and the one complained of in particular. By the end of the history he will have noted any abnormality of conformation, and if swelling is present, whether it is general or local, and if the latter, the precise site. In many instances the history combined with such observations, and essential academic background knowledge, make further examination almost superfluous. But it is indicated to confirm the provisional diagnosis; and that other possibilities are eliminated.

But observation, of course, is not and must not be, limited to what is seen as the patient sits before the examiner while the history is taken. It is a continuous process while the patient lies on the couch with the knees initially extended or later, flexed.

## EXTENSOR APPARATUS

The importance of observation as a method of examination has been stressed. The first action is to compare, standing at the foot-end of the couch, the development of the quadriceps on the two sides. The muscle should be observed first in relaxation and then in contraction, the patient asked to brace his knees against the couch. If a difference is noted it is pertinent, in a youth, to inquire if he is naturally right- or left-footed.

Observe thereafter whether wasting is uniform or whether certain elements are picked out, for example, vastus medialis. Differential wasting involving vastus medialis alone could be the clue to the diagnosis of recurrent subluxation of the patella.

It is at this stage that the existence of a minimal degree of flexion deformity, that is, loss of complete extension, may be evident. If so, the quadriceps will be wasted in some degree by comparison with the other side. If there is no wasting of the quadriceps there is not likely to be very much wrong with the knee.

Inspection of the muscle, particularly in relation to detecting minor degrees of wasting, is more important than measurement. Measurement is applicable to extremes; but not otherwise. A degree of wasting which cannot be measured can be appreciated by the eye. In any event measurement is dependent on the point at which the tape surrounds the limb and the tightness with which it is applied. In general it is useless in the female thigh with its frequent clothing of subcutaneous fat: the muscle may be wasted, the thickness of the fat is constant. Nevertheless, circumferential measurement is necessary if it is only for the maintenance of records.

In assessing wasting related to chronic disability care must be taken in using the muscle of the normal leg as the basis of comparison. The 'normal' leg is not normal. It has undertaken the function of the other leg in such simple everyday activities as rising from a chair, ascending or descending stairs. The muscles are in consequence hypertrophied. The experienced clinician makes a deliberate adjustment in his appraisal of the situation.

In the gross disease processes the condition of the quadriceps should be recorded as:
1. Strong.
2. Weak to resistance.
3. Able to extend against gravity.
4. Able to extend if gravity eliminated.
5. Flail.
See also Chapter 2, Lesions of the Extensor Apparatus.

## PATELLO-FEMORAL JOINT

### Inspection

The derangements of the mechanism, and of many of the disease processes, of the patello-femoral joint are so closely associated with the relationship of the patella to the femoral condyles that the approach to diagnosis is observation first in the erect position and then supine to determine that relationship. The existence of a large flat fat pad, and a discrepancy in form and development of the quadriceps by comparison with the calf muscles, are common clues as to the existence of patella alta.

**Lateral posture of patella.** When the history suggests subluxation of the patella as the possible diagnosis, observation of the joint in flexion in the dependent position may be helpful. The patient sits on the examination couch with the legs dangling relaxed at a right angle over the side. The joints are observed from in front and the direction in which each patella faces noted. Lateral posture of the patella at this angle, if in marked degree, may indicate instability. In any event the cause must be determined. Is it due, for example, to lateral torsion of the femur? In observing the patient in this position due note will be taken of the position adopted by the foot. It is the means of locating the site of medial torsion. Observation of the knees in this position is important because inspection in extension, standing or supine, does not reveal the abnormal relationship of patella to the femoral condyles nor the site of rotational deformity.

**Location of symptoms.** If in the course of taking the history it is established that the symptoms arise within the extensor apparatus, rather than in a component concerned with rotation, the exact site has to be determined.

1. ATTACHMENT OF QUADRICEPS. This location is rarely the site of pathology other than of gross degree, namely, total rupture; but such a possibility must be kept in mind in the middle-aged and the elderly.

2. PATELLO-FEMORAL JOINT. In youth, an abnormal relationship of patella to femoral condyles, in particular, patella alta with the related possibilities, must be considered. In adult life, chondromalacia patellae, and later, patello-femoral osteoarthrosis are the probabilities. In localising pain, as opposed to some mechanical obstruction to movement, it has to be remembered that articular cartilage has no nerve supply. Pain produced by manual pressure on the patella in extension or in hyperextension is likely to be due to compression of synovial membrane; not of articular cartilage (Ch. 2).

3. SUPERIOR ATTACHMENT OF PATELLAR TENDON. In early youth the Sinding Larsen-Johannson disease is a possibility. In later youth the traction lesion of the inferior pole without radiological findings and which lacks a precise pathological description (Jumper's knee) is a possibility.

4. PATELLAR TENDON. Pain located to the tendon may indicate a peritendonitis or teno-synovitis. In the differential diagnosis will require to be considered the possibility of a fat pad lesion or, uncommonly, a retrotendon bursitis.

5. INFERIOR ATTACHMENT OF PATELLAR TENDON. In the adolescent male the traction epiphysitis well-known as Osgood-Schlatter's disease is the probability. In adult life pain and swelling at the site is usually the residue of traction epiphysitis in youth.

## LOSS OF EXTENSION: FLEXION DEFORMITY

The earliest stage of flexion deformity is nothing more than absence of complete extension. Impairment of function implied by flexion is not assessed in degrees but the point in the range of movement at which loss occurs. It is the small flexion deformity which is important. Loss of 5° to 10° at the extension-end of the range eliminates the essential screw-home movement with consequent loss of function out of all proportion to the range of motion involved. But it will be accepted, in a volume which purports to deal with disease as opposed to injury, that perfection of function is frequently unattainable. It is important to appreciate, however, that complete extension is essential to perfection; and that anything less accepts a lower standard. In examination, therefore, whether in injury or disease, the estimation of extension is mandatory.

At the completion of the screw-home or back-lock position it is possible to stand, even on one leg, without external support with the quadriceps relaxed and the patella mobile to passive movement in every direction. Once the screw-home position is reversed, however, and there is slight flexion, the body-weight can be supported only by contraction of the quadriceps and thus with the patella pressed hard against the femoral condyles. This is a situation of considerable practical importance. In osteoarthrosis in general, and patello-femoral osteoarthrosis in particular, symptoms are precipitated not so much by advance in the degenerative process as by an increase in flexion to the point where, in maintaining the erect position, the worn articular cartilage of the patella is pressed hard against the worn articular cartilage of the femoral condyles. The result is pain; and often in considerable degree.

In the course of taking the history a patient should be asked if he has appreciated loss of the ability to extend. Reactions vary in relation to background, intelligence and education. In some, the absence of those few degrees which constitute the screw-home movement is immediately obvious. In others, 15 degrees of flexion passes unnoticed. Such is the variety of attitudes to which the clinician must adjust. The ultimate decision as to loss of extension, if there is any doubt, depends on examination in the supine position.

**Examination supine.** At this stage the patient is lying on a couch in a state of relaxation as indicated to be necessary. The clinician stands first at the foot-end of the couch to observe the comparable development of the quadriceps and then compares extension of the two knees in turn from the side, standing well away from the couch. A flexion deformity of more than a few degrees should be evident; and the reason is to be determined.

The subtleties of the situation are less in evidence in disease than in injury. If, for example, the complete longitudinal (bucket-handle) tear of the medial meniscus is the classical internal derangement of youth it is by no means exclusively so. It occurs at all ages and must be considered as a possibility even with minimal trauma. The tear, extending far into the anterior segment, is a block to the screw-home movement but obstructs extension only in minimal degree.

The initial approach, as it should be, is one of observation: the comparison of the two knees in extension on the couch. If it is not obvious that there is a difference between the two the effect of gentle manual pressure should be compared. A hand is laid first on the normal knee (assuming that it is normal) to effect a standard of extension, and only then upon the joint in question. If the slightest difference is noted, it becomes a matter of explaining the reason for the difference. It is at this stage that general background knowledge of the possibilities in relation to age, sex and circumstances becomes important.

The last few degrees of extension or, as is so often present in the female knee, hyperextension, can hardly be expressed in exact terms. In the more obvious flexion deformities of rheumatoid or other form of arthritis it is important that exact measurements are made and recorded. Such measurements are of value in assessing reaction to treatment whether of increasing the range of movement or of securing a reduction of deformity. The method, generally accepted as standard practice, is illustrated in Figure 1,1.

## LIGAMENTS

In a volume concerned with diseases, as opposed to injuries, the relevance of the examination of the ligaments may be called in question. In any event the matter is dealt with in some detail in IKJ5. In the disease processes, however, the ligaments have assumed a new importance in the context of total replacement (Ch. 6). It is for this reason that an abbreviated form of examination is appended.

### Medial

In the normal knee, if subcutaneous fat is not excessive, the medial ligament is readily palpable. It stands out as a strong band beneath the forefinger in the circumstances of the method of examination to be described:

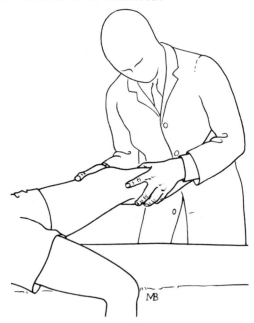

Fig. 1.2. **Examination: ligaments: medial.** To examine the medial ligament one hand fixes the femur above the joint, the other grips the tibia below the joint with the forefinger on the joint line where the ligament is located. By exerting pressure with the elbow on the foot the normal ligament should be palpable under tension; in other circumstances absence, attenuation or overlengthening can be estimated.

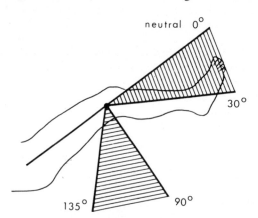

neutral 0°

30°

135°    90°

Fig. 1,1. **Examination.** Standard method of measuring range of motion and/or flexion deformity.

The patient lies on a firm couch, head resting on a pillow, relaxed with hands resting on the chest and fingers interlocked. The surgeon stands on the outer side of the leg. One hand grips and fixes the femur above the knee. The other grips the tibia below the knee with the forefinger placed on the joint line where the ligament is located. The inner side of the elbow is in contact with the medial malleolus. By exerting pressure on the inner aspect of the foot, with the femur fixed, a valgus strain is produced. In the normal knee the ligament is palpable under tension. In other circumstances the ability to open up the joint in varying degree is evident and the absence of a palpable band appreciated (Fig. 1,2).

## Anterior Cruciate

The patient lies on a firm couch, head resting on a pillow, relaxed with arms across the chest and fingers interlocked. In the initial stages *both* knees are drawn up to a right-angle for purposes of comparing the profile of the joint in question with the normal (see below, Posterior Cruciate Ligament and Fig. 1,4).

**Drawer-sign.** The diagnosis of rupture or laxity of the anterior cruciate ligament is based on the ability to demonstrate an abnormal degree of antero-posterior mobility of the tibia on the femur with the knee about right-angled flexion.

The surgeon sits on the patient's toes to fix the tibia in the desired degree of rotation. Both hands grasp the tibial head immediately below the joint. If the muscles are relaxed, as detected by the fingers in the popliteal space, a forward pull reveals the presence or absence of abnormal mobility by comparison with the opposite side. This is the so-called 'drawer sign' drawer forwards (Fig. 1,3). The sign is present in moderate degree in isolated ruptures with the tibia in lateral rotation. It is absent in medial rotation provided the posterior cruciate ligament is intact. The degree of mobility is influenced by the condition of the medial ligament. The sign is most marked in total rupture.

A common error of interpretation leads to the erroneous diagnosis of rupture of the anterior ligament when, in fact, the posterior is at fault. This mistake occurs because the posterior 'drawer-sign' (see Posterior Cruciate), in contradistinction to the anterior 'drawer-sign', appears spontaneously, taking the form of backward sagging of the head of the tibia when the knees are at right angles and the feet on the couch (Fig. 1,4). If this recession of the tibial head

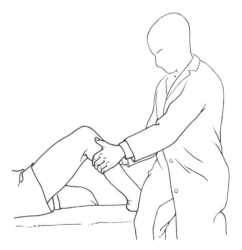

FIG. 1,3. **Examination: ligaments: anterior cruciate.** The surgeon sits on the patient's toes to fix the tibia in the desired degree of rotation. Both hands grasp the tibia immediately below the joint. A forward pull reveals the presence or absence of abnormal mobility. This is the so-called 'drawer sign' drawer forwards.

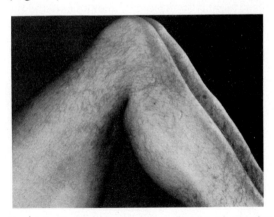

FIG. 1,4. **Examination: ligaments. Rupture of posterior cruciate.** In rupture of the posterior cruciate ligament when the profiles of the knees are compared in right-angled flexion the tibial head is seen to sag backwards on the affected side. The fact that the tibial head can be pulled forward, with the tibia in neutral or lateral rotation (Fig. 1,3), so that the profiles compare should not be interpreted as a positive anterior drawer sign. Forward displacement however beyond the normal profile may be possible in medial rotation.

passes unnoticed—and it is only likely to be noticed by deliberate observation in comparison with the sound side—the fact that the tibia can be pulled forward until the anterior cruciate ligament becomes taut may be misinterpreted as a positive 'drawer forwards' sign.

**Posterior Cruciate**

It is important to recognise that the so-called posterior drawer-sign, whereby rupture of the posterior cruciate ligament is indicated by the ability to push the tibia backwards, is theoretical in conception. Thus the posterior drawer-sign— drawer backwards—is a myth. It is not a matter of pushing the tibia backwards: it sags backwards spontaneously. It is necessary to compare the profiles of the two knees in right-angled flexion with the patient in the supine position; and to appreciate the difference between the two the examiner must stand well away from the couch (Fig. 1,4). Most important of all is not to confuse, in this position, rupture of the posterior with rupture of the anterior ligament. The mistake, and a common one, arises from the ability to pull the tibia forwards. In isolated rupture of the posterior ligament it comes forward in neutral or lateral rotation of the tibia only in so far as the anterior ligament becomes taut and the profile compares with the sound side. On the other hand forward displacement beyond the normal profile is possible with the tibia in medial rotation.

If it is shown by such means that the posterior cruciate ligament is ruptured it becomes neces-sary to determine whether the posterior capsule too is ruptured or, in other circumstances such as quadriceps paralysis, stretched. To do this each limb, completely relaxed, is raised from the couch by the heel and the degree of extension or hyperextension estimated. But a comparison between the two sides is not readily made when the difference between the two is minimal. In such circumstances resource should be made to the method applicable to genu recurvatum.

**Hyperextension.** If the knees hyperextend as in genu recurvatum, comparison of the degree of hyperextension between the two will not be possible with the limbs lying on the couch. To compare hyperextension a hand is placed on the knee over the suprapatellar pouch and the lower end of the femur firmly fixed against the couch by backward pressure. The other hand is now placed beneath the tendo Achillis and the heel raised from off the couch. A comparison is made between the two sides (Fig. 1,5).

**Lateral Side**

To establish the status of the stabilising structures on the lateral side, other than in the acute state, the hip is rotated laterally, the knee flexed to a right-angle and the lateral aspect of the ankle laid on the suprapatellar region of the

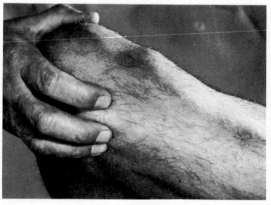

FIG. 1,6. **Examination: ligaments. Lateral stabilising structures.** The hip is rotated laterally the knee flexed to a right angle and the lateral aspect of the ankle laid on the suprapatellar region of the opposite knee. In this position the lateral structures under tension are from before backwards (1) lateral margin of patellar tendon (in front of forefinger); (2) iliotibial band (between fore- and long fingers); (3) lateral ligament; and (4) biceps tendon.

For the further implications of this manoeuvre in examination and in operative treatment see text.

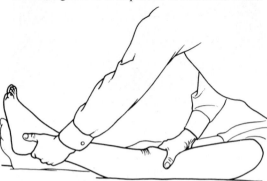

FIG. 1,5. **Examination: assessment of loss of extension or degree of hypertenion.** The knees are compared by fixing the femur to the examination couch with one hand while the other raises the tibia.

opposite knee. If in this position the muscles are relaxed a varus strain is imposed on the joint and the head of the tibia subluxes forward with a gliding action, the condyle becoming markedly prominent. In this position the lateral structures under tension are from before backwards: (1) lateral edge of patellar tendon (in front of fore-finger), (2) iliotibial band (between fore- and long fingers), (3) lateral ligament and (4) biceps tendon (Fig. 1,6).

This position has important implications in other forms of examination and in operative action. The finger tips on either side of the iliotibial band detect that in this position a con-siderable space exists. The manoeuvre can be capitalised in arthroscopy. If the arthroscope is inserted from the medial side of the patellar tendon and the position described adopted the widest possible visualisation of the lateral com-partment is achieved. In operation the same manoeuvre producing a wide gap between femur and tibia permits visualisation of the entire lateral compartment through the limited an-terior incision employed in meniscectomy(IKJ5, p. 169). Reference will be made in Chapter 6 to the utilisation of the manoeuvre to gain access to the postero-lateral aspect of the joint in synovectomy.

## SWELLING

### General

The first point to be decided is whether the swelling is general, involving the entire joint, and, if so, whether it is fluid or soft tissue, i.e. synovial membrane as in rheumatoid arthritis.

A synovial effusion outlines the horse-shoe shape of the suprapatellar pouch and is detected by the experienced at a glance. The test taught to generations of medical students, whereby a hand placed on the suprapatellar pouch raises the patella from off the femoral condyles and permits the 'patella tap' sign to be elicited, is not normally performed. In any event it is not pathognomic for fluid in that pressure on a synovial swelling as in pigmented villonodular synovitis or rheumatoid arthritis has the same effect. Synovial thickening can be distinguished from effusion by finger palpation of the margins of the suprapatellar pouch. Difficulties arise when the effusion contains massive fibrin clots

and in haemarthrosis when clotting has occurred.

The second question to be answered, if it has been decided that the swelling is general rather than local, is whether the entire synovial lining is affected, or whether it is the suprapatellar pouch in isolation. In this regard attention is directed to the 'joint lines', that is to say, the interval between femur and tibia on either side. In a tense effusion, which will be obvious, bulging at these sites is always present and should cause no problems of identification. It is in other circumstances that difficulties arise. If the joint is observed on the lateral side it will be seen, in general synovial thickening of what-ever origin, that the suprapatellar pouch is enlarged. Lower down, and corresponding to the joint line, is a second linear area of swelling.

If it is decided that the swelling is general and affecting the entire lining of the joint, all the

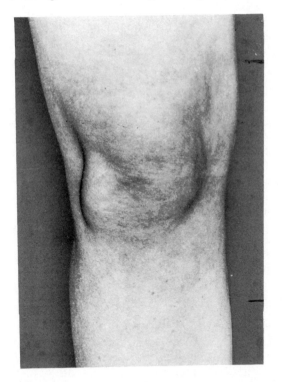

FIG. 1,7. **Examination: inspection.** The weakest area of the capsule, in the female knee in particular, is the gap between patellar tendon and iliotibial band. It is at this site that the extrasynovial fat protrudes in extension as a spindle-shaped swelling in the presence of increased intra-articular tension from synovial effusion or space-occupying lesion in the anterior compartment.

possible diagnoses related to such circumstances must be considered.

**Bilateral.** When the swelling affects both knees simultaneously, possibilities for diagnosis are reduced. The most common cause is trauma, recognised, as in a minor road traffic accident from contact with the dashboard, or unrecognised (see Ch. 3). Thereafter, in the absence of a polyarthritis are such conditions as widely apart as pseudogout and scurvy. When other joints are affected the most common cause is some form of rheumatoid arthritis.

## Local

A soft tissue swelling of firm but compressible consistency within the joint will alter in shape depending on whether the knee is in full flexion, mid flexion or full extension. If, for example, the space-occupying lesion is in the anterior compartment it will be under compression in full flexion and in full extension. The maximum swelling in such circumstances will be at the weakest points in the capsule. The weakest point of all, particularly in the female, is the interval between the patellar tendon and the iliotibial band on the lateral side; on the medial side immediately adjacent to the patellar tendon. The former area, however, is by far the weaker and the maximum localised swelling will occur at this site (Fig. 1,7). The medial capsule is uniformly strong and localised swelling on this side of the patellar tendon tends to be more diffuse.

If there is any doubt as to whether a local swelling is within or without the joint capsule it is merely a matter of asking the patient to raise the extended leg from the couch: an extra-articular swelling is unaffected by such action and remains of the same size and consistency.

Reference has been made already to the most common firm circumscribed swelling of all, namely, cystic degeneration of the lateral meniscus, a characteristic feature of which is the maximum prominence at 45° of flexion.

The most important form of local swelling is of considerably lesser degree and is not circumscribed. Indeed it consists of little more than loss of outline in the area affected. Such local swelling is an important and much neglected sign in diagnosis. It is of particular value in localising

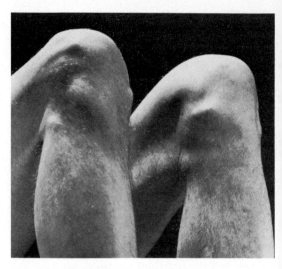

FIG. 1.8. **Examination: inspection/palpation.** The knees drawn up to a right angle for inspection and comparison of the joint lines for the minimal synovial swelling which might indicate, for example, a horizontal cleavage lesion of the posterior segment of the medial meniscus (Ch. 10) and for the purpose of eliciting local tenderness.

internal derangements relative to the menisci and especially in the most common lesion of all, horizontal cleavage tears of the posterior segment of the medial meniscus when it is related accurately to the joint line posterior to the ligament. The sign, whether present on the medial or lateral joint lines, is not readily seen unless the patient is in the supine position with both knees drawn up to approximately right-angled flexion (Fig. 1,8). The swelling is not immediately obvious: it must be sought. It is no more than loss of outline comparing one side of the joint with the other and, if the suspicion arises, with the comparable joint line of the normal knee. Local swelling, however, as a diagnostic sign of major importance in localising an elusive internal derangement, is not necessarily confined to the so-called joint lines. It indicates reaction in a structure with a blood supply, and that structure is synovial membrane. It will thus be seen only in situations where loss of outline is readily observed. Such situations include the medial and lateral sides of the patello-femoral joint and thus might point to such conditions as medial tangential osteochondral fracture, lateral marginal fracture, an anomaly of ossification, etc.

In most instances local swelling in the degree described is also the site of finger-tip tenderness; and this additional sign, carefully elicited, provides confirmatory evidence of localisation of the underlying lesion.

## TENDERNESS

### General

Tenderness, that is to say the ability to produce local pain by finger pressure, should, like manipulations likely to produce pain, be deferred to the termination of the examination.

General tenderness, over a wide area, is present in all forms of acute synovitis but is seldom marked unless the synovitis, or haemarthrosis, is tense. But extreme tenderness is a feature of acute infective arthritis and the condition with which it may be confused, crystal synovitis. If the infection is secondary to acute osteomyelitis it may be of such severity as to obscure the bony tenderness which might otherwise locate the source of the infection. In rheumatoid arthritis tenderness may be present on the entire circumference of the joint at the level of the joint line. In osteoarthrosis tenderness is rarely general but is related to some point of local mechanical interference with synovial membrane. In general, tenderness distributed over a wide area is not of diagnostic significance except to indicate the acute nature of the underlying affection.

### Local

If general tenderness is not of diagnostic significance, local tenderness, within a range of one centimetre, may, in certain circumstances be of such importance as to turn the scale in favour of a particular diagnosis. An example of such a situation in the field of trauma concerns the sprain, as opposed to total rupture, of the medial ligament commonly sustained in skiing. Tenderness in such circumstances is accurately located to the upper femoral attachment of the ligament; and it is largely upon the site of the tenderness that the diagnosis depends. Local tenderness on the joint line is an important feature in the diagnosis of meniscus lesions particularly those based on degenerative changes in the substance of the fibrocartilage.

Tenderness accurately located on the joint line immediately posterior to the medial ligament is invariably present in the horizontal cleavage lesion of the posterior segment encountered in the middle-aged of either sex. Tenderness located on the lateral joint line about the mid-point is found in the cleavage lesion which takes the form of the parrot-beak tear. In the displaced complete longitudinal tear tenderness can be elicited over the anterior horn just as the joint reaches what, in the circumstances, is the limit of extension.

Local tenderness is an important feature of the diagnosis of lesions of the infrapatellar fat pad, and of traction epiphysitis of the patellar tendon in youth, either at the tibia, so-called Osgood-Schlatter's disease, or at the patella, Sinding Larsen-Johannson's disease.

These are but a few examples of the many instances where local tenderness contributes in material degree to the diagnosis. When in doubt, and especially in circumstances of over-reaction, it is well to remember that exquisite local tenderness is virtually impossible in the absence of local synovial or other soft tissue swelling. The exception is meralgia hyperaesthetica, common about the knee, and of which the clinician should be aware.

## OSTEOARTHROSIS

### General

The assessment of the degree of wear-and-tear (osteoarthrosis) is necessary in many circumstances of clinical examination other than when presented as the provisional diagnosis.

Observation will determine whether the deformity, if any, is varus or valgus; and whether unilateral or bilateral. If the latter consideration will be given to the origin: primary varus angulation or, much more serious, medial torsion of the tibiae. Examination is directed accordingly.

It will be at this stage necessary to determine whether a deformity is of recent origin, that is to say, developed in the course of the last few years, or whether it has always been a feature of the conformation of the lower limbs but possibly becoming more noticeable of recent years. The degree of loss of extension, if present, will be noted and compared with the other, possibly normal, side. The clinical impression of the cause of limitation, soft tissue or bony block, is noted. The range of flexion, if limited, is measured and recorded (Fig. 1,1).

If angular deformity is present the importance of weight-bearing antero-posterior radiographs in the assessment of the situation is stressed (Figs. 1,9 and 1,10).

## Detail

In assessing the condition of the articular surfaces it will be remembered that even the most massive exostoses are largely cartilaginous and thus radiotranslucent. Clinical examination by the finger tips rolled over the medial margin of the medial femoral condyle in the manner shown in Figure 1,11 is therefore a more informative method of estimating marginal proliferation, and of comparison with the other knee, than radiographs.

In the absence of complete extension the rotatory action of the screw-home movement is not in evidence. The presence, or absence, of rotation at other degrees of flexion is an indication of the degree of wear; and this should be tested at 45° and at full flexion. The absence of rotation at any point, although not inconsistent with good function, is indicative of considerable degenerative change and reduction of the status of the joint to that of a simple hinge.

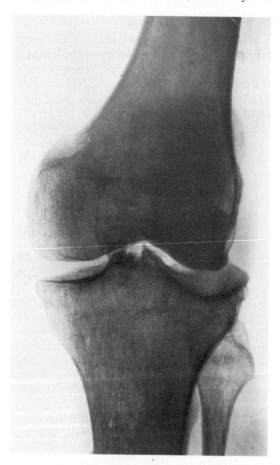 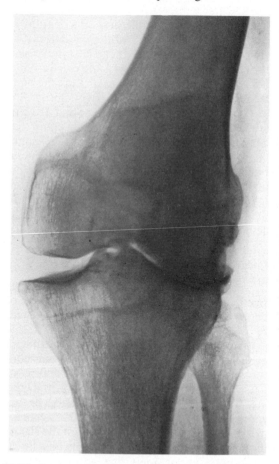

FIGS 1,9–10. **Radiological examination: exposure reflecting biomechanical status of tibio-femoral joint.** Weight-bearing radiographs are essential in assessment of angular deformity. Supine exposure looks relatively innocent (Fig. 1,9).

Weight-bearing exposure demonstrates absence of articular cartilage in the lateral compartment and an angular deformity of 20 degrees (Fig. 1,10).

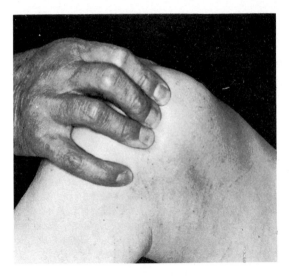

FIG. 1,11. **Examination: osteoarthrosis.** Exostoses are largely cartilagenous and therefore radiotranslucent. Marginal proliferation and the related degree of degeneration is more readily estimated with the fingertips than by radiographs.

## INCREASE OF LOCAL TEMPERATURE

**Method.** In examining skin temperature as an estimate of increase of blood supply, from reaction or other reason, in skin, underlying soft tissues or bone, the hand with the fingers touching is laid gently and delicately to conform to the contours of the anterior aspect of the joint. Comparison is made with the temperature on the normal side.

**Circumstances.** Any condition acute or chronic which entails an increase in blood supply to the part, general or superficial, will produce a local rise in temperature in the joint area. In the acute category is effusion, whether of synovial fluid or blood, from almost any cause, traumatic or infective process. In the chronic category is a wide variety of unrelated conditions. In this range, and with some attempt to record frequency of presentation but without statistical significance, are varicose veins (Fig. 1,12), Paget's disease (Fig. 1,13), pigmented villonodular synovitis, diffuse haemangioma, sarcoma of bone, etc.

**Warm knees and cold feet.** Attention will be directed to the importance of establishing the state of the circulation in a situation in which

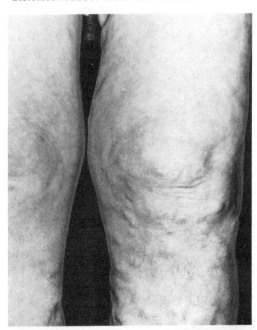

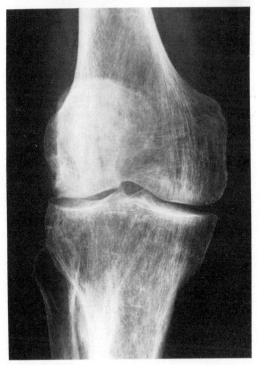

FIGS 1,12 and 1,13. **Examination: warm knees.** Among common causes of increase of local temperature are varicose veins (Fig. 1,12) and Paget's disease (Fig. 1,13). In this unusual example the disease crosses the joint line affecting both femur and tibia.

operative measures are employed in increasingly higher age groups. The existence of a warm knee in the presence of a cold foot should alert the clinician to the possibility of peripheral vascular disease in general and popliteal artery occlusion in particular. In popliteal artery occlusion, as opposed to blockage of the femoral artery above, the collateral circulation is always superficial with consequent rise in the skin temperature about the knee. Gaylis (1966) in explaining the situation calls attention to the fact that when this sign is present the main artery distally is always patent. It is clear that good collateral circulation cannot be established unless the arterial tree beyond the occlusion is reasonably unimpeded (Fig. 1,14).

TRAP FOR UNWARY. Patients seeking examination of an abnormal joint may have been wearing a bandage which they remove, or are required to remove, before entering the consulting room. The possibility that the skin temperature has been increased by the use of a bandage should be considered when there is no other obvious reason and the patient questioned accordingly.

## PERIPHERAL CIRCULATION

In the young athlete with an internal derangement necessitating operation there is the natural assumption that the peripheral circulation is normal. But internal derangements relative to the menisci are no longer confined to young athletes. The commonest tear of all, horizontal

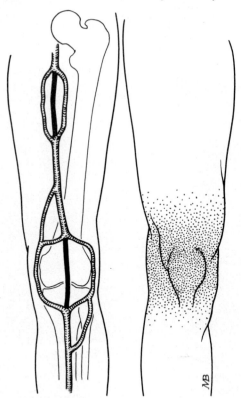

FIG. 1,14. **Examination: warm knees and cold feet.** In occlusion of the popliteal artery the collateral vessels are close to the surface with increase in local heat. In femoral occlusion the collateral vessels are deep and there may be no noticeable increase in local temperature. (After Gaylis.)

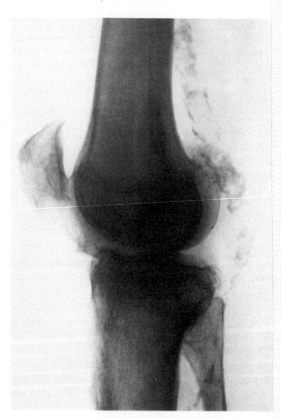

FIG. 1,15. **Examination: warm knees and cold feet.** In this example a good collateral circulation was established. But such a radiograph should alert the surgeon to the hazards of operative action (W.A., male, age 76).

cleavage of the posterior segment of the medial meniscus, is of degenerative origin and occurs in individuals undergoing an ageing process. Meniscectomy for this lesion is undertaken even in the eighth decade.

The assumption that the peripheral circulation is adequate is unjustifiable in the middle-aged or the elderly where the joint is the subject of a disease process possibly necessitating an operation under tourniquet control. It is most important therefore that the peripheral circulation of every patient be checked. If operation is contemplated, a preliminary check should be made of peripheral pulses and the patient questioned in regard to symptoms of intermittent claudication. (See also Increase in Local Temperature.) It is important too, in examining radiographs of patients in these age-groups, that the presence or absence of calcification in the popliteal or other vessels be noted. If there is suspicion of peripheral vascular disease the advice of a colleague with a special knowledge of such matters should be sought before operation is undertaken (Fig. 1,15).

Finally, and particularly in women, there is the question of the importance of varicose veins, previous attacks of phlebitis and varicose dermatitis to be considered in assessing the wisdom of operation in relation to possible complications.

## OTHER JOINTS

In conditions of traumatic origin the affected joint only need be examined using the opposite knee for comparison. In diseases, whether acute, but particularly if chronic, inquiry must be made in the course of taking the history whether other joints are affected and then these joints quickly observed even when no abnormality has been admitted. What appears to be mono-articular may be revealed to be poly-articular and thus point to the diagnosis as in rheumatoid arthritis, to cite the most obvious example. In diseases, as opposed to conditions of traumatic origin, the knee joint cannot be seen in isolation. The condition of the hip, the opposite knee and even the function of the shoulders, elbows and hands requires to be considered and may determine the treatment to be adopted.

## MOTIVATION

When local examination terminates in a decision which involves operative action, or conservative measures dependent on co-operation, an assessment of health in general and, in relation to degenerative disease in particular, physical configuration, overweight in relation to age, sex, etc., is necessary. In relation to chronic disease processes, as opposed, perhaps, to injury, an estimate of motivation is essential. The success or failure of surgical measures, with the possible exception of arthrodesis, is related to the will to recover. Operations dependent on co-operation in the widest sense of the term should not be undertaken in patients with outstanding claims for compensation, with litigation pending, or who otherwise have a vested interest in a continuing disability.

## RADIOGRAPHIC EXAMINATION

### Radiography and Pathological Anatomy: Limitations of Radiography

Perspective. 'The increasing technical excellence of radiography may tempt us to forget that we are still looking at shadows, and that no improvement in tomography or image-intensifying screens will convert them into substance. We may gratefully accept the increasing information they give us about pathological changes in bone or soft-tissue, but would do well to resist the temptation to ask too much of radiological anatomy . . . The study of radiographs is, and will always remain, a practical art, and we could all do well to remember that to expect of such an art the performance of an applied science does not enhance the art but serves only to debase it into quackery.' (Catterall, 1968.)

Radiographs depict bone; not the more important site of joint pathology, articular cartilage. Changes in the latter are advanced before radiological changes in the former are detectable. Considerable experience of the naked eye appearance of joint pathology must be acquired before it is possible to interpret radiographs in terms of what is radiotranslucent. Such skills are acquired only by orthopaedic surgeons.

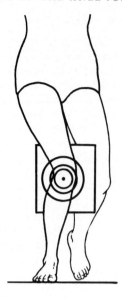

FIG. 1,16. **Radiological examination: projection to indicate biomechanical status of the tibio-femoral joint. Anteroposterior view.** To indicate the true tibio-femoral angle in, for example, osteoarthrosis, the patient must stand with full weight on the affected knee and with the minimal support of the hands. Just standing is not enough. Valgus knees may be touching, and, so placed, convey a wrong impression.

It is unfortunate that the more inexperienced the clinician the more faith he has that the radiographs will reveal the diagnosis he has failed to achieve by examination. The fallacy of reliance on radiographs for diagnosis is illustrated in the most serious injury of all in terms of permanent disability, namely, total rupture of the medial ligament. It has negative findings unless the clinician is thinking of the possibility and the exposure made under valgus strain. But even a fracture is not necessarily depicted unless the gap is 2 millimetres.

In the field of disease processes the fallacies are legion. Sclerosis of bone can be interpreted in terms of ischaemia. But what of a zone of rarefaction? It can be true rarefaction. But uncalcified cartilage, fibrous tissue, and, most important of all, an actual space, have virtually the same appearance. So much for describing pathological anatomy in terms of radiographic findings.

The more experienced the clinician the less he expects from radiographs. They are nevertheless necessary, indeed essential, in a variety of projections depending on the circumstances of the case. They are necessary to eliminate pathology undetectable by clinical means; and it is in such circumstances only that they should alter in material degree a clinical opinion. But there is always the unsuspected tumour, to cite the extreme example, or even osteochondritis dissecans.

These statements and what follows are in no way intended to decry the importance of radiography as an ancillary method of investigation, contributing, often essentially, to the diagnosis, but to place this universal means of investigation in perspective. But the accent, and the word to be repeated, is ancillary. Radiology is not, and never can be a substitute for clinical examination and, at least, provisional diagnosis. There is no radiologist of repute who would not agree.

## Projections Determining Biomechanical Status

This is not the occasion for a treatise on radiographic technique. The attitude of the

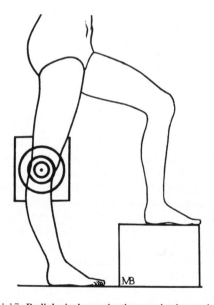

FIG. 1,17. **Radiological examination: projection to indicate biomechanical status of patello-femoral joint.** The relationship of the patella to the femoral condyles in extension can be determined only if the exposure is made in complete extension with the quadriceps in maximum contraction. In addition, the exposure determines the status of the tibio-femoral joint in terms of recurvatus deformity.

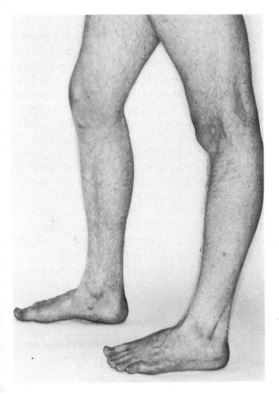

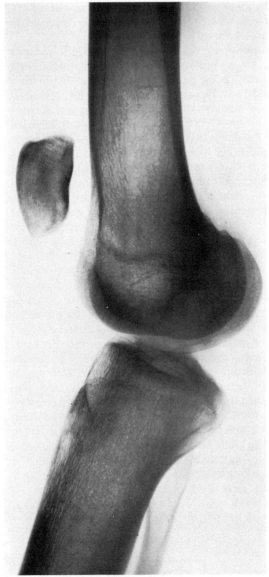

Figs 1,18 and 1,19. **Radiological examination: projection to indicate biomechanical status of patello-femoral joint and tibio-femoral joint in terms of recurvatus deformity.** Weight-bearing view in maximum extension with the quadriceps in maximum contraction (Fig. 1,18). Standard antero-posterior and lateral projections in the supine position would not reveal the biomechanical problems of this example of the patella alta/genu recurvatum complex (Fig. 1.19) (W.T., male, aged 20).

radiologist towards his art differs from that of the orthopaedic surgeon concerned as he is with the ultimate decision. The latter may, in many instances, be interested in the mechanics of the joint rather than the degree of disease process seen in relation to a situation in which many joints are concerned. He may thus be interested in projections which provide information about weight-bearing mechanics. Such projections may not appeal to the radiologist in the

investigation of a single joint but unfamiliar with the total problem as it concerns a particular patient.

The variety of conventional projections appropriate to examination of the joint are well-known and will not be recounted. It is proposed to describe a limited list of projections unrelated to the detection of bone pathology and not in routine use but important to the assessment of the biomechanical status, not only of the patello-femoral and tibio-femoral joints, but of the mechanical problems of angular deformity in the tibio-femoral joint.

**Antero-posterior view.** A straight antero-posterior radiograph of a knee with even a small fixed flexion deformity is a waste of time and material. Flexion, particularly in the presence of osteoarthrosis, entails superimposition of femur on tibia so that the joint space is not depicted. The projection thus conveys no information additional to that obtained from the lateral view.

If the bony outline of the adjacent joint surfaces is required, the beam must be directed in the line of the joint space; and this may not be a simple matter in the hands of a radiographer. It is the recognition of the fixed flexion deformity and the related problem which enables the orthopaedic surgeon who directs his own radiography to obtain the information he requires. Furthermore, even in the absence of flexion, but in the realms of disease processes and particularly osteoarthrosis, the so-called straight antero-posterior view carried out with the patient in the supine position does not convey the maximum information. The angular deformity and related instability which may be the cause of the symptoms is maximal only when the patient is weight-bearing. The antero-posterior view should therefore be taken with the patient's weight entirely on the affected leg. The angle between tibia and femur depicted is the maximum angulation likely to occur in walking as weight is transferred from one leg to the other (Figs 1,16; 1,9 and 1,10).

**Lateral view.** This projection is usually taken with the patient in the relaxed position supine

on the table; and the outcome may satisfy the requirements of the case. But it does not provide the maximum information. It does not indicate complete extension nor, as may be important, hyperextension. If such information is necessary the lateral view should be taken weight-bearing in what, for a particular patient, is maximum extension. This view, too, defines the relationship of the patella to the femoral condyles in extension provided the exposure is made with the quadriceps in maximum contraction, and not, as is possible, standing on one leg, relaxed (Figs 1,17 to 1,19).

If a lateral view is indicated in flexion, as is the routine procedure, it should be taken at an angle of 30°, the position at which movement is eliminated (Fig. 1,20). This gives some yardstick for comparison between knees, but, in any event, permits the distance of the patella from the centre of rotation of the joint in relation to the profile of the femoral condyles to be compared.

## Patello-femoral Joint

The antero-posterior view of the patella, obscured as it is by the femur, reveals little of the pathology present unless it is gross and involves both surfaces as in fracture or anomaly of ossification. The lateral view is more informative. It demonstrates the existence or otherwise of a joint space and thus the existence or otherwise of articular cartilage in the arc of the projection. The views which contribute the maximum information about the level of the patella in relation to the femoral condyles have just been described. In circumstances which direct attention to the patello-femoral joint as the source of the symptoms, tangential or skyline projections taken at 30°, 60° and 90° of flexion are essential not only to determine the shape of the bone but to establish the relationship to the condylar notch throughout the range of movement. If, for example, the symptoms indicate possible instability of the joint it is the relationship of the patella to the femoral condyles at about 30°, the angle at which subluxation occurs, which is of particular interest. To obtain this projection the patient lies prone on the table with the cassette beneath the knees flexed at, say, 50°, and with the feet resting on the

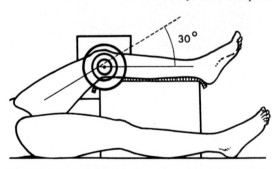

Fig. 1,20. **Radiological examination. Projection to indicate biomechanical status of patello-femoral joint.** The lateral view should be taken in 30° of flexion at which point movement is eliminated and thus provides a basis for comparison.

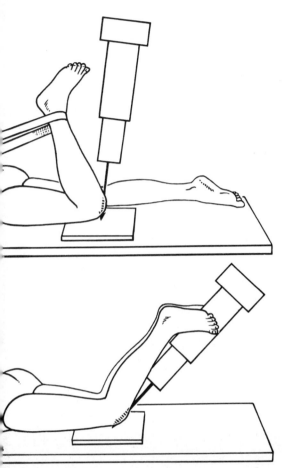

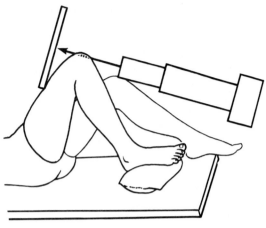

FIGS 1,21–23. **Radiological examination: patello-femoral joint.** Tangential views are necessary to the investigation of suspected pathology in the patello-femoral joint and to convey information not revealed in other projections. Figures 1,21 to 1,23 illustrate the methods to be employed in the various circumstances which may obtain.

tube neutral in respect of rotation of the knee joints. The tube is angled at 45°. The simultaneous projection of both joints on the same plate enables a comparison to be made between the normal and the abnormal in comparable circumstances (Fig. 1,23).

If the radiographer reports the inability to obtain the variety of infrapatellar views required, the existence of patella alta or patella baja should be suspected and the joint mechanics reviewed accordingly.

### Arthrography

If arthrography, using single- or double-contrast media, has any place in the investigation of disabilities of the knee joint it is in the field of trauma and in lesions of the menisci of traumatic origin in particular (see IKJ5). It has little place

in the investigation of the disease processes. The author has in general regarded the method of examination as unrewarding even in the investigation of suspected meniscus lesions. It is employed only in certain specific situations as, for example, to determine the nature, location and dimension of a cystic swelling in the popliteal space (Ch. 4) or giant synovial cyst of calf (Ch. 5).

It will be recognised that in the current scene arthrography as a method of investigation has been largely superseded by arthroscopy as constituting by indirect vision a more scientific method of resolving problems of diagnosis in the traumatic field.

### ARTHROSCOPY

**Background note.** The concept of an instrument for the inspection of body cavities dates back to the invention of the cystoscope by Nitze in 1877. The first arthroscope, based on the cystoscope, was designed by Takagi in 1918. The original instrument, with a diameter of 7·3 mm, was not a practical proposition. But by 1937 Takagi had reduced the diameter to 3·5 mm. In the current scene technical advances have reduced the diameter to as little as 1·7 mm permitting the diagnostic tool to be designated 'needlescope'. Arthroscopes, of which there is now a wide variety available, permit not only photography and cinematography but the introduction of instruments such as punch, scalpel, scissors and cautery.

**Indications.** Some of those who have written about arthroscopy in recent years reveal, perhaps not surprisingly, a singular lack of knowledge of the pathology and pattern of internal derangements. It would seem that arthroscopy, like arthrography, has the greatest attractions for the least knowledgable. Nevertheless it has an established and definable place in the ancillary diagnostic procedures as applied to the knee. It is applicable to a limited range of internal derangements. It is thus more helpful in the injury than in the disease processes. In cases of difficulty the clinician should be able, by history and clinical examination, to reduce the possibilities in diagnosis to two; seldom more. Arthroscopy should be employed to resolve such a situation. It is thus most helpful to the most knowledgable. It should not be used as a routine examination in the absence of provisional diagnosis in the hope that some pathology may be revealed to explain the symptoms. Such examinations cannot be other than misleading in view of the prevalence of subclinical pathology with which the knee abounds.

The procedure is useless in the hands of those unfamiliar with synovial membrane, articular cartilage and meniscus pathology as seen at arthrotomy. Unfortunately even in the hands of the experienced surgeon there is no place for occasional arthroscopy in circumstances of diagnostic uncertainty. To be useful practice of the technique must be acquired; and this is less easy than might first appear. In order to co-ordinate arthroscopic with direct visual pathology patients apparently demanding arthrotomy should be examined immediately prior to opera-

tion adding some 15 minutes to the operative time. With accumulated experience there may be the occasional case saved the necessity for surgical intervention.

In the author's experience arthroscopy has proved useful or likely to prove useful:

1. In determining the nature and extent of pathology within the patello-femoral joint. Reference will be made (Ch. 2) to specific circumstances of use.

2. In the resolution of certain problems of internal derangement relative to the menisci. In youth, is loss of complete extension due to a complete longitudinal (bucket-handle) tear of the medial meniscus? In the middle-aged or elderly, is it due to a flap of meniscus from a horizontal cleavage tear interposed between the condyles?

3. In the post-operative assessment of the results of conservative surgery as, for example, resurfacing (Ch. 10) and osteochondritis dissecans (Ch. 11).

4. In research where it is likely to contribute to our knowledge of the natural history of articular cartilage pathology, for example, the 'split line' or other injury inflicted by uncorrected meniscus pathology and the relationship to the development of osteoarthrosis.

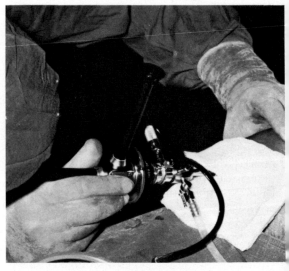

Fig. 1,24. **Arthroscopy.** If the role of arthroscopy is of less potential in the diagnosis and assessment in the disease processes than in internal derangements of traumatic origin it is of importance in assessing the condition of the components of the patello-femoral joint.

**Technique.** The technique of arthroscopy has been described in detail (Jackson and Dandy, 1976) and will not be repeated here.

# ERYTHROCYTE SEDIMENTATION RATE

It is unrealistic and impractical to suggest that the multiplicity of laboratory tests available should be applied to every case in which the diagnosis is not immediately evident by clinical means. It is a matter of reducing the probabilities

TABLE 1

Upper Limits of Normal in Westergren ESR.

| Age (years) | Males (mm in 1 hr) | Females (mm in 1 hr) |
|---|---|---|
| 18–30 | 7 | 10 |
| 31–40 | 8 | 11 |
| 41–50 | 10 | 13 |
| 51–60 | 12 | 18 |
| 60+ | 13 | 20 |

to a minimum and proceeding accordingly in utilising those tests which appear to be indicated to confirm or refute a provisional diagnosis. In this regard it should be recognised that the Erythrocyte Sedimentation Rate (ESR) is by far the most important laboratory test indicating inflammatory activity particularly in the common connective tissue diseases. It is of the utmost value as a screening procedure in the absence of a positive clinical diagnosis in the pressure of sheer numbers of patients imposed by a free health service. In the examination and investigation of the knee, as opposed to certain other joints, the possible diagnoses are legion. The proportion of cases in which a definite diagnosis cannot be achieved at a single examination is high even in experienced hands. In practical terms it is a matter of distinguishing swelling from a simple unspecified internal derangement of traumatic origin which will subside without treatment, from the earliest stage of rheumatoid arthritis, tuberculosis or even malignancy. It is in such circumstances that the ESR screen can identify in one hour those cases requiring more detailed attention and investigation.

# ASPIRATION

This procedure is commonly required in the course of investigation of the contents of the joint; as a therapeutic measure to reduce tension; or to secure replacement by fresh synovial fluid in, for example, infection.

It should be carried out only under aseptic precautions. The possibility of the introduction of infection is not academic theory. It is a practical reality.

**Technique.** The skin is prepared over a wide area with some appropriate antiseptic. The author favours 2 per cent iodine in 70 per cent ethyl alcohol. A minimum period of two minutes of swabbing is required. In the absence of local contraindications the lateral aspect of the joint is the favoured site for entry of the needle: operations are unencumbered by the presence of the other limb; but in any event the medial side is undesirable from the presence of vastus medialis which may be temporarily inhibited if subjected to trauma. The site chosen should permit the needle to be entered beneath the patella towards the superior pole or in the suprapatellar pouch immediately above the superior pole. A weal is raised in the skin with local anaesthetic using a fine needle. The soft tissues down to and including the synovial membrane are infiltrated. The aspirating needle should be of wide bore with a short bevel so that the minimum of injury is inflicted on the synovial membrane: it is desirable to avoid haemorrhage into the joint and contamination of the aspirated fluid by blood. To this end also a hand is placed high on the suprapatellar pouch and backward pressure exerted while the needle is entered. In this way the patella is raised from the femoral condyles leaving a space for the needle and thus minimal trauma to synovial tissue. If a condition such as pigmented villonodular synovitis with abnormally vascular synovial membrane is suspected, the needle should be entered beneath the patella.

When the procedure is completed the wound is sealed and a compression bandage applied.

EXAMINATION. Normal synovial fluid is clear, pale yellow, viscid and does not clot. Gross abnormalities are of diagnostic signficance: blood, or a mixture of blood and synovial fluid in a variety of proportions, is an indication of the degree of severity of an injury to a vascular structure such as ligament or synovial membrane as opposed to injury to an avascular structure, no matter how important, such as meniscus. It may be a matter of distinguishing between *injury* to synovial membrane as opposed to *irritation* of synovial membrane.

In the disease process the presence of blood in high proportion is unusual other than in haemophilia and related diseases; even scurvy. Fat, or fat and blood, is an indication of intra-articular fracture involving cancellous tissue. In infection appearance will vary between cloudiness and frank pus.

Much has been written about the naked-eye appearance of abnormal synovial fluid in regard to cloudiness, as an indication of cell or crystal content, and of physical characteristics such as viscosity, clotting, etc. But in a work concerned with practical considerations it must be accepted that in the present state of knowledge, neither appearance nor the routine analysis of aspirated fluid are of more than marginal value to the clinician confronted with the problem of a doubtful diagnosis. Abnormality of appearance and physical character indicate abnormality of origin; but little more specific than that. On the contrary, cultures, and, with the possibility of tuberculosis in mind, guinea-pig inoculation, are proceedings of proved value. In recent times the identification of specific crystals has increased the ability to achieve a positive diagnosis in gout and pseudo-gout.

The rheumatoid factor can be detected in synovial fluid, but, as in serum, is not specific (Ch. 6).

## BIOPSY

In theory synovial biopsy appears to be the ultimate means of diagnosis in circumstances of difficulty by clinical and biochemical methods. In practice, and regrettably, there is no single histopathological change which identifies rheumatoid arthritis, the major diagnostic problem in the current scene. In other circumstances of difficulty, for example, villonodular synovitis, the experienced surgeon will recognise the condition at the biopsy operation: histological examination is almost superfluous. Even in suspected tuberculosis, biopsy has limitations

in favour of other methods. The attitude to be adopted in chronic 'non-specific synovitis' when all routine investigations have failed to establish a diagnosis and synovial biopsy is the last resort is detailed in Chapter 3.

## ASSESSMENT

In recent years it has been evident that the methods adopted by orthopaedic surgeons of assessing results of treatment, operative or otherwise, by what can only be described as impression, is unsatisfactory. The bona fides of surgeons is not in question. It is a simple matter of human frailty in which so many factors are involved: the essential drive, personality and optimism of the surgeon; the natural wish for improvement, desire to please and to be grateful on the part of the patient.

There are few fields in which the assessment of results have been more difficult than in the conservative surgery of the knee joint particularly in the treatment of rheumatoid arthritis and osteoarthrosis.

It is such considerations which have stimulated, in the North American scene, more scientific methods, if that is the phrase, of assessing improvement or otherwise. The subjective and objective are often at variance. Patient and surgeon have no common baseline. The patient seeks the unattainable. To the surgeon, with his knowledge of surgical pathology, success is achieved at a lower level. The eventual arthrodesis of a tuberculous knee, the site of multiple sinuses, is an achievement for the surgeon; a disaster for the patient who expects a normal mobile joint.

It would be intellectually dishonest to pretend that the author has used these methods of assessment in the cases recorded; but that is not to decry, rather to approve, more scientific methods. On the other hand the pro forma basis of assessment assumes a competence in examination which, in fact, does not exist. The number of times in which patients have been referred for a second opinion on the assumption of a lesion of the anterior cruciate ligament when, on examination, the posterior cruciate ligament was the source of the disability is an indication of the nature of the problem.

TABLE 2

One-hundred point scale for assessment of knee disability (Geens *et al.*, 1969).

| | | Left knee | | Right knee | |
|---|---|---|---|---|---|
| | | Before | After | Before | After |
| A. Function: max. 35 points. | | | | | |
| Does most of housework or job which requires moving about | 5 | | | | |
| Walks enough to be independent | 5 | | | | |
| Dresses unaided (includes tying shoes and putting on socks) | 5 | | | | |
| Sits without difficulty at table or toilet, including sitting down and getting up (reduce if additional aid is necessary) | 4 | | | | |
| Picks up objects from floor by squatting or kneeling | 3 | | | | |
| Baths without help | 3 | | | | |
| Negotiates stairs foot over foot | 3 | | | | |
| Negotiates stairs in any manner | 2 | | | | |
| Carries objects comparable to suitcase | 2 | | | | |
| Gets into car or public conveyance unaided and rides comfortably | 2 | | | | |
| Drives a car | 1 | | | | |
| B. Freedom from pain: max. 35 points. | | | | | |
| No pain | 35 | | | | |
| Mild pain with fatigue | 30 | | | | |
| Mild pain with weight-bearing | 20 | | | | |
| Moderate pain with weight-bearing | 15 | | | | |
| Severe pain with weight-bearing, mild or moderate at rest | 10 | | | | |
| Severe continuous pain | 0 | | | | |
| C. Gait: max. 10 points. | | | | | |
| No limp, no support | 10 | | | | |
| Limp, no support | 8 | | | | |
| One cane or crutch | 8 | | | | |
| One long brace | 8 | | | | |
| One brace with crutch of cane | 6 | | | | |
| Two crutches with or without a brace | 4 | | | | |
| Cannot walk | 0 | | | | |
| D. Absence of deformity of instability: max. 10 points. | | | | | |
| No fixed flexion over 10 degrees with weight-bearing | 3 | | | | |
| No fixed flexion over 20 degrees with weight-bearing | 2 | | | | |
| No fixed flexion over 30 degrees with weight-bearing | 1 | | | | |
| No lateral deformity over 10 degrees with weight-bearing | 3 | | | | |
| No lateral deformity over 20 degrees with weight-bearing | 2 | | | | |
| No lateral deformity over 30 degrees with weight-bearing | 1 | | | | |
| No ligamentous instability | 2 | | | | |
| No locking, no giving-way or extension lag over 10 degrees | 2 | | | | |
| E. Range of motion: 10 points. | | | | | |
| Total amount of flexion-extension degrees (normal 150 degrees). | | | | | |
| Points (one point for each 15 degrees) | 10 | | | | |
| Total Score | | | | | |

TABLE 3

## KNEE FUNCTION ASSESSMENT CHART
(British Orthopaedic Association Research Sub-committee)

**Name** . . . . . . . . . . . . . . . . . . . . . . . . . . . . . . . . . . . . . . . . . . . . . . . . .

Age . . . . . . . . . . . . . . . . . . .        Sex . . . . . . . . . . . . . . . . . . . . . . . .

Hospital number . . . . . . . . . . . . . . . . . . . . . . .

Occupation . . . . . . . . . . . . . . . . . . . . . . . . . . . . . . . . . . . . . . . . .

**Diagnosis** . . . . . . . . . . . . . . . . . . . . . . . . . . . . . . . . . . . . .

Duration of disease        General                           (years)

                           Knee                              (years)

Side . . . . . . . . . . . . . . . .

Previous knee operations . . . . . . . . . . . . . . . . . . . . . . . . . . . . . . . . . . . . . . . . . . . . . . . . . . . . . . . . . . . . .

. . . . . . . . . . . . . . . . . . . . . . . . . . . . . . . . . . . . . . . . . . . . . . . . . . . . . . . . . . . . . . . . . . . . . . . . . . . . . . . .

*Other joints (see Appendix)* . . . . . . . . . . . . . . . . . . . . . . . . . . . . . . . . . . . . . . . . . . . . . . . . . . . . . . . . . . . . . . . .

---

STATE OF OTHER KNEE     Normal
Slightly affected
Moderately affected
Severely affected
Replaced

STATE OF HIPS    RIGHT        LEFT
Normal
Slightly affected
Moderately affected
Severely affected
Replaced

STATE OF FEET/    RIGHT       LEFT
ANKLES             Normal
Slightly affected
Moderately affected
Severely affected
Replaced

**FOLLOW UP (months)**

1. ASSESSMENT  BY  THE  PATIENT
   A. After treatment the patient is:
      (4)  Enthusiastic
      (3)  Satisfied
      (2)  Non-committal
      (1)  Disappointed
   B. Is the patient's present disability due to the affected
      knee?
      (4)  Entirely
      (3)  Mainly
      (2)  Partially
      (1)  Scarcely at all

2. PAIN
   (4)  None
   (3)  Mild pain, not interfering with activities or sleep
   (2)  Moderate pain, either reducing activities or dis-
        turbing sleep
   (1)  Severe pain

3. ABILITY TO WALK

| | *Distance*     OR | *Time* |
|---|---|---|
| (5) | >1 kilometre (unlimited) | >60 minutes |
| (4) | Up to 1 kilometre | 30–60 minutes |
| (3) | Up to 50 metres | 10–30 minutes |
| (2) | 50–100 metres (outdoors) | 5–10 minutes |
| (1) | Indoors only | Indoors only |
| (0) | Unable | Unable |

4. WALKING AID
   (4)  None
   (3)  Stick outside
   (2)  Stick always
   (1)  Two sticks/crutches/frame
   (0)  Unable to walk

5. GAIT
   (4)  Normal free swing
   (3)  Slight limitation of swing
   (2)  Minimal movement
   (1)  Stiff knee

6. FLEXION DEFORMITY
   (5)  0 degrees
   (4)  <10 degrees
   (3)  11–20 degrees
   (2)  21–30 degrees
   (1)  >30 degrees

7. MAXIMUM FLEXION
   (4)  >100 degrees
   (3)  81–100 degrees
   (2)  61–80 degrees
   (1)  <60 degrees

8. EXTENSION LAG
   Additional to flexion contracture if present
   (4)  0 degrees
   (3)  <10 degrees
   (2)  <20 degrees
   (1)  >20 degrees

TABLE 3—*cont.*

9. VALGUS ANGLE
    When the tibia is
    stressed laterally
    (4) 0–10 degrees
    (3) <20 degrees
    (2) <30 degrees
    (1) >30 degrees

10. VARUS ANGLE
    When the tibia is
    stressed medially
    (5) 0 degrees
    (4) <10 degrees
    (3) <20 degrees
    (2) <30 degrees
    (1) >30 degrees

11. ABILITY TO GET OUT OF CHAIR
    (4) With ease
    (3) With difficulty
    (2) Only by using arms
    (1) Unable

12. ABILITY TO CLIMB STAIRS
    (4) Normal
    (3) One step at a time
    (2) Only with a bannister, stick or both
    (1) Unable or only by bizarre method

### APPENDIX
### STATE OF OTHER JOINTS

SLIGHTLY AFFECTED
    Infrequent pain
    Minor stiffness—no functional deficit
    Walking minimally affected. No support required

MODERATELY AFFECTED
    Moderate pain
    Joint stiffness producing some function deficit
    Walking interrupted and support required

SEVERELY AFFECTED
    Severe pain
    Stiffness with marked functional disability
    Unable to walk or walking with difficulty using a major
    support

There is no limit to the possibilities in length, detail and complication of a pro forma. But the collection of minutiae, largely irrelevant to the presenting problem, is unrealistic. Two examples of assessment sheets are included to illustrate the attitude which should be adopted. The first (Table 2) is that of Geens *et al.* (1969). The second (Table 3), somewhat different, was developed by a research sub-committee of the British Orthopaedic Association (Aichroth *et al.*, 1978). The chart has minimal features recorded in a simple way. This has led to compromise and over-simplification but with the advantage that it can be completed by relatively inexperienced members of staff. It records basic parameters. A surgeon with a specific interest in the subject will require additional facts appropriate to his specific needs.

## REFERENCES

AICHROTH, P., FREEMAN, M. A. R., SMILLIE, I. S. & SOUTER, W. A. (1978). A knee function assessment chart. *Journal of Bone and Joint Surgery*, **60B,** 308.

CATTERALL, R. C. F. (1968). *Journal of Bone and Joint Surgery*, **50B,** 3, 455.

GAYLIS, H. (1966) Warm knees and cold feet, *Lancet*, **ii,** 792.

GEENS, S., CLAYTON, M. L., LEIDHOLT, J. D., SMYTH, C. J. & BARTHOLOMEW, B. A. (1969). Synovectomy and debridement of the knee in rheumatoid arthritis. *Journal of Bone and Joint Surgery*, **51-A,** 4, 626.

HILDER, F. M. & GUNZ, F. W. (1964). *Clinical Pathology*, **17,** 292.

JACKSON, R. W. & DANDY, D. J. (1976). *Arthroscopy of the Knee*. New York: Grune & Stratton.

# 2.  Lesions of Extensor Apparatus

## QUADRICEPS MUSCLE: CONGENITAL AFFECTIONS

### PROGRESSIVE FIBROSIS

**Definition.** The condition presents in the infant or young child as progressive loss of flexion in the knee joint due to contracture of elements of the quadriceps muscle.

**Background note.** The establishment of the condition as a clinical entity is attributed to Hnevkovsky (1961), who first stimulated interest by his report of progressive fibrosis of the vastus intermedius. Although clinical manifestations of such contracture were known in congenital recurvatus or dislocation, recent additions to the literature may be due partly to the increase in the use of antibiotics, and partly to recognition of the underlying pathology in progressive loss of knee motion in childhood, and of habitual, as opposed to recurrent, disloca-

tion of the patella in later life (Williams, 1968).

**Aetiology.** In patients presenting at birth the condition is of the same origin, if in a lesser degree, as the form of arthrogryposis which produces congenital genu recurvatum. Those who present in the next few years are more difficult to explain on a congenital basis and the possibility of extrinsic causes arises. In this regard it has been shown that patients in this age group have received intramuscular injections, usually of antibiotics, into the thigh soon after birth [Gunn, 1964; Lloyd-Roberts and Thomas, 1964; Bose and Chong, 1976 (20 out of 38 cases)]. It is known that such injections produce oedema and haemorrhage; and it is likely that this progresses to fibrosis and contracture. In regard to aetiology, however, while the condition is known as 'progressive' fibrosis, it is not

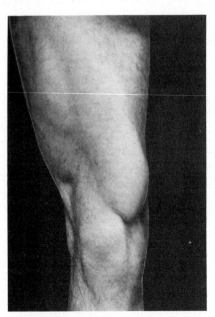

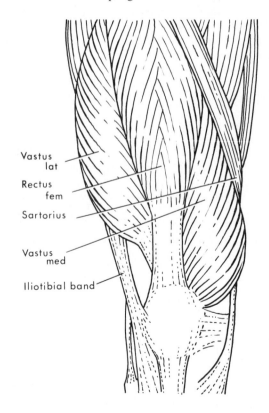

Vastus
lat

Rectus
fem

Sartorius

Vastus
med

Iliotibial band

FIGS 2,1–2. **Extensor apparatus.** Quadriceps of a weight-lifter to show components (Fig. 2,1) and a line drawing identifying them (Fig. 2,2).

the fibrosis which is progressive. It is the growth of the bone which is progressive with consequent increase of flexion deformity.

**Site of lesion.** The condition involves the more lateral elements of the quadriceps, vastus intermedius, rectus femoris and vastus lateralis. Vastus medialis is not implicated. This corresponds to the findings in congenital genu recurvatum; and also to the site of fibrosis following injection or infusion in which the anterior and lateral aspects of the thigh would be likely to be implicated. In the later stages, and possibly for the same reason, the fascia lata may be involved.

**Clinical features.** The child is presented at the average age of three with limitation of flexion in one or both knees. The loss of flexion if kept under observation is progressive. There is frequently a history of prematurity or of the infant having suffered a severe illness after birth.

The limitation of flexion presents in a characteristic way: in active or passive flexion there is a sudden block to movement always at the same point and as if a solid obstacle had been encountered. Movement is not limited by pain; and attempts at forced flexion do not induce pain. At the limit of flexion it may be possible to palpate a tendon-like structure attached to the patella.

**Treatment**

There is no treatment short of operation which has any effect on the natural history of the disease; and it is important that this should be recognised when the diagnosis is made. Failure to restore the situation leads to progressive loss of flexion, patella alta, chondromalacia and finally to habitual dislocation of the patella.

**Operation.** The nature and extent of the operation depends on the pathological findings in the individual case. The object is division, or resection, of the fibrosed elements of the muscle and the lengthening, should this prove to be necessary, of the quadriceps tendon.

**Technique.** The patient is placed in the supine position on the table and a high tourniquet applied. The incision is made along the lateral border of rectus femoris in the lowest third of the thigh. On dividing the deep fascia, adhesion of fascia lata to vastus lateralis, or even of a fibrous attachment to the patella, may be revealed. The vastus lateralis and vastus intermedius are examined and limiting fibrosis located

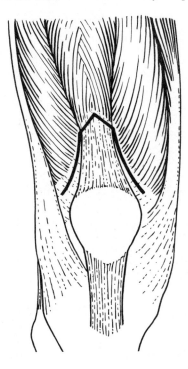

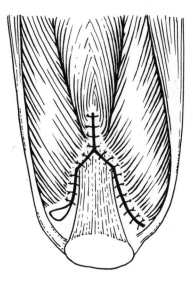

FIGS 2,3–4. **Progressive quadriceps fibrosis: treatment.** If the rectus femoris element of the quadriceps is restricted, the Bennett type of lengthening may be required.

by flexing the knee. Bands are divided, resected or tendons lengthened as the occasion demands. The lateral expansion may require division as also are adhesions in the suprapatellar pouch. If the rectus femoris restricts flexion, Z or the Bennett (1922) lengthening may be required (Figs 2,3 and 2,4).

AFTER-TREATMENT. At the termination of the operation a padded plaster cast with the knee at right-angled flexion is applied. The cast is retained for about four weeks. If lengthening of the rectus femoris has been necessary a considerable extension lag may be expected in the early stages of the return to weight-bearing. In the circumstances of flexion returning with the simple division of vastus intermedius a rapid return to normal is to be expected, particularly in the youngest patients who have not developed secondary changes in the capsule, ligaments or in the articular cartilage of the patella.

**Quadriceps contracture following osteotomy at the hip.** Limitation of flexion in the knee is a not uncommon complication of osteotomy at the hip for osteoarthrosis. It occasions surprise that difficulty should be experienced in regaining flexion when internal fixation has been employed, when the knee is not the subject of osteoarthrosis and has not been immobilised. The rectus femoris, as has been stated, is the only element of the quadriceps which takes origin above the hip joint. Reduction of a flexion deformity places the rectus under tension and the site and displacement of the osteotomy may result in adhesion of the muscle to the bone.

## QUADRICEPS PARALYSIS

### Aetiology

**1. Poliomyelitis.** In the current world scene infantile paralysis (anterior poliomyelitis) is much the most common, but not the only, cause of quadriceps paralysis partial or complete. The fall in the incidence of the disease that followed the introduction of poliovirus vaccines in 1955 is one of the great successes of modern preventive medicine (*Lancet,* 1970). Poliomyelitis is no longer a major public health hazard in the temperate zone so-called developed countries. In tropical and sub-tropical less developed

countries the incidence is increasing (Cockburn and Drozdov, 1970). If this is not the occasion to discuss a matter of such broad implication, it is the place to recognise that paralysis, the result of poliomyelitis, remains a major orthopaedic problem in many countries of the world; and to recognise that a generation of orthopaedic surgeons in the temperate-zone countries have no practical knowledge of the disease and are dependent on the experience of the past.

**2. Nerve root compression.** (L 2, 3 and 4).

**3. Lesions of femoral nerve.** The most common are of traumatic origin, e.g. gunshot wound.

**4. Myopathies.**

### Clinical Problem

The disability which results from paralysis of the quadriceps muscle is severe in the extreme. The knee is completely unstable if the slightest flexion deformity has been allowed to develop. On the other hand the joint may be stable in the presence

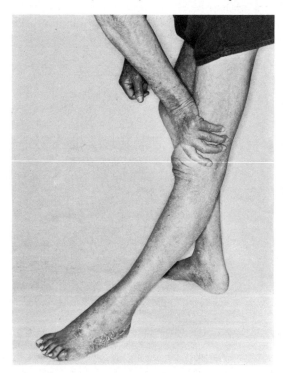

FIG. 2,5. **Quadriceps paralysis: means of ambulation without apparatus.** The hand placed immediately above the knee presses the joint into hyperextension with every step. Note foot placed on the ground in lateral rotation.

of recurvatus deformity if the calf muscles are active; and the means whereby this situation can be capitalised to walk without apparatus are described. If the hamstring muscles are intact there are circumstances in which they can be transferred to reinforce a weak or paralysed quadriceps. In other situations the problem can be solved only by the use of apparatus; or by arthrodesis.

## Treatment

A variety of methods of treatment in total paralysis, and at levels of recovery which will not permit gravity to be overcome, are available.

**Walking without apparatus.** It is not universally appreciated that a patient with a total quadriceps paralysis, and indeed of every muscle below the knee, can walk without the aid of apparatus, crutches or sticks provided there is enough muscle power about the hip region to enable the foot to be cleared from the ground in lateral rotation and the arm on the affected side is normal. This method of progression and of attaining stability is based on the screw-home movement in so far as the joint is stable in extension provided the tibia is in maximum lateral rotation (Fig. 2,5).

Two examples are quoted:

The patients, male and female, live in streets traversed by the author in the course of his work, progress by throwing the leg forward in lateral rotation and then pressing the femur backwards into extension with the hand. In each it is the right leg which is affected. The man keeps his hand in his trouser pocket and has been observed both ascending and descending inclines. In the woman the method of controlling extension is more obvious in so far as she presses her hand back against her skirt with every step.

It is important that the possibility of walking with total paralysis of the quadriceps is recognised, particularly in primitive communities and in the so-called underdeveloped countries where orthopaedic appliances may be unobtainable or impracticable. A patient in such circumstances can be taught to walk merely by utilising the screw-home movement in combina-

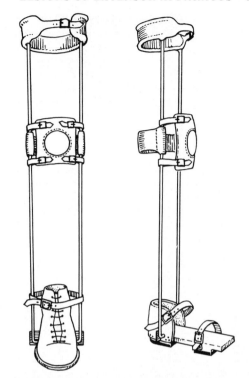

FIG. 2,6. **Quadriceps paralysis: treatment.** Simple calipers suitable for the underdeveloped countries can be mass produced with unskilled labour and local materials at a cost of less than one pound (Huckstep, 1971).

tion with the use of the hand to produce and control extension (Fig. 2,5).

## Apparatus

**To permit ambulation.** In many cases with total paralysis, walking is possible only with the aid of a full length caliper. In developing countries, where the current need arises, elaborate apparatus is unobtainable and, in any event, impracticable. A full-length caliper can be constructed from uprights of the $\frac{5}{16}$ inch (8 mm) mild steel used for reinforcing concrete and let into the heels of wooden clogs. There is a simple cuff-top and knee-apron. It has been shown that such a caliper can be produced by unskilled labour for less than one pound (Huckstep, 1971) (Fig. 2.6). At the opposite extreme, 50 pounds sterling can be expended on apparatus of varieties which compete in ingenuity of design,

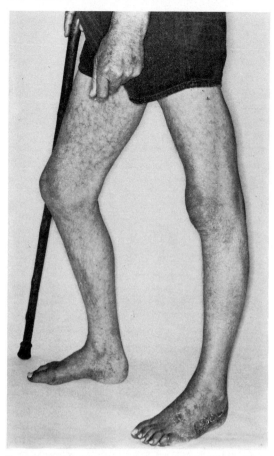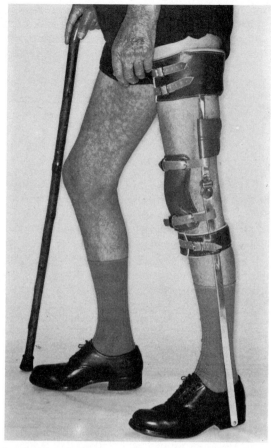

FIGS 2,7–8. **Quadriceps paralysis: treatment.** This patient (J.G., male, aged 68) learnt to walk with the aid of a stick obtaining stability with the foot laterally rotated and the knee in hyperextension. In time however he developed intolerable pain from stretching of the posterior capsule (Fig, 2,7). The hyperextension was controlled by a full length caliper with a knee apron and posterior thigh and calf bands (Fig. 2,8).

lightness and the exploitation of modern materials; but are considerably less robust than the basic splint.

**To prevent hyperextension.** The caliper will incorporate thigh and calf bands; and accurate adjustment is necessary to permit full extension, but limit the hyperextension which induces pain. A knee apron is necessary to prevent the joint from giving way suddenly.

The following is an example of such a case:

The patient (J. G., male, aged 68) suffered a lumbo-dorsal disc protrusion 12 years previously, producing initially a total quadriceps paralysis. A limited recovery occurred to the point where, in the supine position, he could lift his limb from the couch. He had learnt to walk with the knee in extension with the leg in lateral rotation and with the aid of a stick carried in the opposite hand (Fig. 2,7). As the years passed he developed pain in the popliteal space. It occurred only when walking and was clearly the result of stretching the posterior capsule. He was aware that it was hyperextension which produced the pain. He was cured of his symptoms at the cost of having to wear a duralumin jointed caliper which checked hyperextension just short of the point which induced pain (Fig. 2,8).

SWEDISH KNEE CAGE. In general, knee cages are unsatisfactory for the control of instability.

They rarely achieve that purpose and cannot be accurately located anatomically unless attached by a lateral iron to the shoe. Genu recurvatum, the result of quadriceps paralysis, however, poses a different problem. It is the control of a particular movement in a patient who does not demand a high standard of function. In this regard the device known as the Swedish knee cage (Lehneis, 1968), designed for the control of recurvatus, is a simple device worthy of trial in so far as it permits flexion of the knee when sitting. *It is not of value in the presence of angular deformity in the form of varus or valgus or instability of ligamentous origin.* In the control of recurvatus it has the apparent advantages of (1) simplicity; (2) light weight; (3) absence of locking device at knee; (4) natural flexion in the action of sitting; (5) ease of adjustment.

It consists of two aluminium uprights connected posteriorly with a semicircular horizontal bar. It employs the well-known three-point pressure system of controlling deformity (Fig. 2,9) applied anteriorly through two webbing straps fitted above and below the knee, while counter pressure is applied posteriorly through the suitably padded posterior bar.

The anterior straps have a fixed attachment on the medial uprights and are looped over the lateral uprights where they are held in place by a snap button to facilitate application and removal of the appliance. The depth of the posterior pad is adjusted to the size of leg and to the desired degree of recurvatus (Figs 2,10 and 2,11).

**Paralysis with angular deformity.** If symptoms related to hyperextension are capable of solution on the lines indicated, the addition of a valgus deformity complicates the problem. In the paralytic leg which has existed since childhood, stability of the knee is achieved with the tibia in lateral rotation and stabilised against the medial ligament and capsule. But stretching occurs with

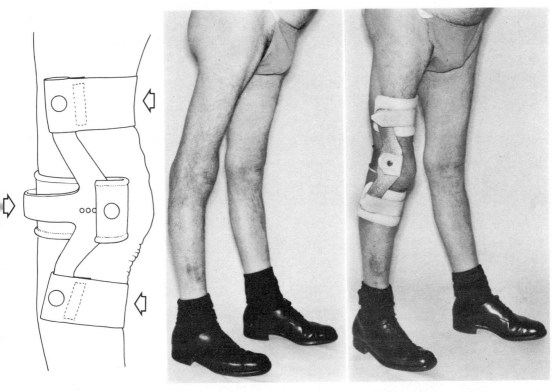

FIGS 2,9–11. **Quadriceps paralysis: treatment.** Use of Swedish knee cage (Fig. 2,9) to control excessive hyperextension on the right side (Figs 2,10 and 2,11).

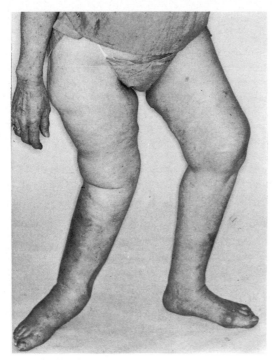

Fig. 2,12

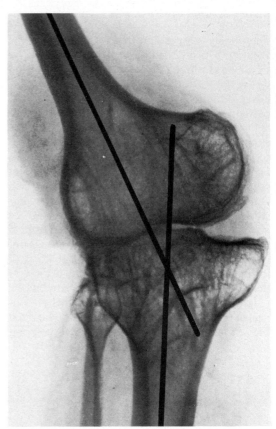

Fig. 2,14

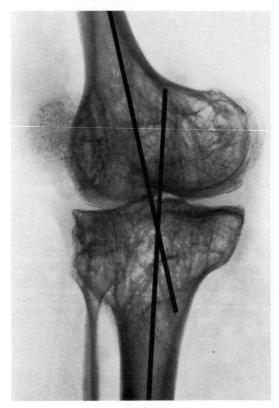

Fig. 2,13

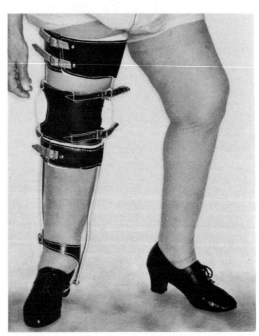

Fig. 2,15

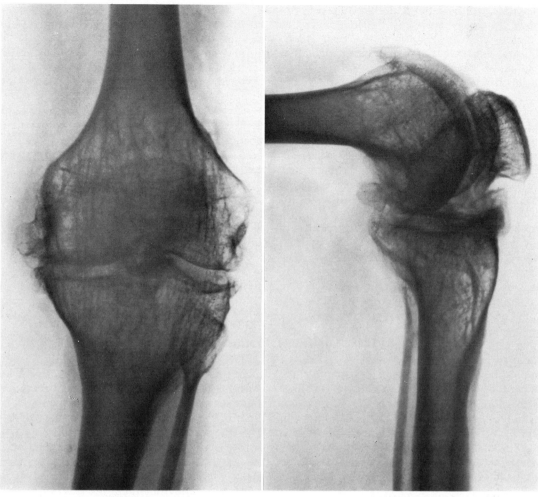

FIG. 2,16                          FIG. 2,17

FIGS 2,12–17. **Quadriceps paralysis.** Total paralysis the result of poliomyelitis in childhood in a patient (D.P.), ambulatory without apparatus and complaining of symptoms for the first time at age 54 as a result of increasing valgus angulation producing pain and instability (Fig. 2,12). The related radiographs in the supine position (Fig. 2,13) and weight-bearing (Fig. 2,14) to demonstrate the increase in tibio-femoral angle so-related. The deformity controlled by full-length cuff-topped caliper incorporating T-strap and knock-knee apron (Fig. 2,15).

**Flexed-knee gait: good (long) leg arthropathy.** Note in Figs 2,12 and 2,15 the flexed knee of the 'good' leg. The patient had walked all her life without compensation for the shortening of the right leg. An osteoarthrosis is evident in the clinical appearance of the joint and shown to be pan-articular in distribution and gross in nature with loose bodies and a bony block to extension (Figs 2,16 and 2,17). (See also 'Good (long) leg arthropathy' Chapter 10.)

the passage of time, particularly if an increase in body weight is involved. Patients with this deformity remain symptomless for many years. There is, however, a critical angle in the valgus angulation beyond which pain and instability occur. If a full length caliper appears to be the solution, it must be remembered that it requires to control both hyperextension and valgus; and to control the latter entails direct pressure against some form of knee-apron. The force involved is not readily tolerated. In certain circumstances the solution to the problem may be arthrodesis; and whether this procedure is acceptable often depends on the condition of the other knee (Figs 2,12 to 2,17).

ARTHRODESIS. Arthrodesis is the alternative in total or almost total paralysis to the wearing of a caliper; or to the progression of hyperextension and related pain as recorded above. It may be indicated in circumstances where apparatus is unobtainable or impracticable. Some patients prefer a stiff knee to the necessity to wear apparatus. When the question of arthrodesis arises it is important that the limitations imposed by inability to flex the knee be appreciated. It is a personal decision for the patient, which is better, the wearing of a caliper with the ability to flex while sitting, or arthrodesis? In order to test a situation in which the decision is irreversible, a trial of a light plaster cast in full extension for a few weeks as a test of the social and domestic acceptability of arthrodesis may be required.

### Tendon Transfer

The muscles available are the biceps femoris, semitendinosis, sartorius and tensor fascia lata. The transfer of biceps and semitendinosis is the operation of choice. The transfer of biceps alone results eventually in dislocation of the patella. Even a weak semitendinosis acts as check.

**Prerequisites** If tendon transfer on the lines indicated above is under consideration it is important that the following prerequisites be fulfilled:

1. ANGULAR DEFORMITY. Flexion contracture of any degree must be corrected and, indeed, from the viewpoint of stability, a minimal degree of genu recurvatum is desirable. Thus preliminary procedures, conservative and operative, for the correction of flexion deformity may be necessary; and even osteotomy of tibia or femur may have to be considered.

2. MUSCLE POWER. There should exist sufficient residual muscle power to warrant the reasonable expectation that in the final result orthopaedic appliances can be discarded.

3. CALF MUSCLES. Normal calf muscles are desirable but not essential. Many patients after operation depend on gastrocnemius for active flexion and for limitation of the tendency to develop recurvatus deformity.

4. HIP JOINT. Deformity, particularly fixed flexion, must be corrected prior to operation.

5. ANKLE JOINT. Equinus deformity of the foot causes compensatory recurvatus of the knee and must be corrected prior to operation.

6. MOTIVATION. The mental ability and will to co-operate in post-operative rehabilitation is essential.

### Operation

**Technique.** The operation is performed in the supine position under the control of a high tourniquet. Three incisions are necessary, one to expose and release the biceps, one to expose and release the semitendinosis and one to effect anterior transfer and reattachment to the patella. The anterior incision extends along the medial border of the quadriceps tendon, patella and patellar tendon to expose the patella and region immediately proximal. The lateral incision extends from about the junction of the proximal and middle thirds of the thigh to a point of some 8 cm distal to the head of the fibula. The lateral popliteal nerve is located immediately medial to the biceps tendon and retracted. The insertion of the biceps tendon is identified and separated from the insertion of the lateral ligament, with which it is closely associated, and divided. The tendon and muscle belly are dissected free in a proximal direction to the origin of the short head and to the entrance of the nerve and blood supply. A subcutaneous tract is established between the two incisions dividing the iliotibial band, fascia of vastus lateralis and the lateral intermuscular septum so that the muscle can pass obliquely towards the patella.

The postero-medial incision extends from the

insertion of pes anserinus below to the junction of the middle and distal thirds of the thigh above. The tendon of semitendinosis is small and round and lies posterior to that of sartorius and gracilus. (Remember: Say Grace before Tea.) It is identified at its insertion and the muscle freed proximally. A subcutaneous tunnel is now established between the postero-medial and antero-medial incisions so that the tendon is rerouted towards the patella. In the final stages the location and pathway of both muscles is adjusted for direction of pull avoiding, as will be obvious, angulation. Attachment to the patella is effected by vertical division of the overlying coverings in the midline and insertion

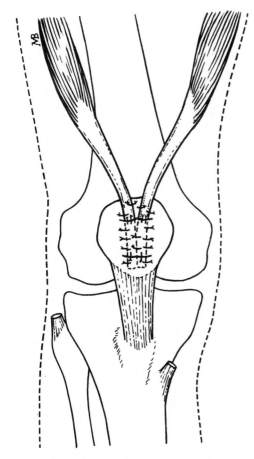

FIG. 2,18. **Quadriceps paralysis.** Transfer of biceps femoris and semitendinosis tendons to patella (after Schwartzmann and Crego).

of the two tendons, suitably adjusted for tension in the context of the circumstances of the case, and secured with multiple sutures (Fig. 2,18).

AFTER-TREATMENT. At the termination of the operation the limb is enclosed in a padded plaster cast extending from the groin to the roots of the toes. The knee is placed in the neutral position in regard to flexion and extension and particular care taken to avoid hyperextension. In bed the leg is supported in a half-ring Thomas bed-knee splint. The patient is nursed supine and the end of the bed elevated but the limb is not otherwise raised to avoid flexion at the hip and reduce tension in the transferred tendons.

The plaster cast is bivalved after three weeks and active exercise begun. The anterior half is discarded at the eighth week. It is about this time that active flexion is encouraged. Splinting is then gradually discarded during the day but the posterior shell retained at night. A return to weight-bearing is eventually permitted wearing a light dural walking caliper adjusted to prevent hyperextension. When sufficient muscle power has been developed to stabilise the knee in extension the caliper is gradually discarded.

#### Complications

GENU RECURVATUM. If a minimal degree of genu recurvatum is desirable as contributing to stability, the development of any considerable deformity constitutes a disability (see below). The danger can be reduced if (1) the operation is avoided in the absence of reasonable power in the calf muscles; (2) equinus deformity of the foot is corrected before the transfer operation or before weight-bearing is resumed; (3) immobilisation in hyperextension is avoided in the immediate post-operative treatment; and (4) every effort is made to improve the power of the remaining knee flexor muscles by exercise therapy.

**Results of operation.** The outcome depends on a number of factors, the extent to which pre-requisites can be fulfilled and upon the stability of the hip and foot. In a review of 134 cases (Schwartzmann and Crego, 1948) it was concluded that hamstring substitution for residual quadriceps paralysis in poliomyelitis is a satisfactory procedure. The best results follow the

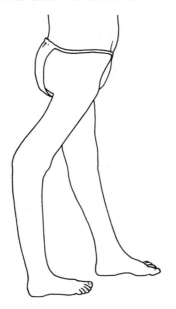

FIG. 2,19. **Paralytic genu recurvatum.** If the deformity is greater than 30° bracing is not effective.

use of biceps femoris in conjunction with semitendinosis. The importance of careful selection of cases and attention to detail in operative technique and post-operative care is stressed.

### Tenodesis

In genu recurvatum of paralytic origin it is seldom that angulation of more than 30° can be controlled by a brace due to the high pressures exerted on the calf and thigh in weight-bearing (Fig. 2,19). In the child, control of the deformity during growth by some means is desirable to prevent secondary deformity of the epiphyses. To this end tenodesis may be a useful method of rendering a patient brace-free or at least making bracing tolerable. None of the procedures so far described have been capable of withstanding the forces generated in the severe genu recurvatum associated with paralysis of the quadriceps. Recently a reconstruction of the lax soft tissues posterior to the joint, done in three layers and thus termed 'triple tenodesis', has been described and with reported encouraging results (Perry, O'Brien and Hodgson, 1976).

**Prerequisites.** If the operation is to be success-

ful three basic principles must be observed:

1. The fibrous tissue mass limiting extension must be of sufficient strength to withstand the considerable stretching forces generated by the paralytic limb. Thus every available tendon must be utilised.

2. The healing tissues must be protected from stretching force for at least one year. In practice therefore the operation is not undertaken without the assurance that a brace will be worn continuously for that time.

3. The alignmnent and stability of the ankle joint must meet the basic requirements of gait. Equinus deformity of the foot which causes compensatory recurvatus of the knee must be corrected by whichever method is appropriate to the situation.

### Operation

**Technique.** The operation is divided into three parts: (1) proximal advancement of the posterior capsule with the joint in 20° of flexion (Fig. 2,20); (2) construction of a midline checkrein with the tendons of semitendinosus and gracilis (Fig. 2,21); and (3) creation of two diagonal straps using the tendon of biceps and the anterior half of the iliotibial band (Fig. 2,23).

The operation takes place with the patient in the prone position. Haemostasis is controlled by pneumatic tourniquet. A large sand-bag is placed beneath the ankle so that the knee is supported in some 20° of flexion.

A lazy S incision is employed. The proximal limb, some 4 cm long, is located on the lateral side adjacent to the biceps tendon. The transverse limb crosses the popliteal space in the central crease. The distal limb is placed to gain access to the pes anserinus. The sural nerve is located beneath the fascia and traced upwards to the medial popliteal nerve which in turn is traced upwards to locate the lateral popliteal nerve. The short saphenous vein, adjacent to the sural nerve, the main neurovascular bundle and the lateral popliteal nerve are all retracted to the lateral side permitting dissection to be carried down to the capsule. The medial head of gastrocnemius is detached in a Z cup preserving a long proximal strap for use in the tenodesis. The femoral attachment of the capsule is divided above each of the condyles and the intervening

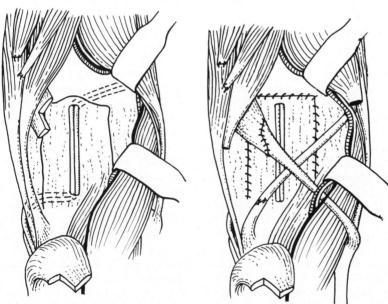

Semitendinosus

Gracilis

Semimembranosus

Sartorius

Biceps

Iliotibial
tract

Capsule

Med head
of
Gastroc

Head of
Fibula

Lat head
of
Gastroc

FIG. 2,20

FIG. 2,22

FIG. 2,21

FIG. 2,23

FIGS 2,20–23. **Triple tenodesis: technique.** The medial head of gastrocnemius is divided in the form of a Z leaving a proximal stump for eventual suture to the biceps tendon (see Fig. 2,23). A broad flap of posterior capsule is outlined and released for eventual advancement upwards (Fig. 2,20).

The semitendinosus and gracilis tendons are sectioned at the musculo-tendinous junction. The tendons are passed through an antero-posterior tunnel in the tibia then vertically across the joint posterior to the capsule and then through an oblique tunnel in the femur to the exterior on the lateral side (Fig. 2,21). The tunnels are seen to avoid the growth plates (Fig. 2,22). On completion of the central strap the posterior capsule is advanced upwards so that it is taut with the joint in 20° of flexion. The cross straps are constructed with the tendon of biceps and the iliotibial band. The biceps tendon is sectioned as high up as possible at the musculo-tendinous junction. It crosses the posterior capsule obliquely deep to the neurovascular bundle to be sutured to the origin of the medial head of gastrocnemius. The iliotibial band is detached from Gerdys tubercle, passed deep to that portion of the track which remains, to the biceps tendon and to the neurovascular bundle to be sutured to the insertion of semi-membranosus (Fig. 2,23). (Redrawn from Perry, O'Brien and Hodgson, 1976.)

notch. Reattachment at a higher level takes place later.

In the next step the tendons of gracilis and semitendinosus are divided at the musculo-tendinous junction, as high up as possible so that the maximum length is available for the midline checkrein (Fig. 2,21). The proximal ends are sutured to sartorius. The drill holes are then made. That in the tibia enters in the midline posteriorly below the growth plate, which it must avoid (Fig. 2,22), and emerges near the insertion of pes anserinus. That in the femur enters in the midline posteriorly proximal to the growth plate, which it must avoid, and emerges on the lateral aspect of the distal end of the femur. The tendons of gracilis and semi-tendinosus are threaded through the tibial drill hole, passed behind the capule, and pulled through the femoral drill hole to emerge on the lateral aspect of the femur. Here, with the knee in 20° of flexion, they are sutured to the periosteum with strong non-absorbable sutures in moderate tension. The divided superior margin of the capsule is now advanced in a proximal direction until it is taut in 20° of flexion and then sutured to the periosteum with non-absorbable sutures.

The final step consists of suturing the tendons of biceps and the iliotibial band in the form of a cross behind the advanced posterior capsule. To this end the biceps tendon is divided proxi-mally and passed across the back of the joint deep to the neurovascular bundle. It is re-attached to the femoral origin of the medial head of gastrocnemius under moderate tension. The anterior half of the iliotibial band is then detached from its insertion and passed deep to the intact portion across the popliteal space deep to the biceps tendon and neurovascular bundle, to be sutured to the semimembranosus insertion on the tibia (Fig. 2,23). If a tendon to be employed has an active muscle attached it is split longitudinally and half only used in the tenodesis leaving the other half attached to the insertion. Suction drainage is inserted and the wound closed.

The operation is said to take approximately two hours. The tourniquet thus requires to be released for five minutes after one hour when any bleeding vessels may be ligatured. The tourniquet is then reapplied.

**After-treatment.** Post-operative management in this procedure assumes a greater importance than in the average orthopaedic case. At the termination of the operation a padded plaster cast is applied in 30° of flexion so that the suture lines are not under tension. The suction drainage is removed after 48 hours. The cast is retained for 6 weeks. At this time the long leg brace, fitted pre-operatively, is reapplied. The brace locks the joint in 15° of flexion and in it weight-bearing is permitted. A night-shell holds the joint in 15° of flexion.

In 12 months time the patient is readmitted to hospital and the flexion contracture corrected to neutral by means of serial casts; when cor-rection has been achieved unrestricted weight-bearing is permitted.

## DIABETIC AMYOTROPHY

**Definition.** Patients suffering from diabetes may develop wasting and weakness of the quadriceps with sensory changes in the thigh indicating a lesion of the femoral nerve (Goodman, 1954; Calverley and Mulder, 1960). In some of these cases the femoral neuropathy may be part of a diabetic mononeuritis multiplex, other individual peripheral nerves being affected. In addition, there is a similar affection with weak-ness and wasting of the quadriceps to which the name diabetic amyotrophy is attached (Garland, 1955, 1960). The exact nature of the neurological lesion in the latter condition remains in doubt. Electromyographic muscle biopsy studies have shown that the wasting and weakness are neurogenic not myopathic. It is thought that the dominant pathological process may be demyelination. It has been pointed out that the rapidity and completeness of recovery of muscle power which occurs in many examples is too great to be explained by reinnervation and suggests that the neurological lesion is reversible (Casey and Harrison, 1972).

**Clinical significance.** The importance of the condition is recognition of the origin. These patients present at an orthopaedic clinic as affections of the knee joint, with wasting and weakness of the quadriceps. Neither the elderly patient nor the referring general practitioner may recognise the association with diabetes;

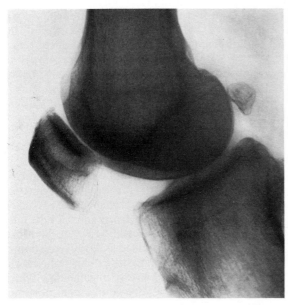

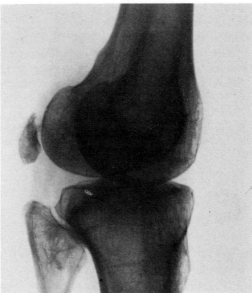

Fig. 2,24

Fig. 2,25

Fig. 2,26

Fig. 2,27

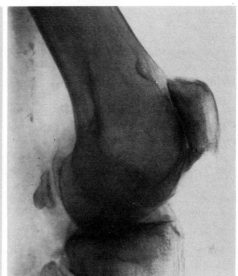

Figs 2,24–27. **Fabella in lateral head of gastrocnemius: abnormalities.** The fabella varies in size. This large one shows trabeculation. It is distinguished from a loose body by site and by the vertical side with subchondral density adjacent to the lateral condyle (Fig. 2,24). The fabella is not without function. Hypertrophy in patient with total quadriceps paralysis who walks without apparatus using gastrocnemius and iliotibial band as extensors of the knee. The size of the fabella indicates the importance of the role of gastrocnemius as an extensor—a posterior patella. The patella which was without function was excised when it was fractured in a fall (Fig. 2,25) (G.F., male, aged 57). Massive hypertrophy, the largest encountered, and presumed due to contact with osteoma of head of fibula (Fig. 2,26). Fabello-femoral joint in osteoarthrosic knee showing evidence of involvement in the degenerative process (Fig. 2,27).

C

and the information may not be offered other than in answer to a leading question.

**Treatment.** The development of this form of neuropathy and its prognosis are influenced by the degree and control of the blood sugar. The condition occurs in patients with uncontrolled diabetes. The first line of treatment, therefore, consists of establishment of rigid control. Active physiotherapy in the form of quadriceps and other exercises as appropriate, help to restore recovery. The temporary use of a light-weight full-length caliper may be indicated.

## FABELLA: SESAMOID IN LATERAL HEAD OF GASTROCNEMIUS: SESAMUM GENU SUPERIUS LATERALE

If the existence of a fabella in the lateral head of gastrocnemius is of interest it is not considered to be important. In selecting a chapter in which its presence and minor clinical significance might be recorded, it was noted to be markedly hypertrophied in quadriceps paralysis in which extension of the knee was undertaken by gastrocnemius. That it has a function when maximum demands are made of gastrocnemius cannot be denied (Fig. 2,25).

**Incidence.** In 800 consecutive radiographs reviewed in the years 1971–72, 114 showed the presence of a fabella, a percentage of 14·25. In a comparable series of 471 patients the percentage was 16·3 (Hessen, 1946).

**Form.** The size of the fabella varies within wide limits from that little more than a speck to a bone of sizeable dimensions (Fig. 2,24). In the large majority of cases the fabella is bilateral but not necessarily symmetrical.

In the course of the investigation a radiograph was noted which showed a bipartite patella on the left side; a normal patella on the right. There was a fabella in the lateral head of gastrocnemius on the same side as the bipartite patella. There was no fabella on the right side.

**Function.** The function of a sesamoid bone is to facilitate the gliding action of a tendon particularly where angulation is involved, acting as a pulley, so to speak. In addition, as in the

patella, it increases the efficiency of the muscle concerned by increasing the distance of the tendon from the centre of rotation of the joint.

If the gastrocnemius is normally regarded as a plantar flexor of the ankle it can be an extensor of the knee. There are circumstances of quadriceps paralysis in which it adopts exceptional importance.

When the gastrocnemius becomes the important extensor of the knee the fabella undergoes hypertrophy. In the case illustrated in Figure 2,25; the patient had complete paralysis of both quadriceps as a result of anterior poliomyelitis. In the early degrees of extension the only extensor was gastrocnemius. In the later range, towards hyperextension, the iliotibial band was active. He gained stability from hyperextension. The salient feature of his radiographs was the exceptional size of the fabellae which took the form of two miniature posterior patellae!

**Differential diagnosis.** If the fabella has any clinical significance it is in the differential diagnosis of a loose body in the posterior compartment of the joint; and errors of interpretation have been known to occur. The fabella articulates with the lateral femoral condyle and is therefore radiologically so related. Moreover because the anterior surface is an articular facet it is flat and shows subchondral sclerosis whereas the posterior surface is rounded (Fig. 2,24). In loose bodies both surfaces are rounded.

**Involvement in disease processes.** In a generalised osteoarthrosis the joint between fabella and lateral condyle of femur is involved in the degenerative process (Fig. 2,27). No case was encountered in which such local osteoarthrosis produced symptoms; nor any instance of isolated radiological osteoarthrosis producing symptoms. Fracture has been described but is a rarity.

It may be noted to be enlarged and irregular on rare occasions in association with Paget's disease affecting the knee joint (Barry, 1969).

**Source of symptoms.** The close proximity of the lateral popliteal nerve is of significance. Occasionally it may be stretched round the medial side of the fabella; this is particularly liable to occur in fractures at the lower end of the femur in which union has occurred with lateral rotation deformity. The following are examples of

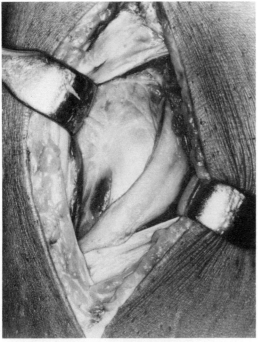

FIG. 2,28

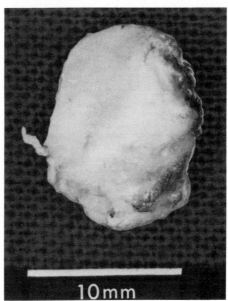

FIG. 2,29

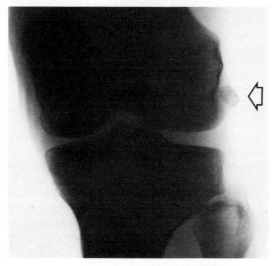

◄ FIG. 2,30

FIGS 2,28–30. **Sesamoid in lateral head of gastrocnemius: source of symptoms.** In this example the lateral popliteal nerve is stretched round its medial side (Fig. 2,28). Excised sesamoid to indicate size and attachment to inferior aspect (Fig. 2,29) (A.H., male, aged 30). In this example the laterally placed fabella (Fig. 2,30) was responsible for giving-way incidents in the popliteal space (I.B., aged 29, ski instructor).

cases in which the fabella was a source of symptoms:

The patient (A.H., male, aged 30), in the course of rehabilitation following a fracture of the shaft of femur, developed pain on the posterior aspect of the joint. On examination there was a visible swelling to the lateral side of the popliteal fossa and palpation revealed tenderness to pressure. It was decided that the palpable mass was the sesamoid, but in view of the unusual circumstances an expectant attitude was adopted. A month later, however, the patient insisted that the pain was such as to interfere with his ability to perform exercises. At operation, the biceps tendon was split revealing a marked prominance in the lateral head of the gastrocnemius close to the attachment to the femoral condyle. To the medial side, and in direct contact with the prominence, was the lateral popliteal nerve (Fig. 2,28). The lateral head of the gastrocnemius was split in the line of the fibres and the sesamoid seen to be attached to muscle inferiorly (Fig. 2,29) and to tendon superiorly and on either side. It was removed by sharp dissection. Examination of the articular surface and that of the opposing lateral condyle showed no evidence of local arthrosis.

On another occasion (I.B., age 29, ski instructor) complained of pain and the recurring sensation of something giving-way in the popliteal space. On examination there was tenderness accurately located to the lateral head of the gastrocnemius where a small mobile mass, evidently the fabella, could be palpated. The radiograph showed that the fabella was much more laterally placed than is normally encountered (Fig. 2,30). It was assumed that the giving-way incidents were due to the sesamoid slipping over the lateral margin of the condyle.

At operation the fabella was readily located by palpation and excised through a small vertical incision at the musculo-tendinous junction of the muscle. The symptoms of pain and the sensation of insecurity were relieved.

## MYOSITIS OSSIFICANS TRAUMITICA: CALCIFICATION AND OSSIFICATION OF QUADRICEPS: CALCIFYING HAEMATOMA

There are three varieties of myositis ossificans:
1. MYOSITIS OSSIFICANS PROGRESSIVA. This is a rare developmental disorder of children, probably of autosomal dominant inheritance, in which there is progressive calcification followed by ossification of fasciae, aponeuroses and muscles. It is characterised by skeletal abnormalities in the form of a short great toe, and sometimes of thumb and fingers present at birth. The condition is ultimately fatal.
2. MYOSITIS OSSIFICANS TRAUMATICA.

This common condition is the result of single-incident trauma or repeated slight injuries of occupational origin. It is of particular relevance to the knee joint in so far as the muscle most often affected is quadriceps femoris.
3. MYOSITIS OSSIFICANS CIRCUMSCRIPTA. This is usually found in paraplegia, chronic infections, burns and poliomyelitis. It may however occur independently of other pathology and without intervening trauma.

### Myositis Ossificans Traumatica

While this work is concerned with disease rather than trauma, myositis ossificans requires mention for the purpose of differential diagnosis. The condition arises generally, but not exclusively, as a result of injury in sport. The quadriceps of the athlete in training can be expected to have a greater blood supply than is normal and thus the haemorrhage as a result of injury is greater than normal.

The name is a misnomer. It is not an inflammatory reaction and it is the connective tissue which ossifies; not the muscle.

The component of the quadriceps most frequently damaged is vastus intermedius. The injury is by direct violence and the usual mechanism is a blow by a kick, knee or head in the course of a football game. Sometimes the incident is forgotten in the course of the excitement of the encounter. Often the patient is able to play on and even complete the game. Later the thigh swells as a result of intramuscular haemorrhage and the swelling may reach considerable dimensions. The potential for prolonged disability is not recognised unless the patient consults an orthopaedic surgeon familiar with athletic injuries. The patient is often treated by massage and other irritative passive measures which increase the swelling and further limit flexion of the knee. With failure to recover, and possibly increasing loss of flexion, further advice may be sought. It is at this stage, say, some three weeks after the injury, that calcification is seen in a radiograph. But a radiograph taken at an earlier date is negative and leads to further confusion.

**Differential diagnosis.** It is most important that this condition is recognised, not only from the viewpoint of treatment, but from a possible

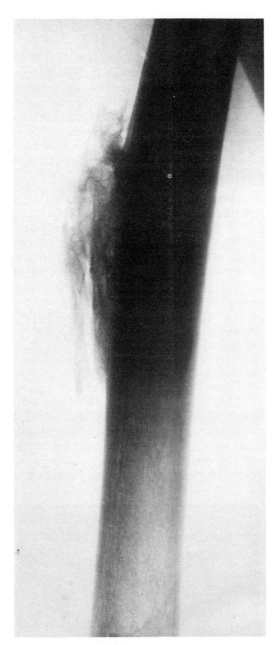 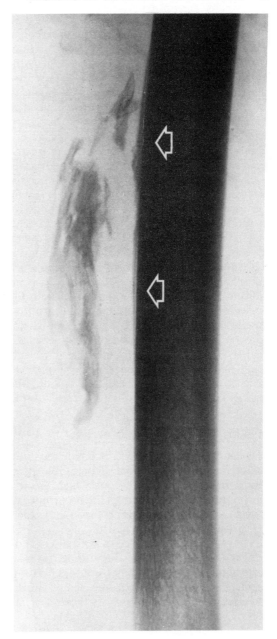

FIGS 2,31–32. **Myositis ossificans traumatica.** The radiological appearance of myositis ossificans traumatica takes many forms. In Figure 2,31 the mass of bone is apparently in continuity with the femur. In Figure 2,32 there is a gap. But note raising of the periosteum. It is this feature which may occasion alarm in the differential diagnosis from osteosarcoma (see also IKJ5, Figs 2,5 and 2,6).

serious misdiagnosis if the appearances are confused with, for example, an osteogenic sarcoma. The shadow tends to be located on the antero-lateral aspect of the thigh in so far as it is the antero-lateral aspect that is most likely to receive the causative blow. Sometimes it is so extensive and, showing elevation of the periosteum is such as to cast doubt as to the origin, that is to say, to raise the possibility of malignancy (Fig. 2,32). **Treatment.** The established condition is treated with rest, possibly bed-rest, and/or a plaster back-shell. Elastic compression to assist absorption of the haematoma is important in the early stages. If deep massage and passive knee movements are employed, such 'treatment' may be responsible for the calcification. When the complication has occurred, all such irritative passive measures and, worst of all, manipulation under anaesthesia or operative action, are contra-indicated. With rest on the lines indicated, the bone tends to undergo spontaneous absorption; but disability may be prolonged; and is not necessarily related to the size of the bony mass. If after an interval of many months or when a completely quiescent state has been reached there is still serious restriction of flexion, the mass should be excised through a lateral incision.

**Myositis Ossifications Circumscripta**

This condition may arise in the quadriceps of a healthy young adult without recognisable intervening trauma and for reasons which are unknown. In such circumstances the occurrence of a progressive swelling with accompanying radiological findings occasions alarm.
DIFFERENTIAL DIAGNOSIS FROM OSTEO-SARCOMA. The gross distinguishing features (Paterson, 1970) are: (1) myositis ossificans is situated over the shaft of the femur whilst osteosarcoma is located towards the end of the bone; (2) in myositis ossificans there is a rapid increase in the swelling initially but thereafter a tendency to diminution in size. The hard consistency, together with the pain which begins early but gradually reduces in intensity is in contrast with that found in osteosarcoma; (3) radiologically the cortex and periosteum are normal in myositis ossificans. The newly formed mass lies parallel to the surface. The cortex is intact. It is broken in osteosarcoma.

## CALCIFICATION OF TENDON OF QUADRICEPS

The tendon of quadriceps may be the site of calcification of degenerative origin such as occurs, but more commonly, at tendinous attachments elsewhere.

The example which follows is recorded as an unusual cause of pain in the knee in middle age as further evidence of the importance of a sky-line radiographic projection of the patella in the investigation of symptoms at this site.

The patient (R.E., male, aged 53) complained of an aching pain, accurately located to the supra-lateral aspect of the right patella, during the previous 18 months. The pain was aggravated by activities such as ascending and descending stairs. The symptoms were not severe but were of more than nuisance value. The reason for seeking advice was that pain was progressively more obtrusive. There was a feeling of weakness in the knee and the record of a single giving-way incident. There was no history of injury nor of symptoms in any other joint.

The outstanding feature of examination was swelling and tenderness at the supra-lateral angle of the patella. Pressure on the patella during movement produced pain in the patello-femoral joint. The clinical diagnosis, in view of the prominence at the supra-lateral aspect of the patella, was an anomaly of ossification and the symptoms were thought to be due to

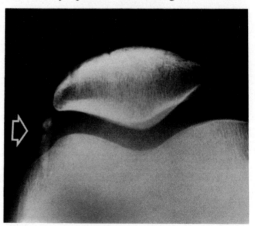

FIG. 2,33. **Calcification in quadriceps tendon.** This unusual cause of pain and swelling was revealed only in the skyline view of the patella.

a related local chondromalacia or arthrosis. It was not until the skyline view of the patella was taken, for the purpose of determining the size and nature of the ossicle that the calcified mass was seen (Fig. 2,33).

At operation the calcified material had the appearance and consistency of tooth-paste and comparable with that commonly evacuated from the rotator cuff of the shoulder joint. The patient made an uneventful recovery.

This is the only example of calcification in the quadriceps tendon encountered. It is presumed to have the same background of degeneration as calcification at tendinous attachments elsewhere. The case is recorded as an unusual cause of pain in the knee in late middle age and as further evidence of the importance of a skyline view of the patella in the investigation of symptoms at this site.

## Osteochondritis of Inferior Pole of Patella

### Sinding Larsen-Johansson Disease

Conditions comparable in every respect with partial separation of the epiphysis of the tibial tubercle (traction epiphysitis or Osgood-Schlatter's disease) are encountered in the patella.

**Clinical features.** The patient, usually an active boy in the 10 to 14 age group, complains of pain in the knee accompanied by limp and the symptoms are sometimes bilateral.

Examination shows tenderness and swelling accurately located to the inferior pole of the patella. Radiographs reveal fragmentation at the inferior pole. The tip may have a bulbous appearance, indicating a possible secondary centre of ossification. The radiographic abnormality, as in traction epiphysitis, is usually bilateral and is not necessarily related to the severity of the symptoms.

The condition, more common at the attachment of the ligamentum patellae, is encountered also at the superior pole (Figs 2,34 to 2,37).

If pathological changes at the attachment of large tendons to growing bones are the result of strain, such conditions might reasonably be expected to occur with greatest frequency in rela-

tion to the most powerful of muscle groups. The condition described may sometimes be seen in acute form in this age group when in the high jump for example, either at take-off or on landing, a shell of cortical bone is avulsed from the inferior pole of the patella.

**Treatment.** This traction lesion, like traction epiphysitis, merits treatment not only on account of the severity of symptoms, but because of possible influence on the future relationship of the patella to the femoral condyles.

The condition heals with rest. A period of 6 to 12 weeks of immobilisation in the cylinder variety of plaster cast has effected a cure in all the examples which have been encountered.

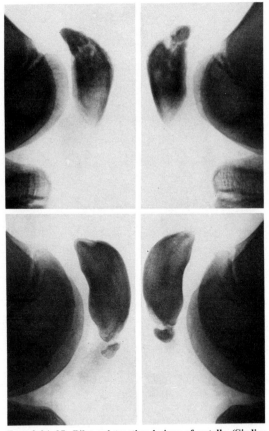

FIGS 2,34–37. **Bilateral traction lesions of patella (Sinding Larsen-Johannson disease): 'osteochondritis'.** Superior pole (Figs 2,34 and 2,35). Inferior pole at later stage of development (Figs 2,36 and 2,37). The former might be responsible for patella baja; the latter for patella alta which indeed is already present (Figs 2,36 and 2,37).

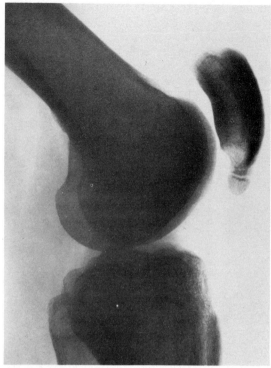
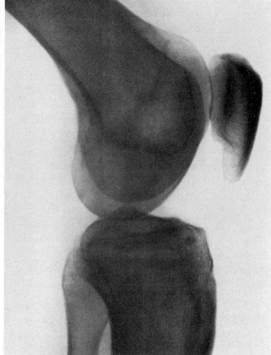
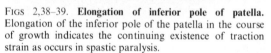

FIGS 2,38–39. **Elongation of inferior pole of patella.** Elongation of the inferior pole of the patella in the course of growth indicates the continuing existence of traction strain as occurs in spastic paralysis.

This example is the subject of a fracture, possibly a stress fracture, and non-union. Note that the elongation has resulted in patella alta (Fig. 2,38). But this does not necessarily occur (Fig. 2,39).

### ADULT VARIETY: JUMPER'S KNEE

There is a variety which gives rise to prolonged and troublesome symptoms in young adult male athletes above the age at which Sinding Larsen-Johansson's disease is active.

The complaint is of pain at the attachment of the patellar tendon to the patella on physical exertion, with pain at the same site on kneeling. Some say they are only free of discomfort with the knee extended and the quadriceps relaxed. Clinical examination reveals tenderness at this site and, in extreme cases, local swelling. In all the examples seen the patient was either tall with long levers acting about the knee joint and/or was engaged in vigorous athletic activities.

The aetiology of this condition is obscure and when it is bilateral and with no objective phenomena or distinctive radiological findings the patient may get little sympathy. But that some

active, if slow, process is present is shown by the fact that patients who have suffered symptoms for years show alteration in the shape of the lower pole of the patella. Furthermore, in the course of this alteration of shape (Figs 2,38 and 2,39), relative decalcification may be noted.

### Treatment

It is the common experience that treatment of this persistent condition is unsatisfactory and discouraging to both patient and physician. Such measures as heat, cold, exercise and support may give temporary relief but have no lasting effect on pain induced in the course of effort. The temptation to inject hydrocortisone should be strongly resisted as liable to contribute to a catastrophic episode in the form of total rupture of the tendon.

The condition, with abandonment of the precipitating activity, is self-limiting. In untreated form symptoms are known to have persisted for as long as four years.

**Operation.** Young men whose athletic activities have been interrupted exert pressure for operative action. In such circumstances the author has inserted multiple drill holes in the inferior pole through a short lateral parapatellar incision in the hope of improving the local blood supply. If this measure appeared to produce a reduction in symptoms it has not been confirmed to be helpful in other hands (Blazina *et al.*, 1973). In the last resort there arises the possibility of resection of the inferior pole with resuture of the tendon as for fracture. The author has no experience of this measure.

### Elongation of the Inferior Pole of the Patella, Stress or Ununited Fracture

Patients who have suffered prolonged symptoms in the course of growth sometimes exhibit elongation of the inferior pole and, in extreme examples, patella alta can result. Occasionally when a lateral radiograph is taken an ununited fracture is revealed. In some instances it may be difficult to determine whether the ununited fragment is the result of an anomaly of ossification, Sinding Larsen-Johansson disease or whether a stress fracture has been superimposed on an elongated inferior pole as the result of ischaemia (Fig. 2,38).

TREATMENT. If symptoms persist treatment consists of excision of the ununited fragment through a short lateral parapatellar incision. The fragment is dissected out from the side with as little damage as possible to the tendon.

## CONGENITAL ANOMALIES OF PATELLA

### FAMILIAL ABSENCE OF PATELLA

Absence of the patella as an isolated congenital abnormality without stigmata of the nail-patella syndrome is rare. Two examples only have been reported (Kutz, 1949; Bernhang and Levine, 1973). In the latter, two brothers had bilateral absence without related disability.

### Nail-patella Syndrome (Hereditary Onycho-osteo-arthroidysplasia)

**Background note.** The syndrome was described

first by Sedgwick (quoted by Little, 1897). It is a hereditary disorder transmitted by a dominant autosomal gene: it never skips a generation and can be transmitted by both sexes.

**Definition.** The condition is characterised by absence of the finger nails accompanied by a dysplasia of the knee joint in which the patella is absent, rudimentary or underdeveloped. There may be other deformities such as genu recurvatum. The knee condition is bilateral but not necessarily symmetrical. There may be other anomalies. Aggarwal and Mittal (1970) describing an Indian family of 57 members with 15 affected individuals noted that every time a family is discovered to have the syndrome new features are added.

### ANOMALIES

A variety of anomalies of congenital origin are encountered, some common such as the bipartite

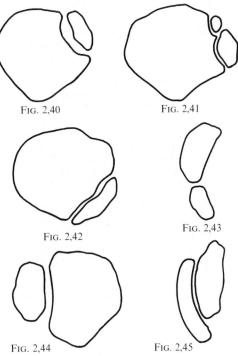

FIG. 2,40          FIG. 2,41

FIG. 2,42          FIG. 2,43

FIG. 2,44          FIG. 2,45

FIGS 2,40–45. **Patella: anomalies of ossification.** The common varieties, bipartite (Fig. 2,40) and tripartite (Fig. 2,41) are located at the supralateral aspect. The other varieties located at the infralateral aspect (Fig. 2,42) and dividing the patella in the transverse (Fig. 2,43), saggital (Fig. 2,44) and coronal planes (Fig. 2,45) are rare.

and tripartite forms (Figs 2,40 and 2,41) and others rare (Figs 2,42 to 2,45).

INCIDENCE. In 500 consecutive cases reviewed in the year 1970–71 there were 18 examples (3·6 per cent) of the various forms illustrated (Figs 2,40 to 2,45).

SEX. In this series there is no significant sex incidence. There were 10 males and 8 females.

**Incidence of related symptoms.** Nine, that is to say, half of the 18 cases presented with symptoms directly related to the abnormality. The other 9 were incidental findings in patients presenting with some knee complaint not related to the patella.

The condition is not necessarily bilateral, or, if bilateral, symmetrical. In 8 cases the radiological finding was unilateral.

**Incidence of varieties.** Fourteen were bipartite at the superior pole. One was bipartite but at the inferior pole. Two cases were tripartite at the superior pole. One example was a combination of supralateral and infralateral anomalies.

The explanation is offered that the predilection for the supralateral angle as the common site is determined by the sparsity of blood supply in this area.

The only example encountered of the anomaly whereby the patella is split in the coronal plane is that illustrated in Figs 2,48 and 2,49 (case of Mr J. F. M. Frew, Inverness, Scotland):

The patient (J. MacN., male, aged 28, carpenter) was the subject of multiple epiphyseal dysplasia. His complaint was of locking in the right knee. When radiographs were obtained it was evident that the locking was taking place between the two halves of the patella which slipped over one another in a limited range. It will be seen that the relationship of the anterior half to the posterior half changes between flexion and extension (Figs 2,48 and 2,49); and that the quadriceps tendon must be attached to the posterior half while the patellar tendon is attached to the anterior.

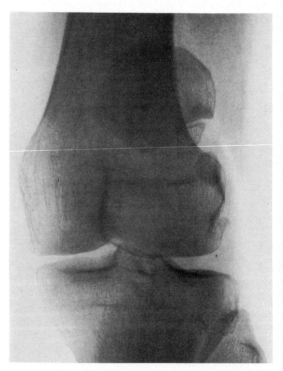

FIGS 2,46–47. **Anomalies of ossification.** When the anomaly is in the supralateral aspect, the common variety, it is recognisable clinically by a visible or palpable prominence (Fig. 2,46) (see Fig. 2,40). If it is located at the infralateral aspect it will only be detectable radiologically (Fig. 2,47) (see Fig. 2,42). In this example the anomaly was bilateral and symmetrical (M.R., female, case of J.H.).

The operation carried out to eliminate the locking incidents between the fragments was patellectomy. With hind-sight, and prejudice against patellectomy, it is possible that excision of the patella might have been avoided by an operation to secure union between the fragments.

The exact outcome in terms of function is not known. The patient lives on a remote island, He is known to be earning his living in his original trade as a carpenter.

The anomaly whereby the patella is divided in the transverse plane (Fig. 2,43) is also rare. One example only, with the certainty of the existence of the anomaly as opposed to an ununited transverse fracture has been encountered. The condition was bilateral and symmetrical. The symptoms were minimal. The patient did not seek treatment.

**Implications of bipartite patella.** Anomalies of the patella are by no means innocent of implications for disability as was formerly supposed. It will be seen that roughly half the common examples encountered were responsible for symptoms; and all the rare gross varieties (Figs 2,43 to 2,45) can be expected to give rise to disability.

The inherent potential disability is illustrated in the extreme form by the following case:

The patient, (R. A., aged 36, professional cyclist, case of J. H.) complained of pain in both knees. It is well-known that of all athletic activities professional cycling is the sport most liable to chondromalacia of the patella, even in normal knees with a normal relationship of patella to femoral condyles. The existence of bipartite patella, if what has been said above is correct, made it certain that symptoms would arise in the patello-femoral joint. It is surprising, in a professional cyclist, that trouble did not occur before the age of 36. Perhaps athletes who take up this activity on a professional basis should have their knees examined. A patient with an anomaly of ossification of the patella certainly should not take up the career of professional cyclist.

The presence of a large fragment unconnected to the main mass of the patella by bone may lead, when the patient is under stress, to a

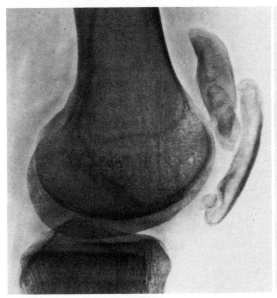 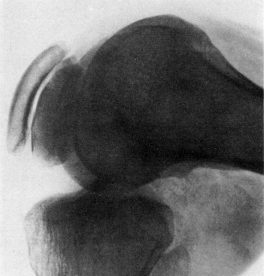

FIG. 2,48                                    FIG. 2,49

FIGS 2,48–49. **Anomaly of ossification.** Patella is bipartite in coronal plane. The relationship of the halves changes in extension (Fig. 2,48) and flexion (Fig. 2,49). It is presumed that quadriceps is attached to the posterior half, patellar tendon to anterior half (J. MacN., male, aged 28, case of Mr J. F. M. Frew, Inverness, Scotland).

feeling of instability or insecurity. The symptoms may thus be confused with those of recurrent subluxation of the patella.

There was one serious error of diagnosis (and of judgement) encountered:

The patient, a girl (M. S., then aged 13) with retropatellar symptoms was misdiagnosed as a recurrent subluxation of the patella and subjected to operation in the form of transplantation of the tibial tubercle. The operation was carried out before the tibial ephiphysis was mature, and the tubercle migrated down the tibia to be responsible for patella baja. Under investigation for gross symptoms in the patello-femoral joint it was discovered

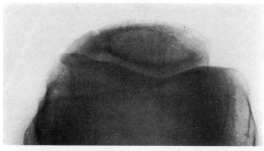

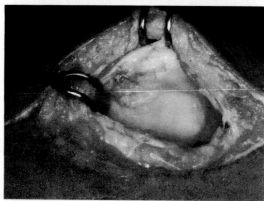

FIGS 2,50–51. **Anomaly of ossification: bipartite patella.** This particular example is illustrated because it is the patella of Figure 2,91 iatrogenic patella baja in which the symptoms relating to an anomaly of ossification had been mistaken for recurrent subluxation. Note difficulty of obtaining skyline view clear of femoral condyles due to patella baja; but it is seen that an angular deformity exists between ossicle and main mass of the bone (Fig. 2,50).

At operation there was gross chondromalacia affecting the articular cartilage of the ossicle (Fig. 2,51). Excision of the ossicle almost amounted to hemipatellectomy (M.M., female, aged 23).

that she had a bipartite patella (Fig. 2,50); and that the symptoms were so related. At operation for excision of the fragment there were gross local changes in the articular cartilage overlying the anomalous ossicle (Fig. 2,51).

The patient was improved, but not rendered symptomless by operation, and the question still remains as to whether restoration of the patella to a more normal location is required. The anomaly in this example was unilateral.

**Pathological anatomy.** If the ossicle projects beyond the mass of the bone the overlying articular cartilage develops, presumably for mechanical reasons, degenerative changes which vary from fibrillation to evident osteoarthrosis, with similar changes on the opposing lateral condyle. Furthermore, because the bone element is joined to the main mass of the patella by cartilage, movement within a limited range is possible. It is under stress that movement occurs; and this is the reason for the giving-way incidents which may be a feature of the symptomology.

**Clinical features.** There may be a history of injury. It is possible that some incident precipitates symptoms of giving-way in so far as a blow or twist disrupts the insecure union between bipartite fragments and the main mass of bone. In general, the symptoms are those of a local chondromalacia or osteoarthrosis with pain and incidents of instability or giving-way located in the patello-femoral joint.

On examination the supralateral angle of the patella is markedly prominent. It appears however that prominence of the supralateral margin can exist but without the necessity for a separate ossicle. It is of interest that occasionally symptoms may be so related. There is pain on pressure over the prominent area and synovial tenderness may be present immediately lateral to the prominence.

**Radiological examination.** Antero-posterior, lateral and skyline projections are necessary. The antero-posterior view shows the anomaly, bipartite or tripartite, located at the supralateral angle. The line of demarcation between the ossicles and the main mass of the bone runs obliquely downwards and laterally (Fig. 2,60), distinguishing the condition from the common

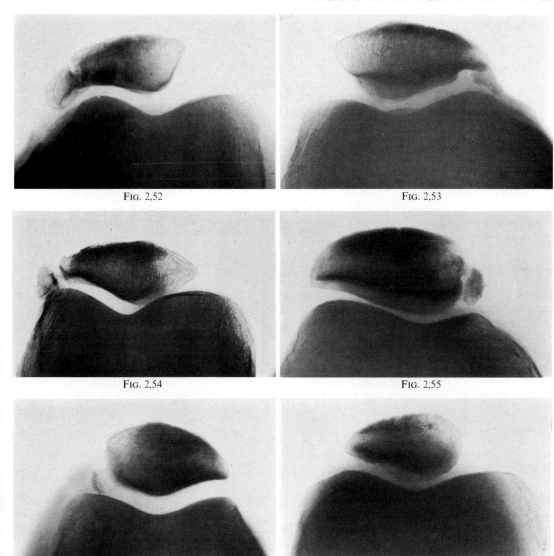

FIG. 2,52                    FIG. 2,53

FIG. 2,54                    FIG. 2,55

FIG. 2,56                    FIG. 2,57

FIGS 2,52–57. **Patello-femoral joint. Variety of pathology as depicted in the skyline view: differential diagnosis.**

Fig. 2,52. **Anomaly of ossification: bipartite patella.** The patient never had symptoms related to the patello-femoral joint. But note congruous opposing surfaces. (M.L., female, aged 52.)

Fig. 2,53. **Anomaly of ossification: bipartite patella.** The existence of a large cartilaginous gap in the radiograph does not necessarily imply related symptoms. But note absence of changes in the opposing joint surfaces. (M.W., male, aged 25, professional football player.)

Fig. 2,54. **Lateral marginal fracture.** This fracture is not only common but commonly missed until unexpectedly revealed in the skyline view. The fracture line is vertical involving the entire thickness of the bone.

Fig. 2,55. **Medial marginal fracture.** In contradistinction to the lateral side, medial marginal fractures are rare. It is differentiated from the medial tangential osteochondral fracture in that the fracture line is vertical (Fig. 2,55) not oblique as in Figure 2,56. (Case of Mr W. E. Tucker, London.)

Fig. 2,56. **Medial tangential osteochondral fracture.** In this complication of recurrent dislocation the fracture line is oblique. It does not involve the anterior surface of the bone.

Fig. 2,57. **Osteochondritis dissecans.** Lesion located towards centre of bone not involving the periphery in adolescent male. It is the result of single-incident trauma or osteochondritis dissecans.

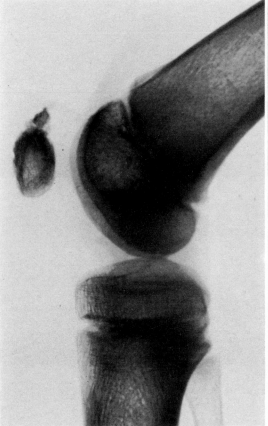
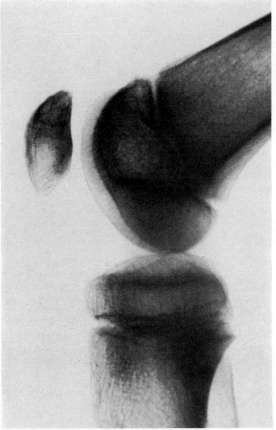

FIGS 2,58–59. **Anomalies of ossification.** A wide variety of appearances are consistent with normality in the growing child (Fig. 2,58). The same patella two years later (Fig. 2,59).

lateral marginal fracture, the direction of which is vertical. The lateral and skyline views not only confirm the curved, as opposed to vertical nature of the line of demarcation, but demonstrate that the ossicles project into the joint beyond the mass of the bone (Fig. 2,61).

Anomalies of ossification should be distinguished from separate ossicles which are the residue of Sinding Larsen-Johannson disease or old or stress fractures at the inferior pole.

**Indications for treatment.** It will be evident from the foregoing that the existence of an anomaly is not an indication for operation: half the cases encountered are symptomless. Even when symptoms can be related with certainty to the anomaly they may be present only at the highest levels of physical activity. In such circumstances all that may be required is abandonment or reduction of the activity involved. Those cases in which symptoms are produced by the activities of every day usually require operation. In children multipolar ossification is common and need not occasion alarm (Fig. 2,58). Separate ossicles usually disappear with the advent of maturity (Fig. 2,59). Sometimes the whole lateral aspect of the patella is the site of multiple bony foci, some of which unite with the main mass of the bone, and others remain separate to constitute an anomaly of ossification.

In the presence of an anomaly, rerouting of the patella as occurs when the tibial tubercle is transferred to a medial, or to a medial and inferior position, will result in the precipitation of symptoms in the form of pain from local chondromalacia or osteoarthrosis. When such an unusual combination of circumstances arise

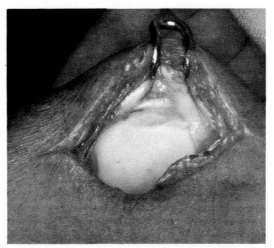

FIG. 2,62a

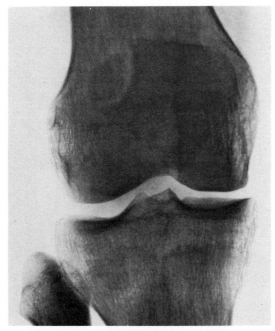

FIG. 2,60

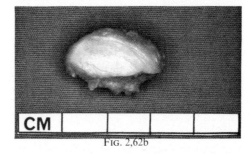

FIG. 2,62b

FIGS 2,60–62. **Anomaly of ossification: treatment.** In this bipartite example there was persistent pain and giving-way incidents on the lateral aspect of the patello-femoral joint (Figs 2,60 and 2,61).

At operation through a short lateral parapatellar exposure a shallow groove is seen between ossicle and main bone; and the connecting tissue was cartilage (Fig. 2,62a). The excised ossicle to show dimensions in centimetres (Fig. 2,62b).

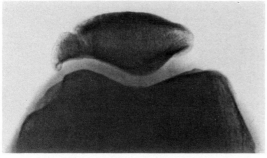

FIG. 2,61

as subluxation in combination with an abnormality of ossification the anomaly should be excised prior to the patellar tendon transplant.

### Operation

**Technique.** The patient is placed in the supine position on the table with the limb in the completely extended position and under the control of a tourniquet. The joint is entered through a short lateral parapatellar incision. The appearance varies at the site of anomaly between intact articular cartilage and local osteo-arthrosis. The line of demarcation on the articular surface will be seen to be a shallow groove; and excision should begin by entering the point of the knife into this groove. The knife, however, cannot be passed through the line of demarcation if it is only for the reason that it is concave in section with the convexity towards the centre of the bone. The best plan, therefore, is to erase the soft tissues from the superficial surface of the patella by sharp dissection beginning at the margin and working centrally as far as the line of demarcation but no further. A gouge with a convexity towards the centre of the bone should now be entered at the inferior pole and made to follow the concavity until the superior pole is reached by which time the fragment is free (Figs 2,60 to 2,62).

AFTER-TREATMENT. At the termination of the operation a compression bandage is applied. It need not be specially tight in so far as there is no wide raw area of synovial membrane and vascular cancellous tissue has not been exposed. When the immediate post-operative pain has subsided straight-leg-raising is initiated. A return to limited weight-bearing is indicated when quadriceps control has been established.

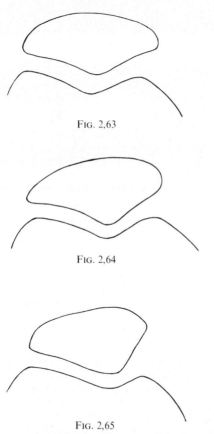

FIG. 2,63

FIG. 2,64

FIG. 2,65

FIGS 2,63–65. **Radiological classification of forms of normal patella in axial view (Wiberg).**
Type I. The ridge is central and the medial and lateral facets of equal size (Fig. 2,63).
Type II. The ridge is located towards the medial side. The lateral facet larger than the medial (Fig. 2,64).
Type III. The ridge is located on the medial side. The lateral facet is large. The medial is small and at right angles to the lateral (Fig. 2,65).

## THE PATELLA

The patella is encountered in a wide variety of shape, size and location consistent with normal function.

**Form.** The classification of normal shape most widely quoted depends on the site of the ridge in

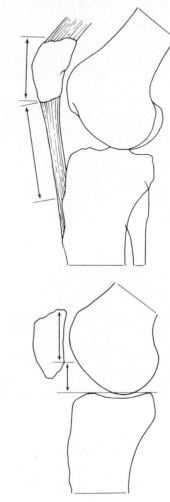

FIGS 2,66–67. **Relationship of patella to femoral condyles: Methods of measurement.** (1) Measurements are made on a lateral radiograph in the manner shown. When the patella is normally located the lengths of patella and patellar tendon are equal. When tendon length exceeds patellar length by more than 20 per cent the patella is located at an abnormally high level (Fig. 2,66). (After Insall and Salvati, 1971.) (2) Measurements are made on a lateral radiograph in 30° of flexion in the manner shown (Fig. 2,67). The ratio 1/2 provides a measure of patella level. The normal ratio is 0·8. In patella alta it is greater than 1·0. (After Blackburne and Peel, 1977.)

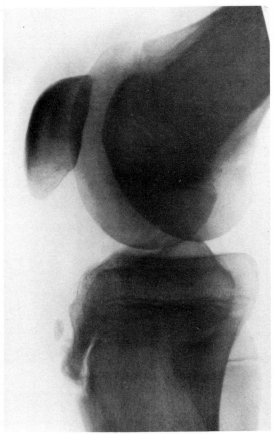

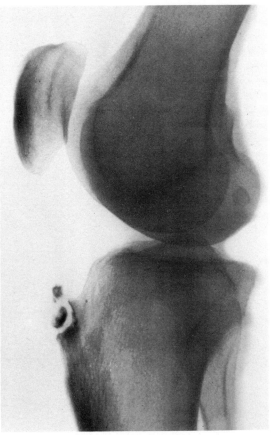

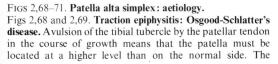

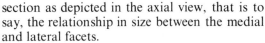

FIG. 2,68

FIG. 2,69

FIGS 2,68–71. **Patella alta simplex: aetiology.**
Figs 2,68 and 2,69. **Traction epiphysitis: Osgood-Schlatter's disease.** Avulsion of the tibial tubercle by the patellar tendon in the course of growth means that the patella must be located at a higher level than on the normal side. The

potential for disability should be recognised at the earliest opportunity and defensive measures instituted (Fig. 2,68). If the condition is untreated patella alta is inevitable in maturity; and with potential for symptoms from ununited ossicles (Figs 2,68 and 2,69). See also Figures 2,70 and 2,71.

section as depicted in the axial view, that is to say, the relationship in size between the medial and lateral facets.

TYPE I. The facets are of equal size (Fig. 2,63).
TYPE II. The ridge is situated towards the medial side (Fig. 2,64).
TYPE III. The ridge is located markedly to the medial side (Fig. 2,65) (Wiberg, 1941).

It follows that a relationship exists between the type of patella and the size of the related femoral condyle. Whether the shape of the patella determines future pathology is a matter of controversy. In Type III, the so-called Hunter's Cap variety, lack of development of the medial aspect may reflect the status of the vastus

medialis component of the quadriceps and particularly the oblique fibres and thus indicate a possible liability to subluxation or dislocation.
**Size.** The size and thickness of the bone affords some indication of quadriceps function. The thicker the bone, for example, the further is the tendon located from the centre of rotation of the joint.

**Location.** The concept of some standard whereby the relationship of patella to the femoral condyle could be measured is attractive. The suggestion that the inferior pole in a normal relationship coincides with the sclerotic line produced by the inner boundary of the femoral condyles in a lateral radiograph taken at 150°

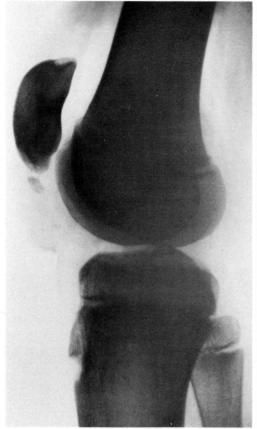

FIG. 2,70        FIG. 2,71

FIGS 2,70–71. **Patella alta simplex: aetiology.**

Fig. 2,70. **Sinding Larsen-Johannson's disease.** If a traction lesion at the tibial attachment of the tendon influences the location of the patella a similar lesion producing elongation of the inferior pole (see Figs 2,38 and 2,39) or fragmentation in the form of Sinding Larsen-Johannson's disease has a similar effect.

Fig. 2,71. **Iatrogenic.** This patient underwent operation for recurrent subluxation of the patella. The tibial tubercle and attached tendon have not been securely fixed. The patella is at an even higher level than originally.

An untreated avulsion fracture of the tibial tubercle would have the same appearance and effect.

(Blumensaat, 1938) has not proved a reliable yardstick.

In the current scene no method of measurement has been evolved which takes into account the variety of factors involved. Two methods merit description. That of Insall and Salvati (1971) compares the length of the patella with the length of the patellar tendon as measured in a lateral radiograph taken in 30° or more of flexion (Fig. 2,66). In the normal knee the distances should be equal, plus or minus 20 per cent. In a method attributed to E. L. Trickey (Blackburne and Peel, 1977), a lateral radiograph

is taken in 30° or more of flexion, which ensures that the patellar tendon is taut. A line is drawn along the tibial plateau and two measurements made: (1) The distance of the lower end of the articular surface of the patella from the tibial plateau and (2) the length of the articular surface of the patella (Fig. 2,67). The ratio 1/2 provides a measure of patella level. The normal ratio is defined as 0.8. In patella alta it is greater than 1.0.

Neither method is without criticism. The former assumes the tibial tubercle, not always readily defined, to be located a standard dis-

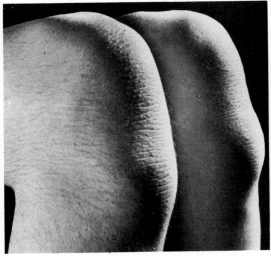
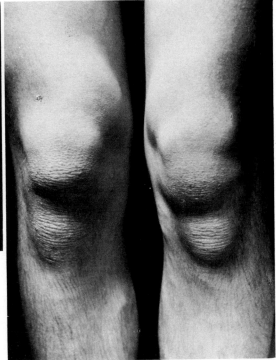

FIGS 2,72–73. **Traction epiphysitis: Osgood-Schlatter's disease.** The clinical appearance of bilateral traction epiphysitis in established form. Note evidence of patella alta in the appearance of the fat pads (Fig. 2,73) (J.L., male, aged 16).

tance below the tibial plateau. Both depend on the size of the patella, the former on total length, the latter on the length of the articular surface. Neither reflect the mechanical status of the joint in the patella alta/genu recurvatum complex.

**Factors determining site.** It is clear that the relationship of the patella to the femoral condyles is determined in the course of growth by the action of the quadriceps. Witness the effect of complete paralysis as in poliomyelitis which produces the extreme examples of patella baja (Fig. 2,88). It appears therefore that a 'normal' degree of quadriceps development is necessary, amongst other things, to determine a normal relationship of patella to femoral condyle. But what is normal development? It is known that quadriceps hypertrophy produced by athletic activity in the course of growth can precipitate traction epiphysitis (Osgood-Schlatter's disease) at the tibial tubercle. In the absence of this condition, or presence in subclinical degree, it is possible that abnormal quadriceps development can in the course of growth locate the patella

at an abnormally high level just as absence of quadriceps influence locates the patella at an abnormally low level.

## PATELLA ALTA SIMPLEX AND PATELLA ALTA/GENU RECURVATUM COMPLEX: AETIOLOGY

### 1. Traction Epiphysitis: Osgood-Schlatter's Disease

**Background note.** The earliest record of traction epiphysitis is of the tibiae of a middle-aged male found in the late Saxon burial ground of St. Catherine, Thorpe, England, dated on archaeological evidence to about the ninth to tenth century A.D. (Wells, 1968). The right tibia is comparable with Figure 2,68 and has the appearance of a prominent tibial tubercle without separate ossicle. The left has a concavity comparable with Figure 2,69 and it can be assumed that originally ossicles existed within the cavity.

**Relationship to patella alta.** If evulsion of the inferior attachment of the patellar tendon takes place in the course of growth the patella is invariably located at a higher level than normal in maturity (Figs 2,68 and 2,69).

Traction epiphysitis is recognised only if it produces clinical signs at the attachment of the patellar tendon, so-called Osgood-Schlatter's disease (Figs 2,72 and 2,73). There is no doubt, however, that the condition exists in subclinical degree; and that this is the explanation of a large proportion of cases of patella alta for which no other reason is forthcoming.

It is not generally recognised that to be exceptionally good at games in early youth, particularly a game such as Association Football, in which players of exceptional skill command exceptional rewards, may be a disaster in the long term. Professional football clubs have talent-spotters who seek out youths of promise. Youngsters play their hearts out as immature Juniors in the hope of being spotted. They are then subjected, usually very willingly, to much training and development of muscles, particularly the quadriceps and calf muscles, to the point of hypertrophy. The effect on the extensor apparatus at the extreme is the development of a traction epiphysitis at the tibial tubercle. But often there are no subjective phenomena with subclinical elevation of the tubercle, lengthening of the tendon, or elongation of the inferior pole of the patella. The consequence is patella alta.

There are other, and worse, possibilities. Excessive training with its effect on quadriceps and calf muscles in the course of growth exerts abnormal pressure on the anterior aspects of the epiphyseal plates of femur and tibia with development not only of patella alta but genu recurvatum. A further example, of less importance because the situation is less exploited, is the tall young jumper of promise. His patellae become located higher and higher as the years pass and when he reaches maturity the promise of youth when they were correctly located is not fulfilled. (See also Jumper's Knee.)

## 2. Sinding Larsen-Johannson's Disease

If a traction lesion develops at the inferior pole of the patella in the course of growth, the patella may reasonably be expected to be located at a higher level in maturity (Fig. 2,70). This condition in established clinical and radiological form is rare and as such unimportant. What may be more important, and pass unrecognised, is the subclinical variety which produces gradual elongation of the inferior pole of the patella (Figs 2,38 and 2,39). If this condition is a source of local symptoms (see below) it is unlikely to be a factor in the overall picture of patella alta simplex.

## 3. Premature Closure of Anterior Aspect of Upper Tibial Epiphysis

If premature closure of the anterior aspect of the upper tibial epiphysis occurs, not only is there a recurvatus deformity but the patella is at a higher level than normal. This is the deformity referred to as the patella alta/genu recurvatum complex. The most common subclinical form is represented by the almost normal recurvatus of the female knee due to the increased pressure on the interior aspect of the growth plate induced by the use of high-heeled shoes. At the extreme is the continuous excessive pressure produced by recumbency in the supine position in any condition necessitating prolonged bed rest.

## 4. Heritable Diseases of Connective Tissue

Laxity of the posterior capsule and ligaments of a degree short of the Marfan or Ehlers-Danlos syndrome are of common occurrence; and the aetiology of the genu recurvatum/patella alta identified as such (see Aetiology of Recurrent Subluxation of Patella).

## 5. Spastic Paralysis

In cerebral palsy with spastic lower extremities, patella alta, as opposed to the common association with genu recurvatum, may accompany flexion deformities. The hamstring muscles are more powerful than the extensors producing fixed flexion against which the quadriceps is constantly acting. The interplay in the course of growth not only locates the patella at a considerably higher level than normal but frequently alters its shape whereby it is elongated or crescent shaped. Fragmentation of the inferior pole with an appearance similar to Sinding Larsen-Johannson's disease is common.

It should be recognised that patella alta in any marked degree is a clinical entity with clear-cut implications for disability.

**Recurrent subluxation of patella.** It will be shown that the most common single cause of recurrent subluxation is patella alta.

**Rupture of patellar tendon.** The stresses imposed on the patellar tendon in the unusual circumstances of a youth with this conformation of joint attaining athletic prowess is shown by the frequency with which so-called spontaneous rupture of the tendon is encountered; so much so that in the event of this unusual injury in youth occurring in the absence of hydrocortisone injections the presence of patella alta should be suspected. The following is an example of a case:

The patient (R. S., aged 23, professional football player) in a leap into the air at the goal mouth to head a ball, sustained a spontaneous rupture of his left patellar tendon. At examination it was clear that he had a patella alta with characteristic large flat fat pad on the 'normal' side. At operation for the repair of the rupture it was demonstrated that even at the age of 23 degenerative changes were present in the tendon. It was assumed that these changes were the result of the stresses imposed by the absence of a functioning patella.

He made an excellent recovery and returned to professional football at the end of six months. He was naturally left-footed and said he had no disability and was playing as well as ever. It was of some academic interest, however, that whereas the quadriceps were of a volume expected in a professional football player of his physique, the vastus medialis was markedly underdeveloped and bore no relationship to the volume of the central and lateral components.

This patient returned with a rupture of the left patellar tendon exactly three years later. He said that he had received a kick but there can be little doubt that it too was a so-called spontaneous rupture.

This is the only example encountered of such a sequence of events. A record of the original rupture was made to illustrate one of the possible complications of patella alta. The validity of the example is shown by the fact that the second tendon too underwent spontaneous rupture.

**Clinical Features**

The symptoms are characteristically vague: and this constitutes a major obstacle to diagnosis. The complaint is of retropatellar ache made worse by physical activity, subsiding with rest. Giving-way incidents may occur and be followed by minimal effusions particularly in the presence of recurvatus deformity.

Examination may reveal no abnormality to the unitiated; and this leads in the teenager complaining of both knees to failure to recognise the source of the biomechanical problem, and thus to misjudgement and injustice. The experienced physician will note the characteristic features of a high, possibly small, patella, long patellar tendon, large flat fat pad, lack of quadriceps development and with wasted vastus medialis but in any event thigh muscles not comparable in conformation to the calf muscles (Figs 2,74 and 2,75).

**Differential diagnosis.** The most common, and serious, error is misinterpretation of the symptoms for those of chondromalacia. In this regard it should be recognised that the pain complained of is based on synovial irritation in the suprapatellar pouch at the superior margin of the femoral condyles from friction and compression by the patella; and that the pain produced by manual pressure on the patella in extension is due to compression of the synovial membrane immediately superior to the articular cartilage of the femoral condyles (Figs 2,76 and 2,77). To oppose articular cartilage to articular cartilage some degree of flexion is essential.

It should be recognised that the biomechanical defects of the genu recurvatum component of the patella alta/genu recurvatum complex render

the joint liable to a greater variety of affections than incurred by patella alta simplex (Fig. 2,78).
**Vulnerability to injury.** The knee of normal conformation, struck from the lateral side in the course of contact games, tends to flex and thus the medial ligament escapes injury. The hyperextended joint in such circumstances cannot readily undo the exaggerated screw-home movement characteristic of the complex (see below) with the result that medial ligament, both cruciate ligaments and the posterior capsule are ruptured.

If, in general, patella alta/genu recurvatum is an inefficient and vulnerable knee for the majority of sports, and in particular contact games, there may be exceptions. It has been suggested, but not confirmed, that the ability to hyperextend may be an advantage in certain swimming techniques, namely the butterfly and back strokes. If this is so it is presumed to be the result of the increase in range of movement beyond normal extension.
**Liability to recurrent synovial effusions.**

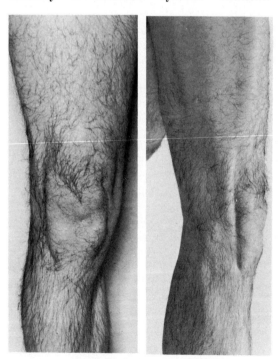

FIGS 2,74–75. **Patella alta simplex.** The typical appearance showing the high patella, long tendon and large flat fat pad (Fig. 2,74). If the patella is functionless as in patella alta the iliotibial band may be used to extend the knee (Fig. 2,75).

Abnormal physical exercise in the form of dancing, long hours of standing, etc., subjects the synovial lining of the fat pad to excessive pressure with resultant effusions which, being bilateral and in the female subject, can be the subject of clinical alarm resulting in a long series of negative laboratory investigations.
**Fat pad lesions.** The result of excessive mechanical pressure is ultimately synovial pain, and possible effusion as above. In women the liability to the premenstrual water retention syndrome is increased in knees with evident hyperextension.
**Lesion of anterior segment of meniscus.** Experience has shown, and for obvious reasons of compression, that the comparatively rare lesions of the anterior segment of the meniscus occur in the female subject with hyperextended knees.

**Clinical Features**
The salient feature of examination is the genu recurvatum rather than the patella alta (Figs 2,79 and 2,80). When examination is carried out in the supine position as described in Chapter 1 and illustrated in Figure 1,5 it is important to note the excessive lateral rotation of the tibia which takes place between the position of extension and hyperextension, in other words, the much exaggerated screw-home movement which explains the vulnerability of such joints to injury in contact games.
**Radiological investigation.** The limitations of the lateral view in 150° extension (Fig. 1,20) in the estimation of the level of the patella has been stressed. Nevertheless, this projection is helpful and should form part of routine investigation. A lateral view in the standing position with the knee in maximum extension, or hyperextension, and with the quadriceps in maximum contraction is essential (Figs 1,17 to 1,19).

It will be evident, for obvious anatomical reasons, that the skyline view (Figs 1,21 to 1,23) may be difficult or indeed impossible to obtain.

If in the course of any investigation of a knee joint complaint, the radiologist reports his inability to obtain a skyline view, suspicion should arise that the patient suffers from a patella alta.

The practical difficulties of diagnosis and treatment are illustrated by the following case:

The patient (J.C.H., male, aged 15) com-

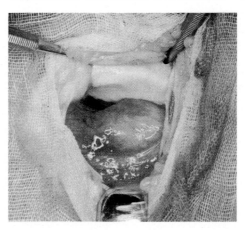

FIG. 2,77

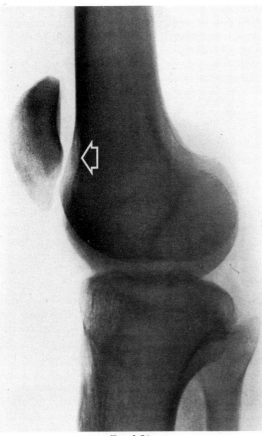

FIG. 2,76

FIGS 2,76–77. **Patella alta.** Retropatellar symptoms in patella alta are most frequently produced by pinching of the synovial membrane immediately superior to articular cartilage of the femoral condyle by the patella in extension. It is most important that this source of symptoms be distinguished from those of chondromalacia patellae. The patello-femoral joint exposed through a limited incision to show the synovial membrane in such a case (Fig. 2,77).

plained that 10 months previously he had developed pain beneath the patella of the left knee. He had not suffered symptoms on the right side. The complaint was, as he described it, a feeling of rubbing beneath the bone, which was later replaced by pain. Initially there had been no effusion. He had been seen by an orthopaedic surgeon who had induced pain on compression of the patella against the femur. The radiograph showed no abnormality. He made a diagnosis of chondromalacia of the patella. He prescribed reduction of athletic activity. The patient stopped cycling to school, a matter of six or so kilometres, and stopped playing games.

At a second examination the same surgeon noted some effusion in the knee and recorded tenderness on pressing the patella backwards with the knee in the extended position. He prescribed a plaster cast of the walking variety; and this had been retained for four weeks.

The patient stated that he had not suffered pain while wearing the plaster cast but after removal and mobilisation of the joint, the pain returned. It is of interest that skyline views of the patella were ordered. The radiographer recorded with regret her failure to obtain the required views.

It was at this stage that the surgeon who originally examined him questioned the diagnosis of chondromalacia patellae and various laboratory investigations for the purpose of eliminating rheumatoid arthritis and tuberculosis were instituted. All tests proved negative. A further attempt was made to obtain skyline views of the patella and these too failed. The symptoms of retropatellar pain continued accompanied by a small

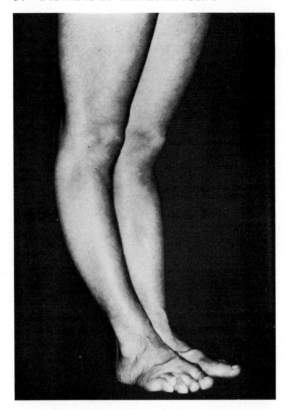

FIG. 2,78. **Recurrent subluxation of patella in patella alta/genu recurvatum complex.** When recurrent subluxation or dislocation is based on the unfortunate combination of patella alta with genu recurvatum, transplantation of the patellar tendon attachment to a lower level may, even in maturity, produce a tension situation with possible stretching of the posterior capsule. This example illustrates patella alta/genu recurvatum in which the dislocation of the patella has been eliminated at the expense of an increase in the recurvatus deformity on the right side.

of the tongue-shaped epiphysis at the upper end of the tibia and thus possibly the cause of the condition: a traction epiphysitis which, symptomless and unrecognised, may have been responsible for the location of the patella at an abnormally high level.

The lessons to be learnt from this case are many:

1. That patella alta as a clinical entity in its own right, so to speak, tends to pass unrecognised.

2. That retropatellar pain in youth is commonly erroneously diagnosed as chondromalacia.

3. That the presence of effusion might have given the hint as to the diagnosis. Effusion does not take place in chondromalacia patellae if it is only for the reason that articular cartilage is involved; not synovial membrane. If effusion is present it must be the result of irritation of synovial membrane. In patella alta, as illustrated by this case, the mechanical irritation of the synovial membrane is immediately above the articular margin of the femoral condyles in the posterior wall of the suprapatellar pouch.

4. The erroneous use of immobilisation in a plaster cast as the treatment of chondromalacia.

TREATMENT. There remains the question of how a case such as this should be managed.

effusion. At the end of a year, with no reduction of symptoms, his mother sought a further opinion; and the case was presented for diagnosis and treatment.

On examination the salient feature was the large flat fat pad and other stigmata characteristic of patella alta: pain on compression of the patella clearly located above the femoral condyles with the knee in extension. There was a slight recurvatus deformity. The radiograph in the lateral view revealed the patella in the expected position above the femoral condyles. In addition it revealed some avulsion

It is to be noted that the patella is located at an exceptionally high level; and may have arisen in traction epiphysitis. It is to be noted also that the epiphysis at the upper end of the tibia has not closed and that further growth potential exists. What then should be done, first to relieve the patient's symptoms and, second, to improve the future function of the knee?

It will be evident that mechanical improvement of this knee can occur only if the relationship of the patella to the femoral condyles can be altered so that the patella is located at a lower level. Any immediate operation to lower the site of attachment of the patellar tendon is precluded by the fact that the upper tibial growth plate remains open. An operation in that region before maturity would interfere with the anterior aspect of the plate and thus

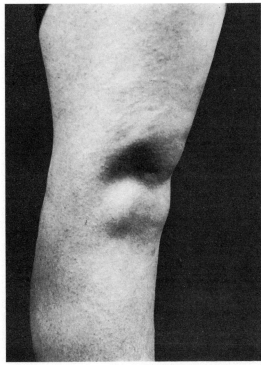

FIG. 2,79

FIG. 2,80

FIGS 2,79–80. **Patella alta/genu recurvatum complex.** The clinical appearance of patella alta/genu recurvatum complex to show high patella, long patellar tendon and large fat pad filling interval between patella and tibial tubercle (Fig. 2,79). Lateral radiograph to show location of patella in extension (it is not known whether this exposure was made in hyperextension and with maximum contraction of the quadriceps): in any event the patella is not in contact with the femoral condyles (Fig. 2,80) (A.W., female, aged 19).

increase the genu recurvatum; but in any event would increase the pressure on the anterior aspect of the plate, increase the recurvatus and thus the height of the patella. There is thus no alternative at this stage to palliative measures of which only the raising of the heels of the shoes can be shown to be helpful. If there is demand for more active measures the reasons for deferring operation should be explained. In circumstances where symptoms are such as to demand relief, experience has shown that excision of the area of synovial membrane immediately superior to the articular cartilage of the femoral condyles effects relief (see below). In general, however, the demand for operative interference should be resisted.

There remains the question as to what should be done when the growth plates have closed. There is a case for transplantation of the attachment of the patellar tendon to a lower level. The problems involved are described later.

## TREATMENT

### Prevention

It will be evident that those varieties of patella alta and patella alta/genu recurvatum which are produced by abnormal development of quadriceps and calf muscles in the course of rapid growth can be prevented. Neither the short, heavily muscled youth nor the tall youngster with long levers acting about the knee should be permitted to carry their enthusiasm for muscle building or athletic prowess to excess during periods of rapid growth. Youths with open epiphyses, no matter how promising, should not be permitted to take part in weight-bearing games in competition with mature

D

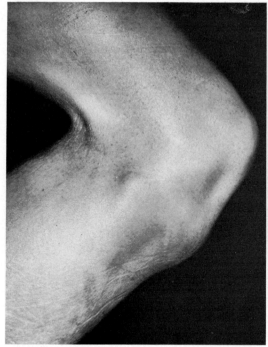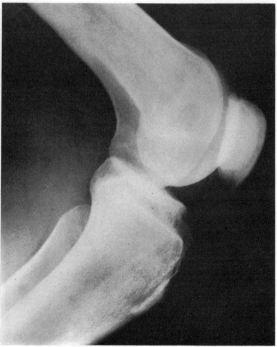

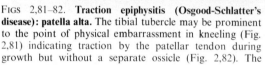

FIGS 2,81–82. **Traction epiphysitis (Osgood-Schlatter's disease): patella alta.** The tibial tubercle may be prominent to the point of physical embarrassment in kneeling (Fig. 2,81) indicating traction by the patellar tendon during growth but without a separate ossicle (Fig. 2,82). The means whereby such a prominence can be reduced and at the same time the patella pulled down to a lower level is described in the text and illustrated in Figures 2,83 to 2,86.

adults. The physiologically permissible exception is non-weight-bearing, namely, swimming.
**Traction epiphysitis: Osgood-Schlatter's disease.** This condition, a well-established clinical entity, while accepted to cause temporary inconvenience and interruption of athletic pursuits in the adolescent male, has not been regarded as potentially disabling. This attitude is erroneous. Attention has been directed above to a clinically undetectable variety of traction strain leading to patella alta. That patella alta results from clinical traction epiphysitis is not in doubt. In unilateral examples where the youth is right-footed the epiphysitis is manifest on the right side and the patella readily demonstrated to be located at a higher level on the right side. If subclinical traction epiphysitis is undetectable, clinical traction epiphysitis is potentially a certain source of patella alta and as such should be taken seriously in the context of preventative medicine as a source of physical disability.

Unfortunately, cases are seldom presented at an early stage; only when symptoms are long established and disabling. The first essential is explanation to the adolescent and his parents of the cause and of the potential for future disability.

The treatment of traction epiphysitis has been described in IKJ5. In brief, and for the sake of completeness, it consists in the first instance of recognition of the precipitating physical activities and cessation of such activities at least on a temporary basis. If this is ineffective immobilisation in a plaster cast for at least three months is necessary. In a large proportion of cases some degree of elevation of the patella will have occurred before the patient is presented for diagnosis. Treatment therefore is aimed at preventing further elevation; and to a degree constituting a permanent disability. It will, at the same time, eliminate the presenting symptom, namely, pain, and limit, but not eliminate, the

accompanying swelling of the tibial tubercle.
**Residue of traction epiphysitis.** In maturity the
residual disabilities produced by traction
epiphysitis are:
PATELLA ALTA. This matter has been considered in some detail. Whether a disability
exists depends on the degree of elevation and
other factors such as the conformation of joint
and whether or not recurvatus deformity is
present; and, of course, whether the most
common serious complication, namely, recurrent subluxation has occurred.
PROMINENCE OF TIBIAL TUBERCLE. Reference has been made to a subclinical variety of
traction epiphysitis which may be responsible
for patella alta of unexplained origin. Sometimes such traction strain is responsible for
marked prominence of the tibial tubercle but
without any history or radiological evidence that
the patient suffered a traction epiphysitis (Figs
2,81 and 2,82). A marked prominence will
invariably be accompanied by patella alta; and
with a dual disability the indications for operation are evident (see below).
PROMINENCE OF TIBIAL TUBERCLE AC-
COMPANIED BY SEPARATE ISLANDS OF
BONE. Patients are encountered who complain
of pain, swelling and tenderness in the region
of the tibial tubercle and are shown, on radiological investigation, to have one or more islands
of bone which have failed to unite with the main
mass of the bone (Figs 2,68 and 2,69). Such
islands arise as a result of traction epiphysitis or
a fracture of the tongue-shaped epiphysis. If this
condition is accompanied by patella alta with
accompanying symptoms the opportunity may
be offered to transplant the tendon to a lower
level (see below). In other circumstances
excision of the ununited fragment will be
indicated (see below).

*Indications for Operation*

**Symptomatic**

**Excision of synovial ridge: local synovectomy.** If
it can be established with a reasonable degree
of certainty that the pain is synovial in origin
and confirmed by the induction of pain by

pressure on the elevated patella in the supracondylar region, excision of the hypertrophic
synovial membrane likely to be present in the
area is effective in establishing a cure.
TECHNIQUE. The suprapatellar pouch is entered
through a short lateral parapatellar incision
centred over the superior pole of the patella. On
entering the joint a ridge of hypertrophic
hyperaemic synovial membrane will be seen on
the posterior aspect of the suprapatellar pouch
immediately above the limit of the articular
cartilage of the condyles. The abnormal synovial
ridge is excised (Fig. 2,77).
*After-treatment.* The site from which the synovial
membrane has been excised is not subject to
direct pressure from a compression bandage:
some degree of haemarthrosis is inevitable.
Suction drainage is therefore introduced at the
termination of operation in addition to the
usual compression bandage. Early quadriceps
exercises are liable to produce irritation of the
area denuded of synovial membrane and exercise
therapy in the circumstances is deferred for
10 days.

**Reconstructive**

In patella alta simplex with the persistence of
symptoms the eventual question is the justification on clinical grounds of simple transplantation of the tibial tubercle and attached tendon
to a lower level. The problem differs from
recurrent subluxation, even if based on patella
alta, in so far as the immediate benefits are less
evident. When the tibial tubercle is prominent
to a point of physical embarrassment (Fig.
2,81) and the patella concomitantly elevated, the
indications for operation with possible dual
benefit are obvious. In patella alta/genu
recurvatum complex it will be evident that
transplantation of the tibial tubercle to a lower
level cannot other than aggravate the mechanical
status of the joint. In the absence of depression
of the anterior aspect of the tibial head readily
correctable by osteotomy (Ch. 9) the solution
to this problem is not immediately evident;
and particularly when based on posterior capsular laxity on a familial basis. If as above there
are indications for operation and in particular
in the obvious example of a prominent tibial
tubercle, the problem is that of transplantation

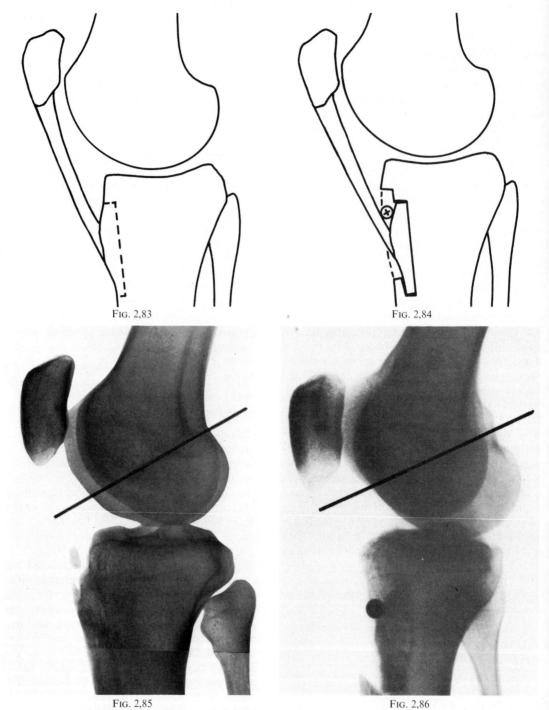

FIG. 2,83

FIG. 2,84

FIG. 2,85

FIG. 2,86

FIGS 2,83–86. **Patella alta: treatment.** Diagrammatic representation of the means of reducing the prominence of the tibial tubercle and at the same time bringing the patella down to a lower level (Figs 2,83 and 2,84). The radiographs of a case in which the technique was followed. Note in Figure 2,85 that the patella alta was caused by traction epiphysitis; and that a separate ossicle is present. The post-operative radiograph shows the patella at a lower level and with the transverse screw maintaining the block of bone in position (Fig. 2,86) (A.M., male, aged 22, case of J.H.).

directly downwards and not downwards and medially as in recurrent subluxation.

TECHNIQUE OF OPERATION. The author's technique, still under trial, is the isolation of the tibial tubercle with attached tendon in the form of a long, narrow rectangle of bone which must include essentially a projection upwards above the attachment of the tendon extending virtually to the joint line. The bed from which the rectangle has been removed is now deepened and the cortex at the inferior limit undermined to accept the lower end of the rectangle. The tibial fragment is then pushed beneath the cortex to the required distance taking into account the fact that the patella will be pulled down not only to the extent of the undermining but to the depth at which the tendon is placed. To lock the rectangle in position a transverse screw is inserted from one cortex of the tibia to the other immediately anterior to and in contact with the upper arm of the rectangle (Figs 2,83 to 2,86).

*After-treatment.* This operation depending on security of fixation on the presence of a screw is not to be compared with the positive locking techniques described for the treatment of recurrent subluxation. If quadriceps-setting can be practised from the outset and the patient made ambulant with patten and crutches at an early date it is doubtful if weight-bearing even with crutches should be attempted before the eighth week. Sound bony union cannot be anticipated before the tenth week and it is questionable if unrestricted weight-bearing should be considered before that time.

## Removal of Separate Ossicle

TECHNIQUE OF OPERATION. The site is approached by a short, lateral incision adjacent to the margin of the tendon. It should not cross the mid-line so that the resulting scar is not subject to pressure when kneeling. The upper limit of the attachment of the tendon is identified and the free tendon above retracted medially. The fragment will be found on the posterior aspect of the tendon attached anteriorly but free posteriorly. It is localised and excised by sharp dissection inflicting the minimum damage to tendon tissue.

## Patellectomy in Patella Alta

If the patella is excised in patella alta there is less loss of function than occurs following patellectomy in a joint in which the relationship of the patella to the femoral condyles is normal. The reason is not far to seek. In patella alta of extreme degree the bone is not exercising the function of carrying the tendon the maximum distance from the centre of rotation of the joint. In such circumstances the lateral expansions and iliotibial tract transmit extensor power to the tibia. Thus excision of a patella which has no appreciable function is not followed by the disability which occurs when a patella of normal position and function is excised.

The following is an example:

The patient, a young man (A.S., aged 22), 18 months previously in the armed forces underwent patellectomy on the right side for chondromalacia patellae. He was thereafter discharged as unfit for military service with a disability of 20 per cent. The occasion of the examination was the assessment of his ability for a post entailing considerable physical fitness.

He claimed to have no disability other than slight weakness of the knee. He stated, in proof, that he played football for a local amateur team.

He had some quadriceps wasting. The patellar tendon was contracting. There was a slight extension lag on straight-leg-raising. The normal side showed patella alta; but not in gross degree. The salient feature was the degree of genu recurvatum; and that he used the iliotibial band for extension.

In view of the occasion of the examination —an opinion as to his physical fitness—he was asked to run and stop suddenly; and this he was able to do even with the right knee. His performance in running was such as to accept the capability of playing football.

The explanation of the ability to run and even to play football lay in the fact that he had, prior to operation, a functionless patella. The disability for which he suffered patellectomy was not chondromalacia patellae, but synovial irritation from a patella alta. The loss of his patella had not materially affected function.

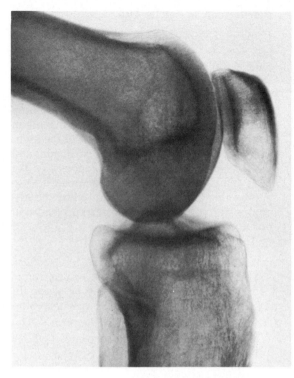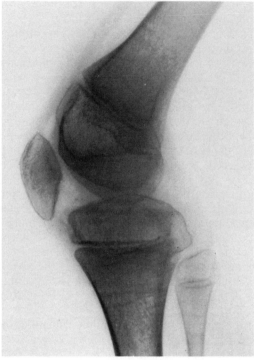

FIGS 2,87–88. **Patella baja: poliomyelitis.** This patient suffered an attack of poliomyelitis in youth producing quadriceps paralysis from which she recovered. The temporary paralysis during growth was responsible for inferior location of the patella (Fig. 2,87) (F.H., female, aged 32, nurse).

Joint of patient who suffered an attack with resultant flail leg. The low position of the patella is determined by the total lack of quadriceps influence since the age of three (Fig. 2,88) (M.S., male, aged 11).

## PATELLA BAJA

### Aetiology

**Rupture of quadriceps.** This injury is normally associated with the middle-aged and the elderly. In youth it occurs in traumatic dislocation of the normally located patella; and when the dislocation is reduced the fact that rupture of the attachment of vastus medialis and even the central elements has occurred is missed. This injury, unless subjected to immediate operative repair, results in an abnormally low patella and a permanently weak joint.

**Paralysis of quadriceps.** Maintenance of normal quadriceps function, but not hypertrophy, particularly during rapid growth, is important for the normal location of the patella. If for one reason or another, but usually as a result of poliomyelitis, the muscle is temporarily paralysed or weak the patella will be permanently located at an abnormally low level even if recovery occurs (Figs 2,87 and 2,88).

**Sinding Larsen-Johannson disease: osteochondritis.** If 'osteochondritis' at the inferior pole can be responsible for patella alta, in theory a similar lesion of the superior pole could be responsible for patella baja.

**Iatrogenic.** If patella alta is the commonest single cause of recurrent subluxation, the commonest error in the operative treatment is to locate the patella at too low a level. The author has made this mistake on more than one occasion. In minor degree there is no serious effect on function. In major degree the effect on function may be such as to necessitate a second operation to restore the situation.

## Treatment

An abnormally low patella for whatever reason is consistent with symptomless function. On the other hand the iatrogenic form, which can be extreme, may demand operative action (Fig. 2,91). The problem which arises then is whether restoration of the abnormal position upwards only is required or whether, as in some examples, it is necessary to restore the patella not only upwards but to the mid-line.

TECHNIQUE. The tendon together with an attached rectangular block of bone is outlined and detached. The superior cortex at the defect so produced is undermined superiorly and the upper part of the rectangle driven underneath; and because this action draws the patella downwards the defect has to be enlarged upwards as far as is possible if the level of the patella is to be raised (Figs 2,90 and 2,92).

If these measures appear simple in theory a limited practical experience has shown that relaxation of the tendon does not restore the height of the patella at the time of operation.

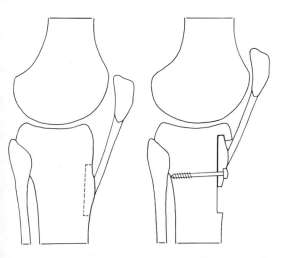

FIGS 2,89–90. **Patella baja: treatment.** To restore the relationship of patella to femoral condyles a rectangular block of bone with detached patellar tendon is outlined and detached (Fig. 2,89). The cortex at the upper end of the defect so produced is undermined and the rectangle driven beneath it. In calculating the distance the patella is to be raised allowance has to be made for the subcortical position of the tendon. A screw is inserted to secure fixation (Fig. 2,90). The operation is the reverse of Figures 2,83 and 2,84. The practical application of the operation is illustrated in Figures 2,91 to 2,93.

This is due to several factors, the most important of which may be that the function of extending the knee has been taken over by the medial and lateral expansions; and they have not been lengthened by the operation. Furthermore, the tourniquet by anchoring the quadriceps in the upper half of the femur does not permit the muscle to take up the slack. The position of the patella may not be altered until quadriceps tone has returned (Fig. 2,93). On the other hand the situation is known to have arisen whereby restoration of the level did not occur until the lateral and medial expansions had been divided. This latter action, however, is not one to be undertaken lightly in a situation of patello-femoral pathology which might lead to the necessity for patellectomy.

# CHONDROMALACIA PATELLAE

**Definition.** Chondromalacia patellae is a degenerative process of the articular cartilage of the patella and of the opposing femoral condyles characterised by fibrillation, fissuring and eventually erosion exposing bone. If it is a pathological entity, in a later form it will be recognised as osteoarthrosis of the patello-femoral joint.

## Aetiology

**Inherent defect in articular cartilage.** It is difficult to explain chondromalacia in the teenager or young adult in the absence of a specific incident of trauma other than on the basis of some congenital inherent defect in articular cartilage; and such has been described (Rubacky, 1963). On the other hand it is not easy to accept in spite of the stresses imposed that the patella only is affected and not other sites.

**Single-incident or repeated trauma.** One variety of chondromalacia is based on trauma. Experience suggests that the gross pathology may be so related (Fig. 2,97). If the articular cartilage of the femoral condyles does not readily tolerate sudden compression forces, which produce split lines of characteristic direction corresponding to site, and reflecting the pattern of collagen fibres, it is probable that sudden

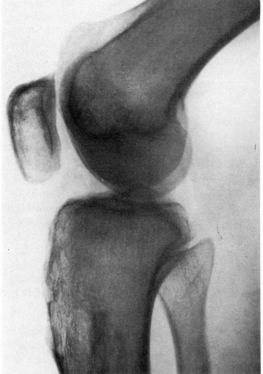

FIG. 2,91

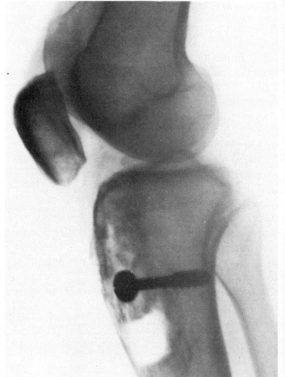

FIG. 2,92

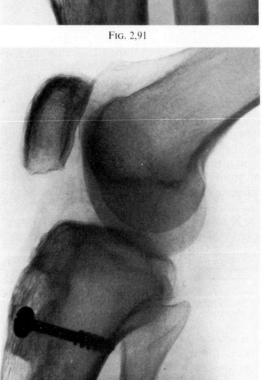

◀FIG. 2,93

FIGS 2,91–93. **Patella baja of iatrogenic origin: treatment.** In the treatment of recurrent subluxation the tibial tubercle has been transplanted too far down the medial side of the tibial head (Fig. 2,91). At operation to restore the situation the tibial tubercle was shifted approximately 2·5 cm upwards and to the lateral side. Note however that in radiographs taken at the termination of the operation the patella is not located at the higher level (Fig. 2,92). Six months later there was evidence of a return to a more normal relationship (Fig. 2,93) (M.M., female, aged 23).

excessive compression force produces a similar effect on the articular surface of the patella and/or opposing femoral condyle. If the course of events based on split lines has not yet been determined it can be anticipated to be degenerative and progressive.

**Overuse.** The concept of overuse is readily acceptable; and the classical example the professional long-distance cyclist.

**Underuse: disuse.** It is probable that disuse in extreme form has a greater influence on articular cartilage degeneration than overuse. In extreme form disuse entails immobilisation in plaster cast or caliper; and evidence has been accumulated that such measures, for one reason or another, result in degenerative changes in the patello-femoral joint and with greater repercussions there than in the tibio-femoral joint. (See Pressure.)

**Pressure.** It is well established that continuous direct pressure has a deleterious effect on articular cartilage. It has been suggested that long-leg plaster casts exert such pressure on the patella and are responsible for degenerative changes in the related joint. Pressure can be avoided by cutting a window in the plaster which allows the patella to protrude (Fowler, 1972).

**Malalignment.** In abnormality of the relationship

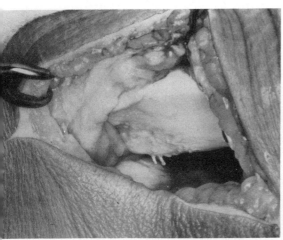
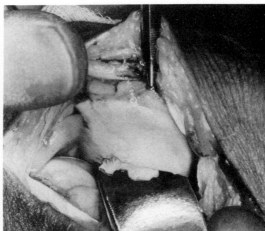
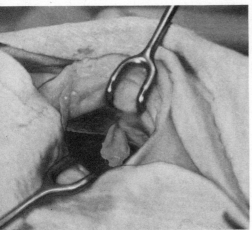
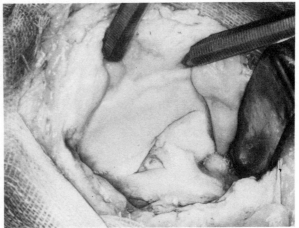

FIGS 2,94–97. **Chondromalacia patellae.** The lesion presents in many forms. It is often local with the remainder of the articular cartilage presenting a normal appearance. Erosion and fissuring (Fig. 2,94). Large tags of articular cartilage interfering with movement (Figs 2,95 and 2,96). Gross lesion probably of traumatic origin (Fig. 2,97).

of patella to femur in the form of patella alta, patella baja or, more commonly, alteration in the Q angle in the form of genu valgum, abnormal stresses are imposed on articular cartilage. In the situations cited, however, the symptoms imposed by the basic pathology are paramount.

**Contact with synovial membrane.** If it is important clinically to distinguish chondromalacia patellae from patella alta the latter condition may in the long term be responsible for the former. Degenerative changes in articular cartilage due to loss of mucopolysaccharide occur for no other reason than prolonged contact with the synovial membrane on the posterior aspect of the supra-patellar pouch.

### Pathological Anatomy

Chondromalacia patellae can be classified into four grades (Outerbridge, 1961):

*Grade I.* There is localised softening, swelling or fibrillation of the articular cartilage.

*Grade II.* There is fragmentation and fissuring in an area 1·3 centimetres or less in diameter.

*Grade III.* There is fragmentation and fissuring in an area of more than 1·3 centimetres in diameter.

*Grade IV.* There is erosion of articular cartilage down to subchondral bone.

**Location of lesion.** This is not a subject on which there is unanimity of opinion. In a recent series of 105 knees, however (Insall, Falvo and Wise, 1976) it is recorded that in 71 per cent the lesion was located within an ellipse passing transversely across the central area of the patella with the superior and inferior thirds of the articular surface nearly always spared. The medial facet alone was involved in 21 per cent and the lateral facet alone in 7 per cent (Figs 2,94 to 2,97).

### Clinical Features

The frequency with which meniscectomy is performed, and in the older age groups, permits the articular cartilage of the patella to be inspected in a wide age range. Experience shows that degenerative changes in the articular cartilage may be present below the age of 20, are invariable over the age of 40 and that gross changes in the older age groups are consistent with symptomless function. What determines the onset of symptoms and why, once established, they tend to persist, remains a mystery.

**Pain.** The presenting feature is pain or ache experienced in or under the patella. It is produced by movements which oppose patella and femur under compression, as in rising from a chair or ascending stairs.

**Interference with motion.** It is a common complaint that the joint is stiff or that there is some obstruction which tends to catch, cause momentary locking or otherwise interfere with smooth movement.

### Examination

**Synovial effusion.** There is no synovial swelling nor effusion. If synovial effusion is a feature it is probable that the diagnosis is wrong because: (1) effusion is the result of irritation of synovial membrane; not irritation of articular cartilage; (2) in any event the symptoms of chondromalacia tend to disappear when for some other reason an effusion occurs: the patella is floated-off the femoral condyles.

**Abnormal mechanics.** The joint is inspected for any abnormal mechanical situation such as patella alta, angular deformity and abnormal patella posture in flexion. The stability is confirmed.

**Crepitus and interference with motion.** The knee is actively flexed and extended with the palm of the examiner's hand laid gently over the patella where it will detect and locate crepitus. The pressure of the hand is then increased so that movement occurs against resistance. In this way momentary obstruction to movement such as might be produced by a tag of articular cartilage is detected. Such catching, if present, is likely to occur in, say, 30° of flexion and to be accompanied by pain. The pain induced by backward pressure in complete extension and particularly when any degree of patella alta is present is due to the compression of synovial membrane.

**Tenderness.** There may be synovial tenderness at the margin of the patella particularly on the lateral side.

**Differential diagnosis.** It should be possible to differentiate the condition from the internal

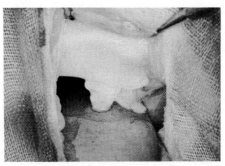

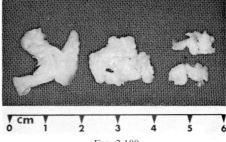

FIG. 2,99

FIG. 2,100

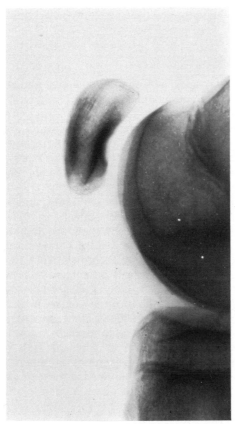

FIG. 2,98

FIGS 2,98–100. **Chondromalacia patellae.** Note defect in patella with sclerosis of bone. It is not osteochondritis dissecans: there is no separating bone (Fig. 2,98).

At operation there was a gross local lesion at the inframedial aspect (Fig. 2,99). Fragments of articular cartilage taken from the site (Fig. 2,100). This is the youngest patient encountered with such a gross lesion (M.L., female, aged 14).

derangements of youth relative to the menisci: there is no interference with rotatory action. It should be possible also to locate the lesion to the anterior aspect of the knee and to the extensor apparatus. Experience has shown that patella alta simplex is likely to be the commonest single source of error. 'Jumper's Knee' and lesions of the fat pad are possibilities to be considered.

**Functional aspects of the problem of diagnosis.** Experience has shown that in youth, male or female, and for reasons not immediately evident, pain is complained of in the patello-femoral joint for which no pathological explanation is forthcoming. In a recent survey (Leslie and Bentley, 1976) it has been shown that 50 per cent only of patients complaining of patello-femoral pain suffer from chondromalacia.

A surgeon prepared to diagnose chondro-malacia in youth should recall that articular cartilage has no blood supply, no lymphatic supply and no nerve supply. Retropatellar pain, as opposed to synovial pain, presupposes pathology of a degree which involves sub-chondral bone. This, of course, is a possibility; but not a likely one.

In the armed services the glamour of Her Majesty's Royal Air Force depicted in recruit-ment advertisements may not in the long term equate with the discipline, monotony and requirements of barrack life. A means of escape, albeit subconsciously, may be sought in terms of an internal derangement of the knee. The pressures in the regular armed services are such that a man cannot be indefinitely 'off work' or otherwise under observation as is the common pattern in circumstances of doubt in civilian life. Such pressures may lead eventually to a surgical operation, the discharge from the services of a young man minus his patella the subject of questionable pathology (Fig. 2,101) and possibly a disability for life which may be rated as high as 20 per cent.

This is not a diagnosis which should be readily assumed. It is often made erroneously by a process of elimination and without positive evidence: no other explanation of the pain has been found. Once the diagnosis has been made tentatively and in the hearing of the patient he may be difficult to convince that there is nothing seriously wrong with his knee. It is in such circumstances that arthroscopy (see below), or even exploration (see below), may be useful.

**Radiological examination.** No abnormality will be detected in lateral or skyline views until such times as the condition is advanced when loss of joint space, sclerosis of subchondral bone and marginal exostoses indicate the transition to osteoarthrosis. There are exceptions even in childhood (Figs 2,98, 2,99 and 2,100).

**Arthroscopy.** It is probable that the most important contribution attributable to arthroscopy is in the visualisation of the pathology of the patello-femoral joint. If there are unsolved problems in the aetiology and in the treatment of chondromalacia of the patella a considerable diagnostic problem of the past has been solved. The site and variety of the pathology is readily determined with the ability to palpate a 'blister' or soft area under vision with the irrigating needle. An important role is the capacity to state with conviction that the articular cartilage of the patella is within the bounds of normal in respect of age, sex, occupation and conformation of joint. It is to be hoped that the ready detection of sub-clinical pathology in, for example, the form of aging articular cartilage, will not lead to more, rather than less, unnecessary patellectomies.

**Exploration.** In general an operation designated 'Exploration of the Joint' and performed in circumstances of doubt cannot be too strongly condemned. In any event, and in circumstances of multiple minimal pathology, it is not likely to be helpful. In the absence of access to arthroscopy in expert hands and in circumstances such as have been described, exploration of the patello-femoral joint through a minimal lateral parapatellar incision may be justified for the purpose of confirming or refuting the diagnosis

and applying whatever measure the situation demands.

## Treatment

**Reassurance.** The origin and 'simple' nature of the pathology should be explained in an effort to reduce or eliminate the 'anxiety' aspect of the symptom complex. The fact that 'rough areas' are rendered smooth with use and the passage of time should be stressed; but if this does not occur a minor surgical procedure can render them smooth. It should be explained that pain is the worst feature of the condition, and with the explanation of the reason, should be accepted. It is not to be interpreted as an indication of the progressive nature of the disease. The purpose of exercise therapy is explained.

**Exercise therapy.** It will be evident that with unexplained pain the limb is likely to be rested with consequent quadriceps wasting. The loss of control so related contributes to the perpetuation of symptoms. In such circumstances redevelopment of muscle power is indicated. It is not, however, a matter of exercises in general as usually indicated but of selecting those unlikely to induce pain and thus inhibit or discourage

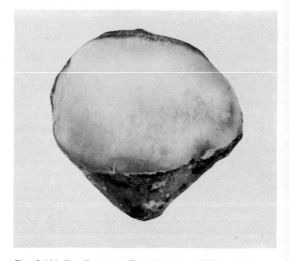

FIG. 2,101. **Patellectomy: For what reason?** This patella was excised for 'chondromalacia'. The superficial marks were inflicted in the course of operation. There is no possibility that pain could have arisen in the articular cartilage. To have excised it, and produced the permanent disability inevitably so related was an act of surgical incompetence (I.K., male, aged 20).

effort. In this regard it should be noted that quadriceps exercises performed by extending the knee from 90° against the resistance of a weight of 9 kg attached to the foot creates a patello-femoral force of 1·4 times body weight whereas straight-leg-raising with a similar load creates a patello-femoral force of only 0·5 times body weight (Reilly and Martens, 1972). Resistance exercises therefore will be avoided in which the patello-femoral joint is heavily loaded and within the range of flexion in which pain or interference with motion is experienced. In particular, exercises will consist of quadriceps setting, straight-leg-raising and progressively loaded straight-leg-raising.

**Immobilisation is contraindicated.** Immobilisation in any form and in particular the use of a plaster cast is irrational and undesirable. If chondromalacia is an indication of the breakdown of nutrition, immobilisation will aggravate the situation. The application of a plaster cast will render the patient symptomless. Removal and mobilisation of the joint results in a return of pain, possibly in more intense degree from related reduction in muscle power.

**Alteration of weight-bearing mechanics in patello-femoral joint.** In some examples the addition of an inside wedge on the sole of the shoe or the use of a valgus insole may effect relief by transferring compression forces from the lateral to the medial side of the joint.

## Operations

**Shaving, or excision, of abnormal cartilage.** The simplest operative measure in common use is the shaving down of an abnormal area of articular cartilage until normal tissue is reached. In the author's hands the results of this operation are unpredictable, varying between the extremes of complete relief of pain and the worsening of symptoms. It has been pointed out (Goodfellow, Hungerford and Woods, 1976) that the shaving process, creating a saucer-like defect, must remove unnecessarily the important tangential zone of superficial cartilage from healthy surrounding areas; and if it appears to produce a smooth surface for articulation it alters precisely matched surface contours (Fig. 2,103). In consequence they recommend the excision of a disc of affected cartilage leaving a crater with

vertical walls such as is recommended in the treatment of certain lesions of osteochondritis dissecans (Ch. 11) and with the same purpose, namely the creation of more congruous opposing articular surfaces (Figs 2,104 and 2,105).

TECHNIQUE. The patient is placed on the operating table in the supine position with the knee in extension or in hyperextension. A short lateral parapatellar incision is made and the articular surface exposed by rotating the bone in the long axis in the manner described (Fig. 2,102). If the shaving procedure is favoured the area affected is so treated until the cartilage 'cuts like an apple'. If excision is favoured a

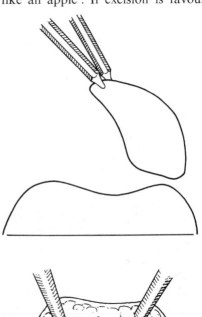

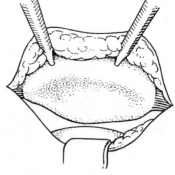

FIG. 2,102. **Exposure patello-femoral joint: operative technique.** A short lateral parapatellar incision is made. Two single-ended straight dental probes are then driven into the cortex and used as a lever to rotate the bone on its long axis to gain access to the articular surface. Care is exercised that the spikes enter cancellous bone and not the bone–cartilage junction lest in exerting a rotation force the articular cartilage is fractured.

circumferential incision is made around the affected area and the cartilage thereafter prised from the underlying subchondral bone (Fig. 2,105). Whether drill holes should be made into the cancellous bone in the base of the crater on the theory that the defect will be filled with fibrous tissue is a matter of debate; and it is in this regard that the follow-up of such cases by arthroscopy may prove helpful.

**Lateral release.** There are circumstances in which clinical examination reveals, and radio-

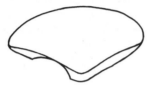

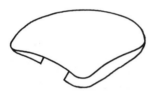

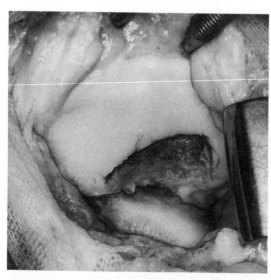

FIGS 2,103–105. **Chondromalacia patellae: treatment.** It is suggested that shaving or saucerisation (Fig. 2,103) produces a greater degree of incongruity of opposing surfaces than a defect with vertical sides (Fig. 2,104). A case (Fig. 2,97) so treated showing vertical sides of the defect exposing cancellous bone (Fig. 2,105).

logical examination confirms, the patella to be displaced laterally and with tightness or contracture of the lateral capsule limiting medial mobility. When this situation obtains shaving of abnormal cartilage may be combined with longitudinal division of the lateral capsule with the purpose of relaxation of tension such as may be effected by the degree of realignment which occurs.

**Realignment.** There are circumstances of abnormality of relationship between patella and femoral condyles, responsible for the degenerative changes, which can be altered only by major realignment procedures. In patella alta, it may be necessary to transplant the tibial tubercle to a lower level; it may be necessary to transplant the tubercle to the medial side, or it may be necessary to transplant the tibial tubercle to the medial side and at a lower level.

**Patellectomy.** There may be circumstances of gross pathology in which in the last resort there is no alternative to patellectomy; but see below.

## PATELLECTOMY: IMPLICATIONS AND CONSEQUENCES

### The Patella is Not Expendable

Patellectomy and arthrodesis are two irrevocable steps in the surgery of the knee joint. Both operations are the final admission of the failure of conservative measures. The operation of arthrodesis is much less likely to be accepted without due consideration by the patient than patellectomy. The consequences of a completely stiff knee can be imagined and indeed a trial of acceptance is possible. The consequences of patellectomy cannot be anticipated by the patient and are rarely explained by the surgeon; rather indeed the reverse. There is a tendency to 'sell' the idea and the consequences, particularly in the young adult, are not appreciated until it is too late.

The most common indication for patellectomy in the young adult, with the exception of fracture, is pain alleged to arise from so-called chondromalacia. Patellectomy exchanges the symptom of pain for the permanent disability of loss of function for which there is no known remedy; and the better the mechanical conformation of the knee in terms of the relationship of patella to the femoral condyles the greater the disability that occurs from its loss. Conversely, the less the function of the patella, as in patella alta, the less is its absence missed. Experience of the surgery of the knee joint recalls that the most common single regret expressed by patients, young and old, is having willingly parted with a patella. Most complain that the full implications and consequences were not explained in the face of pain now long forgotten.

To a young person complaining of inability to play tennis, dance or take part in other physical recreational activities it is often necessary to explain that he has attained a good, or better than average result for excision of the patella but that perfection of function or anything near it is unattainable.

To achieve full extension after patellectomy requires 15 to 20 per cent increase in quadriceps power. In favourable circumstances of youth and in the absence of long-standing disease this increase may be within the functional reserve of the muscle; but seldom otherwise. It is usually impossible to undertake any athletic activity which involves running. It is possible to walk; and thus golf is possible. Nevertheless, as in all aspects of knee surgery, there is the occasional exception: and the reason should be explained lest patellectomy should be deemed desirable (see Patella Alta).

There is in the current scene a reason for conservation of the patella not previously considered but the importance of which should not be underestimated. In total replacement, retention of the patella is an essential feature of the most successful designs. Excision of the patella, like the use of transverse incisions, prejudices the future.

**Technique of operation.** The function of a normally located patella, it is repeated, is to carry the quadriceps tendon the maximum distance from the centre of rotation of the joint. If the patella is excised the tendon is relaxed and extensor force is transmitted to the tibia by the lateral expansions. The technique of patellectomy performed for chondromalacia or osteoarthrosis differs from the operation performed for fracture in so far as the lateral expansions are not torn and do not require repair.

There is no point in attempting to shorten the central tendon to make up for the loss of the patella; rather indeed the reverse. If the central tendon is shortened the lateral expansions are relaxed or overlengthened with consequent extension lag. One of the reasons why manipulation, carried out to improve flexion following patellectomy, is so effective in improving function in general is that the shortened central tendon which is preventing the lateral expansions from transmitting quadriceps action to the tibia, is ruptured. Once this has occurred, and provided the patient exercises freely, the previous overlengthening of the lateral expansions is overcome and function improved even to the extent of eliminating extension lag.

In such circumstances a short transverse incision sufficient only to expose the bone is required. There is a distinct layer of fibrotendinous tissue adherent to the anterior surface and continuous with the quadriceps tendon above, patellar tendon below and lateral and medial expansions. This covering is incised vertically and the bone excised by sharp dissection endeavouring to retain the anterior covering intact. The operation is completed by simple suture of the original vertical incision in the anterior fibro-tendinous layer.

AFTER-TREATMENT. After termination of the operation a compression bandage is applied. There is no suture line under tension: elevation of the limb on an inclined plain is unnecessary. Quadriceps exercises commence as soon as pain has settled and the immediate effects of the operation have passed. In general, a return to weight-bearing after patellectomy should be deferred until straight-leg-raising can be performed. It is usually possible to teach the patient to walk with the aid of crutches by the end of a week.

## Complications

**Rupture of tendon and expansions.** In the presence of extension lag and particularly in the early stages of recovery, giving-way incidents are common. In a fall so precipitated, the central tendon and the expansions may be ruptured and demand immediate operative repair. The necessity for such action is prejudicial to the outcome in terms of loss of flexion.

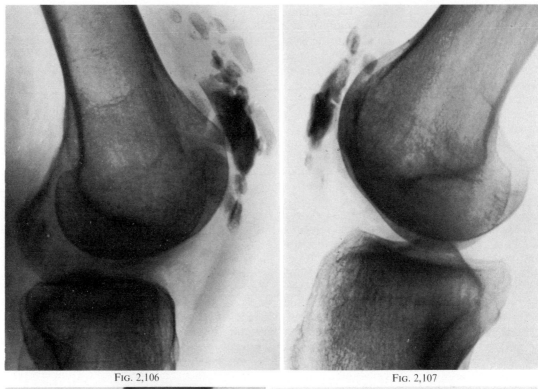

FIG. 2,106                    FIG. 2,107

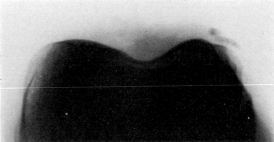

FIG. 2,109

◀ FIG. 2,108

FIGS 2,106–109. **Patellectomy: complications.** Calcification, ossification and regeneration in widely varying degree (Figs 2,106, 2,107 and 2,108) occurs following patellectomy performed for fracture and may be consistent with reasonable function. On the other hand small masses located on the lateral margin of the lateral femoral condyle may produce mechanical incidents (Figs 2,108 and 2,109) (D.G., female, aged 23). If, however, it is the tendon which is dislocating laterally mere excision of the fragment will not effect a cure (see text).

**Calcification/ossification.** Calcification in the capsule or tendon in widely varying degree (Figs 2,106 to 2,109) may occur after patellectomy and be responsible for symptoms. The extent of the calcification, ossification or regeneration and the symptoms produced are not related.

There is a complaint of ache with the possible addition of mechanical incidents due to slipping of the calcified mass or masses over the lateral femoral condyle. In such circumstances there is local tenderness to pressure (Figs 2,108 and 2,109).

When symptoms are accurately located to this source, excision of the fragment responsible may effect a cure. It is important, however, not to attribute symptoms to such masses when, in fact, it is the tendon in which they are incorporated which is dislocating.

**Dislocating central tendon or lateral expansion.** Care must be exercised that symptoms are not attributed to a small calcified mass, which is frequently present, when in fact the fault is dislocation of the central tendon or hypertrophied

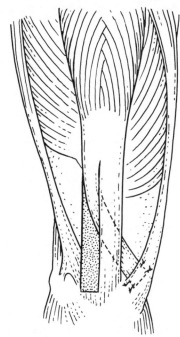

FIG. 2,110. **Patellectomy: complications.** If the tendon or expansion is dislocating laterally there is no reasonable alternative to transfer of the dislocating portion of the tendon to the medial side of the joint after the manner of Goldthwait.

lateral expansion over the lateral margin of the lateral femoral condyle. This is particularly liable to occur when patellectomy has been employed, wrongly in the author's view, in the treatment of recurrent dislocation.

TREATMENT. Symptoms may be of a degree of intensity which demand operative action in which there would seem to be no reasonable alternative to transfer of the dislocating portion of the tendon to the medial side of the joint.

OPERATION. If the Goldthwait operation is not in current use as applied to recurrent dislocation it is relevant in modified form when the patella has been excised.

The joint is entered by excision of the scar of the original operation. The dislocating portion of the tendon is located by flexing and extending the joint. It is isolated by a vertical incision splitting the tendon longitudinally and tracing the lateral portion distally to the tibial attachment where it is divided. It is then passed under the medial portion and out to the exterior through a short vertical incision on the extreme medial side. It is then secured with multiple sutures to the tibial attachment of the medial expansion or to the expansion itself (Fig. 2,110). Suction drainage is introduced to the dead space on the lateral side, the wound closed and a compression bandage applied.

AFTER-TREATMENT. It will be remembered that, in the absence of the patella, contact with soft tissue involves destruction of the articular cartilage of the femoral condyles. There exists therefore, even in a minor degree of haemarthrosis, the risk of adhesion of the expansion to the exposed bone. Early flexion exercises are therefore desirable. Quadriceps exercises, in other than minimal form, are not practised until healing is sound and until some four to six weeks have elapsed. In such circumstances, and in the absence of the patella, redevelopment of muscle power is protracted.

PRECIPITATION OF SYMPTOMS. It has been indicated that even with a satisfactory result the capacity for hypertrophy to deal with changed circumstances is limited. Symptoms of weakness and giving-way may be precipitated by pregnancy and any sudden increase of weight so-related or otherwise. In this situation the reduction of weight will usually result in a reduction of symptoms to a tolerable level.

# RECURRENT SUBLUXATION (DISLOCATION) OF THE PATELLA

## Aetiology

**Patella alta.** An abnormally high patella is the commonest single cause of recurrent subluxation (207 in 286 cases, Andersen, 1958).

The aetiology and clinical implications of patella alta simplex and patella alta/genu recurvatum have been elaborated.

**Angular deformity: genu valgum.** The Q (Quadriceps) angle is the angle of some 15° which exists between quadriceps muscle and patellar tendon. When this angle is increased in an angular deformity in the form of genu valgum the pull of the quadriceps across the concavity tends to produce a dislocation. Some degree of genu valgum is common in the female; and this is one explanation of the incidence of recurrent subluxation in the female.

**Hypoplasia of lateral condyle of femur.** In the femur the lower the lateral condyle in relation to the medial the greater will be the tendency for the patella to slip laterally. In this regard it is important that the height of the condyle be estimated in various degrees of flexion. If the well-known apprehension sign is normally carried out with the patient supine it will be appreciated that subluxation or dislocation seldom occurs in full extension, but in some degree of flexion. The patella posture should therefore be observed by seating the patient on the couch with the legs hanging free. A small degree of lateral posture is not significant, but any marked degree may be of diagnostic value.

**Inadequate treatment of traumatic dislocation.** When a traumatic dislocation occurs in a knee of normal conformation, and particularly one in which the patella is normally located and not a patella alta, it is inevitable that the capsule on the medial side is torn. Views on the treatment of this condition have been stated elsewhere (IKJ5): such cases should be subjected to immediate exploration and operative repair. This opinion, however, is not universally held and in some instances the dislocation is reduced without even temporary immobilisation in a plaster cast. Such treatment inevitably results in weakening of the capsule and particularly of the attachment of vastus medialis to the patella. These cases are liable to recurrent dislocation as opposed to subluxation.

**Abnormal vastus medialis.** If disinsertion of vastus medialis as in traumatic dislocation is a cause of lateral instability of the patella, weakness or abnormal attachment of this component and particularly of the oblique fibres may also be an aetiological factor in subluxation.

**Familial joint laxity.** In an inquiry into the background of 97 patients with recurrent dislocation of the patella (Carter and Sweetnam, 1960) 10 were found to have a near relative with a similar affection. Familial joint laxity was found in 2 of the 10 families with more than one member affected by recurrent dislocation. Familial joint laxity was found also in 2 out of 20 patients with recurrent dislocation of the patella who had no family history of similar dislocation.

**Arthrogryposis quadriceps contracture.** In young children with habitual, as opposed to recurrent dislocation, the possibility of contracture of the lateral elements of the quadriceps in the form of a local variety of arthrogryposus should be considered. It will be evident this situation is a missed sub-variety or late manifestation of genu recurvatum congenitum.

**Abnormal attachment of iliotibial tract.** There is a rare congenital anomaly whereby the iliotibial tract is inserted into the patella or connected to it with a fibrous band (Ober, 1939; Jeffreys, 1963). The iliotibial tract lies in front of the axis of rotation of the joint and passes behind the axis as the knee bends. It follows that if the patella is tethered to the tract by direct insertion or by a fibrous band it must be pulled laterally during flexion. The true incidence of this abnormality is unknown.

Two examples only have been encountered. In the first a band between the iliotibial tract and patella was the cause of a snapping knee. The second was a true malattachment to the patella:

The patient (M.R., female, aged 11, case of Mr B. D. Smith, Lincoln, England) gave a history that a year previously there had been gradually increasing discomfort in the left knee. When examined in hospital it was noted that when the knee flexed the patella dislocated. There was a history of a fall four

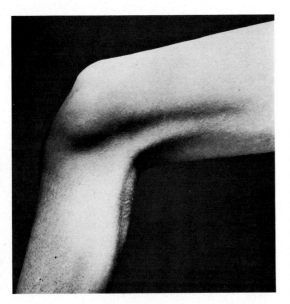

FIG. 2,111. **Recurrent dislocation of the patella: aetiology.** Abnormal attachment of the iliotibial tract of congenital origin. In extension, the patella was in the normal position. In flexion, it dislocated as a result of the abnormal attachment of the iliotibial tract. (Case of Mr B. D. Smith, Lincoln, England.)

months previously; but there was no evidence that the fall had been in any way responsible for the dislocation. The purpose of reference was to seek advice as to what operation would be applicable at the age of 11 in view of the fact that transplantation of the tibial tubercle was out of the question at this age.

On flexion the patella dislocated and it was evident that there was a tight band producing and maintaining the dislocation; and that the structure was attached to the supralateral aspect of the patella (Fig. 2,111). The band corresponded exactly to the site of iliotibial band on the normal right side. The dislocation was relatively symptomless and caused no more than weakness, giving-way and discomfort. The only other abnormality was the marked wasting of the quadriceps and particularly of the medial elements. It was of some academic interest that in the course of taking the history it transpired that as a baby she had suffered from congenital pyloric stenosis.

It was recommended that the abnormal attachment be divided and the quadriceps redeveloped in the hope that no further operation would be necessary. The final outcome is unknown.

## CLINICAL FEATURES

**Sex.** The patient is usually, but by no means always, female; and in the second decade. In the male athlete the incidents occur in the sudden directional change known as 'cutting'. In the female it is the most common cause of internal derangement in this age range. No other diagnosis should be considered until it has been eliminated (see Ch. 12). The invariable complaint is of giving-way incidents usually when she is turning and always in a direction away from the affected side. The incidents may be followed by small transient effusions.

### Inspection

**Erect or supine.** In the most common cause of recurrent subluxation observation of the patient in the erect position, or less obvious supine, will reveal the stigmata of patella alta, namely a small patella located at an abnormally high level with an elongated tendon and large flat fat pad. The vastus medialis is small, and the vastus lateralis by comparison well developed, so-called differential wasting.

**Sitting.** Seated on the examination couch with the knees at a right-angle and the leg hanging free, the patella of the affected, or both sides, may face somewhat laterally rather than almost straight ahead. The position of the patella is observed through the range of movement between complete extension, or hyperextension, and right-angled flexion.

**Apprehension sign.** Lateral mobility, holding the patella between forefinger and thumb, is increased particularly in patella alta. It is this manoeuvre, pressing the patella laterally with the thumb, which produces the almost pathognomonic phenomenon, the apprehension sign (Sir Thomas Fairbank, 1937): the patient recognises the unpleasant sensation immediately preceding subluxation and, by bracing the quadriceps or grasping the examiner's hand, stops the patella from being pushed any further laterally. In eliciting the sign it should be

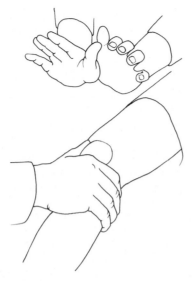

FIG. 2,112. **Recurrent subluxation of patella: 'apprehension sign'.** In applying pressure to the medial aspect of the patella in the course of testing the stability of the joint the patient seizes the examiner's hand to check a manipulation, the unpleasant sensation of which she recognises as occurring at subluxation.

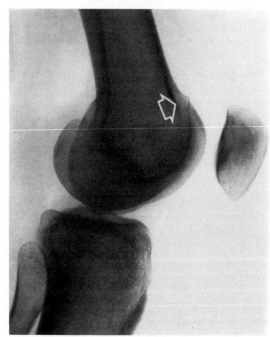

FIG. 2,113. **Recurrent dislocation of patella.** Radiological evidence may exist in dislocation, as opposed to subluxation, in the form of a spur or beak in the immediate supracondylar region. It is the reaction in the abnormal track made by the patella.

remembered that the instability or giving-way incidents do not occur in complete extension but in some 30° or so of flexion; and it is in this position only that the sign may be present (Fig. 2,112).

UNUSUAL PATTERNS. If lateral subluxation occurring in flexion and undergoing spontaneous reduction on extension is by far the most common pattern, the occasional case is encountered in which subluxation occurs medially; and sometimes even the mechanism of subluxation is reversed in so far as lateral subluxation occurs in extension with spontaneous reduction on flexion.

**Radiological examination.** The diagnosis of recurrent subluxation is based on clinical rather than radiological findings. Nevertheless radiological investigation is essential not only to confirm the aetiology, but to determine treatment. To this end: (1) a lateral projection in complete or hyperextension, weight-bearing and with the quadriceps in maximum contraction will determine the biomechanical status of the patellar femoral joint in maximum extension; (2) a lateral projection in 150° will determine the location of the patella at the limit of mobility and indicate the profile of the femoral condyles. In recurrent dislocation, as opposed to subluxation, the characteristic bony projection will be seen indicating reactionary changes in the track of dislocation (Fig. 2,113); (3) skyline views at a variety of angles, not only to determine the height of the margin of the lateral femoral condyle, but indicate, when complete dislocation has occurred, whether or not a medial tangential osteochondral fracture of the patella and/or of the opposing margin of the lateral condyle has taken place.

There are radiological features of bilateral recurrent dislocation in the teenage girl repeated on so many occasions as to constitute a pattern (Figs 2,114 and 2,115).

1. The patella tends to be small and to be located at an abnormally high level.

2. There is apparent loss of modelling at the lower end of the femur. It is not clear whether this apparent failure of modelling is a radiological artefact or due to a rotary deformity of the femur.

3. There is apparent lateral shift of the tibia in relation to the femur.

4. The lateral eminence of the tibial spine is located to the lateral side almost beneath the lateral cortex of the femur.

Patients exhibiting these radiological appearances are frequently the subject of pes cavus in a variety of degrees.

### Differential Diagnosis

**Bipartite patella.** In ordinary circumstances the diagnosis of recurrent subluxation should present no difficulties. There is little excuse for confusing the symptomatology with internal derangements relative to the menisci. A problem arises, however, in the presence of a bipartite patella. If the laterally placed ossicle is mobile, giving-way incidents occur under stress similar to those of recurrent subluxation (see Congenital Anomalies of Patella).

### Arthroscopy

It has been indicated that one of the most fruitful fields of application of arthroscopy is in the investigation of the pathology of the patello-femoral joint. In planning the operative treatment of recurrent dislocation in particular it is important to know the condition of the articular cartilage of the patella in terms of chondromalacia and/or the presence of a medial tangential osteochondral fracture. The former condition cannot be detected radiologically. The latter is misleading radiologically in so far as the minimal bone content gives no indication of the extent of the cartilage lesion. The condition of the articular cartilage as determined by direct vision may not only influence the choice and manner of operation but dictate the necessity for direct action on the patello-femoral joint in addition to any proposed realignment procedure.

### TREATMENT

It has been indicated that recurrent subluxation or dislocation of the patella is seldom a single entity and is thus unlikely to be cured by a single procedure. If the cause can be shown to be due to fibrosis of the lateral expansion such as might be due to contracture of the lateral elements of the quadriceps, as opposed to patella alta, simple division of the lateral capsule might effect a cure. On the other hand it is much more likely that division of the lateral capsule will require to be combined with transplantation of the tibial tubercle to a lower level and/or to the medial side. If it is accepted that treatment is the treatment of the cause, as, to cite another example, an angular deformity of the tibial head requiring opening-wedge osteotomy (Ch. 9), the problem for practical purposes can be resolved into the demands of three age groups: (1) *In the first decade*; (2) *in the first half of the second decade with open epiphyses*; and (3) *in skeletal maturity*.

At all ages and in all circumstances treatment is the treatment of the cause. It is important that it should, if possible, be identified.

### 1. In the First Decade

In infancy the cause is likely to be that of fibrosis of vastus lateralis and the treatment, initially at least, that of excision of the contracted structures.

The condition is common in the mentally defective and particularly in mongols. Permanent dislocation, however, may not be a source of disability in the total scene. No treatment may be necessary or advisable. On the other hand, in recurrent form, the child, constantly falling, may be driven to proceed on hands and knees. Operative action is required to restore confidence in the erect posture.

Multiple pathology is frequently encountered composed of lack of development of the lateral femoral condyle combined, perhaps, with lateral rotation of the femur or of the tibia, genu valgum, and general laxity of the capsular tissues permitting mobility of the patella in all directions.

In a child who is otherwise normal, the restoration of stability and of the relationship of patella to femur is necessary for the normal development of the joint in the course of growth. Furthermore, a permanently displaced patella, by permitting increased mechanical purchase by the lateral elements of the quadriceps, increases pressure on the lateral and posterior aspects of the upper tibial growth plate while relaxing pressure on the medial and anterior aspects. The result is a progressive valgus and

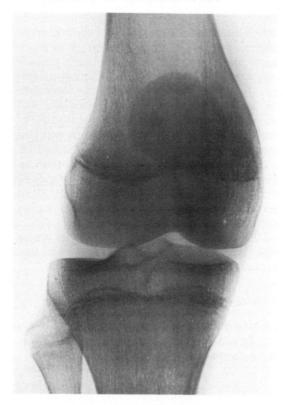

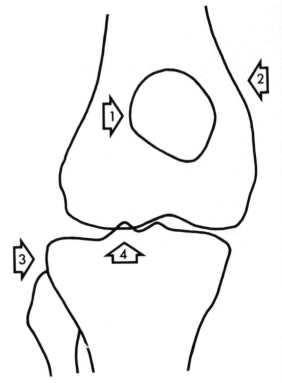

FIGS 2,114–115. **Recurrent dislocation of patella: radiological features in teenage girl.**
1. Patella is small and high in location;
2. Apparent loss of modelling at lower femur;

3. Apparent lateral shift of tibia;
4. Lateral eminence of tibial spine is almost in line with lateral cortex of femur.

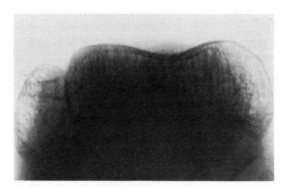

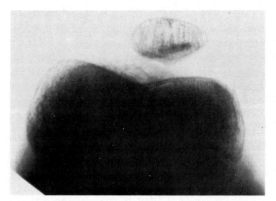

FIGS 2,116–117. **Dislocation of patella in a child.** On the right side the patella lies on the lateral aspect of the lateral femoral condyle (Fig. 2,116). On the left the situation has been restored by lateral capsulotomy (Fig. 2,117). The dislocation however recurred and semitendinosus tenodesis (Figs 2,118 and 2,119) was required. Note relatively small size of patella (Fig. 2,117) (M.H., male, aged 9, case of C.S.C).

flexion deformity. In such circumstances restoration of the situation is imperative; and at the earliest opportunity (Figs 2,116 and 2,117).

At this age it is an essential feature of any operation undertaken that it does not involve, or even expose, the upper tibial growth plate (see below).

## 2. In the First Half of the Second Decade with Open Epiphyses

Recurrent subluxation as opposed to dislocation in the years immediately prior to epiphyseal maturity poses special problems. If there is an obvious cause this must be eliminated or the necessity for operative treatment anticipated. There is, however, the situation of the overweight girl with some degree of valgus in which considerable parental pressure is exerted to 'do something'. The treatment of such a case is expectant but combined with active measures directed to reduction of weight, manipulations and/or splinting directed to the correction of valgus deformity in the interval short of maturity and, of course, quadriceps exercises. A proportion of cases, in the absence of patella alta or persistent genu valgum will stabilise with the advent of epiphyseal maturity. It is important that precipitate operative action, no matter when the parental pressure, be avoided. If it is clear that stability will not be achieved, and the girl is approaching maturity, it is usually possible to defer operation until such time as it is safe to transplant the tibial tubercle. In other circumstances of persistent dislocation a soft tissue operation such as semitendinosus tenodesis (see below) may be necessary to preserve the integrity of the joint.

## Operations

Two soft tissue procedures fulfil the essential criterion of not exposing the upper tibial plate:

## Semitendinosus Tenodesis

**Background note.** This operation was first described by Galeazzi (1921). It has been practised in Toronto for many years but is apparently not in common use elsewhere. The results reported (Dewar and Hall, 1957; Baker

et al., 1972) suggest that it is worthy of greater recognition as probably the best of the soft tissue operations applicable to situations demanding intervention prior to maturity of the upper tibial growth plate.

**Technique.** Two skin incisions are required. The first is situated on the postero-medial aspect of the thigh and locates and identifies the tendon of the semitendinosus. It is stout, at least 13 centimetres long and not to be confused with the flimsy gracilis. It is divided at the junction with the muscle with the object of preserving as much tendon as possible. The distal end of the muscle belly is sutured to the semimembranosus to preserve the power of the hamstrings.

The second incision is medial parapatellar and locates and identifies the insertion of the semitendinosus, the most posterior of the medial hamstrings. The divided tendon is pulled down. The anterior surface of the patella and the quadriceps expansion are exposed by dissection and retraction of the lateral skin flap. The patella is mobilised by division of the lateral capsule. An oblique hole is drilled across the patella in the line of the tenodesis, and the tendon is passed through it from the medial to the lateral side (Fig. 2,118). The patella is pulled strongly downwards and medially and held under considerable tension in this position while the tendon is sewn back on to itself (Fig. 2,119).

AFTER-TREATMENT. At the termination of the operation the limb is immobilised in a plaster cylinder extending from the groin to the ankle. Weight-bearing is permitted after a few days and the patient usually leaves hospital within a week. The plaster cast is retained for six weeks. Recovery of function, with a normal range of joint movement, is rapid. Full activity may be resumed within a few weeks.

**Results of operation.** In the 10 years 1958–68 this technique has been applied in 58 patients in the Hospital for Sick Children, Toronto. Forty-two were traced and reviewed at an average interval of 5 years. Thirty-one had unilateral dislocations and 11 bilateral making a total of 53 operations. The application of the strictest criteria led to the conclusion that 80 per cent of the results could be classified as 'good' or 'excellent'.

In view of the multiplicity of pathology which underlies recurrent or habitual dislocation and

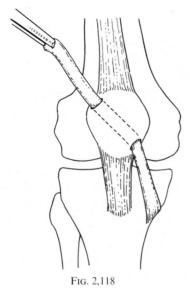

FIG. 2,118

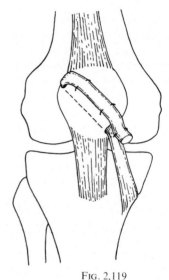

FIG. 2,119

FIGS 2,118–119. **Recurrent dislocation of patella: treatment. Semitendinosus tenodesis.** The tendon of semitendinosus has been passed through an oblique tunnel in patella after division of lateral capsule (Fig. 2,118). The tendon doubled upon itself is sutured under tension drawing the patella downwards and medially (Fig. 2,119) (after Baker et al., 1972).

the variation of length of history encountered, this operation appears to have a serious place in the treatment of recurrent dislocation prior to the attainment of skeletal maturity.

## Transplantation of Patellar Tendon

There are circumstances of rotatory deformity when semitendinosus tenodesis may not be applicable and leave no alternative to transplantation of the patellar tendon to the medial aspect of the head performed as a purely soft tissue operation which does not expose the growth plate.

TECHNIQUE. The curved incision on the lateral side crosses the midline immediately below the tibial tubercle and exposes the tubercle and medial aspect of the tibial head. The tendon is outlined and the inferior limit defined. The tendon is stripped by sharp section from below upwards from off its bony insertion by leaving a thin layer consisting of the most posterior aspect so that soft tissue remains and the epiphyseal plate is not exposed. A contracted lateral capsule is divided. The pes anserinus is then exposed and two parallel incisions made in the direction of the tendons and the tissue between the incisions undermined. The patellar tendon is threaded through the superior incision and out through the inferior incision, flexed upwards and sutured to itself adjustment for tension depending on whether or not it is desirable to pull the bone down to a lower level. The lax capsule on the medial side is plicated.

The operation alters the direction of pull of the patellar tendon at little risk of disturbance of growth by transplantation into the pes anserinus which, in theory at least, will tend to exert influence in a medial direction and thus add an additional mechanical factor preventing lateral dislocation.

Results. This operation has been performed only in mongols and similar situations of gross deformity. It is known to have effected stability in the short and long-term. In the cases ex-

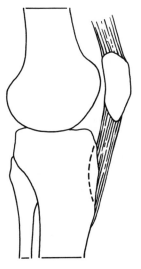

FIG. 2,120

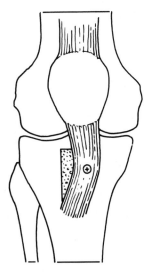

FIG. 2,121

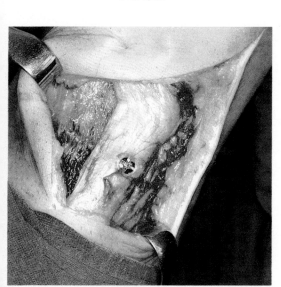

FIG. 2,122

FIGS 2,120–122. **Recurrent subluxation of patella: treatment.** In the simplest distal realignment procedure (Emslie operation) a horizontal osteotomy of the tibial tubercle is performed leaving the distal attachment of the tendon intact (Fig. 2,120). The tubercle is then displaced medially and secured to a prepared cancellous area by a single screw (Figs 2,121 and 2,122).

amined to date no disturbance of growth has occurred which could be attributed to the operation.

### 3. In Skeletal Maturity

**Lateral release.** There is evident attraction in a simple operation which does no more than divide the lateral capsule; and there are circumstances in the affections of the patello-femoral joint in which this procedure is indicated. Division of the lateral capsule is generally accepted to be an integral part of the operation of transplantation of the tibial tubercle downwards and medially (see below). It is unlikely that lateral release as an isolated measure can be effective in a condition based essentially on patella alta; rather, indeed, the reverse (see below). If, however, in the unusual circumstances of dislocation arising solely from contracture of the capsule, division will effect a cure.

### Transplantation of the Tibial Tubercle to Anteromedial Aspect of Tibial Head

The procedure in most common use for the treatment of recurrent subluxation or dislocation of the patella is transplantation of the tibial

E

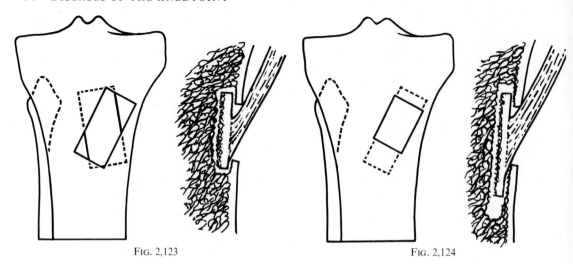

FIG. 2,123                                                    FIG. 2,124

**FIGS 2,123–124. Recurrent subluxation of patella: treatment.** Diagrammatic representation of the means of locking the rectangle of bone with attached patellar tendon beneath the cortex by rotation as practised by the author (Fig. 2,123), and an alternative method said to be easier of execution (see text) (Fig. 2,124).

tubercle downwards and medially as described by Roux (1888) and elaborated and popularised by Hauser (1938). There are a multiplicity of means by which this can be achieved; and these depend on 'driving fit'; fixation by screw, staple or otherwise. Some methods which purport to lock the block of bone in position are not sufficiently positive. In others the tendon cannot be transferred to a lower level. Most have the disadvantage that they necessitate an undesirably long period of immobilisation if bony union is to be achieved and before flexion and extension exercises can be practised. Two methods will be described: (1) that of Elmslie (R. C. Elmslie, 1878–1940, orthopaedic surgeon, St Bartholomew's Hospital, London, 1912–1932, unpublished work) which has the advantages of simplicity and avoids the possibility of displacement of the patella to an abnormally low level or too far medially, but the disadvantage that it depends on screw fixation until bony healing is established. It is most suited to instability in the *absence* of patella alta (Figs 2,120 to 2,122). (2) That of the author which has the advantage of positive locking of the tibial tubercle at its new site and thus the possibility of immediate flexion exercises and weight-bearing in two to three weeks. It has been used with the modifications to be described on more than 250 occasions

between 1940 and 1976. It has the disadvantage of the necessity for accuracy of technique: the margin for error is limited. The precise site, pulling the patella down the exact distance required, but not more, is difficult to determine. It is most suited to instability in the *presence* of patella alta (Figs 2,123 to 2,128).

**Elmslie Tibial Tubercle Transplant**

**Technique.** The operation takes place in the supine position. Haemostasis is controlled by a pneumatic tourniquet. The skin incision begins medial to the patella and extends downwards and obliquely to cross the midline somewhat distal to the tibial tubercle. Vertical incisions are made in the periosteum on either side of the patellar tendon extending downwards to about 1 cm below the tubercle. The periosteum is erased from the medial tuberosity to expose an area of bone rather greater than the width of the patellar tendon. The upper limit of the attachment is located by direct vision from the lateral side. The tubercle, as it merges into the tibial shaft, is located by palpation. The upper limit of the horizontal osteotomy is determined by making a shallow transverse osteotomy a few millimetres above the upper limit of the attachment of the tendon. The tubercle osteotomy in the frontal plane is then performed, the upper limit determined by the transverse cut, the lower leaving the distal extremity of the tendon and the periosteum undisturbed (Fig. 2,120). A lateral release is then accomplished by extending the incision on the lateral aspect of the tendon upwards through the capsule to the side of the patella. This is done blindly with straight blunt-pointed scissors keeping the capsule under tension by downwards traction on the tendon. This action relaxes the tendon and permits selection of the site, in regard to downward and medial displacement depending on the circumstances of the case at which the tubercle will be fixed. The cortical bone at this site is removed and a cancellous area corresponding to the osteotomised tibial tubercle exposed. Fixation is secured with a single screw which engages the opposite cortex (Figs 2,121 and 2,122). The erased periosteum is sutured to the displaced tendon. Suction drainage is introduced and the wound closed.

AFTER-TREATMENT. At the completion of the operation a compression bandage is applied and the tourniquet released. Fixation of the tubercle until healing occurs depends on a single screw. Plaster slabs are therefore incorporated in the outer layers of the bandage.

When the skin stitches are removed on the tenth day a skin-tight plaster cast, well moulded round the superior pole of the patella, is applied. At this time the patient is ambulatory using a patten and crutches. The cast is removed at the eighth week and mobilising exercises begun. Weight-bearing is not permitted until the twelfth week.

## Author's Operation

**Technique.** The operation is performed under tourniquet with the patient supine and a sandbag of such a size beneath the knee that the joint is held securely in 5° to 10° of flexion.

The skin is marked with scratches or dye. A curved incision, the lower extremity of which crosses the midline a short distance below the tibial tubercle, is made on the medial aspect of the joint. When the skin flaps have been dissected, exposing the tibial tubercle and the patellar tendon, an incision is made in the periosteum immediately medial to the tendon and continued downwards below the tubercle and then towards the medial margin of the tibia. A flap is erased to expose the entire width of the bone on the medial side. A rectangle of cortical bone about 32 mm long by 15 mm wide, containing the entire attachment of the patellar tendon, is outlined. It is important that it includes an upward extension free of tendon which can be locked beneath the cortex in the new position (Figs 2,123 and 2,124). To this end the uppermost limit of the attachment of the tendon is determined. A site about 1 cm above this point and just below the joint line is selected and a transverse cut made across the tibia with a fine-bladed osteotome about 1 cm wide. This osteotome may be left in position to act as a mark while the vertical cuts on either side of the tendon are made (Fig. 2,125). On the medial side it is important to keep as close as possible to the tendon so that the maximum area of bone is available on the antero-medial aspect of the tibial head for the cutting of the window.

It is at this stage that the lateral capsule is divided. This is done partly under direct vision, partly blind, and is accomplished by means of blunt-pointed scissors. The capsule is put under tension by exerting traction on the patellar tendon with its attached bone and split vertically exposing the extra synovial fat. The forefinger is passed into the incision to make sure that the restraining influence of the lateral capsule has been eliminated.

This action allows the tibial tubercle to be brought down to a point below the original attachment (Fig. 2,126). It is an important feature that not only is the tibial tubercle transplanted to the medial side, but at a lower level. This is the action which overcomes the commonest cause of recurrent subluxation, namely patella alta. But the action to be taken depends on the aetiology. It may be unnecessary and undesirable to bring the patella down to a lower level; alternatively, to move the tubercle to the medial side. If it is a matter of transplanting it to a lower level in the midline the technique described under 'Patella Alta' is pursued.

It is at this stage that the decision must be made as to the exact position of the window to be cut. This is perhaps the most important part of the operation and the one in which most

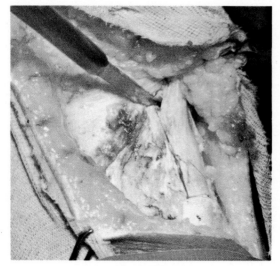

FIG. 2,125

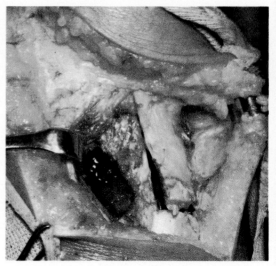

FIG. 2,127

FIG. 2,126

FIG. 2,128

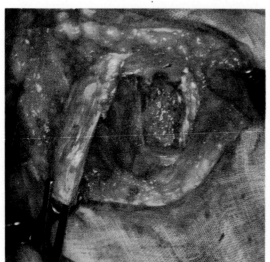

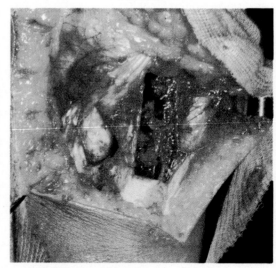

FIGS 2,125–128. **Recurrent subluxation of patella: treatment by transplantation of tibial tubercle to a lower level on the medial aspect of the tibial head.** Steps of operation.

Fig. 2,125. To determine the upper limit of the rectangle of bone, ensuring that sufficient bone free of tendon is present to lock under the cortex (Figs 2,123 and 2,124) and limiting the possibility of entering the joint cavity, a narrow-bladed osteotome is driven transversely across the tibia and left in position until the block is free. Note osteotome in position and the outlined rectangle of tibial tubercle with attached tendon.

Fig. 2,126. When the lateral capsule has been divided the block of bone with attached tendon can be drawn down to a much lower level.

Fig. 2,127. The oblique slot has been cut in the antero-medial aspect of the head of the tibia and the cortex undermined to receive the rectangle of bone which is seen lying at original site.

Fig. 2,128. In the final step the rectangle of bone is passed through the slot and rotated so that it is locked under the cortex (Fig. 2,123).

judgement is required. The detached rectangle of bone should be held against the tibia and then the knee flexed to determine the position the patella will adopt. In deciding the exact point at which the window is to be made it will be remembered that in passing the rectangle of bone through the cortex the patella will be pulled down an additional distance depending on how far it is passed into the depths of the medullary cavity. Allowance for this extra distance is made in deciding the site of the window.

A rectangular opening of approximately the same size as the block of bone is cut in the cortex on the medial side. The long axis of the window is inclined at an angle of about 40° to the vertical. The position is important for it determines the final relationship of the patella to the femoral condyles and the tension on the tendon. The fact that the joint is in some 5° to 10° of flexion, determined by the sandbag in the popliteal space, is not only of assistance in entering the block of bone through the window but ensures a reduction of tension in full extension.

It is useful to remember that if it is not possible to make the block of bone larger, neither is it possible to make the window smaller, thus until familiar with the technique, the block of bone is better to be too big and the opening too small (Fig. 2,127).

Cancellous tissue is excavated from the depth and from under the cortex at the superior and inferior extremities of the cavity producing the effect of overhanging margins. The rectangular block of bone suitably adjusted for size, is now placed in the window, driven through with the knee held in full extension and rotated so that its long axis lies in the axis of the quadriceps. This means that the tibial tubercle and attached tendon are locked under the margins of the opening (Figs 2,123 and 2,128) and at this stage the joint is fully flexed to demonstrate that positive locking has been achieved.

ALTERNATIVE METHOD. There is another method of locking the tibial tubercle in position said to be simpler in execution (J.H.) than the original The tubercle with attached tendon is removed in the manner described. The slot in the antero-medial aspect of the tibia is cut in the line at which the transplanted tendon is intended to pull. The slot is cut very considerably shorter than the detached rectangle with the tendon attached. The cortex is undermined superiorly and inferiorly and cancellous tissue removed. The rectangle is then passed through the slot and downwards then manoeuvred upwards so that the free bone above the attachment of the tendon engages beneath the cortex. It will be clear that the window in the tibia must be short enough so that when the free bone engages superiorly the lower end is also locked beneath the cortex (Fig. 2,124).

No matter which method has been used there remains a large defect from which the tibial tubercle was removed. The free rectangle of cortex from the window should not be used to fill this space for it may fail to obtain a blood supply. The sharp edge at the inferior extremity is bevelled. Suction drainage is introduced to the defect from the lateral side.

AFTER-TREATMENT. At the termination of the operation a compression bandage is applied. When the sutures are removed about the twelfth day the compression bandage can be discarded other than for support. Flexion exercises, progressing to straight-leg-raising, may be started in the next week. Weight-bearing with the aid of crutches is resumed from the fourth to the sixth week.

## Old Dislocations

It has been indicated that permanent dislocation of the patella may not necessarily be a source of serious symptoms. In such circumstances no action may be indicated. The disability most likely to be complained of in middle age from incidents of dislocation is, of course, the falls precipitated and in permanent dislocation, instability. In such circumstances operative action may be indicated.

How rewarding can be the result of transplantation of the patellar tendon coupled with local debridement in dislocation of long standing with osteoarthrosis of the patello-femoral joint in the right patient is illustrated by the following case:

The patient (Mrs I.B., aged 55) complained of gross instability of the right knee. She gave a history of trouble with both knee joints from the age of 15. It appeared that what had originally been subluxations had, in

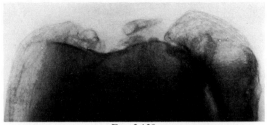

FIG. 2,129

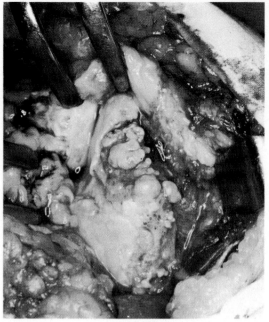

FIG. 2,130

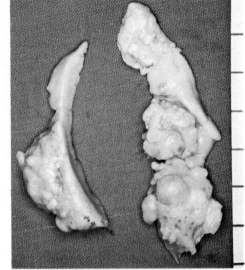

FIG. 2,131

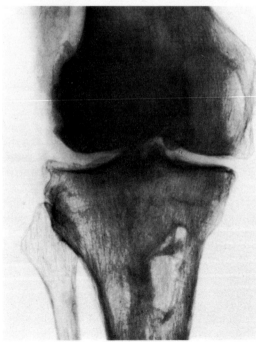

FIG. 2,132

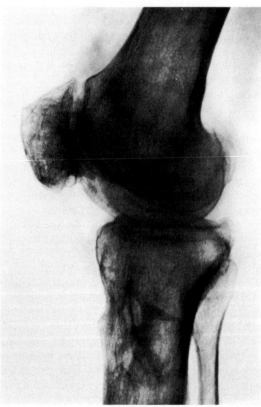

FIG. 2,133

FIGS 2,129–133. **Dislocation of the patella: debridement of patello-femoral joint and restoration of relationship by transplantation of tibial tubercle to antero-medial aspect of tibial head.** Skyline view to show dislocated patella (Fig. 2,129). Medial margin of the medial femoral condyle and adjacent patella (Fig. 2,130). Excised medial margin of patella and exostoses from medial margin of medial femoral condyle (Fig. 2,131). Radiological appearance of the joint after operation. Defect in antero-medial aspect of tibia is slot for transplantation of tibial tubercle. The tibio-femoral joint is relatively normal (Figs 2,132 and 2,133) (I.B., female, aged 55).

the course of time, become permanent dislocations: on each side the patella was lying on the lateral aspect of the joint. Many years previously, as is so often recorded, a normal medial meniscus had been removed in error. In the course of an incident she had sustained a medial tangential osteochondral fracture of the patella. Degenerative changes of radiological degree were present in the medial compartment as a result of the erroneous removal of the normal meniscus. To add to her troubles she was much overweight.

The most outstanding of her symptoms was instability arising from the dislocation. The means of providing relief were not obvious. It was decided to explore the patello-femoral joint and consider the possibility of restoring the normal relationship.

The operation was performed through the medial incision described for recurrent subluxation. When the capsule was incised, medial to the patella, the salient feature was the size and extent of the cartilaginous masses outlining the margin of the medial femoral condyle. The lateral condyle, presumably from limited contact with the patella, was not so affected.

A decision had to be made whether or not the entire patella should be excised. But it was clear that the shape of the condyles was such that the reconstituted tendon would dislocate; and that the end result, in terms of instability, would be worse than before operation. It was decided therefore, in spite of the gross nature of the pathology, to restore the patella to the normal position by transplanting the tibial tubercle to the anteromedial aspect of the tibial head. To this end a debridement of the patello-femoral joint was carried out with a fine-bladed osteotome. Exostoses were removed until the medial margin was congruous with the surface of the condyle (Fig. 2,131). When the tibial tubercle had been transplanted, the opposing surfaces of the condyle and patella were reasonably, but by no means perfectly, congruous (Figs 2,129 to 2,133).

After-treatment, contrary to expectations, was not characterised by pain. Nor were the anticipated difficulties in regaining movement encountered.

The final outcome of operation exceeded expectations. The patient declared herself to have attained, if not a painless joint, at least one which was stable and which enabled her to continue with her work.

She reported six years later asking that the operation, which had been so successful on the right side, should be performed on the left knee.

## COMPLICATIONS OF OPERATION

**Adherent scar.** Reference has been made to the dead space which exists after transfer of the tibial tubercle. The advent of suction drainage has reduced but not eliminated the complications inherent in haematoma at this site.

**Chondromalacia patellae.** It is the common experience that if the result of operative action is to prove unsatisfactory, symptoms are manifest in the short rather than the long term. If chondromalacia patellae is already established, rerouting of the patella can be expected in theory to be responsible for the aggravation of symptoms. In a considerable experience of a variety of circumstances the incidence of symptoms so related has been surprisingly infrequent. If symptoms are encountered in the immediate short term patience should be exercised and no precipitate action undertaken. The patello-femoral joint has the capacity to accommodate to adverse mechanical situations and a new, and stable, tract may be 'rubbed smooth' with use and the passage of time.

In adverse circumstances treatment follows the line of action recommended in chondromalacia patellae.

It is important that the symptoms of chondromalacia patellae are not confused with compression of the fat pad inherent in the biomechanical situation created by the operation (see below).

**Fat pad lesion.** If patella alta is the most common single cause of recurrent subluxation it will be remembered that patella alta is characterised by a large fat pad which must fill the space between tibial tubercle and patella. When the patella is pulled down to a lower level the space available to the fat pad is reduced without concomitant reduction in the size of the fat pad. It may thus be subject to pressure to pro-

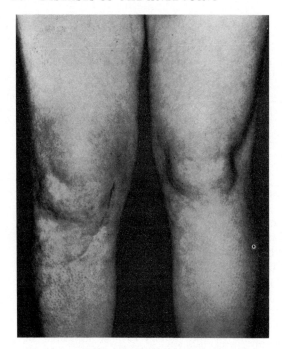

Fig. 2,134. **Recurrent subluxation of patella: complication of operation. Fat pad lesion.** A large flat fat pad is characteristic of patella alta. When the patella is brought down to a lower level the space for the fat pad is reduced. It may be under compression and symptoms may be produced. These symptoms should be distinguished from those of chondromalacia.

Note prominence of fat pad on operated side.

trude through the weak area between patellar tendon and iliotibial band but also on the medial side of the tendon. The typical fat pad symptoms of aching pain in the anterior compartment on exertion possibly accompanied by small transient effusions may be produced (Fig. 2,134).

These symptoms are liable to misinterpretation and are readily mistaken for those of chondromalacia. If they are excessive, or do not resolve with explanation, reduction in the size of the fat pad by the technique described may be necessary.

There may be circumstances in which compression of the fat pad can be anticipated. Such a situation may arise when patella alta is extreme. If such a possibility is anticipated a reduction of intracapsular but extrasynovial fat may be indicated.

**Patella baja.** The utmost care should be exercised in the course of operation to locate the patella at the correct level. To find it situated at an excessively low site is a common fault.

The condition is manifest by, (1) immediate disability after operation; (2) retropatellar pain and crepitus; (3) limitation of flexion; and (4) distal displacement of patella on clinical examination and confirmed radiologically (Blazina *et al.*, 1975). Early recognition of the cause of the symptoms and revision of the transfer is important if irreversible damage is to be avoided. Revision takes the form of the technique illustrated in Figs 2,89 and 2,90.

**Patella baja/genu recurvatum.** It is important that no operation is undertaken which interferes directly or exerts excessive muscular pressure on the upper tibial epiphyseal plate in the course of growth.

If the operation of transplantation of the tibial tubercle is undertaken when the upper tibial plate is open the site will migrate down the tibia not only to produce patella baja but a recurvatus deformity from premature closure of the anterior aspect of the plate. The effect of such an error of timing is illustrated in Figure 2,135.

Every effort should be made to avoid operation of any kind until the epiphyses are mature. The possible exceptions have been indicated. Even in maturity an increase in recurvatus is known to occur. Figure 2,78 illustrates a patient cured of recurrent dislocation at the cost of increased asymptomatic recurvatus.

**Failure of fixation.** If immediate quadriceps exercises and early weight-bearing are contemplated, it is essential that the tibial tubercle be locked positively at the site of the transfer by one of the methods described: a soft tissue suture, the transfer of a plug of bone secured by driving fit, staple or screw no matter how well executed, require at least eight weeks for bony union to occur. Exercise therapy and weight-bearing is not possible, therefore, before union is complete. An example of failure to observe these precautions is illustrated in Figure 2,71. Two examples only in a considerable series have displaced as a result of errors of technique. In one example (case of R.D.M.), the patient, an epileptic, in a fit, fractured the bridge of bone between the original site and that of transfer.

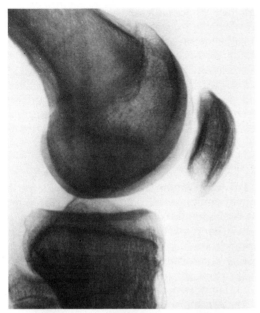

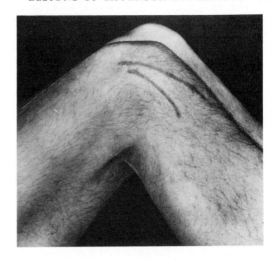

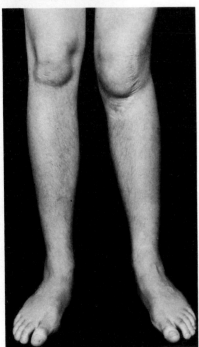

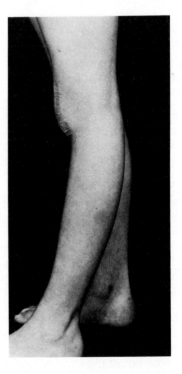

FIGS 2,135–138. **Recurrent subluxation of patella: errors in treatment.** In these examples transplantation of the tibial tubercle was carried out before closure of the growth plate resulting in migration of the tubercle down the tibia and with it the patella, resulting in patella baja and deformity of the tibial condyles (Fig. 2,135). Related knee to show lateral meniscus incision illustrating common error of diagnosis and profile of flexed knee by comparison with normal (Fig. 2,136). In addition valgus angulation (Fig. 2,137) and recurvatus deformity (Fig. 2,138) can result from the same error of judgement in the choice or error of timing of operation.

**Simultaneous extra- and intra-articular operations.** In general it is unwise to combine intra- and extra-articular operations in spite of social and financial pressures. The combination is self-defeating as resulting usually in delay in recovery. In recurrent dislocation the intra-articular procedure of removal of a loose body from a medial osteochondral fracture should not be combined with the extra-articular procedure of transplantation of the tibial tubercle. The removal of the loose body, a minor matter in the content of a separate procedure, should be deferred until mobilisation is complete.

**Timing of operation.** It is common experience that a fall, carrying a recently-born baby, or even a kettle of boiling water, is the final incident which alerts the patient to the necessity for operation. It is important in terms of delay of recovery that a second incident of trauma in the form of a major operation is not superimposed on the damaged tissues until reaction, induced by the fall, has subsided. In other circumstances operation difficulties are increased and recovery prolonged.

## OSTEOARTHROSIS OF PATELLO-FEMORAL JOINT

Osteoarthrosis of the patello-femoral joint occurs in two forms:

**Local.** This is the variety limited to the patello-femoral joint and arising for local mechanical reasons at one extreme, of single-incident trauma possibly in the form of fracture, in other circumstances of long-standing derangement of the mechanics or excessive wear and tear of the joint.

**General.** This is the variety associated with osteoarthrosis of medial and lateral compartments of the tibio-femoral joint, or otherwise of generalised or pan-articular osteoarthrosis. It will be shown (Ch. 10) that this variety in bilateral form is commonly based on the derangement of mechanics inherent in medial torsion of the tibiae and as such poses possibilities of prevention but problems of treatment.

### Local

It is not proposed to repeat the list of factors thought to be responsible for chondromalacia patellae. If chondromalacia merges imperceptibly into osteoarthrosis with the passage of time the majority of cases present as established osteoarthrosis and without previous history. In such circumstances the important aetiological factors will be seen to be the excessive wear and tear imposed by long-standing adverse mechanical conditions of wide variety (see chondromalacia patellae).

### Circumstances Precipitating Symptoms

**1. Driving position.** The situation whereby the patient complains of pain only when driving a car is of common occurrence.

In driving, particularly for long distances, it is important that the thigh of the right leg is resting comfortably on the seat. If the seat is close to the controls, or the patient tall, the thigh is not supported and consequently contraction of quadriceps and hamstrings is required to maintain the foot on the accelerator pedal in the moving vehicle. In such circumstances the patella is pressed hard against the femoral condyles (Fig. 2,139). If the patello-femoral joint is worn the outcome is local pain. This is the reason why patients have to get out of the car to 'stretch their legs' from time to time. The same situation may obtain in degenerative lesions of the meniscus and in tibio-femoral osteoarthrosis.

Sometimes the situation is precipitated by a change of vehicle in which the driver's seat is higher and thus requires a greater degree of flexion of the knee. If a new and unaccustomed arc of the worn joint is utilised pain is induced.

Recognition of the source of the pain together with the explanation may be all that is required for the solution of the problem by raising the seat and/or adjusting the distance from the controls. In extreme situations a change of driving position determined by a change of vehicle may be the only solution to the problem (Fig. 2,140).

**2. Flexion deformity.** Any situation, say a period of bed rest producing or increasing flexion deformity with concomitant loss of muscle tone, may be responsible. The simple explanation is the greater tension required in the worn patello-femoral joint to maintain the erect position.

**3. Removal of lateral meniscus.** Patello-femoral

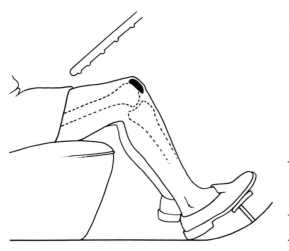

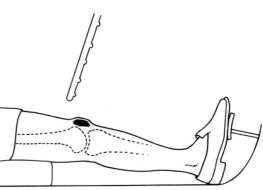

FIGS 2,139–140. **Patello-femoral joint: osteoarthrosis. Diagrammatic representation of the biomechanical problems of driving a car.** In driving it is important that the thigh is supported. Otherwise quadriceps and hamstrings must be contracted with the patella pressing hard against the femoral condyles (Fig. 2,139). At the opposite extreme, with the thigh supported and the leg in extension, the quadriceps are relaxed. The patella is not constantly compressed against the femoral condyles (Fig. 2,140).

osteoarthrosis is most common in the female. The operation most likely to precipitate symptoms is the removal of a thick primitive lateral disc also most common in the female. The effect is to exaggerate a valgus deformity which may already have been present and thus increase the Q angle.

**4. Locked medial meniscus.** The so-called locking which occurs with the complete longitudinal tear eliminates the screw-home movement and precipitates symptoms in the patello-femoral joint the subject of degenerative changes. This situation normally relates to youth, not the subject of wear and tear changes in the patello-femoral joint; but not exclusively so.

**5. Osteotomy of tibial head altering alignment of track.** The opening of a wedge brings the patella down to lower level with possible mechanical advantages but must alter alignment of patella to tibial tubercle. When a wedge is closed the patella is located at a higher level and the alignment of patella to tibial tubercle altered but in the opposite direction.

## Clinical Features

A common subject of isolated patello-femoral osteoarthrosis will be recognised as a short,

overweight, middle-aged woman; and there are reasons why it should be so. It is not just her weight; or her age. It is that extension of the knees is so much more difficult in those of short stature; and it is those of short stature who wear the highest heels. The necessity to walk with the knees flexed wears the cartilage of the patello-femoral joint. Symptoms are precipitated by the increasing weight of middle-age.

The reason for the onset of symptoms is not any sudden advance in the osteoarthrosic process but the advent of a flexion deformity. It will be recognised that normally with the knee screwed-home in extension it is possible to accept the entire weight on one leg with the quadriceps relaxed. Impose, however, the slightest flexion deformity and the body-weight must be supported by the quadriceps with, in osteoarthrosis, a worn patella pressed against worn femoral condyles in which, at the extreme, subchondral bone may be exposed.

**Examination.** The salient feature of examination is that the knee complained of is the subject of slight flexion deformity when compared with the normal side. The patient indicates the site of her pain to be retropatellar or at the margins of the patella, particularly on the lateral side. The manual pressure of the patella against the femoral condyles induces pain. There may be local synovial tenderness; and likely to be located on the lateral side.

### General

In the patello-femoral osteoarthrosis which forms part of a pan-articular osteoarthrosis symptoms directly related to the patello-femoral joint are seldom paramount in the overall situation. If present, they do not differ from those described. In prescribing treatment, however, it should be recognised that the local operative measures which may be indicated in the isolated form may not be applicable in pan-articular osteoarthrosis and, indeed, may be contraindicated.

**Radiological examination.** The antero-posterior projection is not helpful. The lateral view may show the patella to be located at a somewhat lower level than usual. The reason for this is not immediately evident but may be the aetiological factor in so far as a patella so located is under compression through a greater range of motion

than one normally located and the articular cartilage subjected to excessive wear and tear. The joint space is seen to be reduced and with sclerosis of subchondral bone particularly in the patellar element (Fig. 2,141). There is a hypertrophic or proliferative variety in which extension of the articular surfaces is apparent and with massive bony excrescences (Fig. 2,142).

The skyline view is more dramatic and provides more information. The bone is seen to be displaced to the lateral side often with subluxation. Fracture of the overhanging lateral margin is not uncommon (Fig. 2,143). It should be recorded that the most grotesque radiological changes in both the lateral and skyline views are consistent with symptomless function (Fig. 2,144). Decisions regarding treatment, and particularly operative treatment, should not be based on the radiological appearances of the joint.

### Treatment: Conservative

It is important that it should be appreciated as

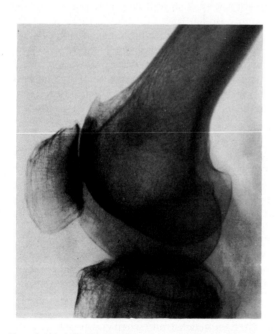

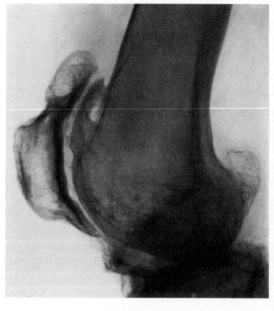

FIGS 2,141–142. **Patello-femoral osteoarthrosis.** The condition in established form showing loss of joint space and sclerosis of opposing joint surfaces. Note patella baja. The tibio-femoral joint is unaffected (Fig. 2,141) (G.S., female, aged 50).

In this gross example of the hypertrophic form the patello-femoral osteoarthrosis is part of a pan-articular osteoarthrosis. Note changes in tibio-femoral joint and bony block to extension (Fig. 2,142).

has been indicated that a very large proportion of patients presenting for the first time with symptoms referable to the patello-femoral joint can be demonstrated to have developed a minimal flexion deformity. If the physical conditions of the joint, and of the tibio-femoral joint are such that no bony block to extension exists, the simple prescription to the physiotherapist of 'Instruct patient in passive stretching to improve extension and in quadriceps exercises' in a co-operative subject results in rapid relief of pain. The means whereby such measures, in progressive form as indicated, are applied will be described in Chapter 6. In many instances it is unfortunate that relief of pain is so readily achieved. In spite of the instructions that passive stretching and simple exercises must be practised permanently if recurrence is to be avoided, human frailty is such that few patients continue beyond the point in time when symptoms are finally, as they think, relieved. Recurrence in such circumstances is inevitable.

## Treatment: Operative

**Debridement.** It is probable that too fatalistic an attitude has been adopted to gross changes in the patello-femoral compartment. There are, for example, occasions when loss of extension is due to the impingement of opposing osteophytes of

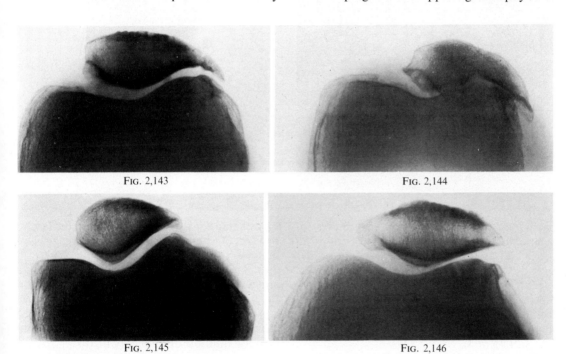

FIG. 2,143

FIG. 2,144

FIG. 2,145

FIG. 2,146

FIGS 2,143–146. **Patello-femoral osteoarthrosis.**
Fig. 2,143. In this example pain was precipitated by the fracture of the lateral marginal exostosis. Note contralateral changes in the femoral condyle.

Excision of the fragment through a short parapatellar incision rendered the patient symptomless.
Fig. 2,144. Gross radiological changes are consistent with symptomless function. This example is one of bilateral symmetrical joints neither of which had ever given trouble. It is clear however that correction of angular deformity in the tibia by altering the mechanics of the joint could transform the situation to one in which serious symptoms could arise.

Fig. 2,145. In this example the joint space is preserved but there are local lateral marginal exotoses and a contralateral lesion in the opposing condyle. Such cases may react favourably to a local debridement.
Fig. 2,146. The patello-femoral joint shows the marked changes in pan-articular osteoarthrosis based on medial torsion. Note lateral displacement, loss of joint space and changes in lateral femoral condyle consisting of decalcified areas interposed with denser bone. It is the constant necessity to produce lateral rotation in gait which is responsible.

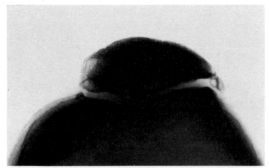

FIG. 2,147

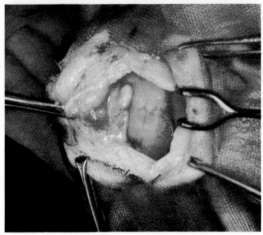

FIG. 2,148

FIGS 2,147–149. **Patello-femoral osteoarthrosis.** Lateral marginal exostosis possibly the subject of fracture and the source of local pain and tenderness (Fig. 2,147). Appearance at operation through a limited parapatellar incision to show exostosis. The contralateral changes in the femoral condyle, as is the usual pattern, are the more marked (Fig. 2,148). The exostosis excised at local debridement (Fig. 2,149).

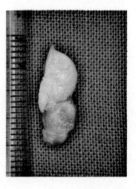

FIG. 2,149

patella and condyle. A common source of symptoms is the projection which develops on the lateral aspect of the patella and protrudes over the articular facet on to the lateral aspect of the femoral condyle. This projection is vulnerable to injury; and a fracture commonly occurs from minimal injury or no injury at all. Examination locates the pain and tenderness to this protuberance (Fig. 2,147).

There are thus circumstances when operative action, consisting of the removal of the excrescences and smoothing of the opposing surfaces through a limited exposure, can result in marked improvement of function.

TECHNIQUE. The bone is exposed through a short lateral parapatellar incision and rotated in the long axis to expose the articular surface of patella and femoral condyle. The multiple pathology is inspected and the mechanics assessed by flexion and extension of the knee. The operation proceeds according to the find-ings. It may consist of debridement of the lateral margin of the patella and/or the margin of femoral condyle. Degenerative changes in articular cartilage are likely to be more extensive and advanced on the femoral condyle than on the patella (Fig. 2,148); and if subchondral bone is exposed resurfacing with fibrocartilage may be indicated by bringing a blood supply to the area through multiple drill holes (Ch. 10).

*After-treatment.* At the termination of operation a compression bandage is applied. Care must be exerted in applying a post-operative compression bandage in patello-femoral osteoarthrosis in so far as pain may be induced by pressing the worn patella hard against the opposing worn femoral condyles.

## Realignment Operations

The simplest method of reduction of compres-

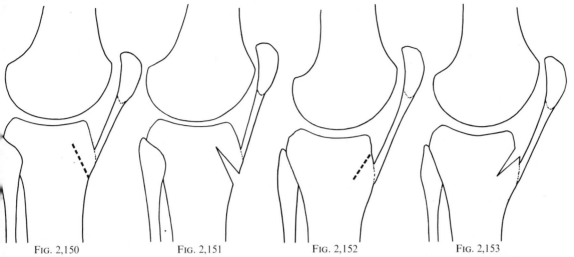

FIG. 2,150         FIG. 2,151                    FIG. 2,152         FIG. 2,153

FIGS 2,150–153. **Chondromalacia patellae: patello-femoral osteoarthrosis: treatment.** Methods of changing the biomechanical status of the patello-femoral joint by altering the compression loading by lengthening (or shortening) the distance from the centre of rotation. Osteotomy below the tibial tubercle raises the patella to a higher level and decreases the load at the patello-femoral joint (Figs 2,150 and 2,151). Osteotomy above the tibial tubercle brings the patella down to a lower level at a greater distance from the centre of rotation and thus decreases the load at the patello-femoral joint (Figs 2,152 and 2,153).

sion forces is by *lateral release*. In a more complex situation may be required some form of *anterior displacement of the tibial tubercle*.

**Lateral release: isolated division of lateral patellar retinaculum and capsule.** This is an operation with a wide range of application in affections of the patello-femoral joint. It has the advantage not common to many procedures that it does not prejudice the future nor preclude any of the more radical measures which may be required.

CONTRAINDICATION. The operation is effective only in situations in which 'there is something to release'. In no circumstances should it be applied as an isolated procedure to recurrent subluxation or dislocation of the patella based on patella alta. The release of compression forces (see below) renders the patello-femoral joint even more unstable.

**Biomechanical basis of operation.** It will not have escaped notice that 'skyline' views of the patella, and for whatever underlying pathology, usually reveal the bone to be displaced to the lateral side. The normal valgus angulation of the female knee makes such findings obvious; but there are other factors less evident. In any event experience of transplantation of the tibial

tubercle in the treatment of recurrent dislocation shows that when the capsule and lateral retinaculum are divided the patellar tendon and attached tibial tubercle can immediately be drawn down to a lower level; and in some instances to a degree responsible for location at an undesirably low level. It follows therefore that division of the lateral retinaculum and capsule performed as an isolated procedure reduces compression forces in the patello-femoral joint. In such circumstances there arises the possibility of relief of symptoms in a variety of pathological situations such as recurrent subluxation (as opposed to dislocation), chondromalacia and osteoarthrosis.

**Operation.** A short lateral parapatellar incision gives access to the site. The capsule is divided 1 cm lateral to the patellar tendon and extended upwards maintaining this distance from the patella. Ideally the capsule and retinaculum are divided leaving the synovial layer intact. In practice this may prove impossible as the incision advances proximally. If a rent cannot be repaired it is ignored. To test the effectiveness of release the knee is flexed to a right-angle and any remaining contractions, which may include the vastus lateralis expansion, divided.

Closure of the wound is completed by suture of subcutaneous tissues and skin.

AFTER-TREATMENT. This procedure differs from most knee operations in that in order to maintain the gap created it is necessary to immobilise the joint in some, say, 30° of flexion. The compression bandage is applied in this position and the flexion preserved by incorporating plaster slabs in the outer layers. The patient is nursed initially on the Braun-type splint but can resume ambulation with the aid of crutches on the fourth day. The flexed position is maintained until the skin stitches are removed on the tenth day. Weight-bearing can be resumed when active control of complete extension has been achieved.

### Reduction of Compression Forces

Elevation of the tibial tubercle with its attached patellar tendon by oblique osteotomy from below (Figs 2,150 and 2,151) or from above (Figs 2,152 and 2,153) alters the compression forces within the patello-femoral joint. The distance the tubercle can be elevated in a forward direction is determined by cosmetic considerations and difficulties of skin closure; 1·5 cm may be the limit so imposed. There is evidence, however, to suggest that little is to be gained in the reduction of compression forces by elevation of the tubercle beyond half an inch (1·5 cm) (Ferguson, Brown, Fu and Ruthkowski, 1979).

Maquet (1969) pointed out that forward displacement of the patellar tendon had the same effect. Originally this was achieved by interposing a graft taken from the crest of the ilium and held in position by wire suture between the patellar tendon and the upper extremity of the tibia. This technique for the cosmetic reasons referred to above, and the occasional absorption of the graft, has been abandoned in favour of elevation of the tibial crest maintained by the interposition of an iliac graft (Maquet, 1976) (Figs 2,154 and 2,155). The revised technique permits rerouting of the patella to the medial side should the occasion demand (Figs 2,156 and 2,157).

Blaimont and Van Elegen (1979) seek to solve the problem in a similar manner by the Elmslie operation, which realigns the extensor apparatus towards the midline, while reducing patello-

femoral compression forces by the insertion of a cortico-cancellous bone block, some 8–15 millimetres thick taken from the adjacent lateral femoral condyle, and inserted beneath the transposed tendon. The author has no personal experience of the outcome of these operations.

**Anterior displacement of the tibial tubercle by elevation of tibial crest: technique.** The incision 10–13 cm long extends downwards from the inferior pole of the patella on the antero-medial aspect of the leg approximately 1 cm posterior to the tibial crest. The periosteum is incised longitudinally and a row of transverse drill holes made through the tibia parallel to and 0·7 cm posterior to the crest. A linear osteotomy is then performed by joining the drill holes with a small

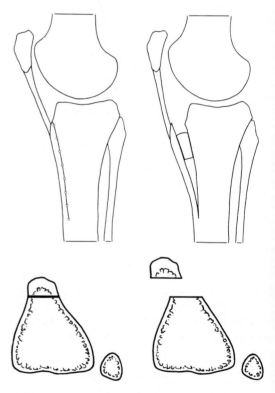

FIGS 2,154–157. **Anterior displacement of tibial tubercle (Maquet).** An osteotomy is performed by joining horizontal drill holes with a fine-bladed osteotome (Fig. 2,154). Anterior displacement is maintained by the introduction of a wedge-shaped bone graft from the crest of the ilium (Fig. 2,155). If it is considered desirable to reroute the patella in the intercondylar groove the tubercle and tibial crest are displaced to the medial side (Figs 2,156 and 2,157).

fine-bladed osteotome (Fig. 2,154). The anterior flap so created remains attached distally and the required elevation maintained by wedge shaped grafts taken from the ilium in the manner described in Chapter 9 (Fig. 2,155). If a fracture occurs at base of the flap fixation with a screw may be necessary. In this regard it should be noted that the operation in addition to anterior displacement of the tibial tubercle permits it to be displaced medially retracking a laterally displaced patella and thus distributing compression forces over a wider area. Such displacement would entail the use of internal fixation in the form of screws. Closure of the skin incision without tension may prove difficult; and to this end medial and lateral relief incisions may be required.

Mobilisation of the joint is undertaken as soon as the patient has recovered from the immediate after effects of the operation.

**High tibial osteotomy combined with anterior displacement of patellar tendon.** Maquet (1969) further pointed out that when osteoarthrosis of the patello-femoral joint is associated with an angular deformity anterior displacement of the patellar tendon is simply achieved by dome, or what he calls barrel-vault osteotomy shifting anteriorly the entire distal fragment and maintaining the correction by Steinmann pins and compression clamps (Figs 2,135 to 2,136).

The author cannot claim any practical experience of these procedures. The underlying theories are attractive. The former operation appears to offer a possible solution to what can be an intractable problem and does not prejudice the future as does patellectomy. The latter operation offers possibilities for relief when the correction of varus angulation by simple linear opening or closing-wedge osteotomy would increase the compression forces in an osteoarthrosis patello-femoral joint by displacing the patellar further to the lateral side.

**Patellectomy.** Recent advances in total knee replacement dictate that procedures which prejudice future options are to be avoided. Patellectomy is such an operation. The age range affected by patello-femoral osteoarthrosis is likely to be considerably higher than that affected by chondromalacia; and thus the contraindications are less well defined except in terms of future possibilities. The indication will

be intractable pain unrelieved by any other measure which may be indicated in the circumstances of the case. It will exchange, as do many orthopaedic procedures, one disability for another. No patient subjected to patellectomy for osteoarthrosis can run, take part in sporting activities and will experience difficulty in ascending stairs. It is generally accepted,

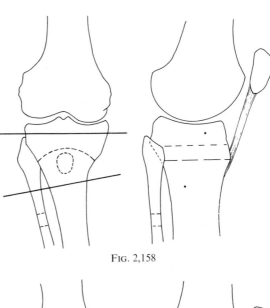

Fig. 2,158

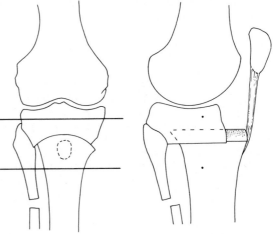

Fig. 2,159

Figs 2,158–159. **Pan-articular osteoarthrosis: treatment.** Correction of angular deformity and anterior displacement of the patellar tendon can be achieved by dome osteotomy of tibial head with displacement of the tibial tubercle controlled by Steinmann pins incorporated in the plaster cast (Figs 2,158 and 2,159) (after Maquet).

however, to be effective in the relief of pain. The technique as applied to osteoarthrosis has been described under 'Chondromalacia'.

## Patello-femoral Joint Replacement

**Indications.** The resurfacing of the articular aspect of the patella by a plastic stud which articulates with the condylar flange of the femoral component is common practice in total knee replacement. There are circumstances of pathology confined to the patello-femoral joint such as osteoarthrosis, chondromalacia, persistence of symptoms following tibial tubercle transplant for recurrent dislocation etc., unrelieved by the methods described whereby isolated replacement of the joint would be preferable to patellectomy. The replacement components available are similar in concept and design. They consist of a shield-shaped femoral groove implant of stainless steel recessed into and cemented to the femur and a matching patellar component of polyethylene which replaces the articular surface of the patella (Fig. 2,160).

The author has no personal experience of the procedure, other than witnessing the operation performed and noting the exacting nature of the technique; nor of the results to be anticipated.

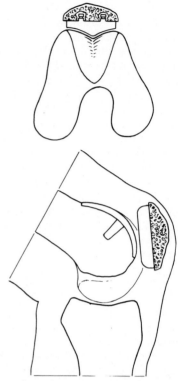

FIG. 2,160. **Patello-femoral joint replacement.** Components consist of a shield-shaped femoral groove implant recessed into and cemented to the femur and a matching patellar component of polyethylene secured by cement which replaces the articular surface of the patella.

## REFERENCES

AGGARWAL, N. D. & MITTAL, R. L. (1970). Nail-patella syndrome. *Journal of Bone and Joint Surgery,* **52B,** 1, 29–35.

ANDERSEN, P. T. (1958). Congenital deformities of the knee joint in dislocation of the patella and achondroplasia. *Acta orthopaedica scandinavica,* **28,** 26.

BAKER, R. H., CARROLL, N., DEWAR, F. P. & HALL, J. E. (1972). The semitendinosus tenodesis for recurrent dislocation of the patella. *Journal of Bone and Joint Surgery,* **54B,** 1, 103.

BARRY, H. C. (1969). *Paget's Disease of Bone.* Edinburgh & London: E. & S. Livingstone.

BENNETT, G. B. (1922). Lengthening of quadriceps tendon. *Journal of Bone and Joint Surgery,* **4,** 279.

BERNHANG, A. M. & LEVINE, S. A. (1973). Familial absence of the patella. *Journal of Bone and Joint Surgery,* **55A,** 1088.

BLACKBURNE, J. S. & PEEL, T. E. (1977). A new method of measuring patellar height. *Journal of Bone and Joint Surgery,* **59B,** 241.

BLAIMONT, P. & VAN ELEGEN, P. (1979). Our experience of the advancement of the anterior tibial tuberosity associated to the recentralisation in the treatment of patellofemoral osteoarthritis. *1st Congress of the International Society of the Knee,* April 24–27, Lyon, France.

BLAZINA, M. E. (1971). Los Angeles, California, U.S.A. (Personal communication).

BLAZINA, M. E., FOX, J. M., CARLSON, G. J. & JURGUTIS, J. J. (1975). Patella baja. A technical consideration in evaluating results of tibial tubercle transplantation. *Journal of Bone and Joint Surgery,* **57A,** 1027.

BLAZINA, M. E., KERLAN, R. K., JOBE, F. W., CARTER, V. S. & CARLSON, G. J. (1973). Jumper's knee. *Orthopaedic Clinics of North America,* **4,** 665.

BLUMENSAAT, C. (1938). Die Lageabweichungen und Verrenkungen der Kniescheibe. *Ergebnisse der Chirurgie und Orthopädie,* **31,** 149.

BOSE, K. & CHONG, K. C. (1976). The clinical manifestations and pathomechanics of contracture of the extensor mechanism of the knee. *Journal of Bone and Joint Surgery,* **58B,** 478.

CALVERLEY, J. & MULDER, D. W. (1960). *Neurology,* **10,** 963.

CARTER, C. & SWEETNAM, R. (1960). Recurrent dislocation of the patella and of the shoulder. *Journal of Bone and Joint Surgery*, **42B**, 4, 727.

CASEY, E. B. & HARRISON, M. J. G. (1972). Diabetic amyotrophy: a follow-up study. *British Medical Journal*, **i**, 656.

COCKBURN, W. C. & DROZDOV, S. G. (1970). *Bulletin of the World Health Organisation*, **42**, 405.

DEWAR, F. P. & HALL, J. E. (1957). Recurrent dislocation of the patella. *Journal of Bone and Joint Surgery*, **39B**, 798.

FAIRBANK, SIR H. A. T. (1937). Internal derangement of the knee in children and adolescents. *Proceedings of the Royal Society of Medicine*, **3**, 11.

FERGUSON, A. B., BROWN, T. D., FU, F. H. & RUTKOWSKI, R. (1979). Relief of patellofemoral contact stress by anterior displacement of the tibial tubercle. *Journal of Bone and Joint Surgery*, **61A**, 159.

FOWLER, A. W. (1972). Chondromalacia patellae. *British Medical Journal*, **ii**, 528.

GALEAZZI, R. (1921). Nuove applicazioni del trapianto muscolare e tendineo (XII Congress Societa Italiana di Ortopedia). *Archivio di Ortopedia*, **1922**, 38.

GARLAND, H. (1955). Diabetic amyotrophy. *British Medical Journal*, **ii**, 1287.

GARLAND, H. (1960). *Proceedings of the Royal Society of Medicine*, **53**, 137.

GOODFELLOW, J., HUNGERFORD, D. S. & WOODS, C. (1976). Patello-femoral joint mechanics and pathology. 2. Chondromalacia patellae. *Journal of Bone and Joint Surgery*, **58B**, 291.

GOODMAN, J. I. (1954). *Diabetes*, **3**, 206.

GUNN, D. R. (1964). Contracture of the quadriceps muscle. *Journal of Bone and Joint Surgery*, **46B**, 492.

HAUSER, E. D. W. (1938). Total tendon transplant for slipping patella. *Surgery, Gynecology and Obstetrics*, **66**, 199.

HESSEN, I. (1946). Fabella. *Acta radiologica*, **27**, 177.

HNEVKOVSKY, O. (1961). Progressive fibrosis of the vastus intermedius muscle in children. *Journal of Bone and Joint Surgery*, **43B**, 318.

HUCKSTEP, R. L. (1971). Orthopaedic appliances for developing countries. *Tropical Doctor*, **1**, No. 2, 64–68; & **1**, No. 3, 108–114.

INSALL, J., FALVO, K. A. & WISE, D. W. (1976). Chondromalacia patellae. *Journal of Bone and Joint Surgery*, **58A**, 1.

INSALL, J. & SALVATI, E. (1971). Patella position in the normal knee joint. *Radiology*, **101**, 101.

JEFFREYS, T. E. (1963). Recurrent dislocation of the patella due to abnormal attachment of the ilio-tibial tract. *Journal of Bone and Joint Surgery*, **45B**, 4, 740.

KAUFER, H. (1971). Mechanical function of the patella. *Journal of Bone and Joint Surgery*, **53A**, 8, 1551.

KUTZ, E. R. (1949). Congenital absence of the patellae. *Journal of Pediatrics*, **34**, 760.

LANCET (1970). Editorial, **iii**, 646.

LEHNEIS, H. R. (1968). The Swedish knee cage. *Artificial Limbs*, **12**, 2, 54–57.

LESLIE, I. J. & BENTLEY, G. (1976). Arthroscopy in the diagnosis of chondromalacia patellae. Paper presented at the Hebeden Society Meeting, London, November, 1976.

LEVY, M., SEELENFREUND, M., MAOR, P., FRIED, A. & LURIE, M. (1971). Bilateral spontaneous and simultaneous rupture of the quadriceps tendons in gout. *Journal of Bone and Joint Surgery*, **53B**, 3, 510.

LITTLE, E. M. (1897). Congenital absence of delayed development of the patella. *Lancet*, **ii**, 781.

LLOYD-ROBERTS, G. C. & THOMAS, T. G. (1964). The etiology of quadriceps contracture in children. *Journal of Bone and Joint Surgery*, **46B**, 3, 498.

MAQUET, P. (1969). Biomechanics and osteoarthritis of the knee. SICOT, XIe Congrès, Mexico, 317.

MAQUET, P. G. J. (1976). *Biomechanics of the Knee*. Berlin, Heidelberg, New York: Springer-Verlag.

OBER, F. R. (1939). Recurrent dislocation of the patella. *American Journal of Surgery*, **43**, 497.

OUTERBRIDGE, R. E. (1961). The etiology of chondromalacia patellae. *Journal of Bone and Joint Surgery*, **43B**, 752–757.

PATERSON, D. C. (1970). Myositis ossificans circumscripta. *Journal of Bone and Joint Surgery*, **52B**, 296.

PERRY, J., O'BRIEN, J. P. & HODGSON, A. R. (1976). Triple tenodesis of the knee. *Journal of Bone and Joint Surgery*, **58A**, 978.

ROUX (1888). Luxation habituelle de la rotule. *Revue de Chirurgie (Paris)*, **8**, 682.

RUBACKY, G. E. (1963). Inheritable chondromalacia of the patella. *Journal of Bone and Joint Surgery*, **45A**, 1685.

SCHWARTZMANN, J. R. & CREGO, C. H. (1948). Hamstring-tendon transplantation for the relief of quadriceps femoris paralysis in residual poliomyelitis. *Journal of Bone and Joint Surgery*, **30A**, 3, 541.

WELLS, C. (1968). Osgood-Schlatter's disease in the ninth century? *British Medical Journal*, **i**, 623.

WIBERG, G. (1941). Roentgenografic and anatomic studies on the femorpatellar joint. *Acta orthopaedica scandinavica*, **12**, 319.

WILLIAMS, P. F. (1968). Quadriceps contracture. *Journal of Bone and Joint Surgery*. **50B**, 278.

# 3. Affections of the Synovial Membrane: General

## Definition

**'Synovitis'.** The reaction of synovial membrane to irritation is effusion of fluid into the joint cavity. The irritation can take several forms: *mechanical* as in trauma, exogenous or endogenous; *chemical/mechanical,* as in 'pseudo-gout'; or *disease process* in the widest sense, general or local.

Synovial effusion is not the universal clinical sign nor the invariable reaction to degenerative disease. The most common 'diseases' affect fibro-cartilage and articular cartilage. Both are avascular structures. Neither involves synovial membrane. Degenerative processes in these structures, whether it is a horizontal cleavage lesion of the posterior segment of the medial meniscus, or chondromalacia of the patella or elsewhere, are not characterised by synovial effusion. It is of importance in the interests of accuracy of diagnosis that these basic facts are recognised.

## SYNOVIAL EFFUSION

### Introduction

There are few diagnostic exercises in ortho-paedic surgery with such a wide variety of possible solutions as a knee joint, the site of an acute, a chronic or a recurrent effusion for which no immediate explanation is evident.

Pain is the symptom which causes patients to seek advice. Many of the conditions produc-ing chronic synovitis are painless at least in the early stages. There is thus a tendency for a painless swelling to have existed for many months before presented for diagnosis. Thus a condition of simple origin may become chronic from the mere passage of time and lack of the appropriate treatment in the early stages.

## DIFFERENTIAL DIAGNOSIS

### Trauma

The most common cause of an effusion of synovial fluid is trauma normally of a degree recognised by the patient. 'Synovitis' is thus a

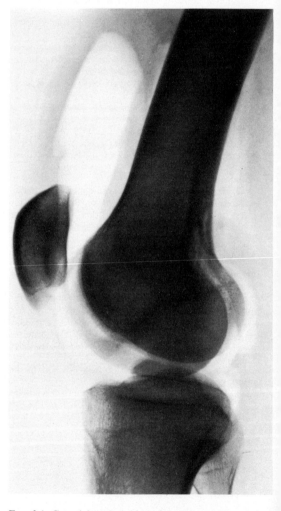

Fig. 3,1. **Synovial cavity.** Air arthrogram to demonstrate synovial cavity and in particular location and extent of suprapatellar pouch.

symptom of trauma. It is not an acceptable diagnosis unless the cause is known. Nevertheless, simple synovitis, with a recognised traumatic basis, treated by bed-rest with the knee flexed over a pillow until the effusion subsides, can constitute a problem. A return to unrestricted weight-bearing with wasted quadriceps results in recurrence of effusion. Further bed-rest results in more quadriceps wasting and progressively less protection for the damaged joint; and so the vicious circle is established (Fig. 3,2). Immobilisation in a plaster cast, the refuge of the clinically destitute, is an addition to the problem of considerable magnitude.

This is a situation which will be recognised by the experienced clinician from the history and, in particular, from the mechanism of injury; from the bed-rest in the absence of compression and exercise; and in an otherwise fit young patient. In other circumstances, a synovitis resulting from, say, a blow on the suprapatellar pouch, and mismanaged in the manner indicated, can constitute a problem of diagnosis in the absence of reaction to every known investigation. It is a condition of innocent origin but with potential for disaster, particularly if the aetiology is a simple industrial or other injury with an outstanding claim for compensation and with a possibly doctor-made situation capable of being capitalised for gain.

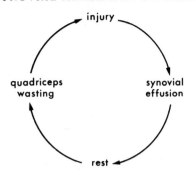

FIG. 3,2. **'Idiopathic' synovitis.** What was originally a simple traumatic synovitis can be transformed into a chronic idiopathic synovitis if the joint is rested without quadriceps exercises. A return to weight-bearing without adequate muscular protection results in recurrence of the effusion.

## UNRECOGNISED TRAUMA

### Exogenous

A single incident of direct trauma or even a twisting injury of a degree likely to result in effusion seldom passes unrecognised. But repeated incidents of so-called microtrauma, such as occur in some habitual action, may not be evident to the patient. The following are examples:

The patient, a young farmer, had sought advice for several years running for an unexplained effusion in the right knee. It occurred in the spring and at no other time. Every investigation had proved negative. When seen during an attack the positive findings, apart from the effusion, were soft tissue thickening accompanied by vague tenderness over the lateral aspect of the joint. The quadriceps muscle was of volume comparable with the sound side. In the course of a detailed history it transpired that in the spring of the year he was engaged in the monotonous task of ploughing many hundreds of acres of land. In the course of this occupation he 'rested' the relaxed knee against the mudguard where it was subjected to repetitive blows as the tractor travelled over the rough ground.

The patient (A.F., female, aged 45, factory worker), complained of a painful, swollen right knee for the past seven months. In the absence of obvious cause, the simple screening test, namely, the ESR was carried out and found to be 27, raised, but not significantly so. In the absence of diagnosis or of serious concern, she was prescribed the standard treatment of non-weight-bearing quadriceps exercises. The effusion persisted.

In pursuing the possibility of trauma it transpired that her work as a machine-operator entailed the compression of a lever with the right heel ten thousand times per shift! The patient was of small stature and the compression of the pedal involved a considerable amount of force. When it was suggested that this action might be the cause she agreed and volunteered the information that it was possible to operate the pedal with the left heel. In two weeks the effusion had subsided.

On the three occasions on which the ESR

was repeated it was 22, 22 and 14 in the first hour. There was no recurrence of the effusion.

It remains to be seen whether she will return sometime in the future with an effusion in the left knee!

INDUSTRY. In the industrial field a trap for the unwary is the continuous use of a knee in the manoeuvring of packing cases, bales of hay, straw, cotton or jute.

Certain industrial actions can be at fault. The 'knee-kicker' or 'knee-stretcher' used by carpet layers is struck repeatedly by the knee in the area of the suprapatellar pouch while in the kneeling position. An excessive amount of work can result in an effusion. Carpet layers, however, readily recognise the nature and source of the effusion.

AGRICULTURE. In the countryside the use of heavy gum boots by the middle-aged to walk or to work in muddy conditions is a common cause of effusion: the feet are fixed by the mud and rotation forces exerted on the wearing joints. If there is a family history of arthritis, rheumatoid or otherwise, the bilateral nature of the condition can occasion alarm and fruitless investigation unless the cause is recognised.

SPORT. In the realms of field sports a similar situation arises when heavy body-wading boots are used by the middle-aged when river fishing. In a strong current the feet are fixed and unaccustomed rotation about the worn knees occurs in the course of casting with a fly rod.

## Endogenous: General

It should be recognised that certain forms of joint, accepted as being within the bounds of normality, are mechanically unsound and fail to withstand prolonged or unaccustomed activity. In this regard the recurvatus deformity of the female knee, when exaggerated, is particularly liable to bilateral effusions. It is presumed that the origin of the synovitis is trauma to the synovial membrane lining the retropatellar fat pad and thus subject to compression in extension. The liability to compression is increased if the unaccustomed physical activity is undertaken wearing low-heeled shoes. It is important that this situation is recognised. A swelling of more

than one joint in the young female subject is liable to misinterpretation.

**Hypermobile joints.** General laxity of joints occurs as an isolated clinical finding in otherwise normal people; and it is known that such findings may have a familial background. The question which arises is whether the condition represents one extreme of a normal variation in joint mobility, or whether it is to be regarded as an incomplete form of a heritable disorder of connective tissue such as the Marfan or the Ehlers-Danlos syndrome. In spite of the familial background, however, these cases do not show the stigmata of the heritable disorders such as hyperelastic skin, easy bruising, high palate or abnormalities of body proportion.

The hypermobility as it affects the knee takes the form of a recurvatus deformity producing a mechanically unsound joint liable to attacks of pain and effusion which occur when the patient is subjected to unaccustomed exercise or long periods of standing. Such a case is illustrated in Figures 1,18 and 1,19. The reasons for the effusion have been referred to above. It is important that this syndrome is recognised and that the recurrent pain and/or effusion has a mechanical background. These patients have usually had numerous biochemical investigations with negative results and had a variety of possible diagnoses in the field of arthritis attached to their complaint.

## Treatment

If there is no active treatment, a confident and acceptable explanation for the pain and recurring effusions is received with relief. It is explained that activities known to bring on symptoms must be avoided. If the maintenance of muscle volume helps to protect the joint, quadriceps exercises are not necessarily helpful in genu recurvatum. The raising of the heels limits hyperextension and by preventing compression of the synovial membrane posterior to the fat pads reduces the liability to effusion.

An example of the problems posed by a synovitis of unknown origin based on unrecognised trauma of exogenous and/or endogenous origin is recorded in the following case history:

The patient (Mrs H.O., aged 29), a nurse, gave a history that during hostilities in the Middle East two years previously, and in an attempt to escape injury, she had fallen on her left knee directly on to a concrete surface.

There had been some swelling immediately following the injury. It was not of a severe nature. She thought little of it at the time. The swelling, however, had recurred at repeated intervals over the past two years, and had been accompanied by pain. There followed thereafter a long history of a variety of treatments including injections of hydrocortisone, short wave diathermy, etc. While she said that she had carried out quadriceps exercises throughout, when asked to demonstrate them the performance was not such as to accept that they had been carried out correctly or conscientiously. The outstanding feature of the investigations, and amongst a large file of documents, were two instances in which her ESR had been raised to 18 and 21, and more alarming, two instances in which the R.A. Latex test was said to have been positive. She was eventually referred for opinion by an orthopaedic surgeon of known competence who said that he had been unable to achieve a diagnosis. He suggested the possibility of chondromalacia of the patella; but, of course, there was the possibility of early rheumatoid arthritis.

On examination there was little difference between the two joints. There was no synovial effusion. She overreacted to palpation of the suprapatellar pouch and to pressure on the joint lines. There was no clinical evidence of chondromalacia. It was noted that there was a degree of genu recurvatum considerably greater than would be regarded as normal in a woman.

The massive documentation was completed by a large packet of radiographs of poor quality, none of which showed any gross abnormality. In the circumstances there seemed to be no alternative to the repetition of investigations. All the common tests were carried out, the most important of which, the ESR, was negative. The possibility of synovial tuberculosis after two years seemed unlikely, and particularly with the normal ESR. The radiographs of the lung fields were negative.

The possibility of brucellosis was eliminated. Radiographs of the knee of good quality including axial views of patella were obtained with negative results other than to confirm the mechanical defect in the form of genu recurvatum.

The patient had travelled 2000 miles for an opinion as to the diagnosis. She was, it is to be noted, a nurse. She had become obsessed with the possibility of chondromalacia patellae, and, of course, was worried with the knowledge that on two occasions her R.A. Latex test had been positive. It was explained that there was no evidence of any serious pathology in the joint. This did not impress her, and her answer was: 'if there is no serious pathology, what is the source of the pain which I have suffered for the past two years?'

It was the author's clinical opinion that the effusions were due to synovial irritation of mechanical origin.

In the circumstances of the distance she had travelled and the fact that she was a nurse and would not accept a clinical diagnosis, it was decided to examine the articular surface of the patella, and if desirable, carry out a synovial biopsy. A short 4 cm incision was made on the supralateral aspect of the patello-femoral joint. There was no excess fluid in the joint. The articular cartilage of the patella was normal. The synovial membrane of the suprapatellar pouch was of normal appearance. There were synovial tags adjacent to the patello-femoral joint both on the lateral aspect and the superior aspect. They showed no evidence of trapping incidents. One tag was excised on the grounds that it might have been trapped, but in any event as a synovial biopsy. The so-called exploration therefore, was negative and only effective in so far as to produce absolute evidence of the absence of chondromalacia patellae. Histological examination of the tag of the synovial membrane did not demonstrate any abnormality.

The explanation offered for the recurrent effusions (if, in fact, such occurred) was the mechanical anatomical conformation and defect in the joint of which the patient was aware. To what extent the conditions of warfare contributed was impossible to estimate.

The patient was reassured from direct

observation that she did not suffer from chondromalacia patellae; that the synovial membrane of her knee was of normal appearance and was reported to 'show masses of mature fat cells covered by a thin synovial lining. There is no evidence of the histological appearances seen in rheumatoid arthritis or of other inflammatory change'. It was explained that the hyperextension of her knees, of which it is repeated she was aware, was the probable cause. The only treatment recommended was quadriceps exercises; and the use of high heels.

She returned to her country in a happier frame of mind. The final outcome, however, is unknown.

## POST-OPERATIVE EFFUSION

In the context 'unrecognised trauma' is trauma sustained in the course of operation and which may be a cause of persistent effusion. Furthermore, and in the same context, is.the return to weight-bearing following operation without adequate quadriceps protection resulting in the kind of vicious circle depicted in Figure 3,2.

### Prevention

**Trauma at operation.** It is important at all times that the tissue concerned with effusion, synovial membrane, is handled with care. The prolonged and forceable pressure of retractors is readily accepted as a source of trauma. What is less well appreciated and possibly more important is the mechanical friction produced by the constant use of dry swabs or sponges. In this regard it is good practice when effusion is encountered in meniscectomy to remove all possible fluid at the outset. The flexed position of the joint will have emptied the suprapatellar pouch in favour of the intercondylar fossa and the posterior compartment from which it will exude throughout the operation. A hand, covered by a towel, is placed in the popliteal space and, exerting forward pressure, evacuates the accumulated fluid which is then removed with moist swabs or sponges wrung-out of normal saline. If this act is performed thoroughly no further flow of synovial fluid should obstruct visualisation of the meniscus.

**Drainage into extra-articular soft tissues.** The pushing of forceps through the roof of the suprapatellar pouch into the adjacent quadriceps at the termination of an arthrotomy in order to permit post-operative effusion to escape into the thigh is barbaric in concept and execution. It is not to be considered.

**Suction drainage.** When suction drainage is employed within the synovial cavity it is in the context of prevention of effusion of blood rather than prevention of effusion of synovial fluid. It is thus applicable to such major procedures as synovectomy or where the site of operation is not subject to external pressure. Suction drainage has not been employed in the prevention of post-operative effusion.

**Quadriceps insufficiency.** In the course of recovery from synovial effusion whether the result of disease or injury, operative or accidental traumatic, the importance of the maintenance of quadriceps volume has been stressed. If a patient is permitted to return to weight-bearing and allowed to 'stand about' with the joint inadequately protected from the stresses and strains so imposed the trauma to the synovial membrane produces an effusion or recurrence of effusion. Weight-bearing should not be undertaken without muscular control. This is not a subject, in a variety of pathological conditions and age-ranges, in which it is possible to generalise. If a rule must be made to cover every eventuality in the course of recovery, no patient should be permitted to return to weight-bearing unless he can lift his extended knee from the bed and maintain it in this position without obvious effort. This will be recognised as the minimal acceptable standard.

## SYNOVIAL EFFUSION: RELATIONSHIP TO MAINTENANCE OF MOVEMENT

### Who has seen a stiff knee with a synovial effusion?

Permanent stiffness rarely follows synovial effusion unless it is an early manifestation of a progressive pathological process. Rather does the reverse obtain. It is the impression, for example, that loose bodies, no matter what the origin, producing an effusion are objectionable;

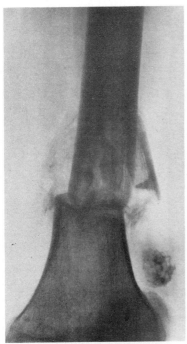
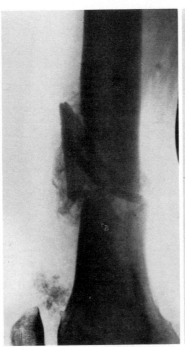

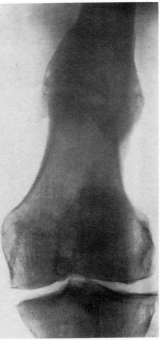

FIG. 3,3                    FIG. 3,4                              FIG. 3,5

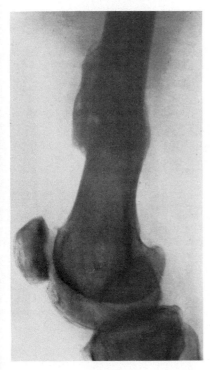

FIG. 3,6

FIGS 3,3–6. **Who has seen a stiff knee with a synovial effusion? Case demonstrating beneficial effect of loose bodies in potentially stiff knee.** Supracondylar fracture of femur in process of healing showing large loose body in supra-patellar pouch (Figs 3,3 and 3,4). The fracture healed and loose body removed. Note degree of osteoarthrosis in joint (Figs 3,5 and 3,6). (See text.)

and it would seem that the possibility of an exception could not arise. But no subject in medicine is without exception. Even loose bodies can have therapeutic value:

The first patient in whom such an effect was noted sustained, in an accident involving gross violence, a supracondylar fracture of the femur with comminution and with considerable soft tissue damage. The fracture was treated by closed reduction in the manner described in IKJ5 and satisfactory alignment obtained. The nature of the injury was such that although callus appeared rapidly, an unfavourable outcome in terms of knee joint movement was anticipated. The prognosis, as far as the function of the knee was concerned, did not seem to be improved by the

F

presence of loose bodies in the suprapatellar pouch (Figs 3,3 and 3,4) and osteoarthrosis of radiologically detectable degree (Figs 3,5 and 3,6). The patient, however, instead of the anticipated delay in restoring movement and possibly of permanent stiffness, regained a full range of flexion within two weeks of discarding his splints and before union was considered adequate for weight-bearing.

The second sustained, in a road traffic accident, the familiar dashboard fracture of the patella well known for slow return of flexion as a result of associated contusion of the soft tissue components of the joint (IKJ5). He too was noted to have loose bodies in the suprapatellar pouch, the effect of which was expected to be detrimental to recovery (Fig. 3,7).

He too, repeated the experience recorded in the first case and regained a full range of movement within two weeks of release from restraint (Fig. 3,8).

What is the explanation of this phenomenon? Is it that the irritation of the loose bodies produces an innocent effusion and the adhesions which would otherwise have occurred are avoided; or is it that as the result of the presence of loose bodies, or of the pathology responsible for them, the synovial membrane is conditioned to injury? These observations are not without therapeutic implications for the future.

In the current scene it will be evident that the situation can be capitalised to the patient's advantage in avoiding a stiff knee in the unusual circumstances of an injured knee being noted to be the site of loose bodies. The clinician should not be precipitate in recommending removal until such time as a full range of movement has been restored.

## SYNOVITIS: MANIFESTATION OF ALLERGIC REACTION

It is alleged, to use a linguistically similar and possibly appropriate word, that a synovial effusion can be the result of an allergic reaction due to sensitivity to food, bacteria or other substances. In one example the offending article of food was identified as 'English walnuts'! (Lewin and Taub, 1936). There exists a

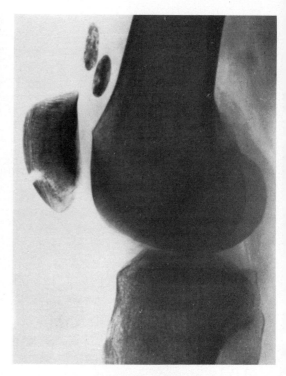

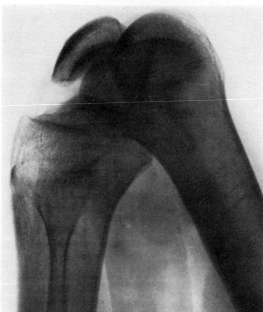

FIGS 3,7–8. **Who has seen a stiff knee with a synovial effusion? Case demonstrating beneficial effect of loose bodies in potentially stiff knee.** Dashboard fracture of patella with loose bodies in suprapatellar pouch (Fig. 3,7). The complete return of flexion was achieved (Fig. 3,8).

considerable literature relating intermittent hydrarthrosis to asthma, urticaria, migraine, epilepsy and a variety of other conditions but the subject has not been expanded or taken any more precise form in recent years.

In this series no case of intermittent or recurrent effusion has been attributed to this cause in spite of the number of problem chronic or recurrent effusions encountered for which no cause was found. It is a condition of evanescent origin not likely to be referred to an orthopaedic surgeon, even one with a known interest in the knee joint. It remains a possibility to be considered as a cause of mysterious recurrent simple effusions.

## MALINGERING: SELF-INDUCED EFFUSION

The circumstances in which a synovial effusion is deliberately induced occur most often in a conscript army in conditions of war. An effusion can be produced by manual trauma in the form of repeated blows to the suprapatellar pouch immediately above the patella continued for say an hour or two. But evidence of the aetiology may exist in the overlying skin. To avoid such evidence the joint has been known to be enclosed in a wet cloth and the trauma inflicted by blows from a hairbrush. No doubt there are other methods. At the extreme, in the author's knowledge, is the injection by hypodermic needle of some noxious substance, said in one instance to have been nicotine from the tobacco of a cigarette, into the joint. This procedure was successful in avoiding an unacceptable situation; but the risks involved must be considerable.

## SYNOVIAL EFFUSION AS MANIFESTATION OF OCCULT MALIGNANT DISEASE

### Hypertrophic Pulmonary Osteoarthropathy

This syndrome, usually manifest as a poly- rather than a mono-articular arthritis, is most commonly secondary to intrathoracic conditions the most important of which is an occult neoplasm. It is more likely to be mistaken for classical rheumatoid arthritis than the mono-articular form in which circumstances the

opportunity to extirpate a tumour may be lost. The presence of clubbing of the fingers will point to the correct diagnosis.

A synovial effusion into the knee may be the first manifestation of malignant disease; and this has occurred on three occasions in the author's experience. It has been recorded elsewhere (Roques, Amigues and Puget, 1974). A mysterious effusion occurring without reason in the knee joint of the middle-aged or elderly should be regarded with suspicion especially when associated with loss of weight or anaemia. In the author's cases the true diagnosis came to light in the course of the routine investigations indicated in such circumstances. In none was the site of the primary tumour located. In the case recorded by Roques et al., the primary tumour was a gastric epithelioma.

## SYNOVIAL IRRITATION BY EXTRA-ARTICULAR FOREIGN BODY

Under the heading 'Unrecognised Trauma' should be recorded the fact that a foreign body in the soft tissues, the presence of which may be unknown or the incident forgotten by the patient, can produce irritation and be the cause of recurrent effusions. The foreign body is often a small fragment of metal from a gunshot wound. The incident may have appeared trivial in relation to the events or major injuries at the time and to have been forgotten (Figs 3,9 and 3,10). The following is an example of such a case:

The patient (R.B., male, aged 46) a schoolmaster, gave a history that for the past two years he had suffered recurring effusions in the knee which on each occasion had subsided with rest and compression in a matter of two weeks. The effusions had been investigated with negative results. It was known that he had sustained minor gunshot wounds of the thigh in World War Two, 15 years previously. The radiographs taken with the purpose of eliminating the possibility of a foreign body in the joint had proved negative. When finally an effusion persisted, the advice of the author was sought. When in the course of examination further radiographic examina-

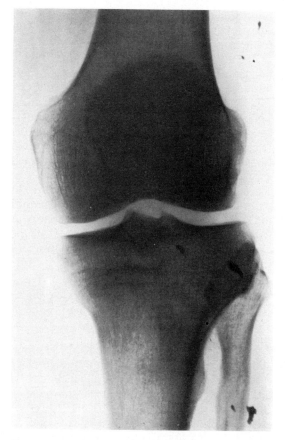

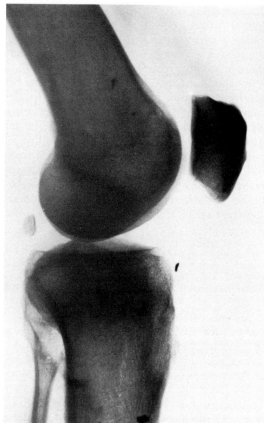

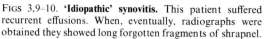

FIGS 3,9–10. **'Idiopathic' synovitis.** This patient suffered recurrent effusions. When, eventually, radiographs were obtained they showed long forgotten fragments of shrapnel.

At the time of injury 30 years previously in World War Two his major wounds elsewhere made the knee wounds trivialities [Capt. H.R., R.N. (retired) aged 62].

tion was advised, the advice was resisted as a repetition of what had previously proved negative. The radiograph, however, which covered a wider field, revealed the presence of a fragment of shrapnel in the quadriceps above the upper limit of the suprapatellar pouch. When it was removed there was no recurrence of the effusions.

## SYNOVIAL IRRITATION FROM ADJACENT DISEASE IN BONE

It is well known that an old, apparently healed, lesion of osteomyelitis, particularly in the femur, can give rise to recurrent effusions; and if the disease has resulted in the alteration of the architecture of the joint, the liability can be all the greater for mechanical reasons. Such

effusions, however, with a history of the disease in childhood, possible deformity and scars, and finally from a radiological examination, occasion no problem of origin. Sometimes however the cause of the recurrent effusions is revealed by the discovery of an unexpected focus of chronic disease in the form of a so-called Brodie's abscess.

## ENDOGENOUS TRAUMA: LOCAL

If tags of synovial membrane in one form or another appear to be a variety of local synovitis they are a cause of synovial effusion and often of a variety extremely difficult of diagnosis and particularly by a clinician unfamiliar with the underlying pathology.

**Pathological anatomy.** It is probable that the most common site at which synovial membrane is subjected to local endogenous trauma is the lining of the infrapatellar fat pad. An attempt is made here to place this lesion in the category of 'Synovitis: Local' (Ch. 4), but one of the clinical reactions is synovial effusion; and thus the matter must be expanded under 'Synovitis: General'.

The next most common site at which tags of synovial membrane are subject to trapping incidents and thus the cause of recurrent effusions is the medial margin of the medial femoral condyle or the lateral aspect of the patello-femoral joint. Examination of the normal knee will often reveal a thin flap of normal synovial membrane at the margin of the atricular cartilage of the medial condyle. Such a flap could be interposed in tibio-femoral or patello-femoral joint to be trapped and be the cause of an effusion. The liability to such incidents increases in the osteoarthrosic joint as a result of the presence of irregular marginal exostoses. Once an incident has occurred hypertrophy of the tag from oedema and haemorrhages takes place and thus the liability to further incidents is increased.

**Clinical features.** The recurrent synovial effusions are small; never to the point of a tension-situation requiring aspiration. Their occurrence is irregular and unpredictable. They are, however, associated with local pain; and the site of the pain, the point at which a tag of synovial membrane, other than posterior to the fat pad, has been traumatised is the clinical clue to the cause.

## CRYSTAL SYNOVITIS

There are two major causes of 'crystal synovitis': (1) *sodium urate crystal deposition disease (gout)*; and, more common and more important in the context of disease of the knee joint, (2) *calcium pyrophosphate crystal deposition disease (pseudogout)*.

**Nature of disease.** It appears that the numbers, shape and size of the crystals involved are the factors essential to irritation of the synovial membrane and to an attack of crystal synovitis rather than the chemical composition of the crystals.

## GOUT

**Mechanism of acute attack.** The events leading to the initial crystallisation of monosodium urate, after an average of 30 years of asymptomatic hyperuricaemia, are poorly understood (Wyngaarden, 1967). The synovial effusion in acute gouty arthritis almost invariably contains crystals of sodium urate. The crystals are seen within the polymorphonuclear leukocytes present in the synovial fluid and are seen also free in the fluid. Duncan *et al.* (1968), from a study of the ultrastructure of the crystal-containing cells have shown that the crystal is not contained within a membrane-bounded vacuole which always surrounds phagocyted material. The initial and critical formation of crystals is probably intracellular. The natural degradation of leukocytes or active extrusion of crystals permits their dispersal in the synovial fluid; and this release of crystals 'seeds' the uric acid-rich synovial fluid and thus induces extracellular deposition of sodium urate crystals. Thus the acute attack may be more directly dependent upon the intracellular level of uric acid rather than the uric acid level in the plasma.

### Provocative Factors

**Trauma.** The metatarso-phalangeal joint of the great toe is liable to microtrauma from unaccustomed physical activity and the footwear so related. In so far as the knee joint is concerned the incidence of trauma is less in evidence than in pseudogout.

**Surgical trauma.** It is common experience that a surgical operation can provoke an attack of acute gouty arthritis. If acute arthritis occurs during the first week after an operation gout should be suspected (Hench 1948).

**Indiscretions of diet.** Dietary excesses including the excessive consumption of alcohol have for long been considered to have precipitated attacks.

**Miscellaneous.** Emotional upsets and other stress situations together with a wide variety of other causes may be implicated.

### Clinical Features

**Disease of males.** Gout is predominantly a disease of the adult male. It has been known since the time of Hippocrates that it is unusual in females.

**Incidence.** Traditionally gout in the acute attack strikes the first metatarso-phalangeal joint and not the knee. When this joint is affected it is seldom in isolation.

**Clinical examination.** See 'Clinical Examination' in 'Pseudogout'.

**Radiological examination.** Punched-out areas, 5 mm or so in diameter, in the subchondral bone in the bases of phalanges, heads of metatarsals or metacarpals are common and may be followed in the late stages by marked destructive changes. Such appearances are shared by other conditions and are not pathognomic. There are no typical changes in the knee joint. Sodium urate deposits in the menisci and elsewhere are radiotranslucent.

### Laboratory Investigations

**Blood uric acid.** An increased serum uric acid level is essential to the diagnosis of gout but may be obviated by uricosuric drugs and even aspirin.

**Erythrocyte sedimentation rate.** The ESR may be raised in an acute attack and a leucocytosis may be found.

**Crystal examination.** Urate crystals are present in aspirated synovial fluid and can be differentiated from those of calcium pyro-phosphate by polarising-light microscopy (see pseudogout).

### Treatment

If there is no known cure for gout, this disease is almost unique among the arthritides, with the exception of infective arthritis, in that there is effective medical treatment for the acute attack. In such circumstances the opportunity is taken in medical textbooks to stress the dramatic effect of drug therapy in the form of Colchicene which, in brief, consists initially of 1 mg by mouth followed by 0·5 mg by mouth at intervals of two hours for 5 to 10 doses; and there are, in the current scene, other drugs.

In so far as the joint under consideration is concerned, aspiration of a tense synovial effusion followed by bed-rest, compression and splinting in the form of a compression bandage are required.

CALCIUM PYROPHOSPHATE<br>DEPOSITION DISEASE:<br>CHONDROCALCINOSIS: PSEUDOGOUT

**Background note.** The screening of synovial fluid for sodium urate crystals led to the discovery that some acutely inflamed joints contained crystals of a different substance now known to be calcium pyrophosphate dehydrate (McCarty and Hollander, 1961); and that patients exhibiting this phenomenon were observed to show radiological calcification of articular cartilage (McCarty, Kohn and Faires, 1962). This radio-opaque material has been shown to have the same chemical composition as the synovial crystals (Kahn, Hollander and Schumacher, 1962). The condition is thus of different aetiology from gout but similar in some respects in the clinical features of the acute attack; and hence the name 'pseudogout'.

**Terminology.** The terminology 'pseudogout' and 'chondrocalcinosis articularis' is unsatisfactory. Calcification of articular cartilage is difficult to detect (Fig. 3,15). Radiographs showing the condition in such marked degree as Figure 3,12 are unusual. On the other hand radiographic calcification of the menisci is a common finding and readily detected because opaque material is superimposed on opaque material in the antero-posterior projection whereas, if the isolated meniscus is exposed the material is seen to be but thinly distributed over a wide area (Figs 3,11; 3,13 and 3,14). Furthermore, the opaque material is deposited in synovial membrane where it is readily seen (Fig. 3,16). In such circumstances calcium pyrophosphate deposition disease, if clumsy, is a better description of what is now known to be a more common disease than gout.

**Incidence.** The knee is the joint most commonly affected as opposed to the first metatarso-phalangeal joint of gout.

### Clinical features

A rapidly developing tense synovial effusion in a middle-aged or elderly patient of either sex apparently otherwise healthy is not necessarily related to trauma although the patient may so relate it. An injury is commonly blamed for human ills; and indeed minimal trauma related to nothing more than undertaking some unusual activity is often the precipitating factor in crystal synovitis. It should be recognised as the most common single cause of an effusion in the knee in the elderly. The condition however is not confined to the elderly and in the familial variety of the disease attacks may occur in the third decade. In retrospect this provides the explanation of tense, painful but unexplained effusions which were encountered in the past but which made an uneventful recovery following aspiration.

The effusion characteristically occurs rapidly, perhaps more rapidly than any other effusion except of blood. The pain is intense partly from the mechanical irritation of the synovial membrane by the crystals, partly from the tension which may be created. The experimental injection of 20 mg of sodium urate crystals in 1·5 ml of saline into the normal human knee produced pain four hours later of an intensity which required 100 mg pethidine hydrochloride for control (Faires and McCarty, 1962). The largest, most tense and most painful effusion ever encountered (G.S., male, aged 67), the right side of a bilateral effusion which occurred some hours after returning from a fishing trip, was later shown by polarised light-microscopy to be crystal synovitis of pseudogout superimposed on chronic gout. The pressure at aspiration, in the less tense joint of the two, was observed to be 43 mm of mercury.

**Radiological examination.** Calcium pyro-phosphate crystals are radio-opaque. In circumstances of a high index of suspicion antero-posterior and lateral radiographs of the knee joint show calcification of the menisci (Fig. 3,11) synovial membrane (Fig. 3,16) or articular cartilage (Fig. 3,12) or of all of these components of the joint.

If, in a general degenerative process, calcification of the femoral artery is bilateral, if not necessarily symmetrical, calcification of the menisci may not be bilateral. Cases may be encountered in which there is gross symptomatic osteoarthrosis of one side without calcification of the menisci whereas the opposite knee, less affected by osteoarthrosis and asymptomatic shows calcification of both menisci. There is thus not necessarily a relationship between radiological osteoarthrosis and calcification of the menisci.

**Arthroscopy.** In cases of diagnostic doubt where the lesion in the early stages is not seen radiologically, nor the presence of the characteristic crystals established, arthroscopy will reveal the white material in the fronds of the synovial membrane, possibly on the superior surface of the menisci if such can be seen, or along the medial margin of the medial femoral condyle.

### Differential Diagnosis

**Simulation of infective arthritis.** An acute attack of crystal synovitis presents an appearance not unlike acute infective arthritis. It is the crystal synovitis of pseudogout, in which the knee is affected, which is most likely to result in an error of diagnosis. In gout the knee is less frequently affected although the combination of gout and pseudogout in the knee is not unknown (see above). The clinician unaware of the manifestations of crystal synovitis may regard the hot acutely painful knee when associated with a febrile reaction, leucocytosis and raised ESR, as an infective arthritis; and the aspiration of cloudy fluid, later shown to be sterile, may appear to confirm the diagnosis.

A clinician familiar with the clinical picture is unlikely to be misled. The routine radiographs which form part of the investigation of an acute monoarticular arthritis will reveal calcification of the components of the joint and radiographs of the 'normal' side will confirm the nature of the radio-opaque material. The microscopic examination of the synovial fluid for the tell-tale crystals is now widely practised as a routine measure.

**Polarised light-microscopy.** Examination of the synovial fluid by polarised light-microscopy provides a rapid and relatively simple method of diagnosis in crystal synovitis. It is an essential procedure in the diagnosis of acute arthritis. Synovial fluid from a joint which is the site of acute crystal synovitis usually contains numerous crystals some of which are intracellular. Crystals can be identified by the simple addition of two polarising filters to a standard laboratory microscope. In such conditions

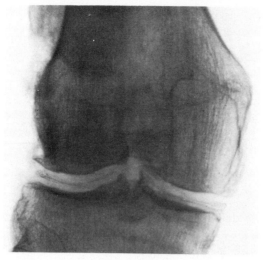

FIG. 3,11.

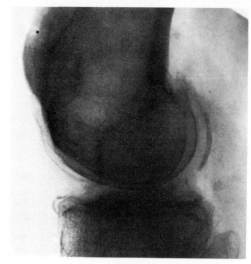

FIG. 3,12.

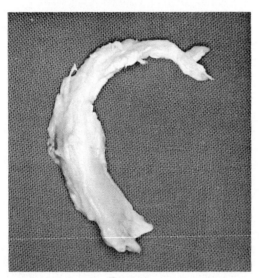

FIG. 3,13.

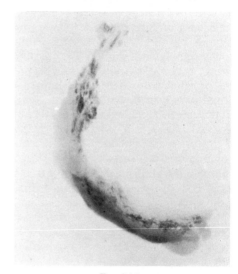

FIG. 3,14.

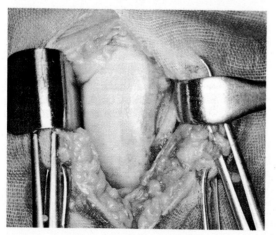

FIG. 3,15.

FIGS 3,11–15. **Crystal synovitis: chondrocalcinosis.** Calcification of the menisci is the most common finding (Fig. 3,11). Calcification of articular cartilage of the degree depicted in this example is unusual (Fig. 3,12). The medial meniscus from such a joint as Figure 3,11 to show calcification on the surface (Fig. 3,13) and the related radiograph (Fig. 3,14). In this example calcification affects the medial margin of the medial femoral condyle (Fig. 3,15). In this degree it will not be detectable radiologically.

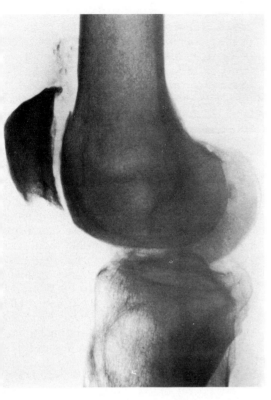

FIG. 3,16. **Crystal synovitis: chondrocalcinosis.** Calcification of the synovial membrane of the suprapatellar pouch in an osteoarthrosic joint. Note also calcification in articular cartilage of posterior aspect of femoral condyle. It is the calcification which may be present in such cases which is responsible for the sudden unexplained onset of effusion rather than the osteoarthrosis.

crystals which exhibit the property of birefringence, such as those of the sodium urate of gout and the calcium pyrophosphate of pseudogout, appear as bright objects. Furthermore, urate crystals can be differentiated from pyrophosphate crystals and thus gout identified from pseudogout. Urates are strongly and negatively birefringent whereas pyrophosphates are weakly positive.

DIFFERENTIAL DIAGNOSIS. Corticosteroid esters recently injected intramuscularly may appear microscopically in synovial fluid as crystals and these require to be differentiated from those of sodium urate or calcium pyrophosphate (Kahn *et al.*, 1970).

## Treatment

**Reassurance.** The most important item of treatment is reassurance that the sudden, alarming and painful effusion has no serious underlying pathological basis, the nature of which should be explained.

**Aspiration.** Palliative symptomatic treatment consists of aspiration, which may require to be repeated, application of a compression bandage and rest. Non-weight-bearing quadriceps exercises are instituted as soon as the acute phase has passed. Weight-bearing with the support of a compression bandage is resumed when the effusion has resolved.

In the present state of knowledge there is no known means of halting the deposition of crystals or of removing those already present.

## CHRONIC SYNOVITIS

### Modified Infective Arthritis

One of the commonest and most perplexing of problems which confront the clinician is the chronic synovitis of many months, or even of years duration, in which no firm diagnosis has been achieved and no rational therapy instituted. In almost all of these cases the pathology had been modified and the problem of diagnosis confused by the effect of various empirical measures, but principally antibiotic and steroid therapy. It is important therefore in the investigation of such cases to determine the exact mode of onset, whether there was systemic reaction, and the nature and the duration of antibiotic therapy prescribed. An unknown proportion of cases of chronic synovitis, or arthritis of indeterminate origin, are in fact examples of infective arthritis modified, but not 'cured', by antibiotic therapy.

There exists however a broad band of overlap between 'synovitis' and 'arthritis'. Reference is made above to the modification of infection by antibiotics. There are a variety of other possibilities. A mysterious effusion in the knee joint may be a minor clinical manifestation of chronic rheumatic fever, as in the case recorded overleaf.

The patient (N.McL., male, aged 15) a schoolboy from a residential private school, reported with pain and swelling of the right knee of one week's duration. He had been playing football immediately before the onset of the swelling but had no recollection of having received an injury. There was no previous history of trouble with the knee. On examination there was an effusion of moderate size but no other abnormality.

Aspiration was carried out and 60 cc of clear fluid obtained. Treatment consisted of a compression bandage and gentle quadriceps exercises. Culture of the synovial fluid was sterile. No organisms were seen and the egg culture showed no acid-fast bacilli. A guinea pig was inoculated, but four weeks after the date of the inoculation the animal was healthy. The final report eliminated the possibility of tuberculosis. The boy was the son of a farmer; and the possibility of brucelossis from milk from the neighbouring farm arose. The agglutination test for *Brucella abortus* was, however, negative. Blood investigations showed his haemoglobin to be 97 per cent. The film was normal. His ESR, however, was raised, being 21/1 hour. The R.A. Latex test was negative.

When the raised ESR was noted, further inquiries were made. It appeared that at the time when the effusion occurred he had suffered a 'sore throat'. This was considered to be a trivial matter, and resolved in a day. It was thought, however, that this aspect should be pursued. A week after his admission a throat swab grew a scanty growth of haemolytic streptococcus Langhan Group A, and a coagulase positive staphylococci. The ASO titre of 166 Todd Units was not thought to be of significance.

The effusion subsided rapidly with bed-rest and progress in redeveloping the quadriceps was achieved. He was discharged from hospital approximately three weeks after admission. He attended thereafter for supervision of his exercises.

It was at this time that he returned to his home for the Christmas vacation. On Christmas day his father telephoned with the knowledge that a tense effusion had returned, accompanied by a swelling of the calf. Examination at that time showed a large effusion; and swelling of the calf was confirmed. The diagnosis was further confused by the fact that since his return home he had fallen from his pony; but denied that an injury to the knee had been sustained. The return of the swelling seemed to indicate that further supervision was necessary and he was admitted to hospital. At no time had the temperature been raised. The joint was re-aspirated and a compression bandage applied. ESR was 24/1 hour—not dissimilar to the first occasion. In view of the previous history the matter of the throat was pursued, but coagulase negative staphylococcus only was reported. It was at this time, however, that the ASO titre was 733 Todd Units—a significant reading at his age. Within 48 hours of admission the remaining effusion had disappeared, and the joint appeared virtually normal. He was discharged to his home 14 days later. His ESR was 11/1 hour. The ASO titre was 833 Todd Units. Fourteen days later his ESR was 8/1 hour; haemoglobin, white cell count were normal, as was his ECG and chest radiograph.

That was not to be the end of the story. The school doctor did not accept the diagnosis. No treatment was administered. Three months later the boy reappeared with recurrence of the effusion. The diagnosis now appeared so evident that he was referred to a consultant physician. He considered that although there was no absolute proof the evidence favoured atypical rheumatic fever. He was of the opinion, in view of the importance of preventing a recurring streptococcal infection, that long-term administration of Penicillin was indicated. It was recommended in the current scene (1971) that 250 mg of Phenoxymethyl Penicillin be administered twice daily; and that this should be continued for five years!

There has been no recurrence of the effusion since the antibiotic was administered.

This case is recorded as an example of effusion into the knee of a schoolboy which was asymptomatic other than as a result of tension. It is an example of the difficulties of diagnosis which arise. In retrospect, the sore throat might have given a hint as to the possible diagnosis at an earlier date, but at that time the ASO titre was not significant. It is probable that the eventual titre of over 800 in this boy indicated that the mono-articular arthritis was related to the streptococcal throat; and that he was an atypical manifestation of rheumatic fever.

## Synovitis: Ankylosing Spondylitis

In the same category is cited an example in which synovitis occurred in a patient known to have suffered from ankylosing spondylitis, thought to be burnt-out and with no subjective manifestations related thereto:

The patient, W.A., male, aged 59, presented with a tense effusion in the right knee of some four weeks duration. The clinical impression and provisional diagnosis in the absence of a history of injury at his age was that of crystal synovitis. There was no clinical evidence of osteoarthrosis in the opposite knee; nor of angular deformity in the knee presented. Arrangements were made for therapeutic and diagnostic aspiration related in particular to the provisional diagnosis; and for radiographs to be obtained. It had been noted, as he entered the room, that he walked stiffly. It was thought prudent to examine his spine. At this stage he volunteered the information that 30 years ago he had received deep therapy for a back condition. On pursuing the matter it appeared that he received radiotherapy to the sacroiliac joints, dorsal and lumbar spine. Seven years later he had received similar treatment to his cervical spine. Two years later the left knee had been treated and a year later the right. After an interval of ten years he had received treatment to both knees. Records from the Radiotherapy Department were not available and as a result the dosages are unknown.

The only other relevant information available was that three years previously his ESR had been 9 in the first hour; and it was presumed on this information that the ankylosing spondylitis was burnt-out.

The ESR, at the time of presenting the swollen right knee, was 23. The radiographs showed decalcification with minimal loss of joint space. The appearances were those of a rheumatoid-like condition rather than those of osteoarthrosis.

The question which arose was whether the effusion was directly the result of reactivation of the ankylosing spondylitis; the result of the radiotherapy; or to crystal synovitis. The patient unfortunately refused aspiration on the grounds that improvement was occurring. The last possibility therefore could not be eliminated. He was treated expectantly with a compression bandage and quadriceps exercises.

The lessons to be learned from this case are: (1) the necessity for meticulous case-taking: this patient did not consider it relevant to mention ankylosing spondylitis nor that he had received radiotherapy; (2) the feature of ankylosing spondylitis affecting the knees as the only peripheral joints affected. The hips were normal clinically and radiologically; (3) the possibility that the knees had not been affected in the first place but, in the diagnosis of ankylosing spondylitis had been involved by implication. In peripheral spread it is unusual for the knees to be affected while the hips remain normal; but the possibility remains.

## CERTAIN DEFINED SOURCES OF RECURRENT SYNOVITIS

If under the heading 'idiopathic synovitis' there are situations which occasionally demand such a radical measure as synovectomy there are a number of clinically defined but pathologically indeterminate conditions to which the clinician should be alerted and which may be innocent in terms of future joint destruction. No doubt there are others in the classification 'idiopathic synovitis' for which the cause may be determined in the future. Examples are recorded:

### INTERMITTENT HYDRARTHROSIS

**Background note.** In the first description of the condition (Moore, 1864) this statement occurs. 'The subject of periodicity, or the tendency manifested by certain phenomena of life to recur after equal or nearly equal intervals of time, is still one of the curiosities of medical science. It has been often observed, yet not explained.' And of the same condition, Garrod (1910) wrote: 'Of periodicity in disease, no more striking example can be quoted than the recurrent effusion into joints with little or no febrile disturbance or local signs of inflammation, which goes by the name of intermittent hydrarthrosis.'

**Clinical features.** The condition is characterised by transient effusion into one or both knee joints at regular intervals. The onset is often sudden. The effusion lasts 2 to 6 days and recurs in cycles of 7 to 11 days. There are reports of extremes of 3 and 30 days (Mattingly, 1957). The duration of the effusion and the length of each cycle are more or less constant in any one patient. In Mattingly's review of the literature it appears that both genders are affected equally, usually between the ages of 20 to 50. The belief, apparently unproved, that young women in particular are affected should draw attention to the possibility that some cases are examples of infrapatellar fat pad lesions in the form of the *premenstrual water retention syndrome* of which previous writers on the subject have been unaware (Ch. 4). Once established intermittent hydrarthrosis may persist indefinitely. The fact that it is subject to spontaneous remissions and relapses makes assessment of treatment virtually impossible.

**Aetiology.** The cause is unknown. In idiopathic intermittent hydrarthrosis the sedimentation rate, Latex test, Wassermann reaction, gonococcal complement fixation test and brucella abortus agglutination tests are all negative. Reference will be made to the possibility of a hormonal origin in young women.

The results of synovial biopsy are unhelpful.

A proportion of patients later develop rheumatoid arthritis.

**Treatment.** There is no known effective treatment. It appears that in contradistinction to rheumatoid and certain other causes of chronic synovitis, permanent damage to the articular cartilage is not inevitable. In the circumstances of a condition in which pain is not an outstanding feature, caution should be observed in the use of radical empirical measures such as radiotherapy and synovectomy which of themselves can be productive of disability.

## PERIODIC DISEASE (FAMILIAL MEDITERRANEAN FEVER)

**Background note.** Periodic disease is characterised by recurrent attacks of non-specific inflammation of serous membranes, peritoneum, pleura and synovium. It is termed familial Mediterranean fever because it is considered a familial disease peculiar to people of Mediterranean origin. Armenians, non-Ashkenazic Jews and Arabs have been prominent in the cases so far recorded. But the disease is not restricted to people of Mediterranean origin (Cozzetto, 1961). The importance of the geographical distribution is unknown. In many areas of the world the disease may pass unrecognised (Makin and Levin, 1965) and indeed was unknown to the author until he read their article on which this section is based. The cause of the disease is unknown but is thought to be a genetically determined metabolic disorder (Sohar, 1964).

**Clinical features.** The disease arises in childhood or adolescence and is characterised by recurrent attacks of abdominal pain associated with fever and a monoarticular arthritis most frequently affecting the knee joint.

**Diagnosis.** There are no specific laboratory aids to diagnosis and synovial biopsy is not helpful. The recurrent monoarticular arthritis dating from childhood associated with abdominal pain and systemic reaction with a possible territorial background are the only clues in what must be regarded as a clinical diagnosis.

JOINT MANIFESTATIONS. If the abdominal and other symptoms tend to be of a fleeting nature those affecting joints tend to be prolonged in the form of chronic synovitis. In the circumstances and in the presence of a raised ESR, a variety of possible diagnoses is raised, in the acute phase, septic arthritis, and later, tuberculosis. The fact that organic joint damage can occur is not widely recognised (Herness and Makin, 1975).

**Treatment.** There is no specific therapy. The treatment recommended is rest in extension with maintenance of the quadriceps until such time as inflammation subsides followed by a gradual return to weight-bearing.

SIGNIFICANCE. It is clear that there exists a condition of unknown origin which simulates in its clinical manifestations acute septic arthritis, rheumatic fever, tuberculosis, etc.

## SYPHILIS

This subject is mentioned briefly under the heading 'synovitis' rather than 'arthritis' in so far as the problem of diagnosis is most likely to occur in a synovial effusion, unilateral or bilateral, of unknown origin.

### Acquired

A synovial effusion occurring in infectious syphilis is rare.

### Congenital

**Clutton's joints.** Bilateral symmetrical synovial effusions of the knee joints as a manifestation of congenital syphilis was first reported by Clutton (1886). The condition is likely to present as a synovial effusion, unilateral or bilateral, of insidious origin.

DIAGNOSIS. In the absence of obvious stigmata of congenital syphilis the diagnosis is difficult and depends on a high index of suspicion and a positive serological test. No example has been encountered in recent years. In the few cases recalled from the past the diagnosis depended on a positive serological test acquired in the course of routine investigation for a painless effusion of unknown origin. The last example recalled (Mrs G., aged 50, Sept. 1950) had every investigation for a chronic unilateral effusion including deep inguinal adenectomy and direct synovial biopsy proved negative. The mystery was solved when eventually the serological test, the Wassermann reaction at that time, was found to be positive.

TREATMENT. Aspiration is characteristically followed by recurrence of effusion; and this situation may persist for years. Management consists of aspiration as required, compression and maintenance quadriceps exercises on a permanent basis.

Antibiotic therapy is not effective.

PROGNOSIS. It is said that even after many years and repeated relapses the synovial membrane and articular cartilage remain relatively unaffected.

## 'Synovitis': swelling of the knee joint in children

The presentation of a child the subject of a swelling of the joint and in the absence of history of accepted single-incident trauma is at all times a problem of diagnosis even to the experienced. It is in this context that the record of 50 knee-joint swellings (Blockey, 1976) is presented (Table 4) not only to illustrate the variety of diagnoses finally established and to which there is reference here and elsewhere in this text, but to the high proportion, virtually 50 per cent, in which no diagnosis was made but in which resolution occurred with the regime recommended below.

### TABLE 4

Diagnosis in 50 knee-joint swellings in children (Blockey, 1976)

| | |
|---|---|
| Haemarthrosis | 4 |
| Anaphylactoid purpura | 1 |
| Tuberculosis | 2 |
| Rheumatoid arthritis | 2 |
| Acute rheumatism | 3 |
| Septic arthritis (proven) | 11 |
| Acute osteomyelitis | 4 |
| Intra-articular fractures | 2 |
| No definite diagnosis | 21 |
| | 50 |

## 'SYNOVITIS': TREATMENT

### General Principles

The essential features of the treatment of acute synovitis from whatever cause involve one or other or all of the following:

**1. Splinting.** This includes *compression,* in the extended position.

**2. Aspiration.** If the volume of fluid is such as to prevent complete extension as above aspiration is required as a therapeutic measure.

**3. Rest.** The degree of rest required depends on the underlying pathology and varies between limited weight-bearing with the support of a compression bandage and bed-rest.

**4. Quadriceps exercises.** If rest from weight-bearing is usually necessary, rest from quadriceps exercises need seldom last beyond the acute phase or longer than four days.

### Compression Bandage: Jones Bandage

'Elastic pressure, to check bleeding or promote absorption without interfering with the general circulation of the limb, can be obtained by using large quantities of cotton wool, and is best done as follows: first swathe the part in wool and bandage firmly over this, taking care that the bandage is running in the right direction to maintain the desired position. Then apply more sheets of cotton wool and continue the bandaging rather tighter than the former. As the swelling goes down the bandages will become loose. Do not disturb the joint by removing the bandage, but keep up the pressure by an additional bandage over everything. This can be removed and reapplied as often as necessary without moving the joint or disturbing the position of the wool padding. The more wool is used the tighter can the bandage be applied without fear of doing harm or hurting the patient.'

This description (Sir Robert Jones, 1915) is more precise than might appear at first sight. In the current scene, as applied after meniscectomy, the most common post-operative situation in which compression is required, it consists of three layers of cotton wool, interposed between which are layers of non-stretchable 6 inch (15 cm) bandage, two of which 6 yards (6 metres) in length, are required. If the cotton wool must be compressible, the bandages must not be stretchable. If crêpe bandages are used intolerable pressures can be created.

Each compression bandage requires 1 lb (0·5 kg) of cotton wool of British Pharmaceutical Codex quality. The cotton wool is usually 12 inches (30 cm) wide and is cut into lengths of about 18 inches (45 cm). When unrolled the wool is compressed and requires to be 'fluffed'. This is achieved by placing the sheets on a radiator or in a heated cabinet. The pieces are then rolled loosely and packed for sterilisation.

The bandages are 6 inches (15 cm) wide and are of a cotton material known as 'domette'. It is possible, however, to use any cotton or linen bandage provided it is not stretchable.

ECONOMICS. The cost of the bandage in the current scene (1971) varies between 120p and 500p depending on whether it consists of hospital material at contract price or bought at retail price in a pharmacy. The economics of the situation is such as to demand research into methods and materials.

**Biomechanical basis of therapeutic action.** The bandage as originally described constitutes the most common and most useful instrument of treatment in swelling of the knee, soft tissue or synovial effusion, of whatever origin. In counteracting stasis it promotes absorption of effusion. In exerting elastic compression it reduces tension pain from stretched soft tissues. In providing physical support it reduces the feeling of weakness which accompanies synovial effusion. Wherein lies the variety of attributes? Is it pressure on the synovial membrane and/or on the soft tissues enveloping the capsule? The splinting effect on the injured joint, accidental traumatic, or operative? Is there some other explanation? Or is the beneficial effect multifactorial?

When the bandage is applied at the termination of operation and the tourniquet removed, the superficial veins in the leg below are visibly distended, as are those of the opposite limb if in lesser degree, presumably by reflex action. When the patient returns to a fracture-board bed and the end is elevated the distension disappears. The pressure exerted initially by the bandage as described is some 40 to 60 mm of mercury, and this rapidly falls off during the next 48 hours when pressure is reduced to 20 to 10 mm (Mills and Smillie, 1979).

It is not the author's practice to extend the compression bandage downwards to the roots of the toes. In theory this is desirable; but it appears that the pressure of the bandage at the knee is seldom so great or maintained for sufficiently long to be responsible for any considerable degree of oedema. In any event such a bandage is uncomfortably hot and prevents observation of the limb. Increase in oedema, accompanied by pain, suggests increase in intra-articular tension and directs attention to the possibility of complication in the form of haemarthrosis.

On the other hand there are occasions when simple oedema is of a degree which demands attention. Some swelling occurs after the use of a tourniquet partly from ischaemia incured by the tissues below the knee and possibly because an operation which is prolonged entails trauma to the soft tissues about the joint even if it is only from the pressure of retractors. If oedema of any considerable degree occurs after the application of a compression bandage, for whatever reason, a crêpe bandage should be applied from the roots of the toes up to the knee bandage; and at the junction between the two cotton wool should be inserted so that no band of tissue exists to which pressure has not been applied.

### Aspiration

The maximum capacity of the synovial cavity is in some, say, 15° of flexion. A flexion deformity is thus the invariable accompaniment of any considerable synovial effusion from any cause. The commonest single cause is trauma; but almost every disease process is accompanied by effusion and/or swelling of the synovial membrane which, in the posterior compartment in particular, has the same effect. Thus swelling of a degree which produces a tension situation and which is permitted to exist for any length of time is liable to produce a deformity which may not necessarily disappear when the original cause is eliminated.

The technique is described in Chapter 1.

### Quadriceps Exercises

**General considerations.** A patient with a painful knee from whatever cause will not in the normal course of events exercise it; rather the reverse! The purpose of non-weight-bearing exercise therapy therefore must be explained and the exercise demonstrated on the normal leg. It is insisted that the exercise is practised for a few minutes every hour, never beyond the point of fatigue, throughout the waking day. The single measure to be described is applicable at the first opportunity and immediately the acute phase has passed. The variety of exercises applicable at a later stage are documented in IKJ5 and, more fully, elsewhere.

STRAIGHT-LEG-RAISING. This is the simplest natural exercise which the quadriceps can perform. It has the widest possible application in the context of the disease processes in the knee. It has the important advantage that the patient is required to do no more than raise his own

leg from the bed, and is not asked to learn anything strange and new at a time when neuromuscular co-ordination is poor. It has the added advantage, not common to other forms of quadriceps exercise, that it can be assisted.

In the early stages of recovery and to initiate contraction it should be performed in the supine position so that rectus femoris, with its origin above the hip joint, can be utilised. The knee should be extended to the maximum possible before the leg is raised.

INHIBITED MUSCLE. There are circumstances of acute pain or recent injury, accidental traumatic or operative, when the patient cannot be persuaded to raise his leg from the bed or otherwise contract his quadriceps. A method, almost invariably successful in initiating contraction, is to disorientate the patient by turning to the prone position, fix the foot by digging the flexed toes into the mattress, and then to raise the knee from the bed.

LOADED STRAIGHT-LEG-RAISING. The popular idea that 'muscles flex best if they have something to pull against' has some basis in fact. The provision of slight resistance, manual or otherwise, may be necessary to initiate straight-leg-raising.

At a later stage of recovery from 'synovitis', operation or the application of a thigh length plaster cast, loading is achieved by the addition of weights, of a series ranging from 1 to 4 kg (2 to 9 lb), attached to an ankle and used progressively as the muscle shows evidence of improvement.

## IDIOPATHIC SYNOVITIS

### Management in Absence of Diagnosis

There are a considerable number of synovial effusions to which no cause can be assigned and no precise diagnosis established. It has been indicated elsewhere that when an immediate provisional clinical diagnosis cannot be achieved, the only test carried out is the simple, rapidly accomplished screening procedure of the ESR; and it is only if the reading is abnormally high that the matter is pursued further. It is not the practice to undertake further laboratory investigations without a lead in a particular direction.

If the ESR is normal and the effusion not excessive a compression bandage is applied and the patient taught simple non-weight-bearing quadriceps exercises which are thereafter performed for a few minutes in every hour. Walking short distances is permitted. Standing for any prolonged period is forbidden. If the effusion is large, aspiration, primarily therapeutic but of possible diagnostic value, is performed prior to exercise instruction.

This regime increases the volume of the quadriceps and eliminates the possibility of an effusion being maintained by quadriceps insufficiency and inadequate protection of the joint from the stresses and strains of everyday use.

**Never apply a plaster cast.** There are no circumstances in which an effusion of unknown origin is treated by immobilisation in a plaster cast. It has been indicated elsewhere that, in general, any form of immobilisation is undesirable. If there is a time when plaster immobilisation should never be used it is in the absence of diagnosis. If a cast is applied the synovial effusion, whether the result of trauma or other pathology, subsides. When the plaster is removed there are no relevant clinical features on which a diagnosis can be based. There is no history, other than that of a possible incident of trauma; and the joint cannot be examined in the absence of flexion which will have been eliminated by immobilisation. In such circumstances, a case, which may have been nothing more than a simple, if unrecognised, traumatic synovitis, becomes a major problem both of diagnosis and treatment. In the current scene there are few occasions where a knee joint must be enclosed in a plaster cast; and an effusion of unknown origin is not one of them.

The irreversible effect of prolonged immobilisation for no valid reason is illustrated in the following case:

The patient (Dr G.I., male, aged 29), at the age of 22 had an internal derangement of the right knee joint diagnosed as a tear of the medial meniscus. This was removed; and while the wound healed by first intention there was post-operative effusion. The effusion per-sisted and was treated by the application of a plaster cast which was retained for some six weeks. At the end of this time, and for reasons not defined, he was fitted with a weight-relieving walking caliper. This he used for one and a half years during which the knee was not moved. He recalled that when the caliper was removed considerable difficulty was encountered in securing a return of flexion.

The complaint was of pain, stiffness after standing in the same position for any length of time or after sitting. Examination showed loss of complete extension and loss of flexion amounting to not more that 10°. The salient feature was the loss of mobility of the patella.

The radiographs showed degenerative changes in the patello-femoral joint related to subchondral bone with loss of joint space. There was decalcification, abnormal trabeculation and evidence in the subchondral bone of overlying degenerative changes in the articular cartilage throughout the tibio-femoral joint.

The treatment prescribed was passive stretching to improve extension, knee flexion exercises and passive mobilisation of the patella.

At the end of six months the mobility of the patella had increased and improvement in extension was evident. He had regained almost full flexion. Improvement in function was freely admitted. He complained still of pain after standing in one position for any length of time and after sitting. The pain, as before, was located to the patello-femoral joint.

This case illustrates the breaking of the rules: (1) the knee joint should never be immobilised in a plaster cast on the basis of effusion without a positive clinical diagnosis and one in which immobilisation is the treatment of choice; (2) the immobilisation of a normal knee joint, for a matter of two years cannot other than be followed by degenerative changes in the articular cartilage; and the longer the period of immobilisation the greater the changes. In this case the degenerative changes involved the entire joint but, in particular, in so far as the immediate symptoms were concerned, the patello-femoral joint. Such changes in a man of this age cannot be other than progressive.

In this example, however, exercise therapy, maintained on a permanent basis, can maintain function if a certain degree of pain is accepted. If, with the passage of time, pain becomes intolerable, it is difficult to know what steps to take for alleviation other than arthrodesis if it is only for the reason that the entire joint, tibio-femoral and patello-femoral, is involved in the degenerative pathology.

**Spontaneous recovery.** It is surprising how many cases resolve with the regime described without the clinician knowing either the reason for the original effusion or the reason why it should subside. It is probable that a high proportion of those in the middle-age range which undergo spontaneous resolution without residual synovial thickening have a simple explanation and are examples of local endogenous mechanical trauma of synovial membrane. In any event, the possible causes of effusion are so many that there is no justification for undergoing every possible investigation which might reveal the cause, but which might, in the end, be of little more than academic interest. Even a synovial biopsy may be reported 'non-specific synovitis'.

It is important, however, that an idiopathic synovitis is not permitted to continue indefinitely. These cases must be reviewed at monthly intervals and further investigations undertaken as indicated.

### Treatment in the Absence of Recovery

It must be admitted that there exists a chronic synovitis in which every reasonable investigation fails to establish a cause but which proceeds to destruction of articular cargilage as in rheumatoid arthritis with irreparable damage to the joint. On the other hand it is common experience that idiopathic synovitis of considerable duration, but not perhaps meriting the label 'chronic', sometimes resolves without treatment and for no apparent reason. Such is our knowledge of the subject in the current scene. There remains the problem of treatment in the circumstances of failure to establish a diagnosis in a situation which must be accepted as 'chronic'. The point at issue, as in rheumatoid arthritis, is the destruction of articular cartilage; and at what point to interfere before changes are irreversible. In this respect some arbitrary time must be selected at which it is decided that resolution will not occur and synovectomy is necessary. It is a decision of considerable difficulty in the absence of a clear-cut diagnosis. It must depend on the judgement of the surgeon in respect of the advance of pathology to the destruction of articular cartilage. Perhaps a year is not an unreasonable time to keep the patient under observation in the hope of improvement.

**Synovectomy.** If synovectomy is contemplated it is important, as in rheumatoid arthritis, that the patient has not only been taught and understands the importance of quadriceps and knee flexion exercises but has already attained the maximum possible extension and flexion. It is for this reason that any surgical interference with the joint necessitating immobilisation, and in particular biopsy, is undesirable, immediately preceding a proposed synovectomy.

The attitude to be adopted, if biopsy is thought to be necessary in the unhappy circumstances of an unknown diagnosis, is to seek the permission of the patient to proceed to synovectomy if, at the biopsy operation, it is clear on inspection that the pathology and condition of the joint is such that the process is likely to be irreversible and eventual synovectomy inevitable. This policy has been pursued on a number of occasions and never with regret.

The following are two examples of so-called idiopathic non-specific synovitis which eventually came to synovectomy:

The patient (Mrs E.S., aged 45) gave a history that she first suffered trouble with her right knee about two and a half years previously, when she sustained a twisting injury while riding a bicycle. At that time there was pain in the joint with considerable swelling. She was treated by her own doctor who applied a pressure bandage and advised her to rest. This measure had some success and within two weeks she was back at work. Approximately four weeks later she again suffered a twist injury to the knee which caused a further exacerbation again with considerable pain and swelling. From this point onwards her knee became increasingly troublesome. Her main symptom was pain which became worse on resting and improved with exercise. The pain was dull aching in type and was present throughout the day. In addition there was considerable swelling of the joint. She maintained that the joint never locked nor did it give way on any occasion. She suffered her symptoms for approximately two years before she was referred to hospital. At that time her symptoms were minimal. The salient feature was a large swelling of the knee (Fig. 3,17).

The outcome of investigations undertaken as an outpatient were: ESR 65 in the first hour.

R.A. Latex was negative.

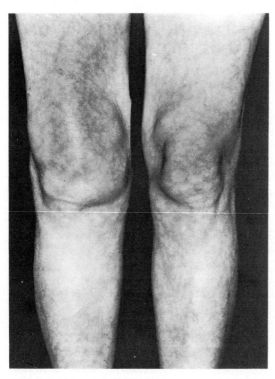

Fig. 3,17. **Idiopathic synovitis.** This synovial effusion and thickening persisted for three years without the cause ever being found. She was eventually subjected to synovectomy by which time considerable damage had occurred to the articular cartilage. A Telflon sheet was inserted at operation. She regained more than a right-angle flexion. The Teflon sheet remains *in situ*. She never returned to have it removed (Mrs E.S., aged 45).

Aspirated fluid was sterile both to ordinary culture and for tubercle.

The ASO titre of 100, haemoglobin 94 per cent and the white cell count 6,700.

Three months later in the absence of improvement she was admitted to hospital for investigation. There was no new clinical findings other than a swollen knee with flexion limited to 45 degrees.

Laboratory investigations showed:

R.A. Latex was very weakly re-active.

ESR 27 in the first hour.

Haemoglobin was 91 per cent.

Radiographs of the knee revealed osteoporosis only.

Exploration biopsy was advised but declined and she was discharged to her home.

Six months later she returned. The condition of the knee was more or less the same. If anything the swelling had become greater.

**Systematic review.** The family history was unremarkable. Parents and one brother alive and well. No history of tuberculosis or rheumatoid arthritis in the family or in close contacts. Her own past medical history was unremarkable. Her weight was steady. Symptoms of renal disease were absent. She had no symptoms suggestive of cardiovascular disease. She did not suffer from any chest complaint. In all her general health seemed to be good and there were no indications of systemic pathology. She had no history of any trouble with other joints. Her occupation was domestic work on a farm. To the best of her knowledge she had no contact with brucellosis.

On examination she was found to be a thin but healthy-looking patient with a tendency to over-excitability. No abnormal findings were discovered in either cardiovascular, respiratory, alimentary or central nervous systems.

**Lymph nodes.** She was noted to have an enlarged gland in the right inguinal region. A deep inguinal adenectomy was advised and accepted. The gland was examined for tubercle and other pathology and found to be negative.

Laboratory investigations were repeated:

Haemoglobin was 82 per cent.

ESR was 38 in the first hour.

White cell count 7200 with a normal differential.

Serum uric acid was 2·5 mg per cent.

R.A. Latex and Rose Waller tests negative.

Mantoux 1 to 10 thousand was strongly reactive with a 1½ inch (3·8 cm diameter zone of erythema and considerable weal formation over an area approximately ½ inch (0·64 cm) in the centre.

Urine culture: 100 000 colonies per ml enterococci.

TB culture of urine and sputum negative.

Repeat radiographs of the right knee show some general osteoporosis but intact articular surfaces.

Synovial biopsy was again recommended. Permission was sought to proceed to synovectomy if the pathology appeared aggressive and destruction of the articular surfaces was occurring. By this time she realised that the recovery was not to take place by natural means. The recommendation was accepted.

**Operation.** The procedure began with a short 5 cm lateral parapatellar incision for the purpose of inspecting the synovial membrane and, if the pathology appeared innocent, limiting the procedure to biopsy. On opening the suprapatellar pouch, however, the synovial membrane was pale and markedly thickened. There was a large quantity of straw coloured synovial fluid with fibrin clots. There was damage to the articular surface of the femoral condyles. It was, however, not advancing from the periphery but involving the central areas. The articular cartilage of the patella was eroded. In this bone, however, the pathology, whatever it was, was advancing from the periphery. The central part of the patella was relatively normal. It was decided in these circumstances, and in view of the length of the history, to proceed with synovectomy. The synovial membrane about the cruciate ligaments was markedly affected. In view of the fact that the patient was a female and most anxious to retain flexion an interposition membrane of Teflon was introduced in the manner described (Ch. 6).

It was noted at the termination of the operation that there was considerable laxity of the quadriceps apparatus due to the stretching which had occurred as a result of the size of the effusion and the synovial thickening.

At manipulation under general anaesthesia 10 days later right-angled flexion was attained with finger pressure only. Convalescence was uneventful. This patient was last seen six months later. She had attained 110° of flexion and had no extension lag. There was slight synovial thickening with a minimal effusion. There was no pain.

It was recommended that she should be admitted to hospital for removal of the Teflon. Arrangements have been made on three occasions for her admission. She has never appeared and has offered no explanation. She is known to be doing full-time domestic work. The Teflon thus remains within the joint.

The pathological report on the synovial membrane was not helpful in solving the mystery of the origin of the condition: It stated 'non-specific synovitis'.

The second (T.D., male, aged 34), a head waiter, gave a history that 10 years previously he had received a minor injury to the knee which settled rapidly. Six months later, however, he developed an effusion and was investigated in hospital where the knee was aspirated and various unspecified investigations, but including synovial biopsy, were undertaken. Apparently it was decided that the condition had an infective background and he was treated with an antibiotic, said to have been terramycin, but with no response. The effusion is said to have subsided in the natural course of events.

It had, however, recurred from time to time. In his job as a waiter he had worked in various cities throughout England and Scotland and visited many hospitals where various investigations, the nature of which he did not know, were undertaken. No firm diagnosis had ever been made and the various forms of treatment he had received had not made any material difference.

Initially he was investigated as an out-patient:

The ESR was 3 in the first hour.

R.A. Latex test was negative.

GCFT was negative.

Serum uric acid was 6 mg per cent.

Serum agglutinans for salmonella, streptococcus and staphylococcus were all negative.

A guinea pig was inoculated for tuberculosis. At 8 weeks the animal was healthy.

A radiograph of the chest was negative. Those of the knee showed slight osteoporosis.

No action was taken other than to inform him that every investigation had proved negative, a situation with which he had now grown familiar. He returned three months later stating that he had reached a stage where he was having difficulty holding down his job; something would require to be done.

He was informed that the only procedure that might help was a synovectomy. He was warned, however, that synovectomy might result in some loss of range of motion. His reply to this was that if he lost any considerable range he would be unable to walk without a limp and thus to hold down his job as a waiter. He was informed that the use of an inter-position membrane at operation would almost certainly result in a least right-angled flexion. He agreed that synovectomy should be under-taken.

At operation, performed through a lateral parapatellar incision, a subacute hyperplastic synovium was removed as completely as possible. Adhesions were encountered only at the site of the previous biopsy. There was erosion of articular cartilage but the actual encroachment was minimal. A Teflon sheet was interposed in the suprapatellar pouch and over the sides of the femoral condyles. It was attached and located by a single staple as described in Chapter 6.

The wound healed by first intention. On the tenth day manipulation under anaesthesia produced 100° of flexion with no more than finger pressure. He was discharged from hospital six weeks after operation with active flexion of 70° and full extension.

Two months later he was readmitted for removal of the Teflon sheet. At this time he had attained 120° of flexion. At operation there was minimal fluid in the joint and the regenerated synovial surfaces were of normal appearance and conveyed a favourable visual impression as opposed to the appearance at synovectomy. A small area was removed for pathological examination.

Removal of the Teflon sheet produced a considerable loss of flexion in the post-operative period. When he was discharged three weeks later he had full extension but had regained only 60° of flexion.

This patient was last reviewed six months later when back at work without pain in the knee and with minimal effusion. He had attained 95° of flexion. There was no thicken-ing of the synovial membrane of the supra-patellar pouch. He was satisfied with the result.

The patient has been sent for on two occasions at six monthly intervals but has never appeared and has been lost to follow-up. His occupation, it is repeated, is that of a waiter. It is not known whether he has moved to another city or whether he has not reappeared for examination merely because his knee is no longer giving trouble. He had become some-what cynical about the inability of doctors to diagnose his condition. He was aware that the medical interest in him was academic.

The reports of the synovial membrane both at the original synovectomy and removal of the interposition membrane were not helpful. They were described as 'chronic synovitis' and one report stated 'there was sufficient evidence to justify the diagnosis of rheumatoid arthritis'.

This is another case of non-specific idio-pathic synovitis the cause of which was never known. The most likely diagnosis seemed to be an infective arthritis modified by the original terramycin treatment, or possibly, monoarticular rheumatoid arthritis. The naked eye appearance of the synovial mem-brane at operation, however, was not that of rheumatoid arthritis. It was more like that seen in the so-called burnt-out stage.

## SYNOVIAL CHONDROMATOSIS (OSTEOCHONDROMATOSIS)

**Incidence.** The condition is uncommon. The knee is the joint most commonly affected; the bursae about the knee, gastrocnemio-semi-membranosus (Figs 4,14 and 4,15) and pre-patellar (Fig. 4,19), less frequently.

**Pathological anatomy.** Synovial chondromatosis arises as a result of metaplasia in the synovial and subsynovial connective tissue. It is regarded as a usually benign but progressive condition

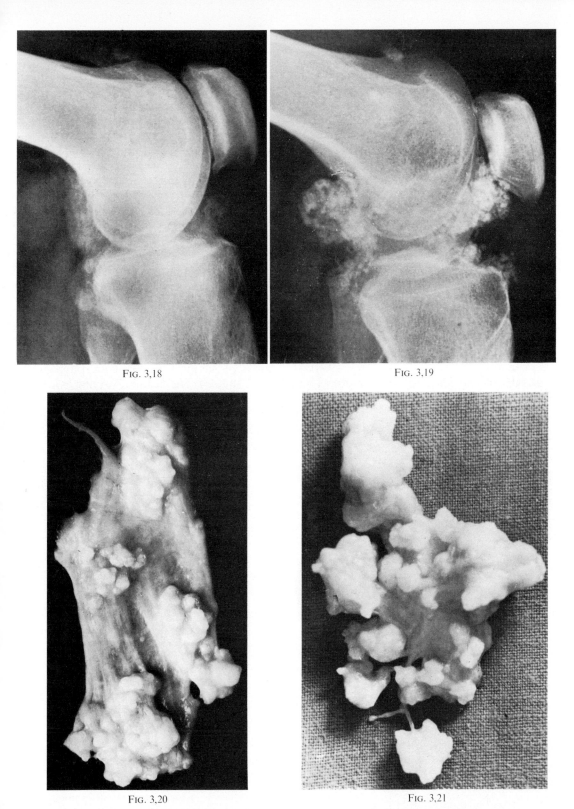

FIG. 3,18

FIG. 3,19

FIG. 3,20

FIG. 3,21

FIGS 3,18–21. **Synovial osteochondromatosis.** The radiological features vary widely (Figs 3,18 and 3,19). But note evidence of osteoarthrosis of patello-femoral joint in both examples. Appearance of masses in synovial membrane from case treated by synovectomy (Fig. 3,20). Specimen from another example to show pedunculated mass with an adjacent peduncle from which the loose body has recently separated (Fig. 3,21).

with a natural tendency to resolution, the origin and natural history of which is not understood. On exploration, an area of synovial membrane, or that of the entire joint including the suprapatellar pouch and posterior compartment, is studded by small firm raised nodules of cartilage (Fig. 3,20). These nodules may undergo calcification and/or ossification, tend to become pedunculated and to separate into the joint as loose bodies even to the extent of some hundreds (Fig. 3,21). If the condition is regarded as innocent it will be clear that pedunculated masses of cartilage and innumerable loose bodies, short of resolution or surgical intervention, inevitably produce mechanical damage to the joint surfaces and an eventual generalised osteoarthrosis (Figs 3,18; 3,19; 3,22 and 3,23).

COMPLICATIONS. Malignant change to chondrosarcoma has been reported (Mullins, Berard and Eisenberg, 1965) but is said to be very rare (Goldman and Lichtenstein, 1964).

**Clinical features.** There are no symptoms and signs specific to synovial chondromatosis. The presenting complaint is likely to be pain, progressive in effect and of long standing, accompanied by swelling, stiffness and possibly locking incidents. On examination there is limitation of movement.

In a limited personal experience mechanical loss of extension has been produced by swelling of the suprapatellar pouch, cartilagenous masses in the anterior compartment and the interposition of loose bodies between the joint surfaces. Flexion is limited for similar reasons and may be accompanied by crepitus. In some cases the loose bodies are palpable and their presence known to the patient. In others of spare build the irregular, firm nodular mass in the suprapatellar pouch can make the diagnosis evident.

**Radiological features.** Whether the condition is detectable radiologically depends on whether calcification or ossification has produced a radio-opaque medium. The typical appearance is of stippled calcification varying widely in form in and around the joint (Figs 3,18; 3,19;

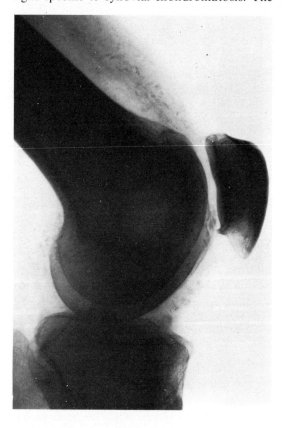

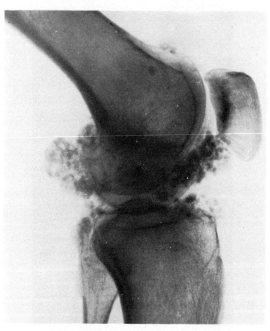

FIGS 3,22–23. **Synovial osteochondromatosis.** The radiological features vary between the imperceptible, even with a dense soft-tissue exposure (Fig. 3,22), and the unmistakable (Fig. 3,23).

Note evidence of patello-femoral osteoarthrosis in both examples.

3,22 and 3,23). The presence of loose bodies in the absence of periarticular calcification is not diagnostic but more than two loose bodies in osteochondritis dissecans is unusual.

**Arthroscopy.** The condition is capable of positive diagnosis by arthroscopy by an orthopaedic surgeon familiar with the characteristic appearance of the synovial membrane.

### Management

The treatment to be adopted depends on the circumstances of the case and thus varies between simple removal of loose bodies, local synovectomy and total anterior synovectomy in the knowledge that the last measure entails the risk of limitation of movement in the final result. That spontaneous regression may occur after subtotal synovectomy or even removal of loose bodies in the knowledge that gross pathological changes exist in the posterior compartment casts doubts on the necessity for synovectomy. The opinion has been expressed that simple removal of loose bodies with the purpose of reducing mechanical damage to the articular surfaces is adequate (Jeffreys, 1967). In the absence of any considerable experience or long term follow-up the treatment of choice has not been determined.

It is of interest to speculate as to the mechanism concerned with the retrogression said to occur following any operative intervention. The known anticomplementary relationship of cartilage to vascularity would suggest that any procedure producing hyperaemia of synovial membrane and/or haemarthrosis might initiate the means whereby abnormal articular cartilage in particular is destroyed. It is a possible means of treatment worthy of pursuit.

### HAEMANGIOMA OF SYNOVIAL MEMBRANE

**Incidence.** The condition is rare. The knee is the commonest joint affected. In reviewing 82 published cases of synovial haemangioma to date, Halborg, Hansen and Sneppen (1968) noted that 80 of them affected the knee joint.

### Pathological Anatomy

There are two types: (1) *diffuse,* (2) *localised,* which differ in pathological anatomy, clinical features and prognosis.

**Diffuse.** The diffuse tumour produces symptoms in the form of swelling, and symptoms of pain from incidents of haemorrhage or thrombosis. They may be a source of stimulation to epiphyses and thus produce overgrowth of the limb. Complete irradiation is difficult if not impossible by orthodox surgical measures.

**Localised.** On the other hand the localised form, particularly when pedunculated, produces mechanical interference with joint function and symptoms of an internal derangement of the knee. When the diagnosis is established, a matter of some difficulty, excision is followed by complete recovery.

MICROSCOPIC FEATURES. Histologically there are four categories (Stout, 1953): (1) capillary; (2) cavernous; (3) mixed cavernous and capillary, and (4) venous.

In the capillary form the vessels grow in a haphazard fashion. If the capillary spaces become widely dilated but still retain the simple capillary wall, the tumour is called a cavernous haemangioma. If the vessels have relatively thick walls and contain smooth muscle cells the tumour is termed a venous haemangioma. Most cases are of the mixed cavernous and capillary types.

A constant feature of histological examination is the presence of thrombosis in various stages of organisation; and these sites presumably correspond to the incidents of pain and swelling which are the salient feature of the clinical features of the diffuse type.

There is no correlation between the histological features, the clinical findings or prognosis.

### Clinical Features: Diffuse Variety

**Age.** The condition is essentially one of youth in as far as the diffuse variety is concerned; but it is rare, and whereas symptoms may arise in early childhood, years may pass in the absence of expert opinion before the correct diagnosis is established. (See example recorded below.)

**Pain.** The history is essentially one of episodes of pain and swelling not necessarily preceded by trauma.

**Swelling.** In the diffuse variety the swelling increases in some degree during episodes of haemorrhage or thrombosis. Resolution to the previous degree of abnormality without treatment is the usual course of events.

A feature of the swelling, almost pathognomonic, is that it is distensible, compressible, and may be made to decrease in size by elevation of the limb.

**Palpation.** The swelling is doughy in character and tenderness to compression varies between vague and exquisite, the latter sensation related to an episode of haemorrhage or thrombosis. A feature of palpation in the diffuse variety is increase in local temperature in the absence of any other sign of an inflammatory process.

**Haemangioma of skin.** A capillary haemangioma of naevus of the skin over the knee and varying from the localised of, say, 1 cm diameter to the widespread (Figs 3,24 and 3,25) has been a feature of cases encountered by the author and when present is almost pathognomonic.

**Overgrowth of limb.** A discrepancy in the length of the leg in the form of overgrowth is a common finding in the diffuse variety.

ARTHROSCOPY. This is a condition in the current scene incurring difficulty of diagnosis which, in inexperienced hands, might be subjected to arthroscopy; and with considerable risk of haemorrhage making visualisation difficult or impossible. In gross appearance, pigmented villonodular synovitis would require to be considered in the differential diagnosis.

**Diagnosis.** Haemangioma is rare and as a result the typical, or relatively typical, features of the diffuse variety are not commonly recognised at an initial examination except by clinicians with previous experience of the condition. In gross appearance haemangioma *in situ* appears as a dark grape-like mass underneath a shining synovial covering (Fig. 3,26).

## Clinical Features: Localised Variety

There are no clear-cut clinical features in the localised variety. It is a post-operative diagnosis (Fig. 3,26). The clinical features are those of a mysterious internal derangement producing symptoms of mechanical interference with joint motion. In particular there is a firm tender swelling which appears without reason from time to time in a situation limited by the length of the pedicle. The pre-operative diagnosis in

the author's experience has varied between cystic degeneration of a meniscus, a torn meniscus with a mobile flap presenting at the periphery and a cartilagenous loose body within a synovial pouch. The pre-operative diagnosis is of academic interest and not important if it is only for the reason that the condition simulated demands operative action and with an equally favourable prognosis.

### TREATMENT

**Diffuse variety.** The condition is rare and experience of treatment is limited. In general the outcome of surgical excision, in what amounts to a limited synovectomy, is unsatisfactory in so far as total excision is impossible and recurrence the common experience. If the condition is limited so that total excision is possible, as in the local variety, recurrence is most unlikely.

The following are examples:

1. The mother of the patient (C.S., female, age 6) gave a history that when she was born a mark was noted on the right knee approximately 1 cm in diameter; but nothing thought of it at the time. There was no abnormality of appearance or function until at the age of 3 when at a nursery school she was thought to have received a knock on the knee; and at that time the joint was swollen and the child unable to walk for a matter of one week. The reason for failure to walk was pain as well as swelling. At that time a radiograph was taken. The diagnosis made was that of a traumatic synovitis. Six months later a similar incident occurred and she was again brought to hospital. On this occasion she saw an orthopaedic surgeon; and it was at this time that the diagnosis was achieved. In the past two years there have been two incidences in which there has been transient incidents of swelling and pain.

The salient feature of examination was the diffuse vascular abnormality in the form of a capillary naevus involving the skin and spread diffusely over the knee in general. The mother said that the naevus had grown in size of recent years and in her opinion was continuing to grow. There existed a vague swelling of the joint particularly of the suprapatellar

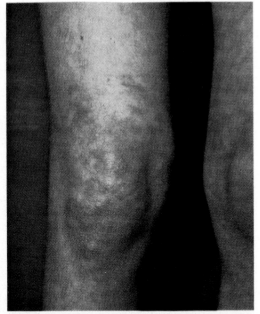

FIG. 3,24

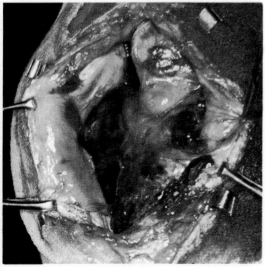

FIG. 3,26

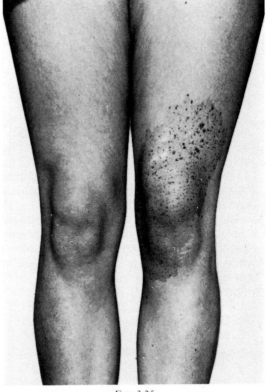

FIG. 3,25

FIGS 3,24–26. **Haemangioma of synovial membrane.** It is not uncommon for diffuse haemangioma to be accompanied by cutaneous haemangioma. In this example the knee will be seen to be swollen. The photograph was taken immediately after an incident of haemorrhage. The swelling subsided in two weeks (Fig. 3,24). (C.S., female, aged 8.)

Extensive cutaneous lesion overlying a diffuse haemangioma. This one is stated to have been little more than a naevus at birth and to have achieved this size on maturity (Fig. 3,25). (E.C., female, aged 23); see text.

In this localised example the haemangioma was situated in the suprapatellar pouch and was extirpated by limited synovectomy (Fig. 3,26). (M.McL., female, case of C.S.C.)

pouch with a distinct increase in local temperature by comparison with the normal side. Wasting of the quadriceps was marked. There was no discrepancy between the lengths of the two limbs.

The case was clearly one of the diffuse variety of haemangioma of the synovial membrane. In view of the questionable out-come of operation it was decided to keep the child under observation; and the reason explained to the mother (Fig. 3,24).

2. The patient, a woman of Turkish nationality aged 25 years, complained of a soft swelling in the suprapatellar pouch which had been present since childhood. From time to time over the last few years the swelling had

G

become much larger and painful. On each occasion various forms of physiotherapy resulted in the firm painful lump disappearing but some swelling always remained. On examination there was a soft flat swelling in the anterior aspect of the suprapatellar pouch. On the skin overlying the pouch was a small bright red naevus about 1 cm square. The quadriceps was markedly wasted. There was no other clinical abnormality. The swelling did not become appreciably larger when she stood upright.

The diagnosis was clearly one of a diffuse haemangioma and the recurrent incidents explained by haemorrhages.

In this example the haemangioma on clinical grounds gave the impression of being less diffuse than that affecting the joint of the child referred to above. The case was seen in consultation as a problem of diagnosis; and, indeed, the possibility of haemangioma had not been considered. It was recommended that the extent of the pathology might be determined by arthroscopy; but, only at the hands of an orthopaedic surgeon experienced in its use and familiar with the appearance of haemangioma. The purpose of arthroscopy was not so much to achieve a diagnosis, which seemed obvious, as to determine the extent of the pathology with a view to the possible elimination by partial synovectomy. The outcome is unknown.

3. The patient (Mrs E.C., aged 23) was first seen at the age of 18, at the beginning of her training as a nurse, when she stated that at the end of the day's work her knee was markedly painful and swollen. The outstanding feature on examination was a swelling of the suprapatellar pouch and a very large pigmented area of the skin (Fig. 3,25). On taking her history it transpired that the pigmented area had been present at birth but was then extremely small and had grown steadily as she grew to reach its present dimensions. There was only one incident in the past. At the age of 16 she had received a blow on the knee and this had caused a large swelling which had taken some weeks to subside. She volunteered the information that the swelling was greatest when standing. At the end of the day when the knee was swollen there was a deep boring ache in the joint. The pain disappeared when she lay down but the swelling remained.

A confident diagnosis of a diffuse haemangioma was made. It seemed so diffuse however that operation was contraindicated. The advice offered was that the situation should be kept under review.

She was not seen again until the age of 23 by which time she had become a State Registered Nurse. She had married and had given up active nursing for a more sedentary occupation. She said that throughout her training she had had trouble with the knee. At the end of a very busy day the swelling was sometimes 'like a melon'. Since abandoning nursing and a standing physical occupation her knee had not troubled her. She thought that the reduction of her weight by 2 stones (23·70 kg) had contributed. Finally, she volunteered the observation that if she attended a cocktail party and drank alcohol, say two or three drinks, the knee swelled and became painful.

The outstanding feature of examination was, as before, the cutaneous haemangioma (Fig. 2,25). There was swelling which outlined the suprapatellar pouch. There was obliteration of the normal contours about the region of the joint line. On palpation the margins of the femoral condyles were comparable with the normal side. There was no clinical evidence of osteoarthrosis.

Radiographs of both knees to determine whether there was decalcification as a result of the abnormal blood supply or evidence of osteoarthrosis were comparable and showed no abnormality.

This case illustrates: (1) the effect of weight-bearing activity on a diffuse haemangioma; and that the patient may require to be restricted in this regard; (2) that it is possible to live with a diffuse haemangioma. In this particular case no deterioration, clinically or radiologically, occurred in the five years in which she was under supervision; and (3) the possible effect of alcohol. This is an interesting observation and might be related to the dilation of peripheral vessels. On the other hand the circumstances in which alcohol was consumed entailed standing for an excessive period of time. It was suggested that the matter might be one for investigation. It would be of some clinical interest if the reason for the swelling could be established with certainty.

# PIGMENTED VILLONODULAR SYNOVITIS

**Definition.** The term pigmented villonodular synovitis was introduced by Jaffe, Lichtenstein and Sutro (1941) to describe a condition of unknown aetiology in which the synovial membrane of a joint is the subject of local or diffuse thickening varying in colour with the content of iron pigment from bright red (Figs 3,27 and 3,29) to brown or yellow. The salient feature of microscopic examination is the marked proliferation of surface cells and of connective tissue together with an extraordinary accumulation of intra cellular and extracellular haemosiderin and lipoid materal associated with an abundance of reticulo-endothelial cells and giant cells.

**Background note.** The condition affects the tendon sheaths of the fingers and the synovial lining of the major joints of which the knee is by far the most important (Byers *et al.,* 1968). It occurs in two forms. The *circumscribed,* nodular or pedunculated was first described by Chassaignac (1852) in the flexor tendon sheaths of the fingers. The same form was first described in the knee by Simon (1865). The early writers

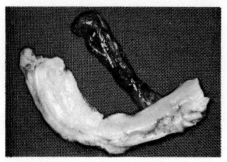

FIG. 3,27. **Pigmented villonodular synovitis: circumscribed form.** This example, which arose on the periphery of the meniscus, from time to time passed under the meniscus to be responsible for incidents of locking and transient effusions.

considered the lesions to be sarcomata. Dowd (1912), who first described the *diffuse* form in the knee, was also the first to question the malignant nature of the lesion. It is now known that it is not malignant. But the true nature of the disease process remains in dispute. Most modern writers favour an inflammatory process. The aetiology is still unknown.

**Clinical significance.** The condition, relatively rare, is, as it affects the knee, a chronic affection of young and middle-aged adults. The diffuse form presents considerable problems of diagnosis. The radiological evidence of bone involvement in particular can mislead the unwary: tuberculosis or malignant synovioma is suspected. It is most important that the benign nature of the pathology is recognised.

## Clinical Features

The condition occurs, as has been indicated, in two distinct forms:

**Circumscribed.** This variety gives rise to internal derangements of mechanical origin in the form of locking or giving-way incidents due to interference with movement. There is frequently a small local swelling the presence of which may be known to the patient. The location of the swelling, if pedunculated, is not necessarily constant nor is it always present (Fig. 3,27). It may be the cause of transient effusions of mysterious origin which result from the trauma to synovial membrane inflicted in trapping incidents. A precise diagnosis is seldom made. The nature of the lesion is discovered at an operation for the relief of the condition it simulates.

DIFFERENTIAL DIAGNOSIS FROM:
*Internal derangements* relative to the menisci.
*Cystic degeneration* of the meniscus presenting on the joint line.
*Radiotranslucent loose bodies* of cartilagenous origin.
*Gastrocnemio-semimembranosus bursa* when presenting in popliteal space. But it cannot be transilluminated.
*Fat pad lesions.*
*Tumours,* in particular, synovioma.

**Diffuse.** The patient presents with widespread synovial thickening. The swelling may be voluminous. The largest and most extensive enlargement of the synovial cavity of the knee ever

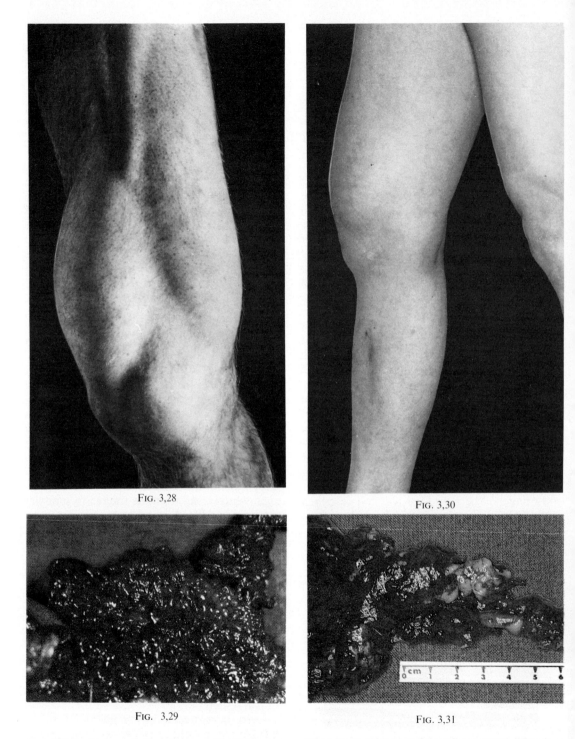

FIG. 3,28

FIG. 3,30

FIG. 3,29

FIG. 3,31

FIGS 3,28–29. **Pigmented villonodular synovitis: diffuse form.**
This is the largest synovial swelling ever encountered. It
had extended under vastus medialis and lateralis far up the
thigh (Fig. 3,28). Appearance of material removed at
anterior synovectomy. The enormous volume of tissue is
not indicated in the absence of scale (Fig. 3,29) (J.M.,
male, aged 24).

FIGS 3,30–31. **Pigmented villonodular synovitis: diffuse form.**
The large synovial swelling mostly related to the suprapatellar pouch had existed for two years when this photograph was taken (Fig. 3,30). The diseased tissue varies
considerably in colour and appearance (Fig. 3,31). Compare
with Figure 3,29 (J.C., male, aged 33).

encountered by the author (Fig. 3,28), a record of which is included below, was of this origin. Pain is not a prominent feature of the clinical picture; and thus patients may not present themselves for two or more years after the onset. The sensation of stiffness may be experienced. Tenderness to palpation is not a feature of examination. Flexion may be limited by the swelling in the suprapatellar pouch. Increase in local temperature may be present and presumed to be due to the vascular nature of the tissue involved and the proximity to the surface.

DIFFERENTIAL DIAGNOSIS FROM:
*Rheumatoid arthitis.* But villonodular synovitis is monoarticular and tests indicating systemic involvement are negative (see below).

*Tuberculosis* does not present in this form at this stage but must always be considered in view of radiological changes. The possibility is capable of elimination in course of investigation.

Tests indicating systemic involvement are negative in villonodular synovitis.

*Idiopathic synovitis* presents a major difficulty in view of absence of systemic reaction; but bloodstained aspirated fluid may provide a hint.

*Haemangioma.* The diffuse variety could give rise to difficulty; but the size of the swelling is related to posture.

*Soft tissue tumours* in particular, synovioma.

*Bone tumours* in particular, giant-cell tumour and aneurysmal bone cyst (see below).

**Laboratory investigations.** The aspiration of bloodstained fluid from a joint the subject of synovial thickening of long duration is suggestive. The sedimentation rate, white count and haemoglobin are all normal. The Rose Waller test for rheumatoid arthritis undertaken in the course of differential diagnosis, is negative.

**Radiological findings.** Radiological changes are unusual (15 per cent of 126 cases at all sites: Byers *et al., 1968*). The changes, however, are important as a source of difficulty in diagnosis or, alternatively, provide confirmation. They consist of single or multiple intraosseous cysts each delineated by a faint line of sclerosis. The surrounding bone is of normal density and the joint space preserved (Scott, 1968). The intracondylar area of the tibia and femur are the usual sites of the cysts.

It is believed that invasion of bone takes place

through the vascular foramina underlying the diseased synovium. Villonodular tissue grows into these foramina alongside nutrient vessels, carrying with it its own blood supply. It expands the foramina and, following the path of least resistance along the course of the osseous vessels, may pass deeply into bone where its growth produces intraosseous cysts by a process of pressure atrophy. No blood supply is obtained from the intraosseous vessels. For growth and survival the villonodular tissue in bone is dependent upon its own blood supply (Scott, 1968). Very occasionally the cystic lesion may be of such appearance and dimensions as to simulate conditions like benign giant-cell tumour and aneurysmal bone cyst from which histiological diagnosis is essential if unnecessarily radial surgery is to be avoided (Jergensen, Mankin and Schiller, 1978).

**Diagnosis.** The fundamental requirement in achieving the correct diagnosis in the diffuse form of pigmented villonodular synovitis is to be aware of the existence and nature of the lesion.

## Treatment

**Circumscribed.** It has been indicated that the diagnosis in this variety is rarely made from the exploratory operation or for relief of the internal derangement it simulates. The pedunculated variety will be excised with part of the structure to which it is attached. In the example illustrated (Fig. 3,27) the meniscus had been mobilised before the nature of the swelling became apparent and thus the entire fibrocartilage had to be removed. In the circumscribed variety it is important that the probable nature of the pathology be recognised. Recurrence is reported (Byers *et al.,* 1968). They are probably due to failure to excise a sufficient margin of synovial membrane around the nodule, or failure to recognise, in a limited exposure that there are other lesions present.

PROGNOSIS. The author knows of no recurrence in his experience limited to four examples of the pedunculated variety in which excision can reasonably be expected to be complete. When it occurs, which is unusual, it is probably due to failure to complete excision in the first instance.

**Diffuse.** The treatment is as complete a

synovectomy as the condition dictates and circumstances permit.

PROGNOSIS. The outcome of operation is less good in the diffuse variety. Recurrence is common and may be related to the advanced nature of the lesion at operation and the virtual impossibility of performing a complete synovectomy in the knee joint. In any event there may be serious loss of flexion such as associated with synovectomy (see below); or a painful progressive arthritis. Two of the author's cases are known to have terminated in arthrodesis for the latter reason; and others are reported (Byers *et al.*, 1968). It is important to recognise in spite of the liability to recurrence that the condition is not malignant. The same writers report two above knee amputations based on an erroneous histological diagnosis of sarcoma.

Two contrasting cases are reported. The first, to which reference is made in the text, with a favourable outcome. The second with evident recurrence.

1. The patient (J.M., male, age 24) a tractor driver, presented with a swelling of enormous dimensions of one year's duration, involving the left knee and thigh (Fig. 3,28). He said he first noticed a swelling in the popliteal space a year ago when he twisted his knee. Since that time swelling of the knee and thigh had gradually increased in size. One week previous to admission he had twisted the joint on rising from the sitting position. At that time he suffered sudden pain in the posterior aspect of the joint; and the entire leg had become swollen. This was the reason for his seeking advice. On examination the swelling was of massive size and extensive dimensions, the largest ever encountered. It involved the suprapatellar pouch but extended high up on the thigh under the vastus medialis on one side and fascia lata on the other. Individual masses, originally thought to be loose bodies, could be palpated in the suprapatellar pouch. There was no other positive clinical finding other than minimal tenderness on the medial joint line.

The matter of the origin of the massive swelling underwent investigation over a matter of four weeks. Three aspirations at intervals of a few days produced on each occasion 6 to 8 oz (170 to 230 cc) of blood-stained fluid. All laboratory investigations proved negative. The radiographs are recorded as negative. They are, however, not available for re-examination at this late date. The author was unaware at the time of the invasion of bone by villonodular tissue; but, in any event, the diagnosis was not known prior to surgery.

At operation the joint was opened through a median parapatellar incision. The content of the suprapatellar pouch was voluminous dark red fatty tissue friable to touch. It was decided that the tissue, conforming to no material encountered previously, might be of neoplastic origin; and that complete excision should be attempted. The pouch extended up under the vastus medialis and vastus lateralis but could be separated readily from these structures and from the anterior surface of the femur. The operation was completed by the excision of diseased synovial membrane from the lateral compartments and from the posterior aspect of the retropatellar fat pad. The total volume of material was greater than had been experienced previously. Consideration was given at the termination of the procedure in view of anticipated stiffening, of the introduction of an interposition of cellophane. It was decided that in unknown pathology, with the suspicion of malignancy, its use would be unwise.

The pathological report included the phrase 'an intermediate zone of hyperplastic polypoid synovia with dense aggregations of macrophages laden with blood pigment' with the conclusion 'the appearances are in keeping with a chronic haemarthrosis'. The author, with the advantage of having performed the operation and seen the tissue involved labelled the case 'pigmented villonodular synovitis'.

The patient was examined one year later. He had attained a symptomless knee but attained only 45° of flexion. He regarded his knee as fit for all ordinary purposes but complained of inability to ride his motorcycle.

The opportunity arose to examine this knee 25 years later. There had been no recurrence of swelling and no disability other than loss of flexion which was limited to 90°. The radiographs were normal other than some evidence of patello-femoral osteoarthrosis presumably related to the limitation of flexion.

2. The patient (J.C., male, aged 33) a Hong Kong Chinese student was first seen at a Casualty Department with a swelling of his knee. The knee was aspirated and a compression bandage applied. No note was made of the quantity or quality of the aspirate. He was discharged from further treatment. Two years later he was referred to the author by his general practitioner because of persistent swelling of the knee. Pain had never been a feature and reflected the delay in reference. Examination revealed a large synovial swelling (Fig. 3,30). There was no tenderness to pressure. The aspirate was deeply blood-stained. The ESR was not raised. A provisional diagnosis of pigmented villonodular synovitis was made. In view of his country of origin and recent visit there the possibility of tuberculosis arose. All tests however including inoculation of a guinea pig proved negative. Anterior synovectomy was performed through two incisions as described in Chapter 6. The presenting synovial tissue was recognised as pigmented villonodular synovitis. It was deeply pigmented and friable (Fig. 3,31) so that difficulty was encountered in securing a

complete clearance of diseased tissue. There was minimal erosion of articular cartilage at the periphery of the femoral condyles. His post-operative recovery was uneventful and he rapidly achieved right-angled flexion. When he left hospital there was still some residual synovial effusion. He was followed at three-monthly intervals for three years. The synovial effusion never completely subsided. When last seen the swelling differed little in size from that which obtained prior to operation. It was clear that the condition had recurred. There was never at any time any complaint of pain; and for this reason he sought no further treatment. He was eventually lost to follow-up. But a request from another country for details of the pathology encountered made it clear that he had been forced to seek further advice.

### Benign Chronic Villous Synovitis

There is a variety of chronic villous synovitis which is benign in terms of articular cartilage destruction and of which the following is an example:

The patient (A.M., male, aged 60) gave a history of increasing pain and stiffness in the right knee for the past 30 years. There was a persistent swelling of the joint particularly at

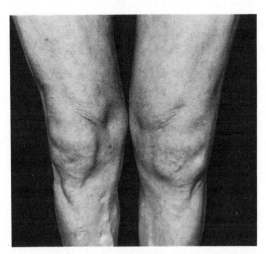

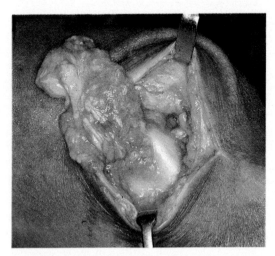

FIGS 3,32–33. **Chronic benign villous synovitis.** This villous synovitis had existed for 30 years! When this photograph was taken the swelling was minimal following a period of bed rest (Fig. 3,32). At anterior synovectomy the articular cartilage of the femoral condyles was of normal appearance despite the long history and reflecting the benign nature of the pathology (Fig. 3,33).

the end of a working day. He was not, however, severely incapacitated. There was no pain or he would have sought advice sooner. His symptoms other than swelling were discomfort amounting to an ache. The swelling subsided but did not disappear with rest (Fig. 3,32). There was no history of injury. The swelling had appeared insidiously. It is of interest and possible significance that he had undergone operation for the removal of a popliteal cyst at the age of 20. There was no special reason for seeking advice. He was, however, entering hospital for a hernia operation and wondered if the knee could be treated at the same time. Examination showed a swelling consisting of swollen synovial membrane rather than fluid. The curious feature of the swelling was that it seemed to involve the suprapatellar pouch rather than the joint in general. There was no swelling nor tenderness on the joint lines. The radiographs were negative. The ESR was not raised. Arthroscopy revealed a massive villous synovitis involving the suprapatellar pouch. The impression was one of inactivity. There was no marginal erosion of articular cartilage. It was evident from the long history and the outcome of investigations that the condition was innocuous. The patient was informed accordingly. He decided, however, that he had lived with his swollen knee too long. At anterior synovectomy, performed through medial and lateral incisions, the inactive nature of the synovial swelling was confirmed together with complete absence of erosion of the articular cartilage (Fig. 3,33).

## REFERENCES

BLOCKEY, N. J. (1976): *Children's Orthopaedics*. London: Butterworths.

BYERS, P. D., COTTON, R. E., DEACON, O. W., LOWY, M., NEWMAN, P. H., SISSONS, H. A. & THOMSON, A. D. (1968). The diagnosis and treatment of pigmented villonodular synovitis. *Journal of Bone and Joint Surgery*, **50B**, 290.

CHASSAIGNAC (1852). Cancer de la gaîne des tendons. *Gazette des hôpitaux civils et militaires*.

CLUTTON, H. H. (1886). *Lancet*, **i**, 391.

COZZETTO, F. J. (1961). Familial Mediterranean fever. Report of four cases. *American Journal of Diseases of Children*, **101**, 52.

DOWD, C. N. (1912). Villous arthritis of the knee (sarcoma). *Annals of Surgery*, **56**, 363.

DUNCAN, H., BLUHM, G. B., RIDDLE, J. M. & BARNHART, M. I. (1968). Synovial urate crystals in acute gouty arthritis. *Clinical Orthopaedics and Related Research*, **59**, 277.

FAIRES, J. S. & McCARTY, D. J. (1962). Acute arthritis in man and dog after intrasynovial injection of sodium urate crystals. *Lancet*, **ii**, 682.

GARROD, A. E. (1910). *Quarterly Journal of Medicine*, **3**, 207.

GOLDMAN, R. L. & LICHTENSTEIN, L. (1964). Synovial chondrosarcoma, *Cancer*, **17**, 1223.

HALBORG, A., HANSEN, H. & SNEPPEN, H. O. (1968). Haemangioma of the knee joint. *Acta orthopaedica scandinavica*, **39**, 1223.

HENCH, P. S. (1948). Rheumatism and arthritis: review of American and English literature of recent years (9th Rheumatism Review). *Annals of Internal Medicqne*, **28**, 66.

HERNESS, D. & MAKIN, M. (1975). Articular damage in familial Mediterranean fever. *Journal of Bone and Joint Surgery*, **57A**, 265.

JAFFE, H. L., LICHTENSTEIN, L. & SUTRO, C. J. (1941). Pigmented villonodular syovitis, bursitis and tenosynovitis. *Archives of Pathology*, **31**, 731.

JEFFREYS, T. E. (1967). Synovial chondromatosis. *Journal of Bone and Joint Surgery*, **49B**, 3, 530.

JERGENSEN, H. E., MANKIN, H. J. & SCHILLER, A. L. (1978). Diffuse pigmented villonodular synovitis of the knee mimicking primary bone neoplasm. *Journal of Bone and Joint Surgery*, **60A**, 825.

JONES, Sir Robert (1915). *Injuries to Joints*, p. 23. London: Oxford University Press.

KAHN, C. B., HOLLANDER, J. L. & SCHUMACHER, H. R. (1970). Corticosteroid crystals in synovial fluid. *Journal of the American Medical Association*, **211/5**, 807.

LEWIN, P. & TAUB, S. J. (1936). Allergic synovitis due to ingestion of English walnuts. *Journal of the American Medical Association*, **106**, 2144.

MAKIN, M. & LEVIN, S. (1965). The articular manifestations of periodic disease (familial Mediterranean fever). *Journal of Bone and Joint Surgery*, **47A**, 1615.

MATTINGLY, S. (1957). Intermittent hydrarthrosis. *British Medical Journal*, **i**, 139–143.

McCARTY, D. J. & HOLLANDER, J. L. (1961). Identification of urate crystals in gouty synovial fluid. *American Journal of Medicine*, **54**, 452.

McCARTY, D. J., KOHN, N. N. & FAIRES, J. S. (1962). The significance of calcium phosphate crystals in the synovial fluid of arthritis patients: the 'pseudogout syndrome', *Annals of Internal Medicine*, **56**, 711.

MILLS, K. L. G. & SMILLIE, I. S. (1979). Compression bandaging of the knee. *Journal of the Royal College of Surgeons of Edinburgh*, **24**, 9.

MOORE, C. H. (1864). *Lancet*, **i**, 485.

MULLINS, F., BERARD, C. W. & EISENBERG, J. H. (1965). Chondrosarcoma following synovial chondromatosis. *Cancer*, **18**, 1180.

ROQUES, C. F., AMIGUES, H., PUGET, J. *et al.* (1974). Metastase synoviale du genou, premier symptome d'un cancer de l'estomac. *Rev. Med. Toulouse*, **10**/3, 235.

SCOTT, P. M. (1968). Bone lesions in pigmented villonodular synovitis. *Journal of Bone and Joint Surgery*, **50B**, 306.

SIMON, G. (1865). Exstirpation einer sehr grossen, mit dickem Stiele angewachsenen Knielgelenkmaus mit glücklichem Erfolge. *Archiv für klinische Chirurgie*, **6**, 573.

SOHAR, E. (1964). The genetic amyloidoses with special emphasis on familial Mediterranean fever. *Henry Ford Hospital Bulletin*, **12**, 343.

STOUT, A. P. (1953). Tumors of the soft tissue, *Atlas of Tumor Pathology*, Section ii, fasc. 11. Washington.

WYNGAARDEN, J. B. (1967). *Etiology and Pathogenesis of Gout, Arthritis and Allied Conditions*. Philadelphia: Lea & Febiger.

# 4. Affections of the Synovial Membrane: Local

## BURSAE

### Introduction

A number of bursae have been described in relation to the moveable structures in the vicinity of the knee joint. The number varies in relation to the interpretation of the term bursa and the detail in which the matter is pursued. In regard to definition: it will be generally accepted that the so-called suprapatellar bursa is not a bursa as such but an integral part of the synovial cavity. There are others, and particularly in relation to the popliteus tendon and lateral ligament, which would carry a similar description. The border line between synovial protrusion and bursa, however, is a narrow one in so far as certain bursae, and particularly the so-called gastrocnemio-semimembranosus bursa, may communicate with the joint.

The bursae are important in so far as they are subject to a variety of pathological processes not necessarily affecting the synovial membrane of the adjacent joint.

### Locations

#### Anterior

**Prepatellar bursa.** This term covers a variety of locations from prepatellar, as the name suggests (Fig. 4,1), to overlying the inferior pole of patella, patellar tendon or even tibial tubercle. This bursa may thus be given a variety of names according to location such as, in the last instance, superficial pretibial bursa. In some examples a single bursa extends from the tibial tubercle to the superior pole of the patella and in such circumstances dimensions as long as 15 cm can be encountered.

**Deep infrapatellar bursa.** This lies between the upper part of the tibia and the ligamentum patellae.

#### Lateral

1. Between head of gastrocnemius and capsule.
2. Between lateral ligament and tendon of biceps.

These and any others may communicate with the joint.

#### Medial

1. Between medial head of gastrocnemius and the capsule with a prolongation between the

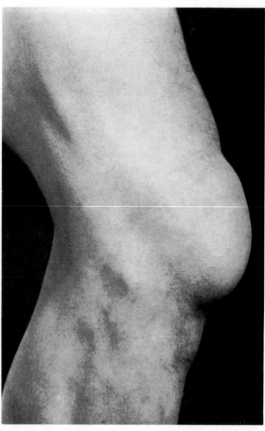

FIG. 4,1. **Prepatellar bursitis.** This large bursa is of interest for the reason that it is 'prepatellar': it is located immediately anterior to the patella.

146

tendon of gastrocnemius and the tendon of semi-membranosus.

These two may coalesce to form the *gastrocnemio-semimembranosus bursa* which may communicate with the joint.

2. There is one superficial to the medial ligament between it and the tendons which comprise the pes anserinus (Figs 4,2 and 4,3).

3. There may be one deep to the medial ligament.

4. There may be one between tendon of semi-membranosus and medial condyle of tibia.

5. Occasionally bursae may be found beneath the tendons which compose the pes anserinus.

## PREPATELLAR BURSITIS

Acute prepatellar bursitis with or without infection is designated an occupational disease under the National Insurance (Industrial Injuries) Act, 1965, in Great Britain. In the revised *Notes on the Diagnosis of Occupational Diseases*, 5th edition, November 1972, Disease Number 32 is described as 'Bursitis or Subcutaneous Cellulitis arising at or about the Knee due to severe or prolonged external friction or pressure at or about the Knee (Beat Knee)'.

In regard to aetiology the condition is described as 'more likely to occur in those unaccustomed to working on their knees, or returning to such work after a prolonged absence, and it is more likely to occur if the skin is wet and sodden. Long-continued or repeated pressure, or minor traumata are important factors, and pivoting on the knee, as in the case of a miner shovelling coal on to a conveyor belt, is a potential cause.'

Under the heading Diagnosis it is said that 'there are two main varieties of "Beat Knee", one in which there is an acute cellulitis of the skin over the knee and upper part of the tibia, and the other in which there is a bursitis with or without infection of the overlying skin. Cellulitis of the skin generally proceeds to suppuration, and may then involve a bursa secondarily. When the first lesion is a bursitis the enlargement may be due to an acute effusion, or to infection of a chronic enlargement. In an acute effusion resulting from a single identifiable trauma, resolution is usually rapid and complete but suppuration and secondary cellulitis of the skin may follow in other cases'.

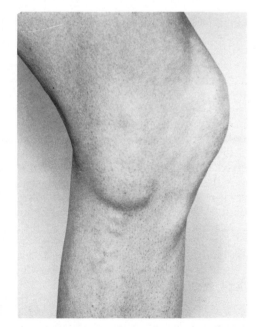

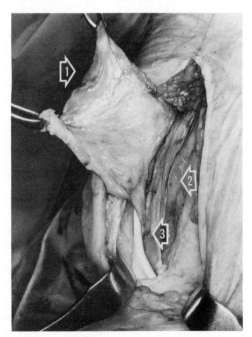

FIGS 4,2–3. **Bursa between medial ligament and tendons of pes anserinus.** Clinical appearance of bursa (Fig. 4,2). Appearance at operation (1) bursa; (2) medial ligament; and (3) tendons of pes anserinus (case of B.C.).

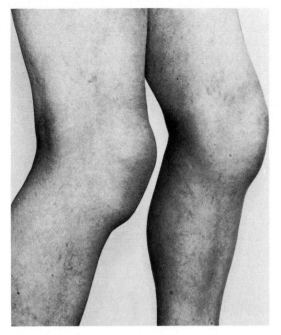

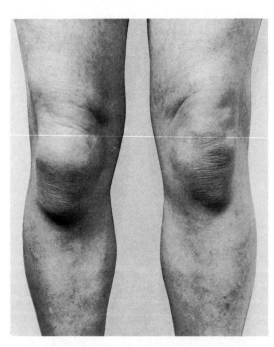

FIGS 4,4–5. **Prepatellar bursitis: chronic.** The bilateral variety occurs in those who work on their knees. It is through the fissures of the skin so-related that infection is introduced (A.R., male, slater, aged 60).

The condition of 'beat knee' is not therefore a clinical entity, but a number of conditions including acute bursitis, with or without infection, and including cellulitis which may precede or be a complication of infective bursitis.

**Clinical features.** The bursa, a fluctuant soft tissue swelling in the mid-line, is normally unilateral. It is likely that those who work on their knees impose the entire body weight on one rather than two using the other leg for propulsion. The exceptions, of course, are floor-scrubbing, and, perhaps it should be said, praying. In ordinary circumstances examination of the knee will show that only one of the two has the hard fissured skin which is the source of the infection in infective bursitis. There are exceptions (Figs 4,4 and 4.5).

The swelling is readily distinguished from an intra-articular synovial effusion in that it remains of the same dimensions and consistency on straight-leg-raising showing that it is outwith the joint.

## TREATMENT

### Acute

**Traumatic.** In an acute attack, the result of a single incident of trauma or unaccustomed kneeling, the condition may resolve with aspiration alone. When the aspiration is completed a pad of sterile orthopaedic felt of suitable size to fit the area affected, and bevelled at the edges, is placed over the site of the bursa and a diverging spica of adhesive elastic bandage applied. Such measures, by keeping the opposing synovial surfaces in contact often result in a cure.

**Haemobursitis.** When the patient gives a history that the swelling, not previously present, occurred within half an hour of some trivial injury, the effusion is blood. Experimental observations in coal miners have shown that in the course of kneeling and shovelling pressures may rise from 0 to 200 lbf/in$^2$ (1380 kPa) at each act of shovelling (Sharrard, 1961). Aneurysmal dilatation of vessels in the bursal wall develop. The bursa may suddenly become enlarged as a result of spontaneous haemorrhage.

A haemobursitis should be aspirated and then subjected to elastic compression to bring the opposing surfaces into contact. If the blood is not aspirated thickening of the walls occurs with a liability to further trouble from kneeling.

**Infective.** If infection is superimposed the appropriate systemic antibiotic will be indicated. Suppuration in such circumstances may sometimes subside with aspiration. If incision and drainage is required the infliction of a mid-line scar, which will be subjected to pressure in kneeling, is to be avoided.

### Chronic

**Operation.** A bursa which fails to subside with aspiration, becomes chronically distended, or is the subject of recurrent effusions, may require to be excised.

In planning the incision it should be remembered that the patients develop the condition working on their knees. Such people do not appreciate an area of anaesthesia. In these circumstances it is probable that a lateral incision is preferable to a medial in that it does not cut the infra-patellar branch of the saphenous nerve. In any event the scar should not cross the mid-line at a point liable to pressure in kneeling.

In dissecting out the bursa it will be found that adhesion to the skin is more in evidence than adhesion to the deeper structures such as patella or patellar tendon. Care may be necessary to avoid button-holing of the skin. The tendency to post-operative haematoma causing skin to become adherent to deep soft tissues can be reduced by the use of suction drainage in addition to the usual compression bandage.

In regard to damage to or adherence of the skin Quayle and Robinson (1976) have pointed out that these hazards can be avoided if only the posterior wall of the bursa is excised (Fig. 4,6). If this technique is practised the anterior wall and the anterior aspect of patella or patellar tendon are scarified before the skin flap with adherent anterior wall are laid back in position.

### BURSA BETWEEN LIGAMENTUM PATELLAE AND TIBIA: INFRAPATELLAR, OR DEEP INFRAPATELLAR BURSA

An anterior bursa of significance is that which lies between the ligamentum patellae and the tibia immediately above the attachment of the ligament (Fig. 4,7). This small bursa is rarely affected by disease or injury, but may become the subject of effusion as a result of a direct blow over the ligament, when difficulty may arise

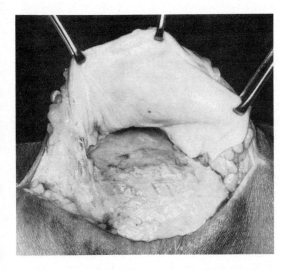

FIG. 4,6. **Chronic prepatellar bursitis: treatment.** To avoid damage to or adherence of the skin flap only the posterior wall of the bursa is excised leaving the anterior wall intact. It is scarified together with the opposing patellar tendon before resuture of the skin flap.

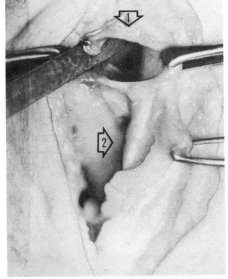

FIG. 4,7. **Bursa between ligamentum patellae and tibia.** The point of the dissector is within the bursa (1) which lies between the ligamentum patellae (2) and the tibia.

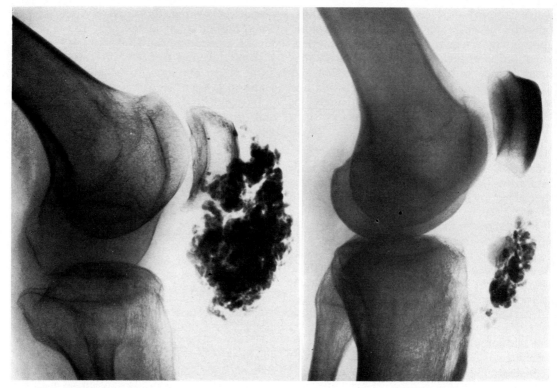

FIGS 4,8–9. **Calcification of prepatellar bursa.** In this example calcification was bilateral but asymmetrical. The patient suffered from osteochondrodystrophy. Note abnormal con- formation of the tibial head (Fig. 4,8). Synovial osteo- chondromatosis has a similar appearance (Fig. 4,9).

in differentiating the condition from haemor- rhage into the retropatellar pad of fat. In both these cases there is pain and tenderness over the ligament combined with inability to obtain full flexion or extension. The swelling which appears on either side of the ligament is fluctuant in bursitis and is usually situated at a lower level, but aspiration is frequently necessary in order to confirm the diagnosis.

### TREATMENT

The condition usually subsides rapidly with rest and elastic compression.

A few cases only (one bilateral) have failed to settle by conservative means and were sub- jected to operation.

### Operation

A vertical lateral incision is made close to the patellar tendon. A medial incision should be avoided, as the exposure, which must visualise the upper inch of the tibia, requires to be rather longer than the normal meniscus incision and would therefore divide the infrapatellar branch of the saphenous nerve. The thin capsule be- tween the patellar tendon and the iliotibial band is divided and the central portion of the capsule retracted to expose the tendon. The bursa is thin- walled and may be opened before it is recognised; it may sometimes be located by the presence of old or recent haemorrhages. It is usually adherent to the posterior aspect of the tendon and in order to excise it in its entirety it is necessary to remove a certain amount of the surrounding extra-synovial fat. The knee joint proper should not be entered. The removal of the bursa, together with part of the retropatellar fat pad, leaves a dead space which must be obliterated by stitching the remaining posterior part of the fat pad to the posterior aspect of the patellar tendon with fine catgut sutures.

# POPLITEAL CYST: GASTROCNEMIO-SEMIMEMBRANOSUS BURSA

**Historical note.** The first reference to a popliteal swelling is attributed to Dupuytren (1829). The first description of a posterior cyst related to an inconstant communication between the semimembranosus bursa and the knee joint is attributed to Adams (1840). The classical description of the cyst which bears his name and relating it to disease within the knee joint occurred in an article by Baker (1877). Current opinion tends to the view that Baker's name should no longer be attached in so far as the condition he described was not a clinical entity but, in fact, a complication of tuberculous arthritis.

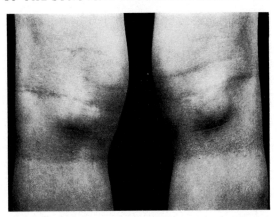

FIG. 4,10. **Popliteal cyst: gastrocnemio-semimembranosus bursa.** The *Primary* variety is seen most commonly in children and is frequently bilateral. The cause is unknown.

## Definition

The most common popliteal cyst is a distended gastrocnemio-semimembranosus bursa which frequently communicates with the joint through the posterior capsule.

There are two varieties: (1) *primary*; and (2) *secondary*.

**Primary.** This variety arises in a joint which is apparently normal. It is seen most commonly in children in whom it may be bilateral (Fig. 4,10) but not necessarily simultaneously and with a tendency to recurrence following excision (42 per cent, Dinham, 1975). It is clear that there is a predisposition to distension of the bursa in some children. The reason is unknown.

NATURAL HISTORY. There is in recent years evidence that a high proportion of primary cysts in children undergo spontaneous resolution (Gristina and Wilson, 1963; MacMahon, 1973; Dinham, 1975). The decreased incidence after the age of 7 is striking.

**Secondary.** In adults and the elderly, popliteal cysts are almost invariably secondary to some irritative lesion usually, but not necessarily, an effusion-producing intra-articular pathological process. The most common internal derangement in this age range is a horizontal cleavage lesion of the posterior segment of the medial meniscus; but there is no specific relationship. This lesion is not normally associated with effusion. The explanation of the apparent association lies in local peripheral synovial irritation (Ch. 10).

## Clinical Features

The complaint is of a swelling of insidious origin in the popliteal space producing mechanical limitation of extension and/or of flexion. Pain is not predominant other than as a manifestation of tension or of the basic pathology in the secondary variety. Occasionally the swelling is such as to obstruct venous drainage and produce oedema of the leg below the knee. On examination the swelling is most prominent in the prone position, the knee extended to the maximum possible, the dorsum of the patient's foot beyond the end of the examination couch. A minority of patients with a valvular connection between joint and bursa demonstrate the ability, by rapid flexion and extension of the joint, to distend the bursa. Passive flexion and extension can produce the same effect. The valvular opening is occluded in full extension maintaining the swelling. Manual compression in flexion, however, results in evacuating the accumulated fluid back into the joint cavity.

## Differential Diagnosis

**Other bursae.** When the swelling presents postero-medially (Figs 4,11 and 4,19) rather than posteriorly it may be confused with one of the bursae associated with the pes anserinus and the medial ligament (Figs 4,2 and 4,3).

**Cystic degeneration of meniscus.** A cyst of a meniscus may be situated some distance from the site of origin. Cysts of the medial structure, which in general tend to be larger than those on the lateral side, may be swept backward in the action of flexion by the medial ligament and present in the popliteal space (Fig. 4,11).

**'Ganglion of knee'.** Soft tissue swellings of similar consistency with which the condition is known to have been confused include lipomata and a 'ganglion of the knee' the origin of which was not revealed (Fig. 4,13).

**Popliteal aneurysm.** It is important to distinguish a bursa from an aneurysm. Popliteal aneurysms are common, but often missed. They are most likely to be confused with cysts secondary to degenerative changes in the joint if it is only for the reason that aneurysms occur in the same age-group with arteriosclerotic changes. There is a similarity too, in so far as popliteal aneurysms

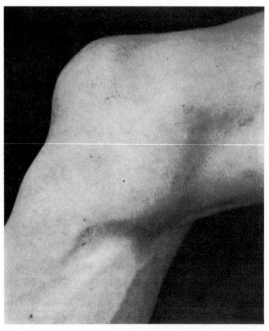

FIG. 4,11. **Gastrocnemio-semimembranosus bursa.** Not all bursae present posteriorly. This swelling on the medial joint line was traced to its point of origin beneath the medial head of gastrocnemius and was shown to be a bursa presenting medially rather than in the usual situation. (See also Fig. 4,19.)

like popliteal cysts are frequently bilateral; and may be symptomless (Eastcott, 1969). In general it can be said that aneurysms present at a higher level than cysts.

The popliteal pulse is not readily palpable in the presence of a swelling. Pulsation palpable over a wide area is probably aneurysmal in origin. A murmur is not necessarily present if the aneurysmal sac is thrombosed.

**Cystic degeneration of popliteal artery.** The aetiology of this condition is obscure. It has been regarded as mucinous degeneration in the adventitial layer of the artery not associated with atherosclerosis. It is believed that repeated minor trauma to the artery may be the cause. The proximity of the lesion to the knee may be so related.

Patients with this condition complain of intermittent claudication in one leg. It may be of sudden or gradual onset and is associated with a cold white foot on exercise.

The fact that the swelling is only occasionally palpable reduces the possibility of error.

**Solitary exostosis with (or without) an overlying bursa.** A single exostosis occasionally presents from the trigone of the femur and there may be a related bursa. There is a relationship between such an exostosis and popliteal aneurysm above (Ch. 14).

This cause of swelling should be eliminated by the radiograph which is mandatory in the course of investigation.

**Popliteal varix.** A swelling other than a cyst may be produced in the popliteal space by the rapid flexion and extension of the knee and which at operation may be revealed to be a varix. This is a further explanation of a negative exploration.

**Rupture or hypertrophy of semimembranosus.** A swelling in the popliteal space may occur as a result of unilateral rupture or bilateral localised hypertrophy (Symeonides and Paschaloglou, 1970) of the semimembranosus muscle. The characteristic feature of the swelling is increase in size on contracture of the knee flexor muscles against resistance. The possibility that the swelling might not be found if an exploratory operation is undertaken under general anaesthesia should be borne in mind; and this is indeed what occurred in the first of the four cases reported by Symeonides and Paschaloglou.

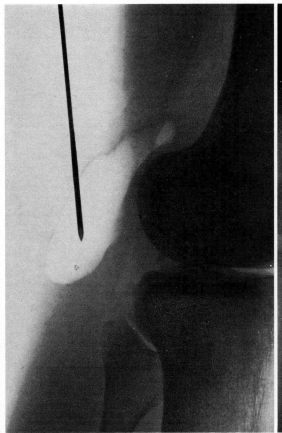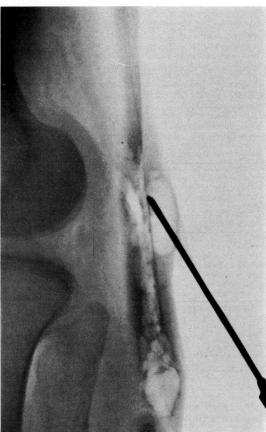

FIGS 4,12–13. **Popliteal cyst.** Aspiration and arthrogram using air as contrast medium can be used to confirm nature, site and origin of bursa (Fig. 4,12). This cystic swelling was multilocular; and it was possible to transfer fluid from one cyst to the other. It did not conform to the pattern of the gastrocnemio-semimembranosus bursa (Fig. 4.12). Aspiration and air arthrogram suggested it was a ganglion (Fig. 4,13). The tissue and site of origin were never determined.

## Complications

**Rupture.** The disease process most likely to be responsible for rupture is rheumatoid arthritis. The influence of corticosteroid therapy, systemic or intra-articular, on the liability to rupture has yet to be determined (see Ch. 6).

**Synovial osteochondromatosis.** The bursa, like the prepatellar bursa (Fig. 4,9), may be affected with synovial chondromatosis in the absence of similar pathology in the adjacent knee joint (Figs 4,14 to 4,16).

Record of a case:

The patient (A.H., male, aged 37, case of W.W.) presented with a firm painless swelling in the popliteal fossa which he first noticed two months previously after doing some heavy work. He thought that the swelling had become larger recently; and this was his reason for seeking advice.

On examination there was a hard swelling in the popliteal fossa at the site usually occupied by a popliteal cyst. Radiography showed the mass to be calcified (Fig. 4,14). No firm pre-operative diagnosis was made.

At operation the mass was found in the position normally occupied by gastrocnemio-semimembranosus bursa and related to semimembranosus and the medial head of gastrocnemius. It was traced to originate in the

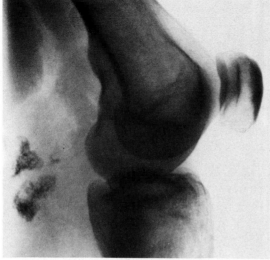

FIG. 4,14

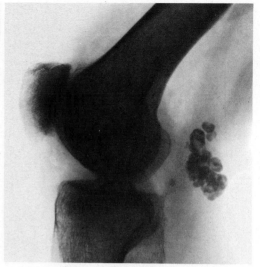

FIG. 4,15

posterior capsule. It measured 6 × 4 × 4 cm and was seen to be partly covered by synovial membrane. On section the central areas were said to be ossified. The histological appearance otherwise was that of a synovial chondromatosis.

### Laboratory Investigations

In view of the fact that a popliteal cyst may be the first manifestation of other pathology, it is prudent when cases present without explanation to have the ESR established. If this simple screening test had been carried out on the case quoted below, an elevated ESR might have given the hint that it was not a primary cyst. Furthermore, and for the same reason, the excised bursa, no matter how simple in appearance, should be examined microscopically.

### Popliteal Cyst as First Sign of Disease Process in the Knee

Sometimes a popliteal cyst, which appears to be of the *primary* variety, is in fact *secondary* and the first indication of disease in the joint:

The patient (Mrs M.S., aged 29) presented with a right-sided popliteal cyst. There was no sign of internal derangement, synovial effusion

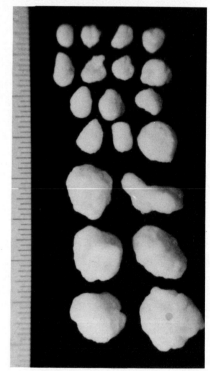

FIG. 4,16

FIGS 4,14–16. **Popliteal cyst: synovial osteochondromatosis.** Gastrocnemio-semimembranosus bursae affected by synovial osteochondromatosis. In neither example was the joint involved (Figs 4,14 and 4,15). The loose bodies from Fig. 4,16 (scale in inches). See also Figure 4,9.

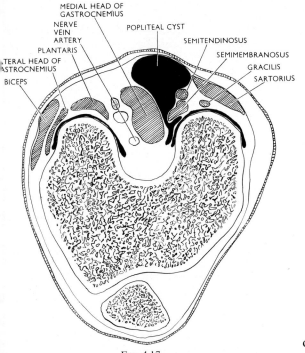

MEDIAL HEAD OF
GASTROCNEMIUS
NERVE
VEIN          POPLITEAL CYST
ARTERY
PLANTARIS          SEMITENDINOSUS
ATERAL HEAD OF          SEMIMEMBRANOSUS
ASTROCNEMIUS          GRACILIS
BICEPS          SARTORIUS

Fig. 4,17

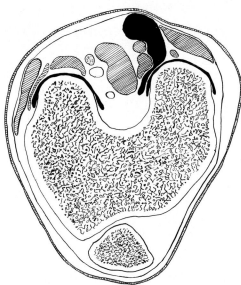

Fig. 4,18

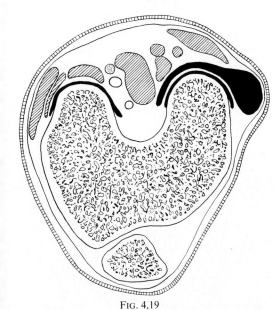

Fig. 4,19

FIGS 4,17–19. **Popliteal cyst: gastrocnemio-semimembranosus bursa.** The distended bursa emerging to medial side of semimembranosus (Fig. 4,17); and to lateral side (Fig. 4,18). The bursa does not always present posteriorly but on the medial joint line behind the condyles (Fig. 4,19) where the swelling may be confused with cystic degeneration of the medial meniscus (Figs 13,2 and 13,3).

or synovial thickening. There were no symptoms in the knee. The reason for operation, both from the patient's and surgeon's viewpoint, was the mass in the popliteal space causing pain and obstructing movement. The cyst was removed and looked like any other cyst. There were no unusual microscopic findings in the section. Eight months later both right and left knees became swollen, the right in considerably greater degree than the left. Examination one year after the original operation showed marked synovial effusion and synovial thickening on the right side and synovial effusion, but in considerably lesser degree, on the left. No other joint was affected.

When it was suggested that admission to hospital for investigation was advisable she stated that she had a gynaecological condition due for investigation. She inquired if the gynaecological and knee swellings could be related.

In hospital a variety of investigations were undertaken including a full blood investigation, ESR, R.A. Latex, *Brucella abortus* titres (in view of the fact that she was the wife of a dairy farmer), uric acid, Wasserman Reaction. In addition, the knee was aspirated. The fluid was clear, straw coloured and of normal appearance. A guinea pig was injected. Every investigation proved negative with one exception: the ESR was 33 in one hour.

In view of the history, a gynaecological opinion was sought. It appeared that she had an ovarian cyst. This was considered a matter of some urgency and she was transferred to the gynaecological department where at operation an ovarian cyst said to be the size of a 'Jaffa orange' and the related right ovary were removed. The cyst was reported to be a 'follicular cyst into which haemorrhage had occurred'.

Two weeks after operation she was reviewed in regard to her knees. The effusions in both knees had subsided. It remained to be established whether the effusions absorbed with rest or whether they were related, as the patient averred, to the ovarian cyst.

This case is recorded to illustrate:

1. A popliteal cyst in the form of a gastrocnemio-semimembranosus bursa presenting as the first indication of some general pathology in the knee. In other words, a cyst removed on the basis that it was *primary*, but shown with the passage of time to be *secondary*.
2. The possible association of bilateral effusions into the knees with an ovarian cyst.

The patient, as stated above, was convinced

that her gynaecological condition and effusions in both knees were related. This suggestion brought to mind the rare condition of Meigs' syndrome (Meigs *et al.,* 1943), whereby ovarian tumours and cysts may be associated with hydrothorax. There has been much speculation as to the mechanism involved; and this raised the possibility that the effusions in the knees might be of similar origin.

When she returned home, however, and resumed her domestic duties, the swellings and pain recurred. It appeared, therefore, that the relationship with the ovarian cyst was fortuitous. Further and even more thorough investigations were undertaken all of which were negative except that her ESR has risen to 48 in the first hour. A rheumatologist to whom she was referred carried out a synovial biopsy which was declared to show a typical 'rheumatoid pattern'.

It was concluded without convincing evidence that she was an example of sero-negative rheumatoid arthritis. When last seen there were marked effusions in both knees and generalised synovial thickening. No other joints were involved. It was decided in such circumstances that she became a possible candidate for synovectomy. Pain, however, was not the presenting symptom. In view of the short history, and the wish to avoid a

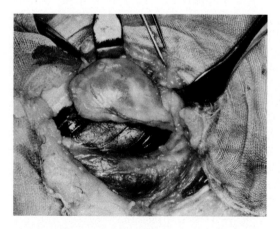 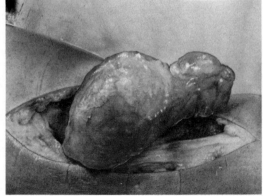

FIGS 4,20–21. **Popliteal cyst: gastrocnemio-semimembranosus bursa.** The distended bursa takes a variety of forms. Small bursa to medial side of medial head of gastrocnemius (Fig. 4,20). Large bursa presenting on division of deep fascia (Fig. 4,21). Bursae under such tension can interfere with venous circulation.

Note erroneous use of straight incision. It should be a lazy S.

destructive operative procedure, it was decided that some little time be permitted to pass in the hope of resolution.

## Treatment

**Primary.** No treatment is indicated in the absence of symptoms. In the presence of pain or interference with movement action may be demanded. Aspiration, repeated as necessary, may be tried on the basis that the bursitis is self-perpetuating in so far as when distended the lining membrane is subject to constant irritation by the movement of the associated muscles.

In the absence of resolution excision is indicated. It should be anticipated that recurrence is common (42 per cent, Dinham, 1975).

**Secondary.** In the young adult the cyst is likely to be secondary to an internal derangement, most commonly a lesion of a meniscus. But any disease process, idiopathic synovitis, rheumatoid arthritis, pigmented villonodular arthritis, synovial chondromatosis, etc., may be responsible; and in some instances the popliteal cyst may be the presenting symptom. In these situations the treatment is that of the cause. It is established that if it is such as to be capable of eradication the bursitis will subside. There remain cases of indeterminate cause and those in which the cause cannot be eliminated. In the former, treatment is determined by the presence or absence of symptoms. In a proportion of cases the mere presence of a 'swelling' is unacceptable and determines the necessity for excision. In osteoarthrosis in the elderly there is seldom any indication for treatment other than by aspiration to reduce tension in a bursa unconnected with the joint. The indications for excision in this age group are rare.

## Operation

When a decision is made in a persistent or recurrent cyst to resort to surgery, if at the time of admission to hospital the swelling is not in evidence, the operation should be deferred. The author has been present in the capacity of assistant at a number of explorations at which the cyst, known to have been present previously, could not be found.

**Technique.** If it is usual to employ a tourniquet it is not strictly necessary in an operation which divides only the deep fascia and is thereafter confined to muscle planes. The operation is carried out in the prone position. A small pillow or sandbag is placed beneath the dorsum of the foot so that the knee joint is maintained in slight flexion in order to relax tendons and muscles and permit retraction to be effected.

The location and type of incision is of importance. A vertical incision is to be avoided as liable to be followed by a keloid scar. A transverse incision within a crease gives limited access. In general, a lazy S, the horizontal portion of which lies in a crease, is to be preferred. The transverse and inferior limit of the S, located on the medial side, may provide adequate exposure.

When the deep fascia is incised longitudinally the tense cyst presents. The dissection takes place on the medial aspect of the medial head of the gastrocnemius. The popliteal vessels and nerves are protected throughout the procedure by retraction of the muscle to the lateral side. No difficulty is encountered tracing the limits of the bursa between the medial head of gastrocnemius and muscular belly of semimembranosus; although occasionally the swelling may present between the semimembranosus and semitendinosus laterally and sartorius and gracilis medially.

The cyst may be found to be closely adherent to the semimembranosus and gastrocnemius; and resection of the superior layer of the latter structure may be necessary to avoid rupture of the adherent wall. If the cyst communicates with the joint it will be found to be adherent to the capsule on the deep surface of the medial head of gastrocnemius. It has not been the practice to close any residual opening; and there is no evidence that this practice leads to recurrence. Nevertheless, there are those who believe that closure is important and accomplished by scarification of an area of the medial head of gastrocnemius which is then fixed to the posterior joint capsule by sutures (Childress, 1970).

AFTER-TREATMENT. A compression bandage is applied which includes a pad of cotton wool accurately placed in the popliteal space. The stitches are removed on the tenth to fourteenth day and ambulation resumed.

## SUPRAPATELLAR PLICA AND SUPRAPATELLAR BURSA IN SIMULATION OF INTERNAL DERANGEMENT

The suprapatellar space has wide anatomic variations of communication between the suprapatellar synovia and the suprapatellar bursa. Eighty per cent of adult human knees have an 'open' communication so that for all intents and purposes it is one synovial compartment. Twenty per cent have a significant remnant of that communication resulting in a synovial fold named the suprapatellar plica (Fig. 4,22). The suprapatellar plica varies from a minor synovial fold, to a valve-like orifice, to a complete membrane separating the suprapatellar synovia from the suprapatellar bursa (Pipkin, 1971).

The advent of the arthroscope has called attention to the plica in recent years. Vague symptoms should not be attributed to its presence in any form. Its principle effect is to influence the localisation of a loose body (Fig. 4,22) and to determine the site at which a loose body attains a synovial attachment or becomes encapsulated within a synovial pouch. If subjected to direct trauma or affected by some undefined pathological process it may undergo fibrosis, shortening and thickening so that a synovial band may ride over the margin of the medial or lateral femoral condyle to produce symptoms on flexion as in sitting for a long time. It may sometimes be palpable with the knee in the flexed position.

The suprapatellar plica when it exists on the medial side in thickened form is alleged to impinge on the antero-medial aspect of the medial femoral condyle and on the medial facet of the patella in flexion. It is thus held to be responsible for the existence of chondromalacia at either side from direct contact with articular cartilage (Patel, 1978). Others believe that such chondromalacia occurs from interference with the normal excursion of the quadriceps mechanism by the bowstring action of the fibrous band (Andrews, 1978).

**Incidence.** In the author's experience symptoms attributable to such a fibrotic band are uncommon. Two recent examples only can be recalled. The diagnosis may have been missed before he was aware of the possibility.

**Treatment.** The band is located through a short para-patellar incision and divided or excised.

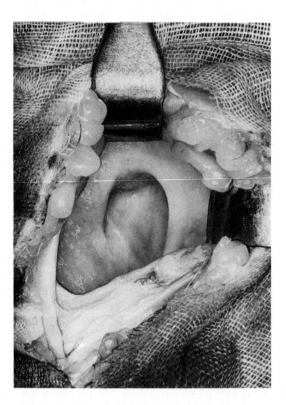

FIG. 4,22. **Suprapatellar plica.** Semilunar fold in suprapatellar pouch. In this example it influenced the location of a loose body.

## HERNIATION OF SYNOVIAL MEMBRANE: EXTRA-ARTICULAR SYNOVIAL POUCH

The synovial membrane can herniate through the capsule of an otherwise normal joint but retaining a communication with the joint as a result of rupture of the capsule, or may herniate, presumably as a result of injury, and become shut off from the joint in the form of an extra-articular synovial pouch (see below). Such swellings particularly when small and productive of symptoms may pose considerable problems of diagnosis. A loose body within a synovial pouch may be located in the extrasynovial fat; and it is presumed that it herniates through the capsule carrying with it a covering of synovial membrane which then becomes shut off from the joint cavity.

The following is an example of massive gravitational herniation of the synovial membrane of the suprapatellar pouch presumed to be the result of a closed rupture of the capsule.

The patient, a coal miner (R.B., aged 29), was involved in an accident in which he received multiple major injuries when he was buried by a fall of roof. He was, a year from the date of the accident, sufficiently recovered to be admitted to the residential rehabilitation unit. Three weeks after his admission he suddenly complained of a swelling in the left knee. The swelling was a most unusual one in so far as when supine on the couch it was not present. Furthermore, even when he contracted his quadriceps as in straight-leg-raising it was not present. If, however, he stood erect within a few seconds a large soft oval swelling appeared on the supramedial aspect of the joint (Fig. 4,23).

Opinion was sought as to the nature of the swelling, not only because the patient was worried about it but because no explanation had been offered. The fact that it came and went in the manner described was particularly puzzling. The explanation offered was that in the mine accident in which he was trapped by a fall of stone from the roof he had received a closed rupture of the vastus medialis and of its attachment to the capsule. This closed rupture gave no trouble until he began his exercise therapy in the rehabilitation centre. The attenuated capsule with exercise became thinner and thinner. When he stood up gravity permitted the synovial membrane of the suprapatellar pouch to herniate through the capsule. The patient was informed that in ordinary circumstances old ruptures of the vastus medialis could not be repaired; but that because the rupture involved capsule there was the possibility that it could be repaired. He stated, however, that he was not suffering a physical disability; but he was worrying as to the nature of the unknown swelling. When told with a considerable degree of certainty the nature of the pathology he was satisfied that no further action was necessary.

## Extra-articular Synovial Pouch

**Aetiology.** If a rational explanation can be offered as to the mechanism whereby a loose body within a synovial pouch can exist outwith the synovial cavity, in for example the fat pad (Figs 4,24 to 4,26) or the extrasynovial fat of the suprapatellar pouch, the origin of a pouch existing in isolation is less easy to explain. It is presumed that synovial membrane is extruded in an incident of direct violence and thereafter shut off from the joint cavity. That a pouch may be related to a mechanical process is shown in case (2) quoted below. The presence of effusion within the pouch is presumed to be related to the mechanical irritation of movement. The condition may be one of some

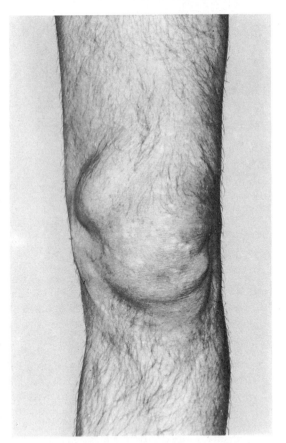

FIG. 4,23. **Herniation of synovial membrane.** This synovial swelling was thought to be due to a closed rupture in the medial capsule of traumatic origin. It appeared when he stood erect and disappeared on straight-leg-raising in the supine position (R.B., coal miner, aged 29).

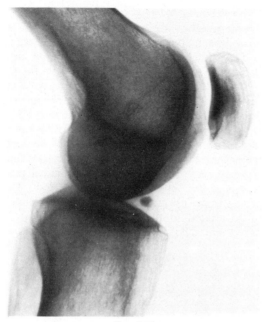

FIG. 4,24

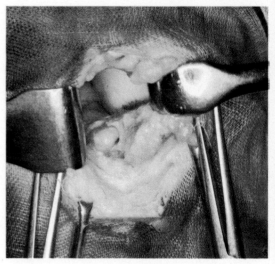

FIG. 4,25

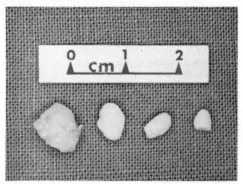

FIG. 4,26

FIGS 4,24–26. **Extra-articular synovial pouch.** This small 'loose' body in the anterior compartment (Fig. 4,24) lies within a synovial pouch within the infrapatellar fat pad (Fig. 4,25). The largest loose body had a synovial attachment. The remainder, which are not seen in the radiograph, were free (Fig. 4,26).

These loose bodies demonstrate the effect of blood supply on articular cartilage. The largest had a blood supply from a synovial attachment. It consisted of bone. There is no cartilaginous covering. The three small loose bodies were free. They consist of cartilage only (Fig. 4,26). (See also Ch. 11.)

rarity; but the fact that a second example was encountered shortly after the first suggests that the condition may have passed unrecognised.

These two cases are quoted:

1. The patient (A.S., aged 23), a professional footballer, complained of swelling on the lateral aspect of the knee after exercise. He said that he could complete a game without difficulty, but afterwards suffered local pain and swelling lateral to the patella. He was kept under observation. On one occasion a soft tissue swelling accompanied by a local increase of temperature was noted. Initially it was thought that the symptoms emanated from the patello-femoral joint. Repeated

observations suggested that whatever the cause it was located in the soft tissues to the lateral side of the patella. An exploratory operation was advised on the basis of a provisional diagnosis of 'synovial tag' or 'local haemangioma'. At operation when the skin was incised a mass presented in the extra-capsular fat. The first impression was that the joint cavity had been entered. Closer examination confirmed that the tissue was not only outside the joint but did not communicate with the joint. The excised mass was reported to be synovial tissue including a cavity lined with synovial membrane. There was evidence of traumatic fat necrosis. The patient made an uneventful recovery. The symptoms of pain and swelling were completely relieved.

2. The patient (R.S., aged 36, case of K.L.G.M.) complained of the presence of a lump on the supralateral aspect of the suprapatellar pouch. The swelling was the source of discomfort after exercise. On palpation a firm but not hard swelling was present which could be moved through a small range in every direction.

It was not radio-opaque and as such was thought to be an encapsulated loose body of fibrous tissue or articular cartilage. At operation, however, the swelling was found to lie posterior to the synovial membrane in the suprapatellar pouch. It was cystic in nature and when opened was seen to be lined with synovial membrane. Attached to the outer wall was the muscle articularis genu. The cyst was excised *in toto* with some fatty tissue and part of the attached muscle. The diagnosis appeared to be one of an extrasynovial articular pouch; and that the lining was synovial membrane was confirmed microscopically (Fig. 4,27).

The interesting feature of this particular example was the speculation as to the origin. The most probable explanation seemed to be that the articularis genu, the function of which is said to be to draw upwards the suprapatellar pouch during extension had, in fact, drawn upwards a local area of synovial membrane which had then been cut-off from the main joint cavity to constitute an extra-articular synovial pouch.

## LESIONS OF THE INFRA-PATELLAR FAT PAD AND RELATED SYNOVIAL MEMBRANE: HYPERTROPHY OF FAT PAD: HOFFA'S DISEASE

**Anatomical note.** The pyramidal space between femur, tibia and the patellar tendon is occupied by the pad of fat which, wedge-shaped and covered with synovial membrane, projects into the cavity to change in shape with every movement up the joint (Fig. 4,28).

It has been shown that the fat pads of the cat are provided with a considerable pain-sensitive nerve plexus system (Freeman and Wyke, 1967). This may apply in greater or lesser degree to the

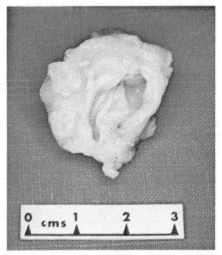

FIG. 4,27. **Extra-articular synovial pouch.** This cystic swelling was located immediately above the suprapatellar pouch and presented as a swelling of unknown origin. It is thought to have arisen as a result of the traction exerted on the synovial membrane by the muscle articularis genu.

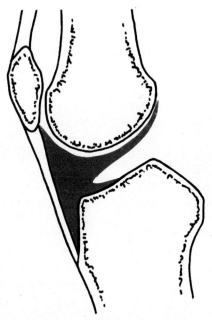

FIG. 4,28. **Infrapatellar fat pad.** The fat pad fills completely the intracapsular extrasynovial pyramidal space bounded by the patellar tendon and the femoral and tibial condyles. It is anchored to the femur by the ligamentum mucosum (semi-diagrammatic).

human subject and with implications of clinical significance.

The synovial lining sends a triangular fold called the ligamentum mucosum (plica synovalis patellaris), containing blood vessels, upwards and backwards to be attached to the intercondylar notch (Fig. 4,29). The clinical importance of the fold, apart from a source of haemorrhage if divided, is that by anchoring the fat pad it may limit expansion in a forward direction when swelling occurs and thus may be responsible for the compression of the synovial membrane.

The free edges of the ligamentum mucosum diverge to include the lateral margins of the fat pad and are called the alar ligaments.

**Biomechanical note.** The infrapatellar fat pad has been considered in the past to be space-occupying but not otherwise of anatomical, physiological or clinical significance. This view is erroneous. If, for example, sub-total excision is performed by an ignorant, inexperienced or incompetent surgeon in the course of access in the operation of meniscectomy, friction occurs between the scar in the capsule and the margin of the femoral condyle with a continuing disability for which no solution is immediately evident. That the volume of the fat pad is important to the function of the joint is shown by the fact that fat at this site is lost only in extreme emaciation and depletion

does not begin until subcutaneous fat has been virtually eliminated (Davies and White, 1961). In less extreme circumstances changes in local conditions, as in the ageing joint, appear to exert little influence on the size of the fat pad. The clinical implications are seen in the pathology encountered.

**Clinical implications.** The existence of internal derangement of the knee joint related to the infrapatellar fat pad has been recognised since Hoffa's original observations in 1904. It is nevertheless a subject to which there is little reference in the literature. But it should be established that it is not, as some would have it, a convenient waste-paper basket for misdiagnosis but a condition with a related symptom complex of some precision readily recognised by the initiated. It is probably second only to recurrent subluxation of the patella as the source of symptoms in the teenage girl (see Ch. 12). It is customary to attribute the symptoms to pathological changes within the fat pad. It will be recognised, in the interests of accuracy, that whereas the basic pathology causing enlargement in the form of oedema, haemorrhage, hypertrophy or fibrosis is located there producing a tension situation, the source of the symptoms may be the related synovial membrane projecting into the joint in the form of villi, fringes or tags to be subjected to endogenous trauma as a result of the swelling. This is the reason for including the subject under 'Local Lesions of Synovial Membrane' rather than some separate heading.

## Pathological Anatomy

The condition is primarily an enlargement, for one reason or another, of the fat pad. Conversely, the space available is reduced in capacity as a result of age-related changes in the articular cartilage of opposing femur and tibia with similar outcome. The general effect is compression of the fat pad which can extrude anteriorly in limited degree on either side of the patellar tendon. There is, however, no possibility of expansion in a posterior direction. Therein lies the source of the symptoms: the synovial membrane is subject to direct compression between femur and tibia towards the completion of extension with resultant pain and possibly

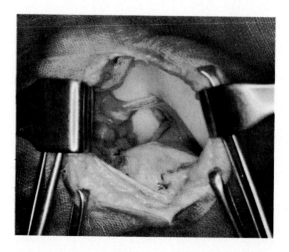

FIG. 4,29. **Infrapatellar fat pad: ligamentum mucosum (plica synovalis patellaris).** The ligamentum mucosum containing blood vessels anchors the fat pad to the intercondylar notch.

effusion. The principal causes of enlargement are:

**1. Trauma.** It takes the form of a direct injury as in a fall (Fig. 4,30). In the current scene, the most common mechanism is contact with the dashboard of a car in a road traffic accident.

**2. Oedema.** The most common source in the female subject is the premenstrual water-retention syndrome (see Ch. 12).

**3. Space-occupying lesion.** The fat pad, it is repeated, fills completely the room available. Any space-occupying lesion will produce anterior extrusion and the liability to a lesion of the lining membrane. It is not generally appreciated that the most common space-occupying lesion is the displaced handle of a bucket-handle (complete longitudinal) tear of the medial meniscus in particular; and examination at operation will invariably reveal a synovial lesion in some degree. If the lesion is unimportant in so far as it resolves when the intruding meniscus is removed, it provides not only an explanation of the tenderness which is a well-known sign of the displaced longitudinal tear

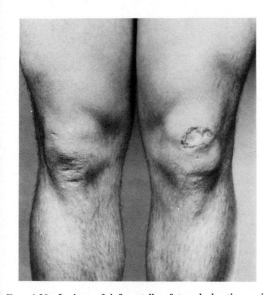

FIG. 4,30. **Lesions of infrapatellar fat pad.** In the male subject a unilateral fat pad lesion is invariably of exogenous traumatic origin. The injury which produced the scar over the patella was responsible also for hypertrophy of the fat pad (Fig. 4,30). Bilateral lesions are rare in the male; common in the female, see Chapter 12. When they occur in the male it is the result of endogenous mechanical trauma the result of recurvatus deformity.

but of, from compression and irritation of the synovial membrane, the small synovial effusion with which the lesion is associated.

**4. Recurvatus deformity.** It will be evident that whatever the cause, the biomechanical status of the joint in terms of recurvatus deformity will increase the liability to occurrence and recurrence. It appears that once the condition is firmly established whereby synovial fronds or villous protuberances have been subjected to trapping incidents with resulting fibrosis the process is irreversible so that symptoms occur with any increase of weight-bearing activity or, in the premenstrual water-retention syndrome, on every occasion in which the fat pad becomes oedematous.

### Synovial Lesion

It is probable that white-tipped tags, if they indicate incidents of trapping and particularly in the ageing joint, are without serious clinical significance. In other circumstances a wide variety of pathology is encountered. Surface haemorrhages, seen at every stage from the acute to the final state represented by deposits of haemosiderin, can be accepted to indicate repeated incidents of trapping (Fig. 4,34). Sometimes the surface is smooth but injected. At the other extreme are injected tags or fringes.

### Clinical Features

**Length of history.** There are few internal derangements so commonly missed or misdiagnosed. The history, therefore, is often of long duration. Patients have been offered so many manifestly incorrect diagnoses and received so much ineffective treatment that the prevailing attitude tends to be one of cynicism. In such circumstances the correct diagnosis may be regarded as one more to add to the list.

**Pain.** The salient feature is pain or deep ache in the anterior compartment directly related to physical activity and always relieved by rest. The pain is worst with the knee in full extension and relief obtained in slight flexion. Female patients are often aware that the use of high-heeled shoes affords relief; and that heel-less shoes induce symptoms.

**Swelling.** There is swelling on both sides of the patellar tendon by comparison with the normal side. It is greatest, occasionally with increase

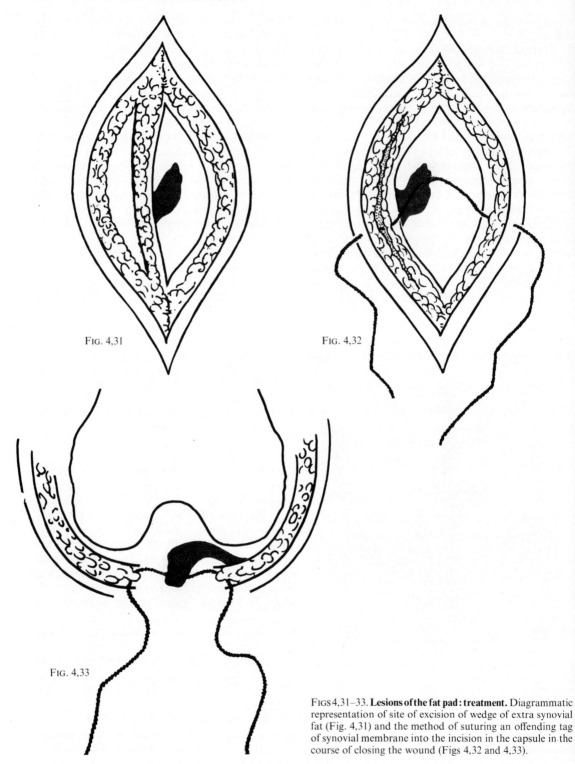

FIG. 4,31

FIG. 4,32

FIG. 4,33

FIGS 4,31–33. **Lesions of the fat pad: treatment.** Diagrammatic representation of site of excision of wedge of extra synovial fat (Fig. 4,31) and the method of suturing an offending tag of synovial membrane into the incision in the capsule in the course of closing the wound (Figs 4,32 and 4,33).

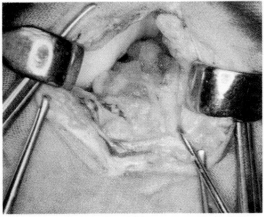

FIG. 4,34

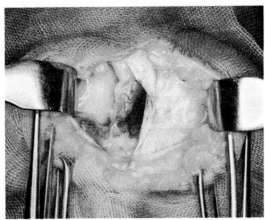

FIG. 4,35

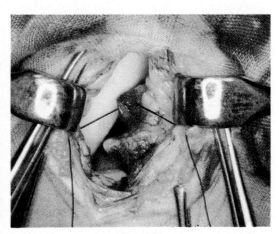

FIG. 4,36

FIGS 4,34–36. **Lesions of the fat pad: treatment.** The joint has been opened through a limited anteromedial incision as for meniscectomy. Multiple lesions of the lining synovial membrane recent and old as indicated by local haemosiderin staining (Fig. 4,34). The bulk of the extrasynovial fat is reduced by excision of a wedge of tissue. From right to left is seen capsule, blood stained area the site of excision of the wedge of fat, margin of synovial membrane and femoral condyle (Fig. 4,35). A suture has been passed through the largest synovial tag and outwards through the capsule on either side. When the suture is tied the tag will be stitched into the incision. Normally the suture is of absorbable material (Fig. 4,36).

of skin temperature, during an attack. A localised swelling to one or other side of the tendon usually has some other explanation.

It should be recognised that the prominent fat pad, in particular the prominence which occurs between patellar tendon and iliotibial band, is most obvious weight-bearing in complete extension; in other words with the patellar tendon pressed hard back against the fat pad and with the joint in hyperextension thus exerting the maximum extruding force. It will be noted that once the patient is under anaesthesia, in hyperextension, even in forced hyperextension, the prominence no longer exists.

**Synovial effusion.** There may be recurrent effusions related to physical activity the direct result of mechanical trauma to synovial membrane. If present, they are small in volume, are not of a size to cause inconvenience and subside rapidly with rest.

**Tenderness.** There is vague tenderness to deep pressure on the patellar tendon. In addition, forced extension by exerting compression on the synovial membrane induces pain or discomfort. Tenderness localised to the joint line usually has some other explanation (see 'Differential Diagnosis').

**Differential Diagnosis**

**1. Any space-occupying lesion.** In the experience on which opinions are based space-occupying lesions simulating swelling of the fat pad which have been encountered at operation include cystic degeneration of the anterior segment of either menisci, lipoma, synovioma and haemangioma.

**2. Internal derangements relative to the menisci.** It ought to be possible to differentiate lesions of the menisci, other than lesions of the anterior segment, and to which special reference is made below, from the fact that there is seldom any complaint other than pain; and the location of the pain is always in the anterior aspect of the joint. There are no symptoms of instability which would direct attention to a rotatory mechanism. Finally, and in view of the frequency with which the condition is encountered in the female subject, the high incidence of errors of diagnosis relative to the menisci should be recalled.

**3. Lesion of anterior segment of meniscus.** Statistics, compiled over the years, show that lesions of the anterior segment of a meniscus are comparatively rare. When they occur it is usually in a joint the site of recurvatus deformity the same conformation liable to a fat pad lesion and for the same reason. In the female knee in particular the possibility of a meniscus lesion should be considered.

Reference has been made (Ch. 1) to the importance of the localisation of tenderness; and that one centimetre or so may make all the difference between one diagnosis and another. A lesion of the anterior segment of a meniscus in the differential diagnosis of fat pad lesions is such an example. In a fat pad lesion the swelling may be on one or other or both sides of the patellar tendon and the tenderness at the same sites or to pressure on the tendon. In the meniscus lesion the tenderness is accurately located to the joint line usually, but not always, to the medial side of the tendon.

**4. Chondromalacia patellae.** (See Ch. 2.)

**5. Jumper's knee.** (See Ch. 2.)

**6. Recurrent subluxation of the patella.** (See Ch. 2.)

Fat pad lesions as a direct complication of transplantation of the patellar tendon are referred to in Chapter 2.

## Fat Pad Lesions in the Male

In the male, as opposed to the female, fat pad lesions are relatively uncommon. The unilateral cases are usually the result of a single incident of trauma of a degree likely to be recalled (Fig. 4,30). In spite of the frequency of road traffic accidents in which both knees come in contact with the dashboard of a car this source of persistent symptom seems to be relatively uncommon. A bilateral variety is occasionally encountered in the teenage male and is frequently the source of misdiagnosis. It is directly the result of the mechanical compression forces imposed by genu recurvatum; and the fact that this deformity is accompanied by patella alta may divert attention erroneously to the patellofemoral joint. In a proportion of these cases the basis of the deformity is a hereditary disorder of connective tissue; and evidence of this should be sought in the metacarpo-phalangeal and elbow joints.

### TREATMENT

**Reassurance.** Reference is made under 'Premenstrual Water Retention Syndrome' in Chapter 12 to the favourable effect which the establishment of a rational diagnosis and explanation of symptoms which, to the patient's resentment, may have been declared to be imaginary. This may be all the treatment necessary. On the other hand there is evidence that fat pad lesions in chronic form may be of more pathological significance than a source of pain in the knee joint. When the lesion has existed for many years it is seen at operation that in addition to fibrous tags and general fibrosis in the synovial membrane posterior to the fat pad, there are opposing changes in the femoral condyles; and these degenerative changes in the articular cartilage appear to be related to the severity of the symptoms and the chronicity of the changes in the synovial membrane.

The following is an example of such a case:

The patient (Mrs E.H., aged 36), was first seen by the author with symptoms of long duration in both knees. Various diagnoses had been attached and various methods of treatment in the form of physiotherapy had been tried without relief. As is so common in bilateral cases in the female without an obvious clinical diagnosis she had received little sympathy. The diagnosis of fat pad lesions was made. No note was made of the possibility of the premenstrual water retention syndrome. If there had been such a relationship it would have been in the more distant past. That the external swelling was of noteworthy size was shown by the record on her case-sheet that the swelling was such as to be capable of photographic record.

The patient, shortly after she was seen, left for another country and did not return until four years later when she again consulted the author. She reminded him of his diagnosis and of the fact that having had the satisfaction of being given a positive diagnosis and the cause of her pain explained, she had accepted the situation and not sought the recommended surgical measures elsewhere. Her symptoms, however, had not subsided and she was now prepared to accept the recommended operation.

Examination showed a markedly large fat pad on the left side which protruded in considerably greater measure than usual through the weak area between the patellar tendon and the iliotibial tract, but was also prominent on the medial side of the patellar tendon. On the right side, that in which symptoms were more severe, the swelling was less evident though the fat pad was abnormally large. There was tenderness to deep pressure on both sides.

At operation the right knee was opened, keeping to the rule of operating on the side with the greater symptomatology first. There were numerous white fibrous tags and a granular fibrotic surface on the lining of the synovial membrane. There was a rough area in the form of chondromalacia on the medial femoral condyle opposing the fibrous tags. On the left side, that of the lesser symptoms, the fibrous tags were even more marked and the degenerate area on the condyle considerably further advanced.

The fat pad lesion was dealt with in the manner to be described.

**Conservative.** There are no effective conservative measures other than quadriceps exercises and the raising of the heels of the shoes. The former will be indicated if rest in excess, leading to quadriceps wasting, has been prescribed. Quadriceps insufficiency renders the joint liable to trapping incidents. Quadriceps exercises will not be indicated in recurvatus deformities. In such circumstances the use of raised heels to prevent hyperextension may be indicated. In the rare instances of bilateral symptoms due to recurvatus deformities in the male, the permanent use of raised heels may be indicated.

**Operative.** The purpose of operation is reduction of the volume of the extrasynovial fat while at the same time protruding synovial tags, if present, are rendered incapable of involvement in trapping incidents. Originally synovial tags were excised; but the raw area so produced was not subjected to compression by the postoperative compression bandage, with the result that a haemarthrosis was liable to occur and consequent retardation of recovery. It is not known whether this hazard could have been overcome by the use of suction drainage. The technique to be described buries a vascular tag or tags in such a manner that the risk of haemarthrosis is virtually eliminated.

TECHNIQUE. The operation is performed under tourniquet with the knee flexed over the end of the table as for meniscectomy. The incisions too, medial or lateral, are those for meniscectomy. On entering the extrasynovial fat, fibrosis, usually indicating a single incident of trauma, is readily distinguished from normal tissue and will in such circumstances confirm a pre-operative diagnosis.

The incision in the synovial membrane extends down as far as, but avoids damage to, the superior surface of the meniscus. The anterior segment of the meniscus is not detached nor mobilised. When the synovial layer is divided, retractors are introduced and the posterior aspect of the fat pad inspected. Lesions of the synovial membrane likely to be responsible for the train of symptoms are readily identified. In other circumstances difficulty may be encountered. It is a matter of deciding whether an error of diagnosis has been committed or whether other pathology exists in the anterior compartment. In this respect reference has been made in terms of differential diagnosis to the possibility of a lesion of the anterior segment of the meniscus. In the circumstances in which such pathology might exist, namely, recurvatus deformity, the anterior segment should be tested for excessive mobility and examined for a possible lesion of the substance of the fibro-cartilage.

The fat pad is reduced in volume by the excision of a wedge of tissue in the area between capsule and synovial membrane (Figs 4,33 and 4,35). In removing the wedge of fat, care should be taken to direct the knife blade laterally rather than towards the centre of the joint. There is the tendency to cut towards the synovial membrane and re-enter the joint cavity.

If synovial tags are present they are not excised but stitched into the incision so that they no longer protrude into the joint cavity. This is accomplished by passing an absorbable suture through the capsule and extrasynovial fat down to synovial membrane, then through the tag and to the exterior again through the extrasynovial fat and capsule (Figs 4,32, 4,33 and 4,36). When the suture is tied the tag, pointing outwards, will be stitched into the extrasynovial fat. The joint is closed otherwise as for meniscectomy.

*After-treatment.* At the termination of the operation a compression bandage is applied. Quadriceps exercises are deferred to the fourth day when the danger of provoking haemarthrosis has passed. Dorsiflexion and plantar flexion exercises of the foot are practised immediately. The operation does not interfere with the mechanism of the joint. Weight-bearing may be resumed on the tenth day. Recovery is rapid.

## OSSIFYING CHONDROMA OF INFRAPATELLAR FAT PAD

**Definition.** An intracapsular or para-articular chondroma occurs from metaplasia in the fibrous capsule or adjacent connective tissue of a joint (Jaffe, 1958). In the knee a common situation is the infrapatellar fat pad where it may undergo degeneration, calcify and even ossify.

**Clinical features.** The patient, an adult, presents with aching or discomfort and a pain from enlarging mass in the infrapatellar region. On examination the mass of bony consistency presents on one or other sides of the patellar tendon. If the mass is large there may be limitation of extension and of flexion. The final diagnosis depends on the appearance of the radiograph in the lateral view (Figs 4,37 and 4,38).

**Differential diagnosis.** The condition is to be distinguished from the many other conditions producing a radio-opaque mass in the region of the anterior compartment of the knee. Among these will be numbered osteochondromatosis of the prepatellar bursa (Figs 4,8 and 4,9), a loose body invaginated into the pad and lying within a synovial cavity (Figs 4,24 to 4,26), calcification of a haematoma, heterotopic bone in patellar tendon, loose bodies in the bursa deep to the patellar tendon and the grosser forms of traction epiphysitis of the tibial tubercle with separation of bony fragments. The differential diagnosis is of academic rather than practical interest: the majority of the lesions if producing symptoms demand the same treatment, namely, excision.

TECHNIQUE OF EXCISION. The operation is performed under tourniquet with the knee flexed over the end of the table as for meniscectomy but with the ability to extend the joint if it is necessary to relax the patellar tendon. The length of incision depends on the size of the mass and is located to the side of maximum prominence. In general the incision need be little longer than required for meniscectomy. The mass is usually intracapsular within the fat pad and extrasynovial; and in such circumstances the joint should not be entered. The necessity to remove one or both menisci to achieve complete extirpation has been described (Mosher, Kettel-kamp and Campbell, 1966).

## OTHER LOCAL LESIONS OF SYNOVIAL MEMBRANE

Local lesions of synovial membrane are most common in the anterior compartment immediately posterior to the fat pad. The mechanical trapping of synovial fringes is, however, by no means confined to this area. They occur at other sites, the most common of which is the medial margin of the medial femoral condyle, the lateral margin of the lateral femoral condyle, the margin of the patello-femoral joint, particularly on the lateral side, and at the superior margins of both femoral condyles where fringes of synovial membrane may be trapped by the patella, particularly in patella alta. These tags take the form of sessile or pedunculated masses of synovial membrane which become the subject

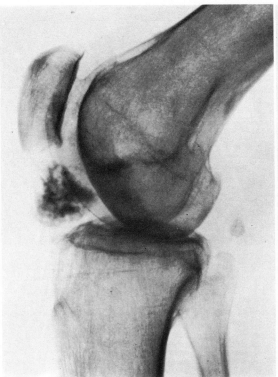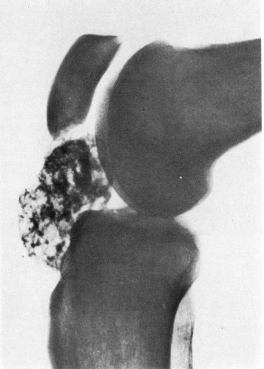

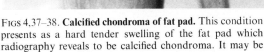

FIGS 4,37–38. **Calcified chondroma of fat pad.** This condition presents as a hard tender swelling of the fat pad which radiography reveals to be calcified chondroma. It may be moulded by the biomechanical forces involved (Fig. 4,37) or may assume massive proportions (Fig. 4,38).

of mechanical trauma and as a result hypertrophy so that, once initiated, the condition tends to the production of progressive symptoms.

The synovial mass which may be located on the supramedial margin of the medial femoral condyle is of particular interest. There is at this site in the normal joint a flap of synovial tissue which overlies the articular cartilage (Figs 4,39 and 4,40). It is not difficult to imagine that such a flap might readily be interposed between patella and condyle in some action of rotation or, rubbing against the prominent margin of the condyle, become hypertrophied (Figs 4,41 and 4,42). Attention has been directed elsewhere (Ch. 6) to the fact that this is the site of the earliest and most marked destruction of articular cartilage in rheumatoid arthritis and with the suggestion that the proximity of this flap of synovial tissue may be a factor in a multifactorial situation.

It will be evident that any condition producing abnormality of synovial membrane in the form of swelling will be more liable to this complication than a normal joint. It is thus a complication of osteoarthrosis, burnt-out rheumatoid arthritis, or even rheumatoid arthritis in active form.

**Rheumatoid arthritis.** In relation to synovial tags producing interference with movement at the margin of the condyles it should be noted that similar mechanical incidents have been ascribed to so-called rheumatoid nodules. The site of the nodule is in the margin of the lateral femoral condyle and may be a source of a mass which appears to jump or slip in and out of position with flexion and extension of the joint. These nodules are said to consist of typical rheumatoid granulation tissue with characteristic necrotic centre surrounded by palisades of fibroblasts which, in turn, are surrounded by a loose infiltrate of plasma cells and lymphocytes (Chamberlain, 1971).

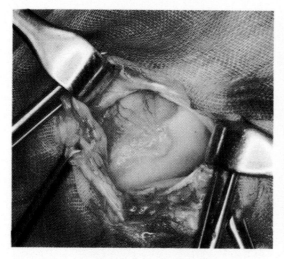

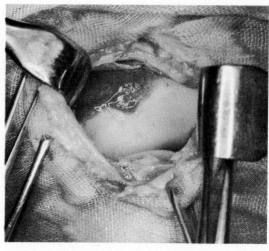

FIGS 4,39–40. **Synovial fringe.** THERE is frequently a fringe of normal synovial membrane at the supramedial aspect of the medial femoral condyle at the anterior limit of the arc of weight-bearing. At this particular site it is liable to be trapped between patella and condyle or between femoral and tibial condyle with resulting pain and local tenderness. Once this has occurred the tag hypertrophies and may be the source of mysterious recurring small effusions. The site is the location of the earliest and most marked destruction in rheumatoid arthritis; and it is postulated that this flap of synovial membrane may be responsible.

Two photographs to show nature of flap and constancy of site, quiescent (Fig. 4,39) and inflamed (Fig. 4,40).

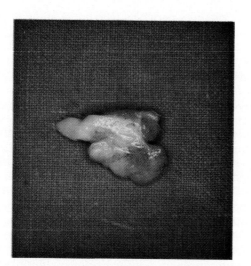

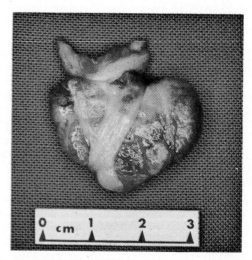

FIGS 4,41–42. **'Simple synovioma': 'localised nodular synovitis'.** Both these pedunculated synovial tumours arose at the supramedial margin of the medial femoral condyle and are thought to have arisen in the constant flap of synovial membrane referred to in Figures 4,39 and 4,40. Both were said to be a 'simple synovioma'. This is a diagnosis unacceptable to Jaffé (see Ch. 13). They are probably the so-called 'localised nodular synovitis'.

CLINICAL FEATURES. The usual complaint is of local mechanical incidents of catching, giving-way or momentarily locking; and the sites located to the margins of the femoral condyles or the patello-femoral joint. Incidents may be followed by a small transient synovial effusion. In these superficial situations the patient is usually aware of the site of the pathology; and some learn the means of disengaging a trapped tag from the patello-femoral joint. In rare instances the offending tag is located internally to be trapped between tibia and femur to produce a situation likely to be confused with lesions of the menisci.

TREATMENT. Excision under tourniquet through a limited exposure can be expected to afford relief even when the local lesion is a complication of more widespread pathology.

## REFERENCES

ADAMS, R. (1840). Chronic rheumatoid arthritis of the knee joint. *Dublin Journal of Medical Science*, **17**, 520.

ANDREWS, J. R. (1978). Arthroscopy of the plicae—synovial folds and their significance. *The American Journal of Sports Medicine*, vol. **6**, no. **5**, 217.

BAKER, W. M. (1877). On the formation of synovial cysts in the leg in connection with disease of knee joint. *St Bartholomew's Hospital Report*, **13**, 245.

BURLESON, R. J., BICKEL, W. H. & DAHLIN, D. C. (1956). Popliteal cyst—a clinical survey. *Journal of Bone and Joint Surgery*, **38A**, 1265.

CHAMBERLAIN, M. A. (1971). Intra-articular rheumatoid nodules of the knee. *Journal of Bone and Joint Surgery*, **53B**, 3, 507.

CHILDRESS, H. M. (1970). Popliteal cysts associated with undiagnosed posterior lesions of the medial meniscus. *Journal of Bone and Joint Surgery*, **52A**, 7, 1487.

DAVIES, D. V. & WHITE, J. E. W. (1961). The structure and weight of synovial fat pads. *Journal of Anatomy*, **45A**, 1241.

DINHAM, J. M. (1975). Popliteal cysts in children. *Journal of Bone and Joint Surgery*, **57B**, 69.

DUPUYTREN, G. (1829). Hydarthrose énorme du genu. La Clinique Hum. de Med. Univ. (Paris), **1**, 251.

EASTCOTT, H. H. G. (1969). *Arterial Surgery*. London: Pitman.

FREEMAN, M. A. R. & WYKE, B. (1967). The innervation of the knee joint. *Journal of Anatomy*, **101**, 3, 505.

GRISTINA, A. G. & WILSON, P. D. (1963). Popliteal cysts in adults and children: a review of ninety operative cases. *Journal of Bone and Joint Surgery*, **45A**, 1552.

HOFFA, A. (1904). The influence of the adipose tissue with regard to the pathology of the knee joint. *Journal of the American Medical Association*, **43**, 795.

JAFFE, H. L. (1958). *Tumors and Tumorous Conditions of the Bones and Joints*, 558–567. Philadelphia: Lea & Febiger.

MacMAHON, E. B. (1973). Baker's cysts in children—is surgery necessary? *Journal of Bone and Joint Surgery*, **55A**, 1311.

MEIGS, J. V., ARMSTRONG, S. H. & HAMILTON, H. H. (1943). Further contributions to the syndrome of fibroma of the ovary with fluid in abdomen and chest, Meigs' syndrome. *American Journal of Obstetrics and Gynecology*, **46**, 19.

MOSHER, J. F., KETTELKAMP, D. B. & CAMPBELL, C. J. (1966). Intracapsular or para-articular chondroma. *Journal of Bone and Joint Surgery*, **48A**, 8, 1561.

*Notes on the Diagnosis of Occupational Diseases* prescribed under the National Insurance (Industrial Injuries) Act, 1965, 5th edition, November 1972. Published by Her Majesty's Stationery Office (SBN 11 760312 0) London, W.C1.

PATEL, D. (1978). Arthroscopy of the plicae—synovial folds and their significance. *The American Journal of Sports Medicine*, vol. **6**, no. **5**, 217.

PIPKIN, G. (1971). Knee injuries: the role of the suprapatellar plica and suprapatellar bursa in simulating internal derangements. *Clinical Orthopaedics*, **74**, 161.

QUAYLE, J. B. & ROBINSON, M. P. (1976). An operation for chronic prepatellar bursitis. *Journal of Bone and Joint Surgery*, **58B**, 504.

SHARRARD, W. J. W. (1961). Haemobursa in kneeling miners. *Proceedings of the Royal Society of Medicine*, **54**, 1103.

SYMEONIDES, P. P. & PASCHALOGLOU, C. (1970). Localised hypertrophy of the semimembranosus muscle simulating popliteal cyst. *Journal of Bone and Joint Surgery*, **52B**, 337.

WILSON, P. O., EYRE-BROOK, A. L. & FRANCIS, J. D. (1938). A clinical and anatomical tudy of the semi-membranous bursa in relation to popliteal cyst. *Journal of Bone and Joint Surgery*, **20**, 936.

# 5.  Infective Arthritis

## OSTEOMYELITIS OF INFANCY

**Background note.** Osteomyelitis of the long bones in infancy at one time incurred a serious threat to life. Green and Shannon (1936) reported a series of 95 cases in which the overall mortality was 21 per cent: 44 per cent of those under the age of 6 months died. If the advent of chemotherapy has reduced this high mortality, by the same token the problems posed by survival have increased in terms of angular deformity and shortening.

The importance of infection of bone at this age, in relation to the future form and function of the joint, is the frequency with which an epiphysis is damaged or destroyed by an abscess or by the complication of suppurative arthritis.

### Pathological Anatomy

Trueta (1959) showed that in infants of 6 months or thereabouts the metaphyseal vessels penetrate the growth plate to terminate as dilated sinusoids within the epiphysis. Infection in the metaphyseal region may thus produce an abscess within the epiphysis and/or result in suppurative arthritis. In the older child the metaphyseal vessels do not penetrate the growth plate and infection tends to remain localised to the metaphysis.

The extent of the damage within the epiphysis is probably determined by the blood supply. Crock (1967) showed that the blood supply to the lower end of the femur and the upper end of the tibia in the infant arises from the medial genicular, lateral genicular and intercondylar arteries. There are thus three areas without vascular communication. The radiological defects in the epiphysis appear to correspond to these areas. The defect may be on the medial or on the lateral side or there may be defects on both sides. In the last, a central area may persist unchanged, probably dependent upon the intercondylar artery (Roberts, 1970). Crock (1967) demonstrated too that the genicular and radiate

epiphyseal arteries are closely applied to the periosteum over the epiphysis. When the periosteum is raised by pus it may be that these vessels are occluded and the related area of epiphysis rendered ischaemic. In certain cases the apparent defect in the epiphysis may be due to ischaemia and not due to an abscess. In these cases regeneration could be almost, if not wholly, complete.

It is important, therefore, to recognise that regeneration of an epiphysis damaged by infection can occur (Figs 5,1 to 5,4). Hall (1954) first reported the case of a child in whom the lower femoral epiphysis, damaged by infection in infancy, showed regeneration at the age of 7 years. Reference will be made later under infective arthritis, and to the regeneration of the femoral epiphysis, recorded by Lloyd-Roberts (1960) which, as will be evident, cannot be demarcated in result from osteomyelitis.

### Clinical Findings

**Interval to onset.** In a recent series of 15 cases (Roberts, 1970) infection is known to have been present within 6 weeks of birth. The shortest interval after birth was 11 days.

**Organism.** *Staphylococcus aureus,* as in suppurative arthritis, is the usual organism encountered. In the Green and Shannon (1936) series, the infecting organism in 63 per cent of the cases was a streptococcus and in 30 per cent a staphylococcus.

**Source.** Septicaemia from umbilical sepsis, bronco-pneumonia or gastro-enteritis, etc. precedes the infection. In other examples the source may not be evident.

**Site.** The lower end of the femur is more commonly affected than the upper end of the tibia.

**Examination.** There is general toxicity and febrile response of considerable degree with swelling about the joint, increase of local temperature and sensitivity to pressure.

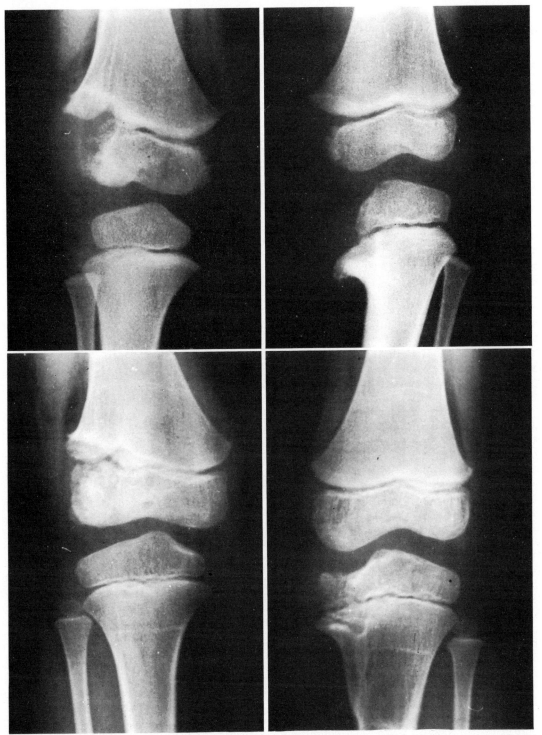

FIGS 5,1–4. **Suppurative arthritis in infancy: osteomyelitis. Sequelae of infection.** Apparent destruction of the lateral half of lower femoral epiphysis on right with partial destruction of medial half of upper tibial epiphysis on left resulting in varus angulation (Figs 5,1 and 5,2). The same knees two years later. The lateral half of the lower femoral epiphysis has regenerated (Fig. 5,3). Partial regeneration of the medial half of the upper tibial epiphysis following osteotomy below tibial tubercle to correct varus angulation (Fig. 5,4) (E.A., male, case of G.M.).

## Treatment

**Immediate.** In the knowledge that the staphylococcus or streptococcus are the most likely organisms involved, the first line of treatment in the current scene is the systemic administration of the appropriate antibiotic.

If destruction of the epiphysis is due to ischaemia rather than the direct result of infection, operative decompression of a tension situation in the form of an abscess within the bone or of suppurative arthritis is imperative. It has been pointed out that in infancy infection subsides rapidly and that sequestra form rarely (Green and Shannon, 1936). At this age bone has a large soft tissue content and, as a result, is less rigid. The cortical bone of the metaphysis is thin and the loose attachment of the periosteum permits decompression of an abscess within the bone. Necrotic tissue is readily absorbed and healing is rapid.

**Late.** It is not possible to lay down hard and fast rules for the treatment of a situation determined by the possibility of recovery of the epiphysis after a delay of several years. The necessity for treatment is determined by the conformation and function of the limb. In the early stages the radiographic appearances may be deceptive and suggest that damage to the epiphysis is irreparable. In such circumstances care should be exercised in regard to radical surgical measures. It has been the author's experience, however, confirmed by others (Roberts, 1970), that plaster casts and/or caliper splints do not control a deformity which may occur as early as 18 months. In such circumstances osteotomy, repeated as necessary, may be required to control a situation, such as depicted in Figures 5,5 to 5,8, and which may terminate in arthrodesis or amputation.

SHORTENING. In all cases there is some shortening of the limb. It is naturally greatest when the epiphyses on both sides of the joint are affected; and in such circumstances may be considerable. When the mature state is reached it is probable that equalisation of leg length by shortening of the normal leg should not be attempted in the presence of a grossly abnormal joint or of arthrodesis. When such conditions prevail, amputation, as was the eventual outcome of the case depicted in Figures 5,5 to 5,8,

may provide a solution acceptable on both functional and cosmetic grounds if an efficient artificial limb service is available.

## OSTEOMYELITIS OF PATELLA

**Background note.** Thirion (1829) was the first to record a case. In the next 100 years only 50 cases were reported (Rocher, 1923). There are occasional cases in the experience of most orthopaedic surgeons and a few have been reported, for example, one, by Kirby-Smith (1942) and five, by Evans (1962). The author, apart from examples the result of a gunshot wound (Fig. 5,9), can recall three cases only, two in children, and one in recent years, the case recorded below.

### Clinical Features

**Age.** The condition is most common between the ages of 5 and 12; and this is explained by the fact that before 5 the patella is cartilagenous and that vascularisation is maximum at 12 to decline at 16 when ossification is complete.

**Aetiology.** Injury has been a feature of a large proportion of reported cases and in the example recorded below.

**Organism.** *Staphylococcus aureus,* as in suppurative arthritis, is the usual organism encountered.

**Complications.** It will be evident that spread of infection to the immediately adjacent knee joint is the common complication. It is said that spread to the joint is more common in adults than in children and explained by the resistance to penetration of the thick layer of cartilage which exists in children between the bony element and the joint cavity.

### Differential Diagnosis

In acute form the patient presents with pain and inflammation over the anterior aspect of the patella. The knee may be held in extension to reduce tension in a swelling anterior to the bone. If there is an associated synovial effusion the joint may be held in slight flexion. There is an acute systemic reaction. The most likely diagnosis appears to be acute prepatellar bursitis;

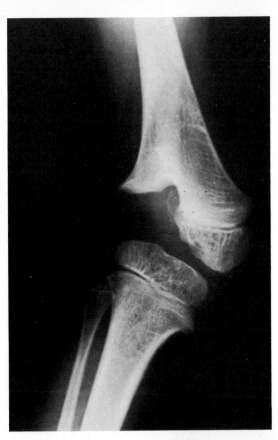

FIGS 5,5–8. **Suppurative arthritis in infancy.** Infection at age 1 month resulted in destruction of the lateral femoral condyle and a gross angular deformity at age 8 (Figs 5,5 and 5,6). This was corrected by osteotomy (Fig. 5,7) and repeated until eventually arthrodesis was performed. At age 13 shortening amounted to 5 in (12·5 cm) (Fig. 5,8). This case terminated with amputation on cosmetic grounds (H.H., male, first seen age 8).

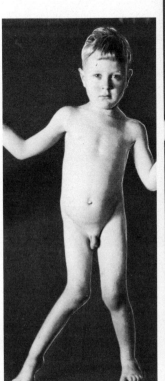

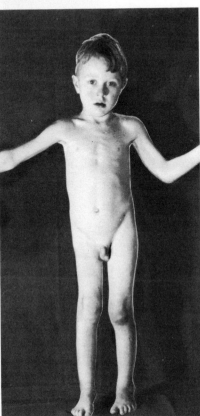

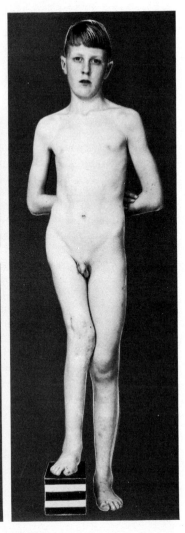

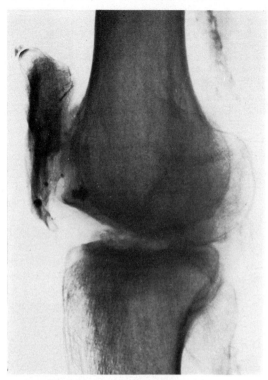

FIG. 5,9. **Osteomyelitis of patella.** Old infective arthritis secondary to osteomyelitis of patella the result of gunshot wound in World War I (G.P., male, aged 72).

and it is only when the condition fails to subside, or radiographs of appropriate projection taken, that the diagnosis is established.

In subacute or chronic form the diagnosis of some form of arthritis is the most common error in a situation which may be masked by the previous administration of antibiotics. The blood supply of the bone is critical and thus the formation of sequestra is common. The true diagnosis may not be established until a skyline radiograph is obtained (Figs 5,10 and 5,11). It is probable that underlying pathology is more often established in children, in whom osteomyelitis is common and prepatellar bursitis rare, than in the adult in whom prepatellar bursitis is common; and this is another reason why infection spreads to the joint in the adult.

## Treatment

An attempt should be made to identify the organism if antibiotics have not been given prior

to presentation of the case. In other circumstances a broad spectrum antibiotic is given. Surgical drainage of an abscess and the removal of sequestra may be necessary. It has been recorded that with antibiotic therapy apparent radiological sequestra can be reincorporated (Evans, 1962). Every effort should be made to avoid the necessity for patellectomy.

The following is the record of a case to demonstrate the delay, difficulty and doubts in diagnosis:

The patient (C.MacK., male, aged 9, case of Mr A. Morrison, Inverness, Scotland) gave a history of having fallen on the ice five weeks previously. Thereafter the right knee was painful and swollen. He rested at home and after a few days, as the joint was still swollen, his general practitioner was called. He found a large effusion in the joint. This was treated with a compression bandage and rest. The

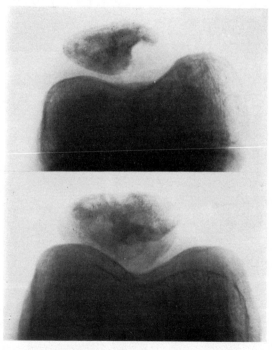

FIGS 5,10–11. **Osteomyelitis of patella.** Appearance of patella one year after original infection (Fig. 5,10). Appearance two years after original infection. Regeneration has occurred and the defect eliminated (Fig. 5,11) (C.MacK., male, aged 9 at time of infection—case of Mr A. Morrison, Inverness, Scotland).

joint was not aspirated. After two weeks the swelling had subsided, but the knee would not fully extend. It was at this stage that he was referred to hospital.

On examination the knee was held in 50° of flexion. It was swollen and hot. The swelling was synovial in origin; not the result of effusion. The quadriceps was wasted; and particularly vastus medialis.

Preliminary laboratory investigations revealed: ESR 101 mm/h. Hb. 85 per cent WBC 7075.

The patient was admitted to hospital with the provisional diagnosis of osteomyelitis of patella. Treatment consisted of traction in a Thomas bed-knee splint and the administration of wide spectrum antibiotics.

On the day after admission aspiration of the knee was attempted under general anaesthesia. No fluid was obtained. The organism was never identified.

At the end of one month doubt was cast on the diagnosis of osteomyelitis of the patella. The radiological appearance was said to suggest post-traumatic osteoporosis. It was at this stage and with doubt cast on the original diagnosis that knee flexion exercises were begun.

Three weeks later 80° of flexion had been achieved. It was at this time that he was permitted to return home. One month later examination showed that flexion had not increased. Extension was limited by 20°. A long leg caliper was prescribed. Three months later flexion had increased to 100°. There was a minimal extension lag. The caliper was discarded.

One year later he was playing football but suffered retropatellar pain (Fig. 5,10). He was last seen two years from the date of the original infection continuing to play football without difficulty. He complained of occasional retropatellar pain (Fig. 5,11).

## ACUTE SUPPURATIVE ARTHRITIS

**Incidence.** The knee is the joint most commonly involved in infective arthritis of whatever origin.
**Organism:** *Staphylococcus aureus* is the infecting organism in the majority of cases. But a wide variety of organisms may be implicated. In a review of 1077 cases of septic arthritis reported between 1905 and 1969, 22 different causative organisms were involved (Nolan, Leers and Schatzker, 1972). Limited reference will be made to the special features of some of the less common infections later in the section.

### Predisposing Factors: General

PRE-EXISTING INFECTION. In the infant, septicaemia arising from umbilical sepsis is the common cause of infection. In the adult such conditions as furunculosis or pneumonia are sources likely to be encountered.
ADMINISTRATION OF SYSTEMIC CORTICOSTEROIDS.
DIABETES MELLITUS.

### Predisposing Factors: Local

TRAUMA. Under this heading is included accidental wounds including gunshot wounds. In less dramatic circumstances is the introduction of infection by needle, arthroscope or operation.

A minor incident of trauma not necessarily involving even an abrasion of the skin is common in children and as always in this age range is a factor difficult to assess.
PRE-EXISTING JOINT DISEASE. The most common disease liable to this complication is rheumatoid arthritis.
INTRA-ARTICULAR INJECTION OF CORTICOSTEROIDS.

### Clinical Features

In the child there is a febrile illness with irritability, pain in the knee and refusal to bear weight. The joint is swollen with effusion and periarticular thickening. It is held in flexion with marked limitation of movement. Gentle palpation reveals an increase of local temperature and acute tenderness to pressure. In general toxicity and febrile response is less than experienced in acute osteomyelitis.
**Differential diagnosis.** In the child, trauma, with which it may be associated and accompanied by acute synovitis or haemarthrosis, is an obvious difficulty. In middle age, gout, pseudogout and

an exacerbation of rheumatoid arthritis, etc. are possibilities to be considered. When the condition occurs in the course of steroid therapy or if antibiotics have been administered before a diagnosis is made the major disorder is masked. Reference will be made to forms of 'chronic arthritis' thought to arise in this way.

**Laboratory investigation.** There is as a rule a polymorphonuclear leucocytosus and a raised ESR.

**Radiology.** Radiographs in the acute stage show no more than effusion and periarticular swelling. In infancy at a later stage there may be appearances suggestive of destruction of epiphysis, epiphyseal plate and extending into the metaphysis (Fig. 5,1). In late or neglected cases findings range through osteoporosis to loss of joint space indicating damage to articular cartilage, eventual destruction of the joint surfaces (Fig. 5,24) and finally bony ankylosis (Fig. 5,15).

**Diagnosis.** In theory diagnosis depends on the identification of the organism from cultures made of fluid aspirated from the joint. In practice the outcome of attempted culture is disappointing due to the prior administration of antibiotics; and this is the reason for the necessity to use a broad spectrum antibiotic in treatment.

ASPIRATION. In infancy and from adolescence onwards a local anaesthetic may be used. Between the ages of 1 and, say, 10, a general anaesthetic is necessary. For technique of aspiration see Chapter 1.

## TREATMENT

The traditional principles on which treatment is based are the administration of antibiotics, immobilisation and drainage. Opinion is unanimous only in the desirability, indeed necessity, for the administration of antibiotics.

### Antibiotics

In the current scene most patients have been given antibiotics on the first suspicion of infection. In general, therefore, a broad-spectrum antibiotic is administered until such time as the appropriate specific antibiotic is established from the result of the culture of aspirated material. This is continued until the ESR has returned to normal or for, say, 6 weeks.

### Drainage

The method to be applied differs widely between repeated aspiration, aspiration and irrigation, continuous perfusion and finally, operative arthrotomy with or without open drainage. Each has advantages and disadvantages. Selection of the method will depend on the requirements of the individual case pursued with the knowledge that in the infant the danger to the growth plate is greater than in the older child; and that at all ages the future function of the joint is dependent on the outcome of treatment.

**Aspiration.** This diagnostic measure is necessary to establish the nature of the invading organism. Repeated therapeutic aspiration, however, is disturbing particularly to a young child due to the number of general anaesthetics which may be required. Such considerations have influenced the use of closed irrigation or continuous perfusion as an alternative.

The technique is described in Chapter 1.

**Continuous perfusion** or **suction irrigation**. This alternative to repeated aspiration, with or without the installation of antibiotics, remains a matter of controversy. It is considered to be a potential source of contamination in open wounds of the joint (Patzakis *et al.*, 1975) but even in the presence of established infection should probably not be continued for more than 5 to 7 days lest a sinus develop.

TECHNIQUE. The largest diameter of polythene vein catheter is used. The needle is inserted under local anaesthetic and, after confirmation of the purulent nature of the contents of the joint, the tube is inserted through the needle and the needle withdrawn. A second tube is inserted in the same manner. The tubes are strapped to the skin to prevent them from slipping or from being pulled out. One is connected to the inflow bottle of saline containing the antibiotic of choice, and the joint perfused with 3 litres every 24 hours. The second is connected to a sterile drainage bottle from which the aspirated fluid can be sent for culture, etc.

Skin traction is applied below the knee and the limb placed in a Thomas bed-knee splint (Galasko, 1966).

**Immobilisation.** The method of immobilisation depends on the method of drainage selected (but see below). In general, it takes the form of skin extension applied below the joint and a light padded gutter splint, or half-ring Thomas bed-knee splint in older children and adults. After 10 to 14 days a plaster cast is applied. Weight-bearing should be deferred until the joint is of normal appearance which seldom occurs until 6 to 8 weeks have elapsed. The systemic antibiotic, whether specific or broad spectrum if the infecting organism has not been identified, should be continued for the same period.

**Open drainage.** If doubt exists as to the adequacy of other methods, open drainage may be necessary. Opinions differ both as to method and management. It will be evident that a joint with a suprapatellar pouch, intercondylar notch, so-called medial and lateral compartments with recesses to either side and perhaps, most obviously, a posterior compartment cannot possibly be drained even with four separate incisions (Cleveland, 1956) when the limb is immobilised with the patient in the supine position. Such considerations prompted, as early as World War I, the breaking with tradition by the use of active movement in the upright position (Willems, 1919). The poor results of treatment, in terms of joint function, by traditional methods have stimulated a revival of interest in drainage by active movement. Ballard *et al.* (1975) believe that the indications for open arthrotomy and early motion are: (1) untreated suppurative arthritis of more than 72 hours duration; (2) an infected knee that has not responded to other forms of treatment; (3) an infected penetrating wound of the joint; and (4) a post-operative infection. In addition, synovectomy is performed if the synovium is found to be: (1) grossly necrotic; (2) grossly thickened to the point of impeding motion or encroaching on articular cartilage; and (3) grossly infected with abscess formation. The method, of which the author has no personal experience, is presented as a possible salvage procedure in the adult knee.

TECHNIQUE. Medial and lateral parapatellar incisions are made from the level of the superior pole to about 1 cm below the joint line. The capsule and synovial membrane is incised in the line of the skin incisions. The infrapatellar fat pad is avoided by curving the inferior limits of the capsular incision backwards. The exudation of purulent material from the synovial membrane as it is incised indicates abscess formation and an indication for anterior synovectomy. To this end the capsular incisions are extended upwards and backwards some 4 cm. The menisci are not removed unless extensively damaged by trauma or by the infectious process. The fat pad is excised only if grossly infected. The final step is irrigation with saline to remove fibrin clots, foreign matter and loose fragments of bone and cartilage.

The wounds are left open on both sides, dressed with fine mesh gauze and a voluminous compression bandage applied.

**After-treatment.** The absorptive bandage is removed after 24 hours in favour of a less bulky dressing held in place by a crepe bandage. It is at this early stage that the patient stands by the bedside and active assisted movements carried out. In the absence of intra-articular fractures weight-bearing, during which the knee is flexed in normal fashion, is encouraged. If after 7 days flexion is less than 70 degrees the joint is manipulated under anaesthesia after which movement, assuming the upright position, is resumed.

**Results of treatment.** The wounds heal by secondary intention usually in 4 to 6 weeks but in some cases take as long as 4 months. In the series of 34 patients treated by the method described 16 had a good result (a painless range of more than 90°); 12 had a fair result (30° to 90° of movement causing some restriction of activity); and 6 had a poor result (less than 30° of flexion with marked restriction of activity). In this last category, 2 came to arthrodesis, 2 to ankylosis and 2 to motion of 20°.

### Suppurative Arthritis of Infancy: Sequelae of Infection

Infantile pyogenic arthritis is not uncommon. The early recognition and successful treatment of the condition may have no more serious consequences than some overgrowth of the limb. In less favourable circumstances some infants develop alarming radiographic appearances suggesting irreparable damage not only to the epiphysis and metaphysis but to the intervening epiphyseal plate. But considerable care must be exercised in the interpretation of these findings and in forecasting the future function of the

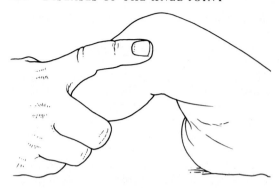

FIG. 5,12. **Suppurative arthritis of infancy.** Palpation may reveal the presence of a femoral condyle, in this case the lateral, apparently absent in the radiograph (after Lloyd-Roberts).

joint. The final shape of the articular surfaces is not dependent on the degree of decalcification of the ossific nucleus or the nearby metaphyses, in which changes are reversible, but upon the damage caused to the epiphyseal cartilage and plate, neither of which can be seen in the early radiographs. The importance therefore of correlating the apparent loss of a medial or lateral condyle with the clinical features of the individual case in terms of range of motion, degree of angular deformity and the ability to palpate the radiologically absent condyle (Fig. 5,12) is stressed. The prognosis may be relatively good and a favourable outcome predicted in spite of the radiological appearances (Lloyd-Roberts, 1960) (Figs 5,1 to 5,4).

### Late Results

Where infection has destroyed the joint surfaces bony ankylosis ensues. In untreated cases flexion deformity is the rule (Fig. 5,13) but not inevitable (Figs 5,14 and 5,15). When infection has taken place in childhood a gross flexion deformity can occur in the course of growth. It is possible for such deformities to be greater than a right-angle. A case has been encountered with such a convexity that the heel touched the buttock following an infection said to have occurred at the age of eight.

### Treatment

Patients with a moderate deformity can walk with a high boot or patten, sometimes with the sound knee slightly flexed (but see 'Good Leg Arthropathy', Ch. 10). If the deformity is considerable, say a right-angle or more, ambulation is possible only on the sound leg with the aid of crutches with the angled knee hanging free (Fig. 5,13). In such circumstances gravity determines that the hip is flexed; and before undertaking operative correction the ability to extend the hip should be checked lest a fixed flexion deformity has ensued.

To determine whether complete correction is possible by a simple wedge osteotomy, or in gross deformities how much correction is possible at a single operation, a paper tracing is made of the outline of the bones as shown in the lateral radiograph. If a wedge is cut from the tracing and the gap closed the resulting correction indicates the outcome of operation or of a single stage of a series of operations. In planning treatment the possibility of interposing a period of skeletal traction between operations should be considered. In any event consideration will be given to the presence of healed sinuses and associated fibrosis and of the pos-

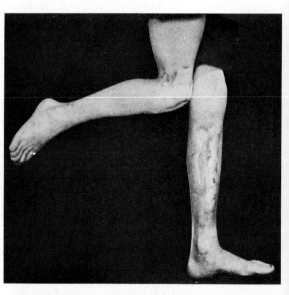

FIG. 5,13. **Infective arthritis.** Knee ankylosed in about right-angled flexion. Note scars of sinuses and evidence of an old healed osteomyelitis in the opposite tibia.

In this example correction of the deformity was accomplished at a single operation removing a large wedge of bone.

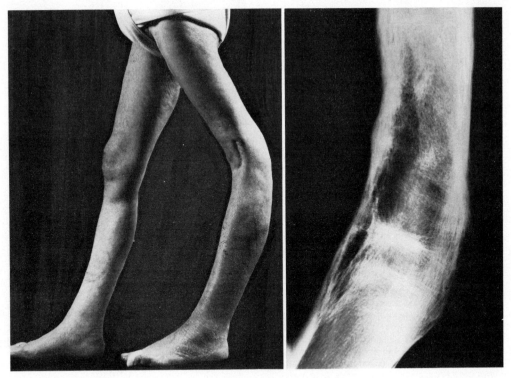

FIGS 5,14–15. **Infective arthritis.** Knee ankylosed in hyperextension (Fig. 5,14). Note absence of patella (Fig. 5,15).

Ankylosis in hyperextension is unusual but has the advantage over flexion deformity in that the patient can walk.

This patient (J.A., female, aged 83) had gone through life with the deformity.

sible effects of correction on circulation. Where a succession of operations is necessary, in the last stage when the limb is extended, an intermedullary nail may be the internal fixation of choice.

If complete correction is achieved with sound union and with hip, ankle and tarsal joints in good functional position, the possibility of equalisation of leg lengths will arise. If the discrepancy is not more than 5 cm shortening of the sound limb in the subtrochanteric region may be considered. If the discrepancy is more and particularly where the function of the foot is poor, amputation may be the operation of choice both on functional and cosmetic grounds and particularly in the female subject in countries where artificial limbs and the related services are developed. In other circumstances and where there is prejudice against amputation it may be a matter of accepting a lesser achievement in the interests of rendering the patient independent (Figs 5,16 to 5,19).

## INFECTIVE ARTHRITIS: MISCELLANEOUS ORGANISMS

There follows a selection of varieties of infective arthritis listed in alphabetical order which in no way indicates incidence or importance in terms of frequency of occurrence or sequelae.

### BLASTOMYCOSIS

**Background note.** The causative organism of North American blastomycosis, *Blastomyces dermatitidis*, gains entrance through the skin or lungs and results in a localised cutaneous lesion or a systemic disorder involving lungs, bone and joints. Involvement of a joint is usually secondary to bone infection but the condition may present as a mono-articular arthritis.

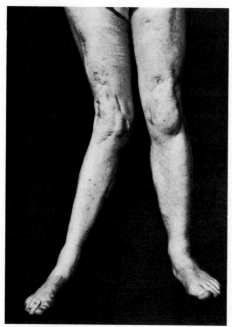

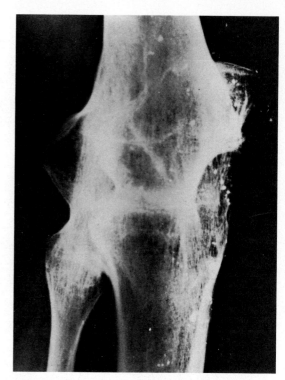

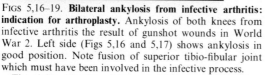

FIGS 5,16–19. **Bilateral ankylosis from infective arthritis: indication for arthroplasty.** Ankylosis of both knees from infective arthritis the result of gunshot wounds in World War 2. Left side (Figs 5,16 and 5,17) shows ankylosis in good position. Note fusion of superior tibio-fibular joint which must have been involved in the infective process.

The right side (Figs 5,18 and 5,19) was subjected to arthroplasty using an interposition membrane of fascia lata as was the practice at the time. It resulted in 50° of flexion under control. There was full passive extension with 20° of valgus angulation. Extension in the absence of the patella was not under quadriceps control. The procedure, however, was successful from the patient's viewpoint in so far as it enabled him to drive his car. The point at issue when these photographs were taken was consideration of revision of the arthroplasty and correction of the valgus deformity (J.S.J.S., male, aged 51).

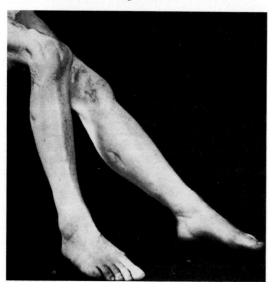

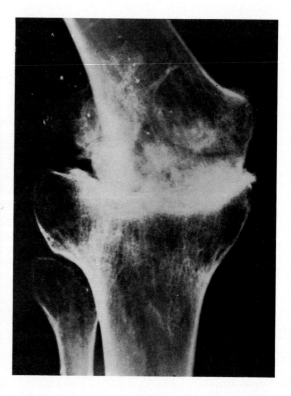

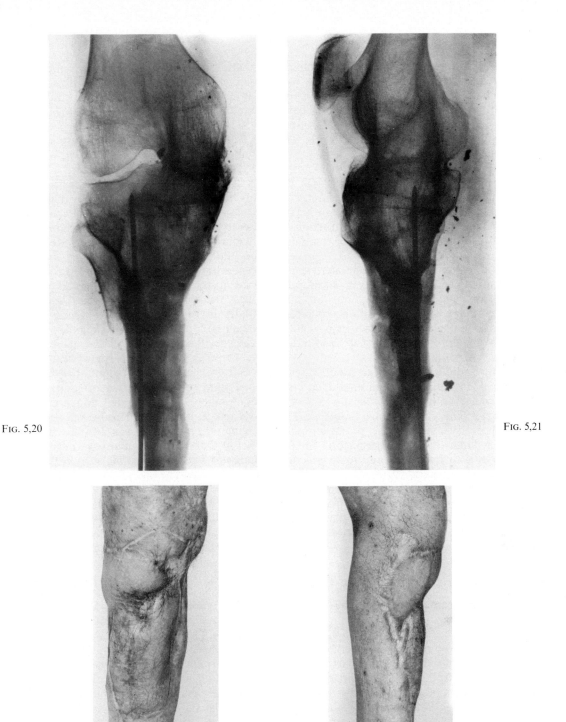

Fɪɢ. 5,20

Fɪɢ. 5,21

Fɪɢ. 5,22

Fɪɢ. 5,23

Fɪɢꜱ 5,20—23. **Ankylosis from infective arthritis: unusual form.** In the current world scene a penetrating wound from a missile remains the commonest cause of infective arthritis. In this case (M.A.P.N.P., male, 32) the result of the detonation of a landmine in Mozambique, ankylosis affected the medial compartment only and the patello-femoral joint was mobile (Figs 5,20 and 5,21). The patient was referred in view of the latter finding as a possible candidate for total knee replacement. There is, however, an absolute contra-indication to such a procedure in the widespread scarring adherent to bone including a large skin graft taken from the abdominal wall (Figs 5,22 and 5,23).

**Clinical features.** In a recently reported example in which the knee joint was affected the case presented as a chronic infective arthritis in which the salient feature was the difficulty and delay in establishing the identity of the causative organisms (Liggett and Silberman, 1970). The condition it is most likely to simulate is tuberculosis which was the provisional clinical diagnosis in the case described. Although the infection reacted dramatically to Amphotericine B therapy, in spite of the longstanding nature of the pathology and extensive destruction of bone and soft tissue, the outcome of treatment was ankylosis.

RADIOGRAPHY. The lesion is characteristically osteolytic with punched-out areas sharply delineated from adjacent bone.

**Differential diagnosis.** The condition as has been indicated is difficult to diagnose. In particular it mimics tuberculosis both clinically and radiologically.

**Diagnosis.** There are no characteristic clinical features. A mycotic infection should be considered whenever there is a chronic osseous, pulmonary, skin and systemic infection. To attain an early diagnosis the physician must exhibit a 'high index of suspicion' in the presence of a chronic bone and joint infection (Liggett and Silberman, 1970).

The specific diagnosis depends on the identification of *Blastomyces dermatitidis* from smear and culture. A skin test using the blastomyces vaccine and the complement fixation test are usually positive.

## Treatment

In the current scene Amphotericine B is the treatment of choice.

**Prognosis.** If the reaction to Amphotericine B therapy is prompt it is unlikely that the diagnosis is established before destruction of the joint has occurred. In such circumstances ankylosis is to be anticipated. It is important therefore that the joint is splinted, initially in a plaster cast, and later in a full-length walking caliper, in a position compatible with optimal function.

### BRUCELLOSIS

**Background note.** Brucellosis is primarily a disease of animals but is often transmitted to man either by drinking raw milk; by direct contact through the broken skin or the conjunctiva; or by the inhalation of infected dust.

Bone and joint infection is rare and most frequently implicates *Brucella melitensis*. In Britain almost all infections are caused by *Brucella abortus*. Until recently (see below) there was no slaughter policy for infected animals in Britain. Where segregation of an infected animal was required evasion was common. In the current scare when positive cultures are obtained the authorities have no power to compel pasteurisation of the infected milk. Since brucellosis in man is not notifiable it is difficult to assess the true incidence of the disease particularly in rural communities where only unpasteurised milk may be available. There is evidence that the disease is increasing in incidence or alternatively more readily diagnosed. In many parts of Britain it is thought to be a more common cause of joint infection than tuberculosis (Adam, Macdonald and Mackenzie, 1967). In 1967, however, a voluntary scheme of eradication was introduced, and by 1971 it was made compulsory (including the slaughter of infected animals) in certain parts of Scotland by The Brucellosis Area Eradication (Scotland) Order (1971). The Brucellosis (Scotland) Order (1972) gave the authorities power to pay compensation for animals slaughtered.

By September 1976 98·2 per cent of the total testable herds were taking part in one of the schemes, and of these 91·7 per cent were fully accredited. In so far as the UK as a whole is concerned, 71·2 per cent of total testable herds were in eradication schemes at the same date, and of these 62·6 per cent were fully accredited.

**Incidence.** The condition is considered to be rare but the incidence is unknown. There is evidence that local manifestations are more common than is generally accepted. It is of interest in the context of the present work that infection of the prepatellar bursa has been described (Johnson and Weed, 1954).

**Pathological anatomy.** The exact pathology of the lesion in the joints is not known. Whether sensitivity plays a part in the lesion can only be surmised (Adam *et al.*, 1967). In the case described below the minimal joint reaction was considered to be related to the proximity of the bone lesion.

**Laboratory investigations.** Unequivocal evidence of brucellar infection requires isolation of the causative organism. This is unlikely to be achieved in the localised form of the disease. A positive blood culture is unusual. Diagnosis therefore depends on high concurrent serum agglutinin titres by comparison with controls of the same age and from the same district.

## Clinical Features

Brucellosis is notoriously a protean disease. The classical features of the bacteriaemic form are recurrent fever, night sweats and general lassitude. In the localised form there may be little if any constitutional upset and the diagnosis is consequently difficult.

In the recorded cases the history is of short duration. It consists of pain, limping and swelling of the knee. On examination there is synovial thickening accompanied by increase in local temperature. Effusion into the joint is of minimal degree.

It will be evident, in circumstances of the commonest of situations about the knee in childhood, that the diagnosis will not be achieved by examination other than by suspicion of the possibility in the rural conditions which have been outlined; or by chance in the course of routine investigation of a condition of unknown origin in which such a possibility is considered, an example of which is recorded below.

The patient (D.C. a male, aged 15, case of W.W.) was referred by his general practitioner with a history that 10 days previously he had been engaged in a gymnastic display. Two days after this activity he complained of pain on the lateral aspect of the left knee. He could not recall any injury. When the general practitioner examined him he noted tenderness at the upper end of the fibula; and that his temperature was 101°F. He made a provisional diagnosis of osteomyelitis. When admitted to the ward there was a swelling over the head of the fibula. Movement of the knee joint was complete. His ESR was 45/1 hour. There was no leucocytosis. Blood culture was negative. Aspiration of the soft tissue abscess revealed bloodstained fluid from which no growth was obtained. He was treated empirically with antibiotics. No radiological change was detected. He was symptomless when he was discharged from hospital three weeks later.

At his follow-up examination radiographs revealed an osteolytic lesion in the upper end of the fibula. There was local swelling and tenderness. The knee joint was slightly swollen but movements were full and free. The label of chronic osteomyelitis in the form of a Brodie's abscess was attached. It was decided, in view of the proximity of the joint and the possible danger of infection, that the abscess cavity should be drained. He was therefore readmitted to the hospital some five months from the onset of his original symptoms.

At operation, through a short lateral incision, the cavity was entered and the contents evacuated and the wall curetted. The material evacuated grew no organisms. The wound healed in the normal time.

It was at this stage that serious consideration was given as to the nature of the condition. The possibility of tuberculosis or of typhoid osteitis arose. The agglutination tests for typhoid and paratyphoid were negative.

When the possibility of brucellosis was raised it was found that: standard agglutination was 0; indirect agglutination was 640; complement fixation test was negative.

This finding, in conjunction with a review of the histology of the material obtained from the cavity, was considered by the pathologist to be consistent with the chronic variety of brucellosis infection.

## Treatment

In the presence of bacteriaemia which is unusual in the localised form the appropriate chemotherapy is indicated. In other circumstances bed-rest with splinting in the form of a compression bandage results in resolution of the infection.

**Prognosis.** It is known that the organisms of brucellosis have a tendency to remain latent in the tissues for prolonged periods and to induce hypersensitivity. In the present state of limited knowledge of brucellosis in local form therefore it would seem prudent to follow the progress of cases for a prolonged period.

## CANDIDA

**Background note.** Acute candida arthritis is rare; but candida infections of all types are on the increase and bone and joint involvement may become more common in the future (Umber, Chapman and Drutz, 1974).

### Clinical Features

Candida infections develop in severely debilitated patients. The symptoms and signs are those associated with an acute pyarthrosis.
**Diagnosis.** Identification of the organism.
**Treatment.** In describing the successful treatment of a knee infected with *Candida guilliermondi* with the oral antifungal agent 5-fluorocytosine, Umber *et al.* (1974) point out that while it is simpler and safer to administer than amphotericin B its use requires laboratory support at the highest level.

## CLOSTRIDIUM BIFERMENTANS

**Incidence.** In presenting a case of post-operative septic arthritis occurring after meniscectomy (Nolan *et al.*, 1972) it is reported that no previous case has been recorded in which *Clostridium bifermentans* alone was isolated.

### Clinical Features

The salient feature of this unexplained post-operative infection was the prolonged incubation time characteristic of clostridial infections. It is observed that post-operative septic arthritis may be a relatively late occurrence. A tense, painful swollen joint developing in the post-operative phase and during the course of mobilisation must be shown to be sterile before the effusion can be attributed to overactivity. It is pointed out that rest will not cure septic arthritis.
**Treatment.** In the case reported intensive antibiotic therapy supplemented by arthrotomy followed by closed irrigation for six days appears to have resulted in a complete restoration of function.

## CLOSTRIDIUM WELCHII

**Background note.** *Clostridium welchii* is most commonly associated with the classical form of gas gangrene. This fulminant disease is a clostridial myositis, which unless prompt and adequate measures are taken, results in systemic collapse and death. In addition to infection of lesions of traumatic origin the organism has been recognised as the causative of many other and varied entities.

**Mode of infection.** In three of the cases there was a penetrating wound of the joint. In two of these, both children, the wound was accidental. The third was the result of gunshot wound. In the fourth the infection occurred spontaneously without injury to the joint. To 1975 5 cases only of acute septic arthritis had been described (Lovell, 1946; McNae, 1966; Torg and Lammot, 1969 and Korn *et al.*, 1975) and all affected the knee joint.

In the fifth there was a supracondylar fracture entering the joint.

### Clinical Features

The symptoms and signs were those associated with an acute pyarthrosis. There were no special features.
**Diagnosis.** Identification of the organism.
**Treatment.** Surgical drainage, immobilisation and systemic penicillin in adequate dosage resulted in restoration of function with minimal evidence of articular cartilage destruction in the cases described. The case recorded by Korn *et al.* (1975) was successfully treated with antibiotics and hyperbaric oxygen without arthrotomy.

## COCCIDIOIDES IMMITIS

**Background note.** It is said that 45000 new coccidioidal infections occur yearly in the United States (Rhangos and Chick, 1964). The majority of cases of primary or disseminated coccidioidomycosis are seen in the endemic areas of California and certain other southern states.
**Relevance.** The knee is the joint most commonly affected (18 out of 25 cases) (Winter *et al.*, 1975).
**Surgical pathology.** The condition is a villonodular granulomatous synovitis. The fungus spreads to the joint by direct extension of adjacent haematogenously seeded osseous foci. A pannus may be formed which slowly erodes the articular cartilage.

## Clinical Features

The condition presents as recurrent episodes of painful synovial swelling of the joint.

**Diagnosis.** In endemic areas such circumstances will engender the suspicion of coccidioidal infection. The ultimate diagnosis depends on the identification of the fungus. In this regard the better source of material for culture is synovial tissue rather than synovial fluid which frequently fails to yield the organism (Pollock, Morris and Murray, 1967).

**Treatment.** The clinical course is widely variable. Neither spontaneous cure nor spontaneous ankylosis has ever been demonstrated in the adult. There is no effective agent available in the current scene. Amphotericin B, with considerable side effects, is fungistatic but not fungicidal. It is indicated in the patient with signs of disseminated disease or a rising complement of fixation titre that exceeds 1 : 16 (Winter *et al.*, 1975). In the patient with a solitary articular focus it is reasonable to avoid the side effects of amphotericin except for a brief course at the time of surgery. The surgical measures indicated vary widely between synovectomy, arthrodesis and amputation.

## FILARIASIS: CHYLOUS ARTHRITIS

**Background note.** It is said that 45 000 new anatomical sacs resulting from lymphatic obstruction are recognised in such entities as chyle thorax, chylous ascites and chylous hydrocele. The occurrence of joint swelling as a result of filarial infection is well known but the cause less well established. Napier (1946), describing synovitis of the knee and hip joints as a complication of systemic filariasis, suggested the possibility of rupture of a lymph varix into the synovial cavity. Das and Sen (1968) investigating 25 cases of this form of arthritis conclude that the mechanism of production is the same as in collections of lymph at other sites, namely 'chyle reflux'. It is upon their work that this section is based.

## Clinical Features

The attack is initiated with acute systemic manifestation in the form of high fever and toxicity. After two to three days the joint becomes acutely painful and grossly swollen with increase in local temperature and extreme tenderness. The inguinal lymph glands are enlarged and tender. The aspirated fluid is thin, creamy yellow and resembles pus. The features are those of acute septic arthritis from which it must be differentiated. The temperature falls in three to five days and with the use of a compression bandage the swelling subsides in a further ten days. There is a full return of painless movement. In the limited number of patients whose progress has been followed for up to two years there has been repeated recurrence of effusion but without the systemic manifestation of the first attack. After three or four attacks permanent nodular thickening of the synovial membrane is recorded and the picture that of a painful chronic arthritis.

**Pathological anatomy.** Lymphographic studies show the constant presence of demonstrable lymphectasia, stasis and varicosity in the popliteal system of lymphatics with short bland channels leading to the joint and abnormal collaterals closely related to synovial reflections. Some of the appearances suggested the possibility of lymphatic fistulation into the synovial sac. They considered that the high concentration of lipids in the synovial fluid tended to confirm the occurrence of such fistulae.

**Laboratory investigations.** Night blood smears were positive for microfilaria in 8 only of the 25 cases. Blood culture was negative and the fluid aspirated from the joint sterile for pyogenic organisms in all the cases.

**Diagnosis.** The lipid content of the synovial fluid is one and a half to three times the normal blood level; and it is upon this finding that the diagnosis depends.

**Treatment.** The importance of the condition is recognition and differentiation from septic arthritis. The possibility should be considered in areas where filariasis is endemic.

## GONOCOCCAL ARTHRITIS

**Background note.** Gonococcal arthritis is not common in Britain at the present time. The majority of patients with polyarthritis associated with genital infection are examples of Reiter's syndrome and do not have true gonococcal arthritis (Ford, 1961; Wright, 1963). Nevertheless, Partain, Cathcart and Cohen (1968) described 10 cases of definite gonococcal arthritis in Boston during a 4-year period.

Gonorrhoea may soon become the commonest notifiable infectious disease in the world. It remains an intractable problem in modern society. The medical and social factors which have produced the situation are likely to continue to operate in the future (Catterall, 1970).

In such circumstances an increase in the incidence of the disease is to be anticipated and with it an increase in the incidence of arthritis.

## Clinical Features

Involvement of the knee joint is usually part of a polyarthritis; but not necessarily so. It develops 10 days or so after the onset of the urethritis. The joint is painful, swollen and with a rise in local temperature. The diagnosis is readily achieved in the male if the possibility has been considered. It is more difficult in the female, half of whom have no symptoms of the original infection.

**Diagnosis.** The ultimate diagnosis depends on growing the gonococcus (*Neisseria gonorrhoeae*) from fluid aspirated from the joint. The complement-fixation test is unreliable. A reliable serological test that can be used for mass screening is urgently required (*Lancet,* 1970). Investigations to develop such a test are in progress.

**ESR.** It is said that ESR is invariably raised in gonococcal arthritis and falls dramatically with clinical and bacteriological cure (Murray, 1979).

**Treatment.** In spite of the existence and spread of resistant strains of *N. gonorrhoeae* throughout the world, penicillin in large doses remains the treatment of choice for reasons of low cost and low toxicity. Investigations continue on the antibacterial activity of other drugs or combination of drugs.

## GUINEA-WORM ARTHRITIS

**Background note.** It is estimated that more than 50 million people in the Middle East, Russia, Africa, South America and India are infected with *Dracunculus medinensis* (Stoll, 1947). A not uncommon manifestation of the disease is the entry of the worm into the knee joint causing synovitis (Reddy and Sivaramappa, 1968). The first report of a case is attributed to Gandhi in 1962.

**Pathological anatomy.** The condition occurs in three forms:
1. A synovitis the result of mechanical or allergic reaction related to the presence of an adult worm in the adjacent soft tissues.
2. An acute arthritis following the discharge of larvae into the joint; and
3. An acute septic arthritis the result of ulceration of the adjacent skin permitting infection of the joint cavity. This is said to be the commonest form (Greenwood, 1968).

True guinea-worm arthritis (2) above is the variety related to entry of the worm into the knee joint and discharge of the uterine contents into the joint cavity. It appears that the cause of the synovial irritation is neither the presence of the worm nor the larvae but chemical in origin due to the uterine secretions of the worm (Sivaramappa *et al.,* 1969).

## Clinical Features

The majority of cases described have been males from areas where guinea-worm infection is endemic. A previous history of infection is the common finding. There are prodronal allergic symptoms of a general or local rash and itching three to four days before the swelling of the joint. The onset of swelling is sudden with an increase in local temperature, synovial thickening, tenderness and effusion. A radiograph may reveal calcified guinea-worms from a previous infection in the adjacent soft tissues.

**Diagnosis.** The diagnosis depends on the demonstration of guinea-worm larvae in the synovial fluid aspirated from the joint.

**Treatment.** Early arthrotomy to remove the offending products of the worm, and if possible the worm itself, is the treatment of choice. Irrigation through a wide bore needle is apparently unsatisfactory (Sivaramappa *et al.,* 1969). The possibility that diagnosis and treatment might be achieved with the arthroscope inserted into the suprapatellar pouch has not been considered at the present stage of knowledge of the pathology or development of the technique.

**Operation.** Under tourniquet control with the joint in the extended position the suprapatellar pouch is entered through a short antero-lateral incision. In nine cases in which the worm was visible it was lying free on the femoral surface of the pouch or partly embedded in synovial membrane. In the latter circumstance an area of synovial membrane must be sacrificed (Sivaramappa *et al.*, 1969). The joint cavity is then irrigated with normal saline to remove all exudate from the surface of the membrane. The wound is then closed and a compression bandage applied.

AFTER-TREATMENT. Antibiotics are indicated only in those cases in which there exists the danger of secondary infection because of guinea-worm ulcers elsewhere in the leg. Quadriceps exercises begin when the patient has recovered from the immediate effects of the operation. The stitches are removed on the tenth day when weight-bearing is permitted with the local support of the compression bandage.

**Prognosis.** In this form of the affection the cases described attained a full range of movement within 12 weeks and returned to heavy work. A follow-up, ranging from 8 months to 2 years, showed no residual synovial thickening or effusion. It will be evident that those cases with secondary infection differ in no respect in treatment or prognosis from septic arthritis. The outcome is dependent on the rapidity with which the diagnosis and therapy are instituted. It is evident that untreated cases, terminated in ankylosis with flexion deformity (Greenwood, 1968; Johnson, 1968).

### HEMOPHILUS INFLUENZAE

**Background note.** *Hemophilus influenzae* is an aerobic pleomorphic Gram-negative coccobacillus which was first isolated and described by Pfeiffer in 1892. In the past it has been accepted as constituting one of the less common organisms producing septic arthritis in children. It is suggested (Almquist, 1970) that a changing pattern may be emerging as a result of the widespread use of antibiotics. In a series of 50 cases during a period of 18 years, a rising influence of the organism as the infecting agent was noted.

**Relevance.** The knee is the joint most commonly affected.

**Age range.** Passive immunity is acquired *in utero* and protects the infant in the first few months of life. Later immunity is lost. In the series referred to above the patients in whom the organism was identified were in the range 7 months to 4 years. In older children and in adults actively acquired immune responses produce high bactericidal levels. The condition is therefore rare in adults. Ten cases only have been reported (Raff and Dannaher, 1974).

### Clinical Features

The symptoms and signs are those associated with an acute pyarthrosis.

**Diagnosis.** The age range affected should engender suspicion of the organism involved. The ultimate diagnosis depends on the identification of the organism.

**Treatment.** Prompt and accurate etiological diagnosis and the rapid institution of appropriate therapy such as has been described as applying to infective arthritis in general is necessary to prevent destruction of the joint. In the circumstances of the common age range it is reasonable to anticipate the bacterial investigation in the selection of antibiotic. In the current scene amphicillin is the drug of choice because of the dangers of chloramphenicol.

### REITER'S DISEASE: REITER'S SYNDROME

**Definition.** If a definition is possible, the condition may be described in brief as a disorder characterised by arthritis associated with genital inflammation and with eye involvement in the form of conjunctivitis and iritis.

**Background note.** Arthritis after dysentery has been recognised for many centuries. It is probable that the first description of the syndrome of urethritis together with arthritis in association with dysentery was recorded by Stoll in 1776. In 1818 Sir Benjamin Brodie, to whose clinical acumen and writings reference has been made elsewhere (Chapter 12), described five cases of what was then thought to be a new syndrome. His original began:

'A gentleman, 45 years of age, in the middle

of June 1817 became affected with symptoms resembling those of gonorrhoea. There was a purulent discharge from the urethra . . . On the 23rd June he first experienced some degree of pain in his feet. On the 24th the pain in his feet was rather increased . . . There was some appearance of inflammation of his eyes.'

Reiter (1916) redescribed the condition to which his name is attached in similar terms with the exception that his case had the 'dysenteric' background with which the original was associated.

**Aetiology.** In the current scene the aetiology of Reiter's syndrome is not known. But it is known to be associated with the following diseases: (1) Bacillary dysentery; (2) diarrhoea of non-dysenteric origin; (3) gonorrhoea with or without an associated non-gonococcal urethritis; (4) non-gonococcal urethritis with or without venereal contact. There is thus a strong suggestion of an infective origin.

## Clinical Features

Reiter's syndrome occurs most commonly in young adult males. It presents, in so far as joint manifestations are concerned, as an acute or sub-acute polyarthritis with a predilection for the weight-bearing joints in the knees, ankles and feet.

**Diagnosis.** The most common presenting symptom is urethritis; the second most common is arthritis, and usually, for obvious reasons, in weight-bearing joints, often the knees. It is in the latter circumstance that an orthopaedic surgeon may be consulted. It is in the latter circumstance also that the diagnosis may be missed in the early stages unless the possibility has been considered and particularly if the genito-urinary symptoms are concealed. The iritis, as in ankylosing spondylitis, may be the symptom which draws attention to the underlying pathology.

The diagnosis presents no difficulty in the form of the classical triad of urethritis, arthritis and conjunctivitis. In other circumstances and in the absence of specific or diagnostic laboratory procedures problems of differential diagnosis from other mysterious forms of arthritis arise;

in particular gonococcal and rheumatoid arthritis.

**Treatment.** The arthritis usually demands bed-rest in home or hospital during the acute phase. The condition is self-limiting in the acute attack and resolves in a matter of weeks or months. The most important part of the treatment is reassurance of the patient to this effect coupled with the warning of possible recurrence and relationship to sexual promiscuity. In the current scene it is generally recommended that Tetra-cycline 250 mg four times daily be administered for seven days. The antibiotic has no noticeable effect on the arthritis (Propert, Gill and Laird, 1964) but is said to influence the urethritis. In a condition of possible weeks or months duration and liable to recurrence it is important that the principles governing the prevention of flexion contracture be observed and hourly quadriceps exercises practised.

The following is an example of a case:

The patient (M.McC., male, aged 26) was admitted with pain in both knees, and with marked swelling of the left knee. The presenting symptom was in the knee. He complained also in the course of history-taking of dysuria and conjunctivitis. The latter two complaints in this particular example gave an immediate lead to the probable diagnosis. On direct questioning he admitted to a promiscuous sexual contact six weeks prior to admission.

## Family History

No family history of rheumatoid arthritis, ankylosing spondylitis, psoriasis, colitis, diabetes mellitus, pernicious anaemia, goitre, or asthma.

## Examination

Conjunctival vessels injected especially on left side.

RS:     normal.

CVS:     pulse rate 70/min sinus rhythm. BP 150/80. Normal heart sounds. No murmurs.

AS:     normal.

CNS:     normal.

GUS:    three small superficial ulcers on anterior aspect of glans penis just behind meatus.

## General Investigations

Radiographs of chest, sacro-iliac joints and lumbar spine were negative.
ECG:    normal.
ASO titre 200/units/ml.
Blood WR: negative.
RPCFT:    negative.
RA Latex:    negative.
LE Latex:    negative.
Blood film showed nothing of note apart from neutrophil leucocytosis.
Haemoglobin 93 per cent (13·6 g/100 ml).
White cell count 10 900/cmm.
ESR 60 mm/1 hr (Westergren).
Throat swab: sterile.
Urine culture: no growth.
Urethral swab and film: no intracellular Gram-negative diplococci seen.
Urea and electrolytes normal.

## Joints

The left knee was the subject of a tense synovial effusion with marked increase of local temperature. At a single aspiration for the purpose of reducing tension and investigation 40 ml were removed.

No other joint was affected by swelling or effusion. Examination of the fluid showed: protein 4·9 g per cent. Microscopy showed polymononuclear leucocytes and a few lymphocytes. There was no growth on culture.

**Radiographs.** Those of the left knee showed marked effusion; but apart from minimal decalcification there was no other abnormality.

## Treatment

**General.** Tetracyline 500 mg q.i.d. was administered over a period of one month.
**Local.** The knee was treated by aspiration for obvious therapeutic and diagnostic reasons. One aspiration only was necessary. Immobilisation was provided by an extensive compression bandage.

**Progress.** At the time of discharge from hospital the origin of the arthritis was explained and the possibility of recurrence made clear. The importance of the completion of the course of antibiotic treatment was stressed.

He had been taught quadriceps exercises while in hospital and it was explained to him that he must practice these exercises hourly until the knee became symptomless and he was no longer aware of its presence.

## SALMONELLA

**Incidence.** Infective arthritis is a rare complication of salmonella infections. It is usually mono-articular affecting, in particular, the knee. It tends to affect infants and young children and may be the first manifestation of the disease. It is rare in adults.

**Diagnosis.** The identification of the organism from synovial fluid culture is necessary to establish the diagnosis. There is usually a high agglutination titre in the blood. The radiographs may establish the existence of a juxta-articular osteomyelitis (see below).

**Treatment.** Aspiration, repeated as necessary, and the parenteral administration of suitable antibiotics is the treatment of choice. The prognosis, if the case recorded below is any guide, is poor.

Report of a case:

The patient, Mrs G., aged 50, was first seen by an orthopaedic surgeon (C.S.C.) in a medical ward in a state of delirium with a temperature of 100·5°F on account of a swollen painful knee. When she had recovered sufficiently to take a history it was found that the knee had been swollen and painful for some two weeks. On examination there was soft tissue swelling and effusion. An outstanding feature was a curious blue-purple hue of the overlying skin. There was no increase in local temperature; and this was possibly one of the reasons why attention had not been directed to the joint previously. On aspiration pus was found; and it is recalled that the appearance of the pus gave the impression of similarity to that evacuated from a cold abscess. *Salmonella enteriditis Gartner* was isolated from the pus. The organism, one of food poisoning, was investigated at the Salmonella Institute which enquired immediately if the patient was so affected. On investigation there was no food poisoning in the area. Enquiries were then made as to the possibility that the organism had been acquired from a rat poison then in current use. No connection was established. The origin of the condition remained a mystery. It was at this stage that radiographs showed the possibility of an underlying osteomyelitis. The question which arose was whether the appearance of osteomyelitis was secondary to the infection of the joint or whether it was the primary focus. The localisation to one point, however, suggested that the osteomyelitis may

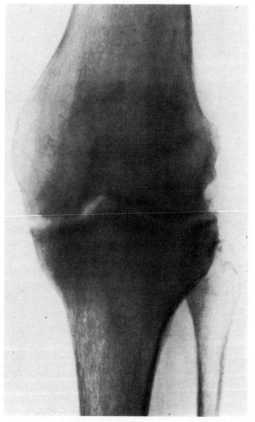

FIG. 5,24. **Infective arthritis:** *Salmonella enteriditis Gartner.* The articular surfaces have been destroyed by the infection resulting in a stiff painful knee with a fixed flexion deformity which eventually came to arthrodesis (Mrs G., aged 50, case of C.S.C.).

have been the original focus. Treatment consisted of repeated aspiration and at that time systemic Chloromycetyn. At one time it was under consideration whether open drainage would be necessary; but the condition settled with aspiration and antibiotic therapy. It was evident, however, from the appearance of the radiographs that the joint surfaces had been destroyed (Fig. 5,24). The outcome was a painful stiff knee which after an interval of 2 years came to arthrodesis (not included in Table 7, Ch. 6).

## SARCOIDOSIS

**Relevance.** It is said that 5 to 15 per cent of patients with sarcoidosis develop monoarticular arthritis although acute transient polyarthritis is the more common manifestation (Pfeifer, 1976).

**Clinical features.** In recording the case of a female aged 28 with monoarticular arthritis of the knee joint, Pfeifer noted an absence of positive findings with the exception of enlarged hilar glands in the chest radiograph. The mother of the patient had suffered pulmonary sarcoidosis and a monoarticular arthritis of the ankle joint.

**Diagnosis.** The ultimate diagnosis depends on the demonstration of the histological features of sarcoidosis in a synovial biopsy.

**Treatment.** In the case recorded above recurrent episodes ceased following synovectomy.

## SPOROTRICHOSIS

**Background note.** Sporotrichosis is a granulomatous fungal infection usually confined to the cutaneous tissue of the extremities. It was first described by Hektoen and Perking in 1900 and encountered in South Africa in epidemic form among gold miners handling timber between 1941–44. Sporotrichosis involving a joint is rare.

**Organism.** The pathogen is *Sporotrichum schenki* which is a diphasic, aerobic fungus thriving on living or dead vegetation. It is present also in the normal intestinal tract, oral cavity and tracheobronchial tree.

**Joint incidence.** The knee is the joint most commonly affected.

**Mode of infection.** In so far as the knee joint is concerned the most likely mode is direct infection from a penetrating wound most commonly by a thorn; and this was the aetiology in the case recorded by Kreft and Amihood (1972) on whose observations this section is based.

**Diagnosis.** The condition should be suspected when an acute or subacute infectious arthritis fails to respond to current antibiotic and other treatment. The arthritis in indolent form is characterised by slight pyrexia, mild leucocytosis and a raised sedimentation rate. If in such circumstances repeated aspiration and culture prove negative, the possibility of a fungus infection should be raised.

**Treatment.** The most efficient agent in treatment is potassium iodide continued for at least six weeks. Sulphonamides, in particular sulphur dimethoxine, to which the fungus is sensitive, are a safe alternative (Kreft and Amihood, 1972).

**Prognosis.** It is evident that an infective arthritis in which the cause is not established before three months cannot have other than a poor prognosis in terms of return of flexion.

## TUBERCULOSIS

**Incidence.** In the decade 1945–55, 80 cases of tuberculosis of the knee joint were treated in the orthopaedic hospital in the author's charge (Stewart, 1955). Twenty-four of these were treated finally by arthrodesis (Moore and Smillie, 1959). By 1960 the number of arthrodeses performed for this condition had increased to 28. It is of some interest, but not statistically significant in view of the advent of chemotherapy, that by 1971, more than 10 years later, the number had increased by 1 case only to 29 (Table 8).

In the current scene in Britain tuberculosis of the knee joint is a condition of some rarity. The classical description in the textbooks of a warm, slightly flexed, diffusely swollen joint accompanied by wasting and spasm of the thigh muscles, is now almost unknown. In many countries of the world tuberculosis is epidemic and tuberculous arthritis a common disease. Even in Britain, it is not extinct. It is one of the number of possibilities to be considered in a chronic or recurrent synovitis of unknown origin. But the pattern is such that patients are often in an older age group than formerly.

Involvement of the knee joint comes third in order of frequency after the spine and hip and accounts for some 10 per cent of all bone and joint lesions. The condition is usually monoarticular; but not necessarily so. Ghormley and Brav (1933) in a series of 168 cases noted involvement of two joints in 13 per cent and in more than two joints in 5 per cent.

**Pathological anatomy.** The condition develops as a metastatic diffuse synovitis which proceeds by a pannus of granulation tissue which spreads over and under and eventually destroys the articular cartilage. If not controlled it advances to invasion of bone at pressure points and may produce large areas of necrosis and eventually leading to complete destruction of the joint. If the infection remains closed the natural outcome is a flexion deformity or unsound fibrous ankylosis. If an abscess discharges and sinuses with secondary infection develop, the outcome may be bony ankylosis in a position determined by the presence or absence of splinting.

The progress of the pathological anatomy has considerable bearing, in a situation determined by chemotherapy, on the treatment to be adopted. In the stage of synovial involvement and early invasion of cartilage, drug therapy in combination with the general principles of treatment listed below can be expected to arrest the process. When caseation, abscess formation and necrosis of bone have taken place, control of infection is not to be expected other than with the addition of surgical intervention.

### Clinical Features

The presenting symptoms are pain and/or swelling and stiffness of insidious origin. The swelling is synovial thickening rather than effusion. There is increase in local temperature and tenderness to pressure. The quadriceps are markedly wasted. It is a diagnosis to be considered in the adult in any persistent swelling of the knee of insidious origin. In circumstances of suspicion radiographs of the chest are likely to be helpful in so far as some 75 per cent of cases show chronic pulmonary tuberculosis. The ESR is likely to be raised. A negative tuberculin test will tend to preclude the diagnosis. Initial examination of synovial fluid is marginally helpful and shows a leukocytosis in which polymorphs predominate. The glucose content is markedly reduced.

In Britain, with her considerable recent immigrant population, the child most likely to develop tuberculosis of the knee is a contact who did not receive *Calmette-Gulrin bacillus* (B.C.G.) in infancy or one in later childhood whose immunity has worn off. The infection is likely to be secondary to a chest infection and to be of human type contracted from an aged relative. The joint will have a cool, firm swelling with marked muscle wasting. The presence of involvement of other joints renders the diagnosis of tuberculous arthritis extremely unlikely (Blockey, 1976). It must be recognised, however, that the clinical diagnosis is one of increasing difficulty particularly in countries where tuberculosis has been reduced almost to the status of a rarity and where a generation of doctors exists unfamiliar with the arthritic manifestations of the disease.

## Diagnosis

It is within the author's professional experience, before the advent of chemotherapy, that the practice existed of treating a joint by prolonged immobilisation on a clinical diagnosis, unconfirmed by histological section, bacteriological examination or other means. There remains the vivid memory of the opportunity to release a number of children from their plaster casts and the inevitable damage to growing joints which unjustified and unnecessary immobilisation implies, from an institutional environment and from the social stigma imposed by the diagnosis at that time.

In no circumstances should treatment be undertaken on a clinical diagnosis whether by chemotherapy, and/or immobilisation, synovectomy, conservative surgery or more radical measures without positive proof of the existence of the disease.

The diagnosis depends on the identification or growth of the organism from the joint fluid, synovial membrane or deep inguinal lymph node, as shown by the demonstration of tuberculous tissue, of epithelioid cells and lymphocytes in characteristic configuration, with or without the presence of necrosis and foreign-body giant cells, or from the inoculation of guinea pigs.

**Radiological examination.** The radiographs are not characteristic in the early cases nor in late cases with advanced destruction. In cases of moderate duration there is decalcification of bone (Figs 5,25 and 5,26), marginal erosions and interruption of the articular cortex. The joint space is usually well preserved until the late stages of the disease as a result of the resistance of the articular cartilage to destruction.

**Arthroscopy.** The principal role of arthroscopy is the ability to perform biopsy from selected areas of synovial membrane.

**Inguinal lymphadenectomy.** The knee joint enjoys a favourable position for this examination by reason of the anatomical arrangement of the regional lymph glands and the frequency with which they are involved. In the decade 1945–55 referred to above, 36 inguinal adenectomies were performed on the author's cases (Stewart, 1955). The procedure was applied only to those cases in which positive proof of the diagnosis was lacking. Inguinal adenectomy was positive 15 times out of 18 operations on proved tuberculosis of the knee or tarsus. Inguinal adenectomy was negative on 18 occasions and in none of these cases did tuberculosis develop subsequently. It is of interest and importance that in the three negative biopsies (Table 5) a possible technical explanation was offered. The final diagnosis in the negative cases is shown in Table 6 to illustrate the wide range of conditions with which tuberculosis can be confused.

TECHNIQUE: POSSIBLE FALLACY. Inguinal adenectomy is a useful diagnostic procedure in doubtful cases of tuberculosis of the knee. But the operation is not one to be undertaken lightly

TABLE 5

Inguinal lymphadenectomy.
Results of 36 biopsies

|  | Positive | Negative |
|---|---|---|
| Cases of proven tuberculosis (18) | | |
| Knee | 13 | 3 |
| Tarsus | 2 | 0 |
| Other cases (18) | 0 | 18 |

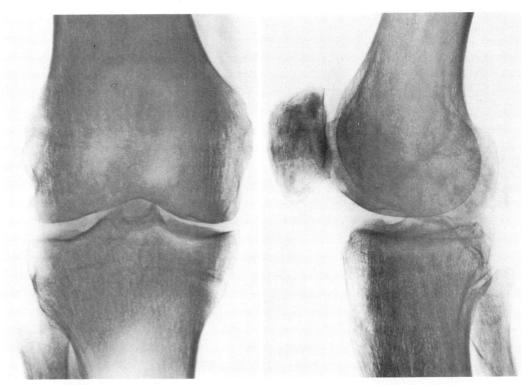

FIGS 5.25–26. **Tuberculosis.** The radiological features are not specific. In this example of moderate duration there is widespread patchy decalcification.

or by the inexperienced. The possible fallacy lies in the hands of the surgeon: only a deep inguinal node is of diagnostic value. The superficial inguinal glands are not concerned in the lymph drainage of the knee joint.

### Treatment

**General.** The advent of powerful chemotherapeutic agents has produced revolutionary changes in treatment and prognosis from the time when prolonged immobilisation and radical surgery were the only measures available.

The current treatment of tuberculous arthritis of the knee and of the ability to undertake conservative surgery, is entirely dependent on chemotherapy in the form of streptomycin, para-aminosalicylic acid (PAS) and isoniazid (INH).

In general a combination of agents is to be preferred on the basis of synergistic action and of delay in the advent of drug-resistant bacilli. It is not proposed in a changing scene to advise which drugs or dosages should be used or of the potentialities for toxic effects except to stress the importance of the maintenance of therapy for a minimum of one year, preferably for 18 months and in certain cases for longer.

TABLE 6

Inguinal lymphadenectomy. Final diagnosis when negative. 18 cases

| | |
|---|---|
| Traumatic synovitis | 6 |
| Rheumatoid arthritis | 3 |
| Pigmented villonodular synovitis | 3 |
| Infective arthritis | 1 |
| Chondromalacia patellae | 1 |
| Hysteria | 1 |
| Malignant synovioma | 1 |
| Subacute non-specific polyarthritis | 1 |
| No final diagnosis (at two months) | 1 |

Tuberculosis, it will be remembered, is a general infection and arthritis of the knee a metastatic lesion. In a condition the treatment of which has been revolutionised by chemotherapy, the principles of the past when recovery depended on the resistance of the patient still obtain and should not be neglected. Bed-rest, a nutritious diet and immobilisation of the joint are still important elements in a situation in which the outcome of resistance to chemotherapy eventually depends on the resistance of the host.

**Local.** Treatment is determined by the stage to which the disease has advanced, in terms of involvement, of the components of the joint, before the diagnosis is established.

STAGE 1. There is a synovial effusion with possible thickening of the synovial membrane. There is normal range of flexion, restricted, possibly, by the size of the effusion.

The radiographs shows a normal joint space. There is no evidence of a focus within the bone nor of destruction or erosion.

TREATMENT. When the disease is early and limited to the synovial membrane, systemic chemotherapy combined with the basic

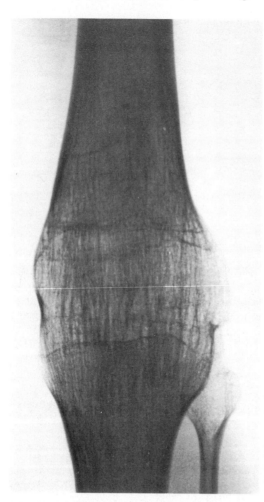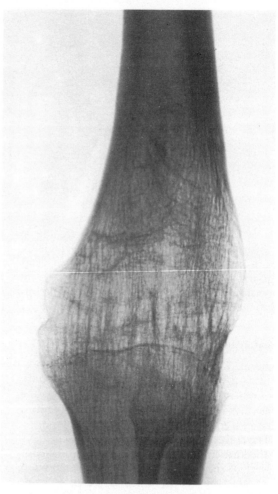

FIGS 5,27–28. **Tuberculosis: Treatment.** This knee joint was arthrodesed at age 7 by the author for gross tuberculous infection. Alignment in both antero-posterior and lateral planes has been maintained (Figs 5,27 and 5,28) showing that deformity at the epiphyseal plates does not necessarily take place when arthrodesis is performed at an early age (D.L., male, aged 31).

principles of bed-rest and immobilisation may result in resolution of the disease and retention of a full range of movement.

STAGE II. There is a long history, with varying degrees of thickening and fibrosis of the synovial membrane but with no effusion. There may be limitation of flexion. In the radiograph the joint space has been maintained and there is no evidence of involvement of bone.

TREATMENT. If the infection of the synovial membrane is extensive the possibility of partial or subtotal synovectomy under chemotherapeutic cover should be considered with the prospect of retaining a mobile joint. The outcome of operation will depend on the degree to which articular cartilage is involved and in this regard the possibilities of inspection by arthroscope have yet to be exploited. In any event it is wise before undertaking operation to obtain the patient's permission to proceed to arthrodesis if the condition of the articular cartilage is such as to preclude a successful outcome (see case reported below).

For the technique of synovectomy see Chapter 6.

STAGE III. There is obvious synovial disease complicated by a bone focus within the tibia, femur or patella. It is to be presumed that such a focus has communication with the joint.

The radiograph reveals that the joint space has been preserved and that the joint surfaces are intact.

TREATMENT. There is, even at this late stage, the prospect of retaining a mobile joint by synovectomy, curettage of erosions of articular cartilage, block resection or curettage of a bone focus with packing of the residual defect with bone chips.

STAGE IV. There is an advancing arthritis with gross limitation of movement.

There is in the radiograph diminution of the joint space and destruction of opposing bone surfaces.

TREATMENT. If destruction of articular cartilage and bone is of a degree which precludes the possibility of restoration of function arthrodesis is the operation of choice (Figs 5,27 and 5,28). For technique see Chapter 6.

*Timing of operation.* If surgical measures in the form of synovectomy, or synovectomy together with the elimination of necrotic bone, with or without arthrodesis, are to be undertaken the timing of the operation is of some importance. The operation should take place as soon as the general condition is stabilised under the protective cover of drug therapy but before resistance to such therapy has had a chance to develop. The interval will vary with the circumstances of the case but it is probable that at least four weeks should elapse before intervention.

The following case summary is quoted as an example of the problem of diagnosis in the current scene:

The patient (A.R., male, aged 55, an iron moulder) complained of pain, stiffness and swelling in his right knee of three months' duration. On examination there was swelling consisting of synovial effusion together with synovial thickening. Flexion beyond a right-angle was painful. There was tenderness on the joint line on the medial side. At the initial out-patient examination there were two other findings of possible significance. It was noted that there was a scar of thoracotomy on the left side. In addition there was swelling and tenderness at the inferior radio-ulnar joint together with swelling of the proximal interphalangeal joints of the third, fourth and fifth fingers on the right side. The patient's disability related to the knee joint was such that he was unable to work. It was decided, therefore, to admit him to hospital for investigation. Investigation in relation to the two possible diagnoses showed:

**Tuberculosis history.** One of his sisters died from pulmonary tuberculosis. He had been followed in a Chest Clinic for some five years at the end of which time a radiograph showed a focus at the mid-zone of his left lung. He had been admitted to hospital and given antituberculosis therapy. It was significant that the therapy consisted of streptomycin, 1 g daily, isoniazid 300 mg daily and PAS 18 g daily over a total period of 25 weeks. Three weeks after the institution of this treatment he underwent thoracotomy at which resection of the affected part of his left lung was carried out. He was discharged at the end of six months, apparently well and free of symptoms. His condition had been followed for a period of four years and there was no recurrence. He was consequently discharged. His general health had remained good with the exception of an incident five years previous to his present admission when he had suffered a haemoptysis. When this occurred he attended his family doctor but no further investigations had been carried out and he had not reported back to the Chest Clinic. On close questioning he admitted suffering night sweats during the past year and to lethargy and the loss of energy during the same period. His ESR was 35 in the first hour, his haemoglobin and white cell counts were within normal limits. Cultures from his sputum, urine and from fluid aspirated from his knee all failed to produce any growth. The 1–1000 Mantoux test was strongly reactive. The agglutination test for brucellosis was negative. A radiograph of the chest revealed a shadow in the second right interspace anteriorly. Films recalled from the Mass Miniature Radiography Unit of four years previously showed that the lesion was present at this time and to be identical in conformation.

**Rheumatoid arthritis history.** This swelling and conformation of the swelling of the right knee was consistent with the diagnosis of rheumatoid arthritis. Extension of the right wrist was limited by synovial swelling and there was pain and tenderness to pressure. The third, fourth and fifth fingers were stiff with a spindle-shaped swelling at the proximal interphalangeal joints. There was considerable limitation of flexion at these joints. He had symptoms, if in lesser degree, in both elbows, both shoulders and neck. The ESR as reported above was 35 in the first hour. The R.A. Latex test from both blood and effusion from the knee were positive.

It was at this stage he was examined by a tuberculosis physician who gave his opinion that the condition was rheumatoid arthritis.

The problem was to differentiate between the possibility of tuberculosis of the knee joint in a patient who had received inadequate chemotherapeutic treatment at the time of his active lung infection and who, with a haemoptysis five years previously, had an active lesion in the lung. On the other hand there was evidence, clinical and from the

positive Latex test, that he suffered from rheumatoid arthritis. Here was a case in which an inguinal adenectomy might have produced absolute evidence of origin. In considering the problem, however, it was decided that the diagnosis was of academic interest in so far as treatment of the knee was concerned: the condition had existed for considerably longer than the three months that the patient was prepared to admit. It had not settled with rest, was undergoing deterioration with destruction of articular cartilage. Whatever the diagnosis he was a candidate for synovectomy.

The diagnosis was settled finally when it was reported that the guinea pig which had been infected had died after four weeks and was found to be suffering from tuberculosis.

On the establishment of a positive diagnosis he received intensive chemotherapy. If his general condition improved the knee continued to show considerable synovial thickening and no increase in range of beyond some $40°$ of flexion. After eight weeks synovectomy was proposed. The patient agreed that if, at operation, destruction of articular cartilage was such as to preclude a favourable result in terms of flexion, an arthrodesis should be performed. At operation considerable invasion of the articular cartilage of the femoral condyles and patella were noted. In view of his age and long history of ill-health it was decided that the appropriate measure in all the circumstances was arthrodesis and resulted in sound fusion, using the compression method, in four months.

It is of some interest, and possibly of significance, that when this patient returned for review six months after his arthrodesis, and still under treatment by antituberculous therapy, he offered the information that the swelling of the joints of his wrist and fingers had disappeared and that he could now close his hand without difficulty, which he had been unable to do before treatment. He demonstrated that he had regained full movement in the elbows, shoulders and neck.

The interest and reasons for recording this particular case are (1) the problems of diagnosis which arise in the current scene; (2) in relation to (1) the emergence of a generation of doctors in all specialities, including tuberculosis, to whom the disease is unfamiliar; (3) the possible, even probable, record of an example of the controversial condition *tuberculous rheumatism* (see below) which it will be noted contributed to the problem of diagnosis; (4) the possible sequelae of the inadequate treatment of pulmonary tuberculosis, admittedly in the early stages of the advent of chemotherapy in this example; (5) the attitude in the current scene to the maintenance of function in the form of a mobile joint by chemotherapy and/or synovectomy, but which in this particular case terminated in arthrodesis.

## 'Tuberculous Rheumatism'

**Definition.** When tuberculosis was common it was long recognised on the continent of Europe, as opposed to Britain and the United States, that a polyarthritis with the appearance of rheumatoid arthritis existed in the presence of a major tuberculous lesion in a joint or elsewhere. The aetiology of the condition was controversial with toxins, attenuated bacilli or allergy cited as the possible cause.

**Background note.** Brav and Hench (1934) in a historical review of the condition recorded that Bonnet, in 1845, noted that frequently joints which were the seat of chronic atrophic polyarthritis presented a gradual change to 'white swelling'. In 1864, Charcot described a large number of patients with polyarthritis (unclassified) who later succumbed to pulmonary tuberculosis. *Lancereaux and Lackerbauer, in 1871, described a patient with tuberculosis of the knee joint, who previously had had generalised arthritis which disappeared except for localisation of arthritis in the knee.* (Author's italics, see case recorded above.) Gubler, in 1874, denied the necessity of finding definite tubercles in the joints in order to prove the tuberculous aetiology. In 1878, Bouilly noted the development of 'tumeur blanche rhumatismale' among children following attacks of atrophic arthritis. Grocco, in 1892, led the way to further clinical and laboratory studies in these cases when he insisted that patients with tuberculosis might present a form of arthritis unassociated with tubercles or abscess, similar to what is now called rheumatoid arthritis. It remained for Poncet, of Lyon, in 1897, to describe the clinical picture of the 'rhumatisme tuberculeux' with which his name is associated.

## *VIBRIO FETUS*

**Background note:** Infection with *Vibrio fetus* is well-known to veterinary surgeons as a cause of abortion in cattle and sheep. Human infection is rare. Three cases only have been described involving joints and all have concerned the knee.

### Clinical Features

It is impossible to establish a pattern in a condition of such rarity. All three cases described were elderly persons, all had a history of trauma of considerable severity at some time in the past. All had suffered recent trauma, two directly to the knee affected. In no instance was exposure to livestock noted nor was the portal of entry of the organism established (Kutner and Arnold, 1970).

**Diagnosis.** The isolation of the organism *Vibrio fetus* from fluid aspirated from the joint is necessary to establish the diagnosis.

**Treatment.** Aspiration, repeated as necessary, and the parenteral administration of a suitable antibiotic is the treatment recommended. In the case described by Kutner and Arnold, the antibiotic was ampicillin and resulted in a complete return of function.

## REFERENCES

ADAM, A., MACDONALD, A. & MACKENZIE, I. G. (1967). Monoarticular brucellar arthritis in children. *Journal of Bone and Joint Surgery*, **49B**, 4, 652–657.

ALMQUIST, E. E. (1970). The changing epidemiology of septic arthritis in children. *Clinical Orthopaedics and Related Research*, **68**, 96.

BALLARD, A., BURKHALTER, W. E., MAYFIELD, G. W., DEHNE, E. & BROWN, P. W. (1975). The functional treatment of pyogenic arthritis of the adult knee. *Journal of Bone and Joint Surgery*, **57A**, 8, 1119.

BLOCKEY, N. J. (1976). *Children's Orthopaedics—Practical Problems*. London: Butterworth.

BONNET, A. (1845). *Traité des Maladies des Articulations*. Tome Second, Paris: Baillière.

BOUILLY, G. (1878). *Comparaison des Arthropathies Rhumatismales, Scrofulueuses et Syphilitiques*. Paris: Baillière.

BRAV, E. A. & HENCH, P. S. (1934). Tuberculous rheumatism. *Journal of Bone and Joint Surgery*, **XVI**, 839.

BRODIE, B. C. (1818). *Pathological and Surgical Observations on Disease of the Joints*, p. 55. London: Longman, Hurst, Rees, Orme and Brown.

CATTERALL, R. D. (1970). The problem of gonorrhoea. *British Journal of Hospital Medicine*, **3**, 55.

CHARCOT, J. M. (1868). *Leçons sur les Maladies des Vieillards*. Paris: Delahaye.

CLEVELAND, M. (1956). *Orthopedic Surgery in the European Theater of Operations*, pp. 305–317. Washington D.C. Office of the Surgeon General, Department of the Army.

CROCK, H. V. (1967). *The Blood Supply of the Lower Limb Bones in Man Descriptive and Applied)*. Edinburgh & London: E. & S. Livingstone, Ltd.

DAS, G. C. & SEN, S. B. (1968). Chylous arthritis. *British Medical Journal*, **ii**, 27–29.

EVANS, D. K. (1962). Osteomyelitis of the patella. *Journal of Bone and Joint Surgery*, **44B**, 2, 319.

FORD, D. K. (1961). *Arthritis and Rheumatism*, **4**, 237.

GALASKO, C. S. B. (1966). Septic arthritis. *South African Medical Journal*, **40**, 906.

GANDHI, N. J. (1962). *British Medical Journal*, **i**, 1206.

GHORMLEY, R. K. & BRAV, E. A. (1933). Resected knee joints. *Archives of Surgery*, **XXVI**, 465.

GREEN, W. T. & SHANNON, J. G. (1936). Osteomyelitis of infants: a disease different from osteomyelitis of older children. *Archives of Surgery*, **32**, 462.

GREENWOOD, B. M. (1968). *British Medical Journal*, **1**, 314.

GROCCO, (1892). Quoted by Brav & Hench.

GUBLER (1874). Quoted by Brav & Hench.

HALL, R. McK. (1954). Regeneration of the lower femoral epiphysis. *Journal of Bone and Joint Surgery*, **36B**, 116.

HEKTOEN, L. & PERKING, C. F. (1900). *Journal of Experimental Medicines*, **5**, 77.

JOHNSON, M. F. (1968). *British Medical Journal*, **1**, 314.

JOHNSON, W. J. & WEED, L. A. (1954). Brucellar bursitis. *Journal of Bone and Joint Surgery*, **36A**, 133.

KIRKBY-SMITH, H. T. (1942). Acute osteomyelitis of the patella. *Journal of Bone and Joint Surgery*, **24**, 942.

KORN, J. A., GILBERT, M. S., SIFFERT, R. S. & JACOBSON, J. H. (1975). *Clostridium welchii* arthritis. *Journal of Bone and Joint Surgery*, **57A**, 555.

KREFT, E. & AMIHOOD, S. (1972). Sporotrichosis of the knee joint, *South African Medical Journal*, **46**, 1329.

KUTNER, L. J. & ARNOLD, W. D. (1970). Septic arthritis due to vibrio fetus. *Journal of Bone and Joint Surgery*, **52A**, 161

LANCEREAUX, E. & LACKERBAUER, M. (1871). Atlas d'Anatomie Pathologique, p. 501. Paris: Masson.

LANCET (1970). Gonorrhoea, **i**, 280.

LIGGETT, A. S. & SILBERMAN, Z. (1970). Blastomycosis of the knee joint. *Journal of Bone and Joint Surgery*, **52A**, 1445.

LLOYD-ROBERTS, G. C. (1960). Suppurative arthritis in infancy. Some observations upon prognosis and management. *Journal of Bone and Joint Surgery*, **42B**, 706.

LOVELL, W. W. (1946). Infection of the knee joint by Clostridium welchii. *Journal of Bone and Joint Surgery*, **28**, 398.

McNAE, J. (1966). An unusual case of Clostridium welchii infection. *Journal of Bone and Joint Surgery*, **48B**, 512.

MOORE, F. H. & SMILLIE, I. S. (1959). Arthrodesis of the knee joint. *Clinical Orthopaedics*, **13**, 215.

MURRAY, D. (1979). ESR in gonococcal arthritis. *British Medical Journal*, **i**, 22.

NAPIER, L. E. (1946). *Principles and Practice of Tropical Medicine*, p. 674. New York: Macmillan.

NOLAN, B., LEERS, W. D. & SCHATZKER, J. (1972). Septic arthritis of the knee due to Clostridium bifermentans. *Journal of Bone and Joint Surgery*, **54A**, 6, 1275.

PARTAIN, J. O., CATHCART, E. S., COHEN, A. S. (1968). *Annals of the Rheumatic Diseases*, **27**, 156.

PATZAKIS, M. J., DORR, L. D., IVLER, D., MOORE, T. M. & HARVEY, J. P. (1975). The early management of open joint injuries. *Journal of Bone and Joint Surgery*, **57A**, 8, 1065.

PFEIFER, M. (1976). An interesting knee. *Journal of Bone and Joint Surgery*, **58B**, 386.

POLLOCK, S. F., MORRIS, J. M. & MURRAY, W. R. (1967). *Coccidioidal synovitis* of the knee. *Journal of Bone and Joint Surgery*, **49A**, 7, 1397.

PONCET, M. (1897). De la polyarthrite tuberculeuse déformante ou pseudo-rheumatisme chronique tuberculeux. Assoc. Franç. Chir., 11ᵐᵉ Congrès, Paris, Procès-Verbaux, p. 732.

PROPERT, A. J., GILL, A. J. & LAIRD, S. M. (1964). *British Journal of Venereal Diseases*, **40**, 160.

RAFF, M. J. & DANNAHER, C. L. (1974). *Hemophilus influenzae* septic arthritis in adults. *Journal of Bone and Joint Surgery*, **56A**, 2, 408.

REDDY, C. R. R. M. & SIVARAMAPPA, M. (1968). Guinea-worm arthritis of knee joint. *British Medical Journal*, **1**, 155.

REITER, H. (1916). *Deutsche medizinische Wochenschrift*, **42**, 1535.

RHANGOS, W. C. & CHICK, E. W. (1964). Mycotic infections of bone. *Southern Medical Journal*, **57**, 664.

ROBERTS, P. H. (1970). Disturbed epiphyseal growth at the knee after osteomyelitis in infancy. *Journal of Bone and Joint Surgery*, **52B**, 4, 692.

ROCHER, H. L. (1923). Ostéomyélite de la rotule. *Journal de Médecine de Bordeaux*, **95**, 921.

SIVARAMAPPA, M., REDDY, C. R. R. M., DEVI, C. S., REDDY, A. C., REDDY, P. K., MURTHY, D. P. (1969). Acute guinea-worm synoitis of the knee joint. *Journal of Bone and Joint Surgery*, **51A**, 1324–1330.

STEWART, I. M. (1955). Inguinal lymphadenectomy: diagnostic accuracy in skeletal tuberculosis. *Tubercle*, June, 185–187.

STOLL. (1776). Cited by Paronen, I., in *Acta medica scandinavica*, 1948, Suppl. 212.

STOLL, N. (1947). This Wormy World. *Journal of Parasitology*, **33**, 1–18.

THIRION (1829). Successful extirpation of the right patella for caries. (Abstract). *Lancet*, **ii**, 399.

TORG, J. S. & LAMMOT, T. R. (1968). Septic arthritis of the knee due to Clostridium welchii. *Journal of Bone and Joint Surgery*, **50A**, 1233.

TRUETA, J. (1959). The three types of acute haematogenous osteomyelitis. *Journal of Bone and Joint Surgery*, **41B**, 671.

UMBER, J., CHAPMAN, M. W. & DRUTZ, D. J. (1974). Candida pyarthrosis. *Journal of Bone and Joint Surgery*, **56A**, 7, 1520.

WILLEMS, C. (1919). Treatment of purulent arthritis by wide arthrotomy followed by immediate active mobilization. *Surgery, Gynecology and Obstetrics*, **28**, 546.

WINTER, W. G., LARSON, R. G., HONEGGAR, M. M., JACOBSEN, D. T., PAPPAGIANIS, D. & HUNTINGTON, R. W. (1975). Coccidioidal arthritis and its treatment—1975. *Journal of Bone and Joint Surgery*, **57A**, 8, 1152.

WRIGHT, V. (1963). *Annals of the Rheumatic Diseases*, **22**, 77.

# 6.   Rheumatoid Arthritis

**Introduction**

This is a situation which does not demand consideration of rheumatoid arthritis in general but of the problems of the knee joint. The occasions, however, when *disease* of the knee can be seen in isolation are limited; least of all in rheumatoid arthritis. The condition is by nature an inflammatory disease which affects general health producing anaemia, loss of weight, poor appetite and disturbance of the sense of well-being. It causes inflammatory changes in from one to virtually every joint in the body. These changes may remit in days, weeks or months, remit and then relapse from time to time, or continue relentlessly until death.

**Diagnosis**

'The absence of specific and reliable diagnostic tests leaves rheumatology as one of the few remaining havens for clinicians. Care and time spent in history-taking and examination reap greater rewards than laboratory and even radiological investigations; laboratory tests interpreted inflexibly often lead to diagnostic disaster.' (*British Medical Journal*, 1977.)

The clinical picture of typical rheumatoid arthritis is well-known and does not require description. In the less typical varieties the criteria for diagnosis have been established by the American Rheumatism Association and have been repeated in related textbooks. The problem of diagnosis as it confronts the orthopaedic surgeon is not so much in poly-articular arthritis as in the mono- or bilateral forms affecting the knee in the absence of peripheral joint involvement.

The questions which arise are: (1) Is this established rheumatoid arthritis? In the presence of a raised ESR and a positive RA Latex test the diagnosis is not in question; but (2) What if the ESR is raised but the Latex test negative? Is it sero-negative rheumatoid arthritis, chronic non-specific arthritis or a form of one of the many conditions of infective origin listed in Chapter 3?

**Biopsy.** In rheumatoid arthritis synovial inflammation is the salient feature of the clinical picture and is the earliest and most constant pathological finding. It requires to be established, however, that synovial biopsy is almost without value in diagnosis:

1. There is no correlation between the changes seen in the synovial membrane and the duration, stage of progression, or activity of the disease.
2. Different areas in the same joint may show fibrosis without inflammation or inflammation without fibrosis.
3. There is no single histopathological change that identifies rheumatoid arthritis.

The most characteristic miscroscopic changes are:

1. Hypertrophy of the synovial membrane and villi.
2. Hyperplasia of the lining cells.
3. Massive lymphocyctic and, at times, plasma-cell infiltration with large focal collections in the villi.
4. Inflammatory hyperaemia and oedema varying in degree.

'Every characteristic feature of the morbid anatomy of rheumatoid arthritis may be demonstrated in joints which are not obviously involved in rheumatoid arthritis.' (Sherman, 1951.)

LYMPHOCYTE INFILTRATION. If no single pathological change in the synovial membrane in rheumatoid arthritis is specific there is some evidence that the findings may be of prognostic value. There are two major features which appear to vary independently of one another. These are: (1) synovial lining-cell proliferation and (2) infiltration with inflammatory cells, predominantly lymphocytes. It has been shown that extensive joint damage is associated with a synovial picture of marked lining-cell proliferation and a sparsity of lymphocytes. Cases with heavy lymphocyte infiltration tend to show less damage to articular cartilage and bone despite a similar duration of disease (Muirden and Mills, 1971).

### Pathological Anatomy: Visual

At operation a wide variety of appearances are encountered not necessarily related to the duration or systemic activity of the disease. They range from flat highly vascular aggressive tissue (Fig. 6,1) spreading over the articular cartilage through a hypertrophic villous synovitis to a joint lined with smooth tissue (Fig. 6,2) but filled with fibrin clot of massive dimensions. The variety is such as to raise doubt in the minds of some as to whether they are observing different stages of the same disease or different diseases.

The earliest gross lesion of articular cartilage to which most attention is directed is located transversely on the medial femoral condyle (Fig. 6,3); and the reason for the site is the subject of speculation. It will be recalled (Ch. 4) that reference is made to the presence of a fold of synovial membrane on the medial aspect of the medial femoral condyle (Figs 4,39 and 4,40); and that it is subject to pathological changes and the source of trapping incidents. In Chapter 10 attention is directed to a site on the medial femoral condyle denoting the limit of extension and liable to both degenerative and related reactive changes. It will be recognised that this is the same site as that of the most marked changes in rheumatoid arthritis. It is postulated that the reason for the location of the lesion is multifactorial. It is the site of a fold of synovial membrane involved in the disease process and in contact with articular cartilage and, at the same time, the site of major compression forces in the normal joint. The combination of these two factors alone could explain the location of this major articular lesion in the rheumatoid knee.

It is necessary to establish some criteria of damage to the joint if it is only for the purposes of record:

Grade 1. There is an inflammatory process of the synovial membrane. The articular cartilage and bone appear normal.

Grade 2. There are early erosions along the bone-cartilage junction. The articular cartilage appears normal.

Grade 3. There are extensive erosions with thinning of the articular cartilage.

Grade 4. There are extensive erosions and damage to articular cartilage. The joint structures are the subject of irreversible changes.

## TREATMENT

### General Considerations

It is impossible to approach the subject of the treatment of rheumatoid arthritis from the view point of the orthopaedic surgeon without evident oversimplification. The stage, variety and combination of circumstances encountered are infinite. Each case is an individual problem. No rules can be formulated. Nevertheless if treatment is to be defined and described in the written word some means of classification is necessary. It is appreciated that classification is without inherent merit; only of practical convenience. If these constraints and restrictions are accepted, rheumatoid arthritis affecting the knee joint presents in one of four forms. It is not proposed to differentiate between knee joint disease in polyarticular arthritis and knee joint disease in mono- or biarticular form although it is recognised that the existence of peripheral disease may determine decisions:

1. **Painful active synovial disease without angular deformity.**
2. **Painful active synovial disease with angular deformity in the form of varus, valgus and/or flexion.**
3. **Flexion deformity, the result of misdiagnosis, mismanagement or neglect.**
4. **Quiescent or burnt-out disease presenting as pan-articular osteoarthritis.**

### Mental Attitude in Rheumatoid Arthritis

There is repeated reference in this work to 'motivation'—the will to get well. There is no surgical speciality in which this is more important than 'arthritis'. No arthritis more important than rheumatoid arthritis.

Patients with severe rheumatoid arthritis are afflicted by a continuing disease process, frequently progressive. That there are effects on the psyche is not surprising when it is considered that the disability is compounded of pain,

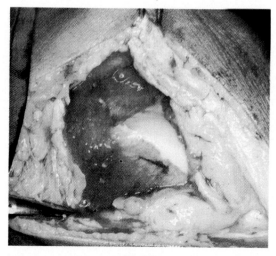

FIG. 6,1

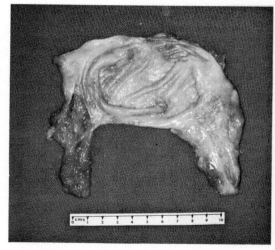

FIG. 6,2

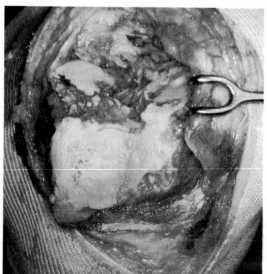

FIG. 6,3

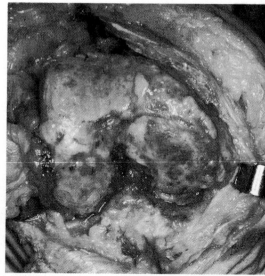

FIG. 6,4

FIGS 6,1–4. **Rheumatoid arthritis: pathological anatomy.** The aggressive vascular synovial membrane seen in the course of synovectomy. The photograph depicts the posterior aspect of the suprapatellar pouch and the lateral aspect of the lateral femoral condyle. There are early erosions along the bone-cartilage junction. The articular cartilage is otherwise of normal appearance (Grade 2) (Fig. 6,1). At the opposite extreme is smooth atrophic synovial membrane of the suprapatellar pouch seen at the burnt-out phase of the disease (Fig. 6,2).

Advanced disease to show the typical site of the major lesion of articular cartilage on the weight-bearing aspect of the medial femoral condyle at the point approaching complete extension (Fig. 6,3). Reference is made (Chapter 4) to the existence of a flap of synovial membrane at this site (Figs 4,39 and 4,40).

In the osteoarthritis of the burnt-out state both compartments of the tibio-femoral joint (Fig. 6,4) as well as the patello-femoral joint are affected. There is no mechanical benefit from correction of angular deformity such as obtains in mono-compartmental osteoarthrosis. The joint surfaces must either be replaced or eliminated.

stiffness, limitation of movement, anaemia and general constitutional upset. It is essential to assess the individual in relationship to her environment before embarking on conservative measures such as synovectomy, which demand courage and fortitude if the optimum result is to be obtained.

The recognition that psychosocial problems exist is important. An interview by a medical social worker may disclose concealed domestic or vocational problems which require attention. 'Treat the patient and not just her disease' is a medical platitude, but is none the less true. The knee joint can often be seen in isolation; but, it is repeated, not in rheumatoid arthritis.

The author learnt his first lesson in such matters at an early age:

> The patient, a single woman in the fourth decade, was admitted to the orthopaedic department of a capital city hospital from a distant mining village in an aura of some publicity. She suffered from quiescent or burnt-out rheumatoid arthritis and had been 'bedridden for years'. The only serious physical problem was that of right-angled flexion deformities of both knees. Turn-buckle plaster casts followed by serial back-shells achieved almost complete extension within six weeks and weight-bearing was resumed. In the next six weeks the degree of recovery was such that crutches had been discarded in favour of sticks, employment had been arranged and she was to return to her home. It was at this stage that she suddenly realised that no longer would the bedridden martyr to rheumatoid arthritis be the centre of attraction in the village. No longer would she be waited upon by her mother and sisters. No longer the weekly visit of the priest. No longer the flowers, candies and cakes handed through the open window where she lay. She was not cured. She would return home to suffer in bed. She would change her doctor for someone who would understand her case. At this level of inexperience it was a shock to encounter a bedridden young woman who did not appreciate the efforts expended on her behalf and without the will to get well.

**Stage of referral.** The results of synovectomy, and indeed of any of the salvage procedures, depend to a large extent on the stage, and age, at which patients are referred. Physicians vary widely in their attitudes to the disease. Many fail to recognise how little influence they exert on the natural course of events. Some adopt the attitude 'If I can't cure the patient, nobody can'. They refer patients only after years of unsuccessful treatment with little faith in the ability of doctors to improve their lot, who are broken in spirit as well as in body and thus unsuitable for procedures in which the end result depends on fortitute and the will to recover. The enlightened appreciate that while synovectomy is an undesirable destructive operation, it is, in the present state of our knowledge, perhaps the only procedure capable of modifying favourably the course of the disease.

## Surgical Management

In the management of rheumatoid arthritis surgical intervention may be indicated at one or all of three stages.
**Early,** in which the object is the prevention of further damage;
**Intermediate,** in which the object is the preservation of function;
**Late,** in which the object is the reconstruction or arthrodesis of an irreparably damaged joint.

Treatment is considered under these headings:

## EARLY

### PAINFUL ACTIVE SYNOVIAL DISEASE WITHOUT ANGULAR DEFORMITY

### Synovectomy: Background Note

The first subtotal synovectomy, performed for tuberculous infection of the knee joint, is attributed to Volkmann (1877). Mignon (1900) performed what is now known as anterior synovectomy for 'chronic traumatic arthritis' and achieved a return to normal function.

In the current scene surgical synovectomy is recognised to be a crude attack on the integrity of the knee joint; and, in any event, can never be complete. Until more is known about the aetiology and pathology of rheumatoid arthritis, or until chemical synovectomy can be achieved, it is the only method known with a material effect on the local course of the disease.

## Rationale of Operation

**Therapeutic.** The operation is accepted to result in relief of pain in a high percentage of cases. The elimination of pain permits redevelopment of muscle power and consequent improvement of function.

**Prophylactic.** There is evidence that eradication of aggressive vascular synovial membrane from abnormal contact with articular cartilage and from invading subchondral bone prevents or retards destruction of the joint.

The following case is recorded as an example of the prophylactic value of synovectomy. It is of clinical interest in the unusual circumstances of occurrence:

The patient (G.J., male, aged 56) presented with a history that 12 years previously he suffered from rheumatoid arthritis in active form affecting, amongst other joints, both knees in equal degree. A decision had been made that both knee joints should be subjected to synovectomy; but, as a result of gastric haemorrhage, only on the left side was the operation completed. It was at this stage in the history that the author recalled having acted as assistant at the operation, the circumstances of the unrelated complication and then the advent of the Second World War which precluded further treatment. Thus, 12 years later when the disease was 'burnt-out', it was possible to compare, as the result of an unusual combination of circumstances, the effect of synovectomy with a control joint known to be affected in comparable degree in which the synovial membrane had been retained. The knee in which the pathological synovial tissue had been removed was relatively normal in function and radiological appearance (Figs 6,5 and 6,6). That in which the synovial membrane remained was the subject of gross osteoarthritis and was the reason for seeking advice (Figs 6,7 and 6,8).

## Indications for Synovectomy

There are no absolute indications for syno-

vectomy as applied to the rheumatoid knee. Each joint must be assessed individually in relation to the other knee, in relation to the disease process in general and to the effect on other joints in particular.

**1. Pain.** The principal indication for synovectomy is pain.
**2. Persistent synovial swelling** with a raised ESR for a period of, say, one year despite an acceptable regime of medical treatment.
**3. Early involvement of the second knee** in the presence of advanced destruction of the first.
**4. Minimal systemic reaction.**
**5. Minimal radiological changes.**
**6. No limitation of flexion** other than as a result of synovial swelling.
**7. No serious involvement of other weight-bearing joints.**
**8. A patient imbued with the will to recover.**

## Other Indications for Synovectomy

If, in the current scene, rheumatoid arthritis is the most common reason for synovectomy, there are other disease processes for which it may be indicated. The following is a list of conditions for which 'subtotal' or anterior synovectomy has been performed:

1. Rheumatoid arthritis.
2. Chronic non-specific synovitis.
3. Ankylosing spondylitis.
4. Pigmented villonodular synovitis.
5. Synovial chondromatosis.
6. Tuberculosis.
7. Haemophilia.

## Timing of Operation

Rheumatoid arthritis is a stress-related condition and may subside when the stress situation is removed. Spontaneous regression or complete remission is common in the early stages of the disease. It is in the early stages therefore that care is necessary regarding synovectomy: the stress situation may be resolved before irreparable damage has occurred to the articular cartilage. On the other hand there is some evidence that the earlier the operation is performed before any destruction of articular

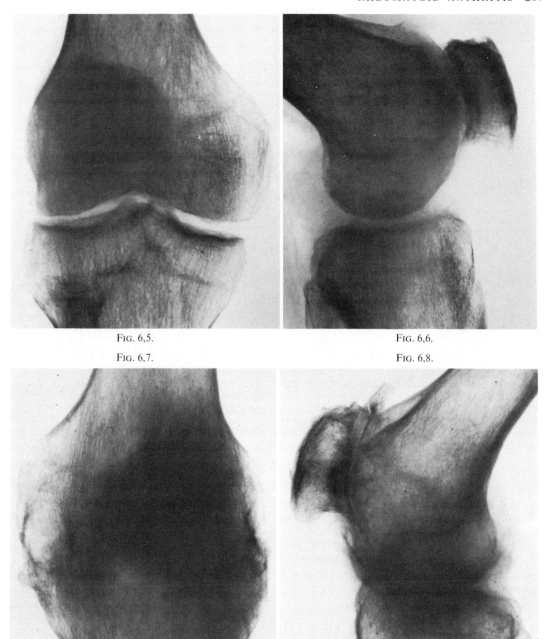

FIG. 6,5.

FIG. 6,6.

FIG. 6,7.

FIG. 6,8.

FIGS 6,5–8. **Synovectomy.** Effect of synovectomy on the development of osteoarthritis in rheumatoid arthritis. The knee joints were equally affected. Synovectomy was performed on right side. Figs 6,5 to 6,6 show state of joints 12 years later. The disease is burnt out. That in which synovectomy was performed is relatively normal (Figs 6,5 and 6,6). Osteoarthritis in marked degree has developed on the side on which synovectomy was not performed (Figs 6,7 and 6,8).

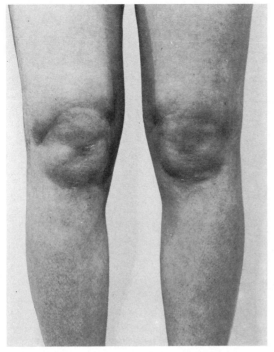
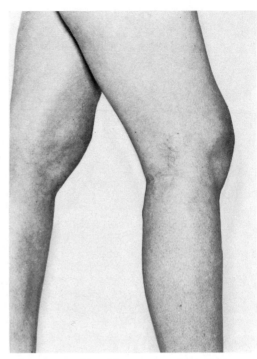

Figs 6,9–10. **Synovectomy? The dilemma.** When these photographs were taken this bilateral sero-negative rheumatoid arthritis had existed for two years. The rheumatologist whom she consulted recommended synovectomy. A patient suffering pain readily accepts the possible consequences of operation. But this patient had no pain and no disability; only synovial swelling. The prospect of two major operations culminating in possible loss of flexion had little attraction for her. This is the patient whose disease presented eight months before the bilateral synovial swelling as a popliteal cyst erroneously considered to be primary (see Chapter 4) (M.S., female, aged 31).

cartilage has occurred the better the long-term result. If the condition has existed for longer than some arbitrary period, say, one year, damage to the articular cartilage will be beginning and permanent disability thereafter inevitable. If the condition has existed for, say, two or more years, and there is no evidence of resolution, the decision to recommend synovectomy if cartilage destruction is not too far advanced is considerably less difficult.

### Consequences of Operation

**Loss of flexion.** If synovectomy is a rational procedure in terms of removal of pathological tissue it is irrational in terms of motion in that it involves excision of opposing gliding surfaces in the suprapatellar pouch and elsewhere.

The operation cures pain, a symptom readily forgotten, and arrests the progress of the disease,

the benefits of which the patient is not in a position to estimate, all at the possible loss of a considerable range of flexion, the disadvantages of which, to a woman in particular, are only too obvious. Thus the earlier synovectomy is done as a prophylactic measure the less may be the subjective benefit for the patient; rather, as indicated, the reverse. In some countries social habits are such that a full range of knee flexion is most important. Such considerations may determine the attitude adopted to synovectomy (Figs 6,9 and 6,10).

In the recovery of movement the angle at which loss of motion no longer obtrudes in the simple demands of everyday life is in the region of right-angled flexion. The majority of patients with rheumatoid arthritis are satisfied with a range of 90°. It enables them to negotiate stairs and to sit without exhibiting disability. But once right-angled flexion has been attained the opportunities for further improvement are considerable in any reasonable situation of conformation of the opposing joint surfaces.

It should be recognised that there is more in return of flexion than social convenience. The return of a range of flexion as great as or greater than a right angle is important if only for the reason that deterioration of articular cartilage occurs in the arc unused in movement; and the greater the loss of flexion the greater is the area of cartilage which will deteriorate.

## Contraindications: Absolute

**Advanced disease.** It is irrational to perform synovectomy in the presence of advanced destruction of articular cartilage as shown by any considerable radiological loss of joint space. The purpose of the operation is prevention of destruction: the damage has already been done.
**Burnt-out disease.** There is no point in carrying out anterior synovectomy in burnt-out rheumatoid arthritis: the damage has been done. Nor should anterior synovectomy be performed at the same time as debridement, hemiarthroplasty or other salvage procedure; indeed rather the reverse in so far as it increases the liability to loss of flexion.

## Contraindications: Relative

**Exacerbation of disease.** Operation should be deferred in circumstances of local exacerbation associated with generalised systemic manifestations if it is only for the reason that the patient may be incapable of the essential co-operation. In this regard some clinical judgement, if on an empirical basis, is necessary. To await the remission which might never occur is to permit destruction of articular cartilage to progress. When in doubt it should be recalled that world literature suggests that most surgeons regret the late stage at which operation is undertaken if the optimum results are to be achieved.

## Preoperative Care

**Anticipating loss of extension.** *Loss of the active control of extension is the most common single source of disability after major surgery of the knee.* If an extension lag is present following

operation, whether it is synovectomy or arthroplasty, there is little chance of the patient being able to walk without the aid of sticks or crutches. The fact that the knee does not extend fully does not necessarily indicate extension lag. It is important to distinguish between loss of extension of mechanical origin from an extension lag.

Extension lag is particularly liable to be present after synovectomy performed in rheumatoid arthritis for a number of reasons existing prior to surgery:

**1. Quadriceps wasting.** Pain is by far the greatest cause of decreased function in rheumatoid arthritis. Decreased function results in muscle atrophy.

**2. Synovial swelling.** Prolonged stretching of quadriceps and patellar tendons from synovial swelling in the suprapatellar pouch and elsewhere results in overlengthening of the extensor apparatus.

**3. Patella alta.** If for one reason or another but particularly for those outlined in (2) above patella alta is present prior to operation, extension lag thereafter will be increased.

If flexion deformity and/or extension lag exists prior to operation the mere removal of synovial membrane will not improve the mechanical situation; rather, indeed, the reverse. It is necessary therefore to anticipate; after operation it is too late.

Patients selected for operation will of necessity be motivated. The purpose and importance of exercise therapy after operation both to regain control of extension and to secure the maximum range of flexion is explained. If pain is not excessive the maximum possible degree and control of extension is achieved in the immediate pre-operation period. It is most important that the existence of patella alta, for whatever reason, is noted prior to surgery so that the steps of the operation can be planned accordingly. The presence of patella alta is an indication for transplantation of the tibial tubercle to a lower level. In other circumstances extension lag is inevitable.

## Technique of Operation

There is no standard technique and this is to be

K

accepted in the variety of conditions to which it is applied including rheumatoid arthritis. If it is agreed that *total* synovectomy is desirable in rheumatoid arthritis, it will be agreed also to be technically, and for practical purposes of return of flexion, impossible. It becomes then a matter of the degree of 'subtotal'. The concensus of opinion tends towards a parapatellar incision with a total excision of the suprapatellar pouch and the synovial tissue surrounding the articular cartilage of the femoral condyles, and as total as is possible in the limited time available, of the lateral expansions and of the intercondylar fossa and cruciate ligaments where signs of activity are usually evident. Few surgeons are prepared to approach the posterior compartment through an additional incision at the original operation.

There are others who adopt a different approach, ignoring the suprapatellar pouch, and through limited medial and lateral incisions remove only the synovial membrane adjacent to articular cartilage and otherwise within reasonable compass of the incision (Marmor, 1966). Such is the diversity of opinion in an operation of wide application but of empirical basis as applied to the most common indication, rheumatoid arthritis.

The author varies his approach according to the circumstances of the case determined by the presence or otherwise of patella alta and the necessity to transplant the tibial tubercle to a lower level. In the latter circumstance a long lateral parapatellar incision is favoured as interfering least with the musculature controlling the joint and with the blood supply of the patella. In other circumstances two incisions are indicated as inflicting the minimal trauma on the integument of the joint (Fig. 6,23). If a lateral incision has been indicated the next step is the location and isolation of the patellar tendon and its attachment. A rectangle of bone is then outlined in the manner described in Chapter 2 and illustrated in Figures 2,83 and 2,84.

Detachment of the patellar tendon provides wide exposure and the operation proceeds by sharp dissection to determine a line of cleavage between capsule and synovial membrane of the suprapatellar pouch and otherwise extended to the margins of the condyles. If two incisions are made (Fig. 6,23) the dissection proceeds as far as

possible on one side and then transfers to the other. It is important in terms of recovery of motion that the fatty layer posterior to the suprapatellar pouch be preserved. The synovial membrane is removed as far as is possible from the lateral expansions and from the cruciate ligaments and intercondylar fossa. In the latter situation the use of a pituitary rongeur is of considerable assistance. The menisci are retained or removed depending on the situation prevailing. It is at this stage, in the circumstances indicating excision of the lateral meniscus, that the hip should be flexed and rotated laterally to permit inspection and possible access to a considerable area of synovial membrane in the posterior compartment.

The time available under tourniquet is not unlimited. The operation should be recognised as a subtotal synovectomy. It should be performed with deliberation avoiding meticulous attention to unnecessary detail. The tibial tubercle, if detached, is returned to a lower situation and locked in position (Fig. 2,84) so that extension exercises can be practised in the immediate post-operative period. Before doing so, but in all circumstances, the articular surface of the patella should be inspected and, if necessary, smoothed as contributing to the rapidity with which the quadriceps can be redeveloped.

Suction drainage is introduced and located in the suprapatellar region. The capsule is then closed with interrupted sutures. The final manoeuvre before skin closure should be production of full flexion so that the surgeon can satisfy himself that manipulation is possible without disruption of the suture line.

**Use of mechanical barrier to adhesion formation.** The most common single source of complaint following synovectomy is loss of flexion (see below). The use of an inert, flexible mechanical barrier to the obliteration of the suprapatellar pouch and opposing gliding surfaces on the medial and lateral aspects of the femoral condyles by adhesions has theoretical attractions and practical advantages. The use of the substance cellophane to form such a barrier is attributed to McKeever (1943).

Initially the material was used to avoid adhesion between iliotibial tract and vastus lateralis, between various elements of the quadriceps and femur and within the suprapatellar pouch. In recent years teflon, a more robust material, has been preferred. No doubt there are other substances equally suitable.

It should be clearly understood that experience of the method is to a large extent confined to chronic non-specific synovitis in which reconstitution of the suprapatellar pouch and peripheral aspects of the femur has been noted to consist of reaction-free replacement of synovial membrane. It has been used also in the less common conditions of synovial chondromatosis and pigmented villonodular synovitis with the retention of flexion greater than a right-angle and similar naked-eye appearances at re-operation. The condition in which it would be most useful in maintaining motion is rheumatoid arthritis. Unfortunately experience is limited; and only to cases which would be classified as Grades 2 to 4. It has not been used to date in an early example. The impression gained, not unexpectedly, is that while right-angle flexion is retained even in late cases the appearance of the 'lining' of the suprapatellar pouch has not been encouraging. It is recognised that the undefined pathology in rheumatoid arthritis is a continuing process and the disease general; not local. The utmost caution therefore has been exercised in its use.

It should be recorded that two patients with chronic non-specific synovitis in which teflon was employed were so satisfied with the result that they refused to have it removed. It is assumed that no serious trouble ensued.

**Technique.** In the present stage of development teflon, 1/2000th of an inch thick and of a sheet size $25 \times 15$ cm and sterilised by autoclave, is employed. At the completion of operation and before introducing suction drainage the material is cut to a width corresponding to the lateral condyle to which it is to be applied. The edge is then folded over two or three times and secured to the side of the femur with a small stainless steel staple (Figs 6,11 and 6,13). The material is then led up into the suprapatellar pouch and down the opposite side of the knee and cut to the shape illustrated (Fig. 6,12). One point only of fixation is employed. The termination of the membrane on the medial side is free (Fig. 6,14).

REMOVAL. The sheet is removed at some arbitrary period, say, three months, when it is thought to have served its purpose, that is to say, flexion has reached a right-angle or more and progress adjudged to be satisfactory. To remove the membrane a short section of the original incision immediately opposed to the staple is excised to gain access to the synovial cavity. The staple is located and removed together with the related teflon sheet.

AFTER-TREATMENT. A limited experience suggests that removal of the membrane results in a temporary reduction of flexion which is rapidly regained in a motivated patient.

## Post-operative Care

At the termination of operation a compression bandage is applied and the tourniquet released. In ordinary circumstances haemarthrosis can be expected to be a complication of synovectomy and as such liable to contribute to residual stiffness. Suction drainage virtually eliminates this particular problem. A synovial effusion, when such occurs, is not a problem and indeed can be beneficial as likely to contribute to the return of flexion. 'Who has seen a stiff knee with an effusion?'

The limb is nursed in a half-ring Thomas bed-knee splint with the end of the bed raised. In the post-operative period and until the patient has recovered from the immediate effects of the operative trauma dorsiflexion-of-the-foot exercises only are practised. On the fourth day straight-leg-raising and flexion exercises within the confines of the bandage are begun and are practised on an hourly basis thereafter. On the seventh or eighth day the massive compression dressing is changed in favour of a crêpe bandage so that flexion is not unduly mechanically restricted. It is about this time that the necessity for manipulation will be considered.

**Manipulation.** The critical time for manipulation under anaesthesia seems to be about the tenth day; and this is the interval from operation recommended unless progress of flexion is so evident as to make intervention unnecessary.

Manipulation should not be deferred until such time as lack of progress is obvious. It is known to have been completely ineffective, exerting the maximum force permissible, on the twenty-first day.

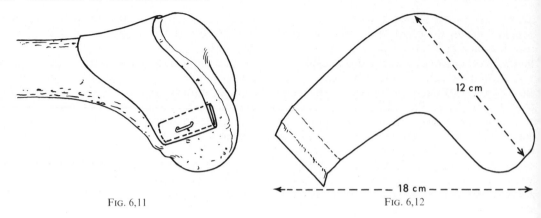

FIG. 6,11                                            FIG. 6,12

FIG. 6,13                                            FIG. 6,14

FIGS 6,11–14. **Use of interposition membrane as barrier to adhesion formation in synovectomy.** Method of application and stapling of teflon sheet to lateral aspect of femur (Fig. 6,11). The general shape of the sheet. This one was removed from a male knee. The dimensions are approximate (Fig. 6,12). The teflon sheet in course of application. It has been stapled to the lateral femoral condyle and is about to be introduced into the suprapatellar pouch (Fig. 6,13). The operation has been completed. The teflon sheet lies stapled to the lateral condyle. It lies free in the suprapatellar pouch and on the medial aspect of the medial femoral condyle (Fig. 6,14).

EFFECT OF INTERPOSITION MEMBRANE. It is probable that manipulation is unnecessary where a barrier to the formation of adhesions has been introduced. In the circumstances in which an interposition membrane has been used, other than in rheumatoid arthritis, the return of flexion has been imperative: routine manipulation has been carried out on the tenth day. In all cases to date right-angled flexion has been attained with no more than finger pressure.

**Resumption of weight-bearing.** Recommendations which cover every eventuality cannot be made in the variety of circumstances which obtain in rheumatoid arthritis. In general, the rule that weight-bearing is not permitted until the extended leg can be raised from the bed should be applied.

## Exercise Therapy

It is appropriate that some reference be made to exercise therapy in the after-treatment of synovectomy rather than elsewhere if only for the reason that it is the operation which imposes on a joint, often with an almost complete range of motion, the serious risk of permanent loss of flexion of socially disabling degree. In injuries and internal derangements it is usually possible to concentrate almost entirely on quadriceps redevelopment and allow the return of flexion to occur in the natural course of events. A different attitude must be adopted in the disease processes. In synovectomy, for example, the avoidance of extension lag by every possible means has been stressed; but not to the exclusion of the muscles on which the return of flexion depends.

It is not proposed that exercises should be listed or detailed but to indicate the underlying principles. It will be evident that the involvement of the patient in her own recovery is essential and to this end examples of the means are described and illustrated; and of simple variations applicable to the home and not dependent on the apparently sophisticated resources of a hospital physiotherapy department. Quadriceps exercises in a variety of forms have been described in IKJ5. Examples of exercises applicable to synovectomy, and to other disease processes in which reduction of

the limitation of flexion is paramount, are appended:

**Passive stretching.** An example of a method applicable after a reasonable range has been attained is to place the foot on a chair and then exert longitudinal pressure in the line of the femur with the hands placed round the thigh immediately above the knee. Such stretching, performed by the patient herself, is not likely to be pursued beyond the point of stimulating reaction (Fig. 6,15).

**Active resisted exercises.** A measure for developing the hamstrings and at the same time increasing the range of flexion is to lie on the floor with the foot on a chair and then exert pressure on the heel so that the lower back is raised from the floor (Fig. 6,16).

### Auto-assisted Exercises

**Skate.** A skate with a roller, say, 10 cm in length and, say, of 3 cm diameter located at the heel and with attached cords controlled by the hands, is a simple method of involving the patient actively in her recovery of flexion. The roller, as opposed to wheels on a narrow base, prevents the possible imposition of rotary forces on the recovering knee. The roller is applied to a plywood board so that resistance is reduced to a minimum (Fig. 6,18).

**Flexion assisted by extension.** A simple pulley system particularly applicable to rheumatoid arthritis in which both knees may be involved is so arranged that extension of one knee is utilised to assist flexion of the other. It necessitated no more equipment than a pulley fixed firmly to the wall at a suitable distance above the floor or bed. Fixation above and below both ankles is effected and a cord attached and adjusted for length so that active extension of the better knee exerts passive flexion on the recovering joint (Fig. 6,17).

**Stationary bicycle.** A bicycle mounted on a stand is a simple method of exercising the quadriceps and increasing extension and, with adjustment of the height of the saddle, applicable to joints with limitation but interest in increase of flexion. There are on the market specially designed stationary bicycles which indicate resistance, speed, incline and distance. There are levels of society in which the very sophistication and expense of such models ensure that they are used (Fig. 6,19).

In this regard a Scots patient (L.R., male, aged 56) equipped with such a device and instructed in daily maintenance exercises became so interested in his mileage accomplishment that he wrote, in the course of Christmas greetings, to say that he had just passed Istanbul and was heading for Ankara in the course of his journey to the Far East!

**Rowing machine.** A method applicable in the later stages of rehabilitation but at a higher level of recovery than is usually attained in rheumatoid arthritis, and to those with a knee

FIGS 6,15–20. **Exercise therapy.** A variety of methods in order of complexity, suitable, after instruction, for use by the motivated patient in the home.

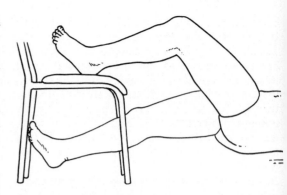

Figure 6,16. Pursuing the matter of passive stretching (Fig. 6,15) to development of the knee flexors, raising of the buttocks from the floor in the manner indicated is simple and effective.

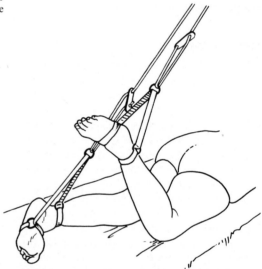

Figure 6,17. A simple pulley system enables extension of one knee to assist flexion of the other.

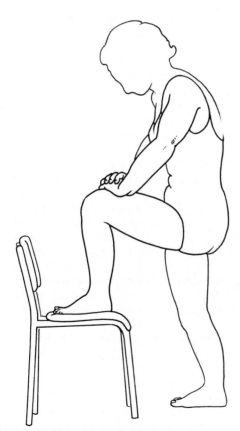

Figure 6,15. When right-angled flexion has been achieved pressure exerted in the line of the femur can be utilised to increase the range of movement.

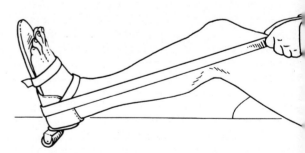

Figure 6,18. A skate with a roller at the heel and with attached cords for control by the hands is an effective method of involving the patient in her own recovery of flexion.

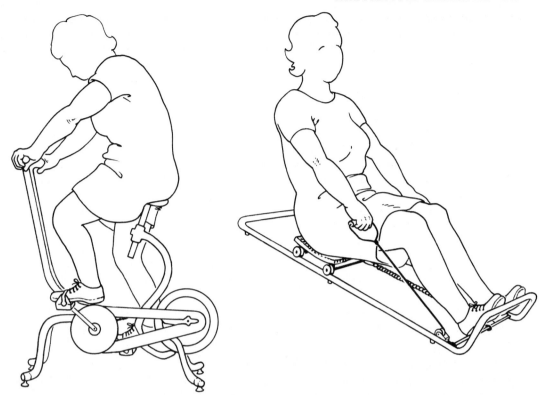

Figure 6,19. The stationary bicycle is applicable to exercise therapy on a maintenance basis and is a method open to improvisation.

Figure 6,20. In the later stages of recovery, and with a view to exercise therapy on a permanent basis, a simple rowing machine is applicable to both flexion and extension and to the skeletal muscles in general.

problem on a permanent basis, is the simple rowing machine which has the advantage of simultaneous exercise of both quadriceps and hamstrings as well as skeletal muscles in general (Fig. 6,20).

### SYNOVECTOMY: RESULTS OF OPERATION

The clinical results of synovectomy are well documented. It is generally accepted that 80 per cent of patients are relieved of pain. Loss of flexion is the most common cause of complaint; and reference has been made to the means whereby this can be minimised.

**Duration of improvement.** The longer the follow-up the lower the percentage of satisfactory results. Paradies (1969) recorded a reduction to 65 per cent at two years and a further reduction to 40 per cent after three years. There is thus evidence of recurrence of disease activity in certain cases with the passage of time.

**Cause of clinical deterioration.** It has been shown that the rate of clearance of radioactive xenon from the joint ($^{133}$Xe) by the blood vessels in the synovial membrane in one to three months following synovectomy is significantly lower than before operation, presumably indicating a reduction in the vascularity of the regenerated tissue after operation. One year later, however, the rate of clearance did not differ significantly from before operation suggesting that regeneration of synovial membrane with abnormal vessels had occurred by this time. It is of interest that these results were not related to an unsatisfactory clinical result. In a group of patients studied two to three years after synovectomy clearance rates did not differ from those obtained in classical rheumatoid arthritis; but at this stage a high proportion of patients still regarded the result of operation to be satisfactory. It was concluded that regrowth of synovial membrane with abnormal vasculature occurs early but that clinical deterioration is deferred. It is suggested that long-term follow-up studies may indicate whether the timing and severity of clinical deterioration is predictable from the blood flow values (Dick *et al.*, 1970). These preliminary findings however may indicate the possible necessity for re-synovectomy in selected cases if irreparable damage is to be avoided.

## Unsatisfactory Results

In this series unsatisfactory results have been attributed to:

1. OPERATION AT WRONG TIME. In retrospect it has been evident that operation in circumstances of local exacerbation are not conducive to return of flexion whatever may be the outcome as a prophylactic measure. There are evident advantages in the ability to concentrate on a single joint to the exclusion of others and of a systemic problem.

2. ADVANCED DISEASE. If the disease has progressed to the stage of advanced destruction of articular cartilage the benefits to be obtained from synovectomy are limited.

3. UNCONTROLLED PROGRESSION OF GENERALISED RHEUMATOID DISEASE. If in the immediate post-operative period the progression of the disease is uncontrolled the possibilities of benefit are markedly reduced.

4. LACK OF MOTIVATION. It will be evident that this is an operation in which co-operation by a motivated patient is essential if a return of a reasonable degree of flexion is to be achieved.

## Re-synovectomy

When occurrence of pain and swelling occurs after synovectomy the indications for surgery are largely the same as for primary synovectomy. If the patient already has a stiff or almost stiff knee on the other side, re-synovectomy can prove beneficial.

The case history which follows is recorded to illustrate the problems which arise in the course of synovectomy for rheumatoid arthritis and in particular the effect of errors of judgement in the timing of procedures on both the short-term and final result:

The patient (Mrs M.M., aged 58) was referred by a rheumatologist of international status for consideration of bilateral synovectomy. The remaining joints did not pose a physical problem. The ESR was 28. The R.A. Latex test positive. She was active, intelligent and motivated. She was aware of the purpose and probable benefits of synovectomy and knew of the consequences in terms of loss of flexion. She was anxious about loss of movement as likely to interfere with social activities. It was decided to proceed with the left, the more swollen and more painful joint. It was noted prior to operation that complete extension could not be achieved despite considerable effort. The inability to extend was attributed to the large synovial swelling. The operation was performed through a lateral parapatellar incision and was uneventful. It had been the intention to introduce a teflon sheet. A considerable layer of fatty tissue remained on the femoral surface after removal of the suprapatellar pouch; and in the absence of experience in the use of the material in rheumatoid arthritis and in an attitude of caution its use was omitted. Suction drainage was employed.

The immediate post-operative period was uneventful. It was noted, however, and with some concern, that control over extension had decreased. Fifteen to 20° of flexion was achieved almost immediately. The physiotherapist continued to report favourably on progress and co-operation until the twentieth day. At this stage it was questioned whether any real increase of flexion had occurred in the past week. The patient, it should be stated, expressed her complete satisfaction: the synovial pain had disappeared completely after the reaction to the surgery had subsided. Examination revealed a range of flexion no more than 15° but with some improvement in the original extension lag. It was decided therefore that manipulation under anaesthesia was indicated. It was with surprise, and concern, that no further range of flexion could be obtained despite exertion of the maximum force justifiable in the circumstances. No material progress has taken place since then. Four years later she had a painless, normal-looking joint but with flexion limited to 15° and with the disability of function so-related.

It had been the original intention to proceed immediately with the second knee. The patient, however, although satisfied with the result of the first operation in terms of absence of pain, was most dissatisfied in terms of loss of motion. She could not contemplate a second knee similarly affected. The surgeon was not in a strong position to promise any better result. In the circumstances the second, the right knee, was permitted to progress in term of pain, swelling and loss of function until it became evident to all concerned that operative action was imperative. At operation it was clear that the disease had been permitted to advance to a stage at which considerable destruction of articular cartilage was evident and for purposes of record classified as Grade 4. A promise had been extracted that measures would be taken that would almost guarantee the preservation of flexion at least to a right-angle. A teflon sheet was therefore introduced in the manner described. It had not been anticipated that the disease would be so far advanced; and in the absence of the promise of right-angled flexion a teflon sheet would not have been employed at this stage. It has been indicated that post-operative manipulation may not be necessary in the presence of an interposition membrane. In this case the promise of a considerable range of flexion made manipulation essential. On the tenth post-operative day right-angled flexion was achieved under general anaesthesia with no more than finger pressure. The subsequent progress was satisfactory and a range of movement greater than a right-angle was attained. Some degree of extension lag continued in spite of considerable effort. It has never been completely eliminated. It is considered to be multifactorial in origin. In retrospect not the least of the factors concerned was patella alta (Fig. 6,21).

The teflon sheet was removed four months later. At operation it was noted that the presumed regeneration of synovial membrane was smooth but considerably inflamed and not to be compared with that encountered after chronic non-specific arthritis. A range of

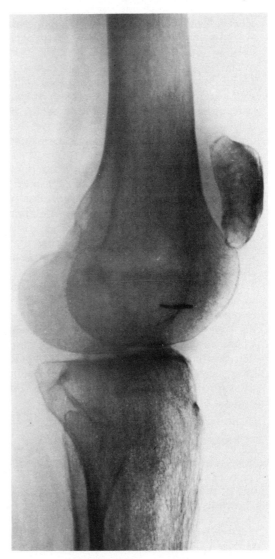

FIG. 6,21. **Synovectomy: error of judgement and technique.** The patient had a marked patella alta with consequent extension lag. She regained flexion of 105° following the use of a teflon interposition membrane; but control would have been established at a much earlier date if the tibial tubercle had been transplanted to a lower level to overcome the patella alta. (See Figs 2,83 and 2,84.) Note location of staple fixing teflon interposition membrane in the lateral condyle.

movement rather greater than a right-angle was rapidly regained.

This patient two years later remains a problem. The left knee is painless and normal in appearance; but flexion remains limited to a range of little more than 15°. The right knee has a range of movement rather greater than a right-angle. There is pain, not excessive, but evident recurrence of synovial swelling and effusion.

The lessons to be learnt from this case are:
1. Failure to recognise the existence of patella alta when overshadowed by gross synovial swelling; and to appreciate the influence of patella alta on recovery: in both knees the tibial tubercle should have been transplanted to a lower level.
2. The importance of the timing of a post-operative manipulation. In this case the failure to detect cessation of progressive increase of flexion until it was too late: If manipulation is to be performed it should take place at the tenth or so day; not at the twenty-first day when it was obvious that progress has ceased; and it may be too late.
3. The mistiming of the operation on the second knee. It will be evident that the failure to regain flexion on the first knee influenced the timing of the operation on the second which was undertaken when it was obvious that destruction was progressing. It should have been undertaken as a prophylactic measure despite the loss of flexion at the original operation.

### SPONDYLITIS ANKYLOPOIETICA

Synovectomy may have a dramatic effect both on pain, clinical appearance and probably on the future of the joint in spondylitis ankylopoietica as shown by the following case:

The patient (W.F., male, aged 47, case of R.D.M.) presented with the history that, when aged 38, he noticed stiffness in his upper back and neck with a developing stoop and increasing difficulty in looking upwards. Some months later he suddenly realised that he was unable to turn his neck sufficiently to look over either shoulder. It was at this stage he first sought medical attention. At no time was

pain a significant feature of his case until his knees became involved.

Three years later a course of deep X-ray therapy was prescribed. The spine, hips and knees were irradiated. He was not having trouble with the knees at that time. At no stage had he received steroid therapy.

Three years ago the right knee became uncomfortable and started to swell following a minor twisting injury. The swelling was intermittent but never subsided completely. The left knee began to swell some months later. At all times the salient feature has been synovial swelling. Restriction of movement had never been of disabling degree. There was stiffness after sitting for any length of time. Pain could not be described as severe rather of the nature of a constant ache.

At synovectomy of the right knee the gross

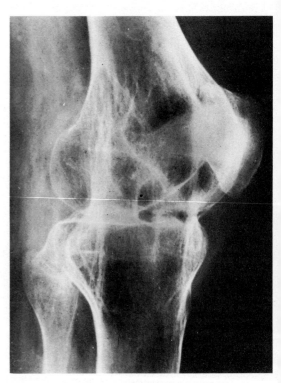

FIG. 6,22. **Spondylitis ankylopoietica.** The radiological appearance of a knee joint ankylosed by spondylitis ankylopoietica. The other knee was similarly affected. Such joints are unlikely to react favourably to arthroplasty. Can ankylosis be avoided by timely synovectomy? (See Figs 6,23 and 6,24.)

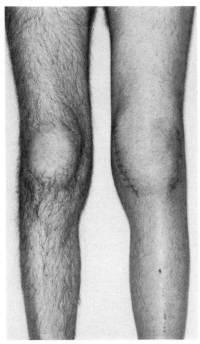

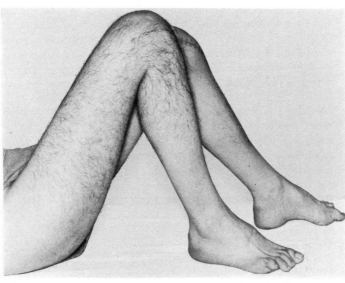

FIGS 6,23–24. **Spondylitis ankylopoietica.** The result, in terms of motion, of synovectomy in spondylitis ankylopoietica. The right knee was virtually normal three months from the date of operation. The left knee demonstrates the range attained six weeks after synovectomy (Fig. 6,24). Note double incision used at operation (Fig. 6,23) (W.F., male, case of R.D.M.). It is possible that timely synovectomy can avoid the disaster of ankylosis illustrated by Figure 6,22.

appearance of the synovial membrane was similar to that of rheumatoid arthritis. The aching pain was relieved immediately. The final result was a complete return of flexion. He regarded the outcome as a virtually normal knee at three months from the date of operation (Figs 6,23 and 6,24). The left knee remained swollen and painful. If anything the ache was worse than that which he suffered on the right side. He had been only too happy to accept a second synovectomy.

At operation of the left knee through two incisions (Fig. 6,23), as on the right, similar conditions were encountered. The immediate result of operation was relief of the aching pain with which he had become familiar. The final outcome on the short term basis of three months was a return to what he considered, by standards determined by the past, to be a normal knee. He had, on examination, complete extension and a full range of flexion.

## PSORIATIC ARTHRITIS

The arthritis which is associated with psoriasis varies widely in definition and in form.

The following case record embodies many well-known features of the disease which in this example presented as a mono-articular sero-negative rheumatoid arthritis affecting the knee:

The patient (Mrs M.I., aged 37) gave a history that two years previously she had injured her left knee. At that time she was just beginning her training as a teacher. After a long period of standing she developed pain in the lateral side of the joint. There was slight swelling. She was treated by heat and a supporting bandage but without improvement. When examined by the author there was tenderness and swelling located to the joint line laterally. There was thus some suspicion that she might have been suffering from a congenital discoid meniscus. On the other hand, with such a long history, and in the female subject, the possibility of rheumatoid arthritis arose. The ESR screening test was established to be 24/1 hour. The Latex test was found to be negative. She was admitted to hospital with the possibility of lateral meniscectomy in view. When reviewed in hospital the joint was generally, but only very slightly, swollen. There was tenderness on the medial joint line as well as on the lateral. Radiographs were negative except that there was a suspicion of decalcification by comparison with the opposite side. The ESR repeated was 18/1 hour. The Latex test was again negative. It was decided to aspirate the joint and have a guinea pig inoculated for the purpose of eliminating the possibility of tuberculosis.

The result of the guinea pig inoculation was negative. In the absence of a definite diagnosis she was labelled mono-articular idiopathic synovitis and kept under observation.

One year later the condition had not materially changed. The ESR was 15/1 hour.

Her case was reviewed at monthly intervals. On one occasion, 13 months after she was first seen, in the course of questioning her again and still in the absence of a diagnosis, she revealed for the first time and with reluctance that her mother had rheumatoid arthritis and had recently had a synovectomy. The diagnosis therefore was changed to mono-articular sero-negative rheumatoid arthritis.

She received no treatment other than observation and the maintenance of her quadriceps. Pain was never severe and, indeed, only troublesome after any long period of standing.

It was approximately two years from the date on which she was first seen that she volunteered the information that she had developed a peculiar condition in the nails of her hands and feet; and that her general practitioner was treating her for a fungus infection. The appearance of the nails, however, was that of psoriasis. She was questioned closely as to whether she had any evidence of the condition elsewhere. This she denied. Eventually it transpired that she had recently developed a condition of the scalp which had

been labelled dermatitis. Examination revealed a patch of psoriasis.

Re-examination at this time showed no evidence of any symptoms or swelling of other peripheral joints. Her ESR was 11/1 hour. All investigations including radiographs of her sacro-iliac joints were negative. The label was therefore changed to mono-articular psoriatic arthropathy.

No treatment was thought necessary other than to keep her under observation; and to encourage her in the maintenance of complete extension and of quadriceps tone. When last seen some five years after the onset of symptoms the appearance of the joint in so far as swelling is concerned and the related symptomatology had not materially changed.

The case illustrates:

1. Apparent mono-articular sero-negative rheumatoid arthritis which later developed psoriasis.
2. Mono-articular arthritis associated with nail changes in the virtual absence of skin lesions.
3. The familial background to sero-negative rheumatoid arthritis.
4. The less extensive and benign nature of the disease presenting in mono-articular form. At the time of development of the nail lesions the arthritis demanded no more than review at regular intervals, the maintenance of extension by passive stretching and quadriceps exercises.

## PAINFUL ACTIVE DISEASE WITH ANGULAR DEFORMITY

If angulation, usually valgus, antedates the onset of rheumatoid arthritis, deformity tends to progress rapidly, presumably as a result of softening of the condyle under compression. In such circumstances early tibial osteotomy by one of the methods described in Chapter 10 may be required (Fig. 6,25).

If synovectomy is indicated the immediate question which will arise is the order in which the procedures should be undertaken. In general, and in so far as rules can be formulated, osteotomy should proceed synovectomy if it is only for the reason that there is some evidence

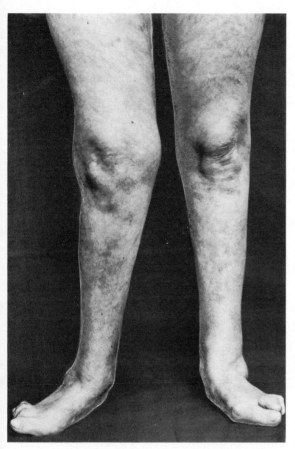

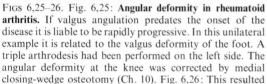

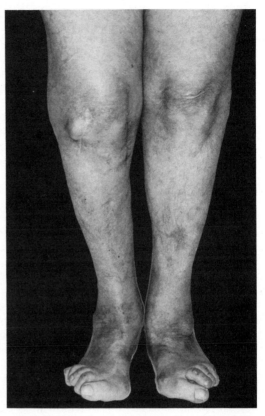

FIGS 6,25–26. Fig. 6,25: **Angular deformity in rheumatoid arthritis.** If valgus angulation predates the onset of the disease it is liable to be rapidly progressive. In this unilateral example it is related to the valgus deformity of the foot. A triple arthrodesis had been performed on the left side. The angular deformity at the knee was corrected by medial closing-wedge osteotomy (Ch. 10). Fig. 6,26: This resulted in reduction, but not elimination, of synovial swelling. Pain was less and with considerable improvement of function. The situation gradually deteriorated over the next three years. Eventually total replacement in the form of the Stanmore hinge prosthesis was necessary to eliminate the intolerable level of pain. (Mrs. I.W., aged 55.)

that osteotomy has a favourable effect on synovial proliferation; and that subsequent synovectomy may not be required.

The division of the tibia in the form of a high osteotomy correcting angular deformity has an apparent effect, for whatever reason, on synovial thickening in osteoarthrosis (Wardle, 1964). In a review of his results he stated: 'At an interval of two years the disappearance of synovial thickening is a striking feature.' Division of the femur and tibia without displacement, for whatever reason, has an effect on the synovial membrane in rheumatoid arthritis (Benjamin, 1969). In this series there were 21 knees which were considered to be affected primarily by rheumatoid arthritis, and of these, 15 showed evidence of active disease at the time of operation. In Trickey's (1969) independent assessment of the result of double osteotomy it is stated: 'The operation appears to be equally effective in osteoarthritis and rheumatoid arthritis. The proliferated synovium of the active rheumatoid knee regresses rapidly following operation.' It was left to question why double osteotomy is followed by regression of synovial proliferation.

## INTERMEDIATE

### FLEXION DEFORMITY THE RESULT OF MISDIAGNOSIS, MISMANAGEMENT OR NEGLECT

**Introduction.** A fixed flexion deformity preventing ambulation is the common outcome of the neglect or mismanagement of many of the disease processes of the knee joint in the acute state. In the current scene in the temperate zone so-called developed countries it is probable that rheumatoid arthritis is the most common cause of such a situation. In tropical and sub-tropical less developed countries poliomyelitis and various forms of infection remain the more usual cause. It is appropriate that the treatment of flexion deformities should be considered under the heading rheumatoid arthritis because it is in this condition that the most difficult situations, mechanical and otherwise, arise not only that the condition may be bilateral but that a multiplicity of other joints may be involved to say nothing of a motivation problem which seldom obtains in poliomyelitis or sepsis; rather indeed the reverse. Moreover, only in minimal examples is it a matter of simple increase of flexion. A deformity of any considerable duration is accompanied by loss of the normal relationship of tibia to femur in so far as posterior subluxation of the tibia occurs. In addition lateral rotation of the tibia is present, said in rheumatoid arthritis to be due to peroneal spasm and related valgus position of the foot (Fig. 6,25). In extreme examples rotation is such that the lateral condyle of the tibia is displaced behind that of the femur accompanied by varying degrees of valgus angulation.

The principles underlying treatment are the same no matter what the underlying disease process. The approach requires modification depending on the background and circumstances of the individual case.

**Biomechanical implications of flexed-knee gait.** The quadriceps force required to stabilise the knee is 75 per cent of the load on the femoral head at 15°; 210 per cent at 30° and 410 per cent at 60°. It is evident that no mechanical problem exists in minimal deformity. Progression to visible deformity however, say 30°, changes the situation to one of high stress (Perry, Antonelli and Ford, 1975).

## Treatment

**Prevention.** The capacity of the synovial cavity of the knee is maximal in slight flexion. A joint the subject of an inflammatory process and/or effusion producing tension will automatically adopt this position in the interests of reduction of pain. In the supine position a pillow will be placed beneath the knees 'to make the patient comfortable'. This error is probably the most important single cause of a flexion contracture in the pathology of the joint and particularly in the disease processes with a chronic course the most common of which is rheumatoid arthritis. The function of the most grossly damaged joint can be shown to be excellent for all ordinary purposes provided extension is complete and quadriceps volume maintained. It is thus essential that every effort be made to prevent, in the acute phase of any disease, the development of even the minimum flexion deformity. At an idealistic level complete extension is the difference between perfection of function and a considerable disability.

If an effusion distends the synovial cavity aspiration is indicated and should be followed by the application of a compression bandage incorporating, if necessary, a light gutter splint. In no circumstances, as has been indicated, should the joint be flexed 'comfortably' over a pillow.

If the tendency to flexion is produced by synovial thickening a light plaster back-shell extending as high up on the thigh as possible and incorporating a right-angled foot-piece is necessary and secured with a removable elastic-stretch bandage, not only permits the joint to be inspected, but allows removal one or more times daily, once the acute phase has passed, for active exercises for the maintenance of movement. Isometric quadriceps exercises are practised hourly if possible, from the beginning of the illness. With evidence of progress to recovery the back-shell can be discarded during the day but re-applied at night when some flexion is the natural position during sleep. In no circumstances should weight-bearing on tiptoe with a flexed knee be permitted in the acute phase nor a return to weight-bearing in any form permitted until straight-leg-raising can be performed without difficulty; and this is the target at which to aim. If recovery is likely to be complete the mechanics of normal gait should be taught. In other circumstances it is better to bear weight on the extended knee, with or without a splint or caliper, than permit an abnormal means of progression to be established on a flexed knee.

In other circumstances of progressive pathology the necessity to maintain extension, and the reason for so doing, is explained to the patient and the methods in combination with quadriceps exercises demonstrated.

The long term effect of permanent gait on a *normal* but flexed knee joint is described in Chapter 10.

## Selection of Method of Reduction in Established Deformity

In considering the methods of reduction available it will be recalled that in the normal knee only the first 20° or so of flexion consists of hingeing. The remainder of the range consists of gliding movement. It will be evident, therefore, that a flexion deformity much greater than 20° cannot be reduced by simple manipulation or by serial or wedge casts. Measures must be adopted which incorporate this gliding motion. An additional problem of even greater mechanical complexity and to which reference has already been made is the fact that in the development of flexion deformity the normal relationship of tibia to femur is altered in so far as posterior subluxation is of common occurrence (Figs 6,27 and 6,28).

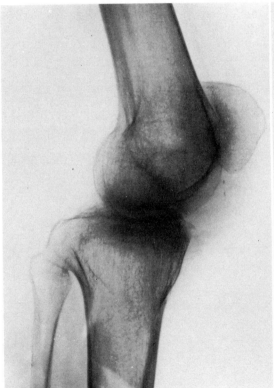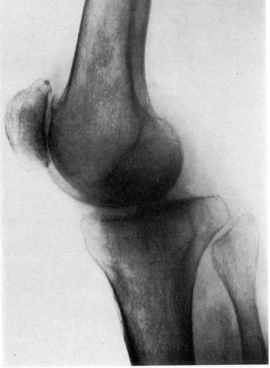

FIGS 6,27–28. **Rheumatoid arthritis: flexion deformity.** Posterior subluxation of the tibia in some degree is a common accompaniment of flexion deformity in rheumatoid arthritis and its existence recognised before undertaking corrective measures. It will be evident in either of these two examples that forcible extension by any method prior to reduction of the posterior subluxation, at best will not achieve reduction of the flexion deformity, at worst is fraught with danger.

A word of caution, therefore, is necessary in relation to the reduction of flexion deformities. The surgeon should not embark on complicated traction-counter-traction systems, turn-buckle plaster casts, etc., without experience of the method and possible complications and without the certain knowledge that the hour-to-hour nursing care which is necessary has the essential skills. In other words the selection of the method may depend on the quality of the nursing care available. The complication of a pressure sore in the heel region or paralysis of the lateral popliteal nerve may be a worse disability than the deformity.

Failure to achieve an objective produces disappointment and loss of confidence. Before embarking on the long, painful and expensive exercise of correction of a flexion deformity the surgeon should ask himself:

**1. Is reduction possible by conservative means or is operative division of contracted structures necessary?**
**2. What is the object of the reduction?**
   A mobile joint?
   A limb capable of being fitted with a walking caliper?
   A prelude to surgery, say, synovectomy, arthrodesis or arthroplasty?
   If arthrodesis, is reduction necessary prior to operation?
**3. Will the method selected achieve the objective?**

### Classification

A possible arbitrary classification of flexion deformities into (1) **mild** (2) **moderate** and (3) **marked** without defining angles may help to indicate that even such a classification is an over-simplification of a situation which in terms of difficulty of reduction or otherwise depends on a multiplicity of factors which include age and sex of patient; causative pathology; duration of disease, and of deformity; involvement of hip, ankle and other joints; whether ambulatory or bedridden, etc; and, of course, motivation.

### METHODS OF TREATMENT

### Mild

Flexion deformities of slight degree occur in two forms: (1) those which in the course of disease of whatever origin have never been more than mild, and (2) those which were moderate or marked but which as a result of treatment of one kind or another have reached a stage somewhat short of the target of complete or almost complete extension.

It is not proposed to catalogue the methods available to this and greater degrees of flexion but to select a variety applicable to this degree of flexion in rheumatoid arthritis and other causes of deformity.

**Manual stretching.** The simplest method of the reduction of flexion is manual stretching by a

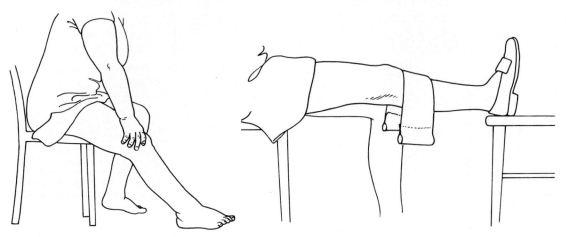

FIGS 6,29–30. **Flexion deformity of soft tissue origin: treatment.** The simplest method of reduction is manual stretching in the manner indicated (Fig. 6,29). Passive stretching of contracted posterior soft tissues can be achieved by the application of an extensor force in the form of a weight to the anterior aspect of the limb (Fig. 6,30).

co-operative patient. She sits on the edge of a chair with her legs extended, the foot plantar flexed to relax the calf muscles. The hand is placed and exerts pressure immediately above the patella so that no direct pressure is exerted on a possibly worn patello-femoral joint. This measure, practised hourly in combination with quadriceps exercises can be most effective. The potential for improvement of function in a flexion deformity of moderate degree by passive stretching, provided there is no bony block to extension, should not be underestimated.

The occasion is recalled when a domiciliary visit was paid to a woman with quiescent rheumatoid arthritis, house-bound because of flexion deformities of both knees. She got about supporting herself with her hands on adjacent furniture. She was offered admission to hospital with the prospect of arthrodesis of the worse joint and the possible retention of mobility in the other. She was warned that delay was inevitable in the circumstances which prevailed at the time. It was noted that her morale was high and with a strong will to recovery. It was suggested, therefore, that the interval before admission might be employed by passive stretching to increase extension and mobilising exercises; and the means were demonstrated (Fig. 6,29). It was with surprise bordering on astonishment that on admission to hospital four months later she had attained virtually complete extension in both knees combined with a flexion range greater than a right-angle and was walking without support.

**Passive stretching.** The patient sits on a chair and places her heel upon another chair. A weight of, say, 5 kg (10 lb) attached to a broad band, is suspended to produce an extension force on the joint. The band is located below or above but not directly over the patello-femoral joint. The stretching is undertaken say, three times a day and quadriceps exercises practised during the course of stretching (Fig. 6,30).

Two further examples of passive stretching are

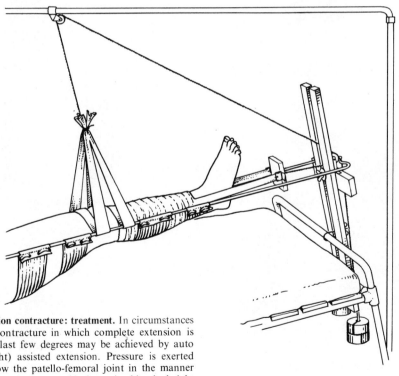

FIG. 6,31. **Flexion contracture: treatment.** In circumstances of soft tissue contracture in which complete extension is attainable, the last few degrees may be achieved by auto (patient's weight) assisted extension. Pressure is exerted above and below the patello-femoral joint in the manner illustrated. The pressure exerted is determined by the height to which the end of the bed is raised.

described, one applicable to bed-rest, the other, at the opposite end of the scale, to ambulation. Both aim at the return of function envisaged in complete extension.

**Weight-assisted correction.** Detachable skin extension is applied below the knee and the limb placed in a half-ring Thomas bed-splint which is fixed to the foot of the bed by the splint-rest illustrated in Figure 6,36. An extension cord is attached and carried through the under aspect of the pulley on the horizontal support of the splint-rest. Strips of 7·5 cm (3 in) orthopaedic strapping are stuck together, opposing the adhesive surfaces, to form lengths of double thickness. Direct pressure on the patello-femoral joint is undesirable. One strip is passed above the patella and under the lateral bars of the Thomas splint, the other below the patella in a similar manner. All four ends finally meet in front of the joint and

are secured to the original extension cord which has been passed through a pulley attached to an overhead beam. The end of the bed is then raised so that the body weight exerts traction while counter-traction produces pressure on the flexed joint. The rapidity of reduction, within the limits of the patient's endurance, is controlled by the height to which the foot of the bed is raised (Fig. 6,31). Quadriceps exercises are practised in the intervals between stretching sessions.

**Corrective walking caliper.** It is possible to produce a corrective extension force with a full-length walking caliper by introducing a spiral spring (Fig. 6,33) into the uprights opposite the centre of rotation of the joint (Fig. 6,32). The method is useful when a caliper is indicated for some other reason. The spring is loaded by flexion of the knee. When the leg is raised and weight transferred to the other foot, the spring

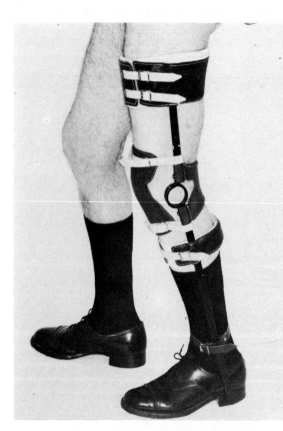

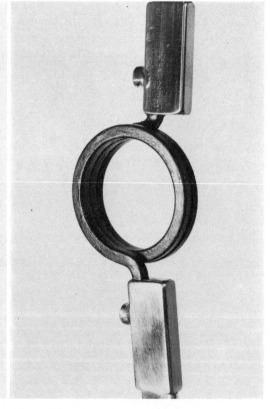

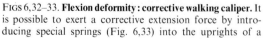

FIGS 6,32–33. **Flexion deformity: corrective walking caliper.** It is possible to exert a corrective extension force by introducing special springs (Fig. 6,33) into the uprights of a walking caliper (Fig. 6,32). The method is applicable only if extension is limited by soft tissue contracture and there is no bony block to extension.

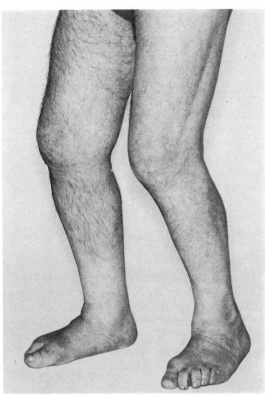

FIG. 6,34. **Rheumatoid arthritis.** Typical flexion deformities of rheumatoid arthritis at a stage when correction can be effected by serial plaster back-shells and, in this example, as a prelude to synovectomy.

FIGS 6,35–36. **Flexion deformity: reduction.** Serial posterior plaster shells are of universal application and the safest form of reduction in general use. In the method favoured the posterior V of the flexion deformity is filled with cotton wool or tapered layers of felt as in the line drawing (Fig. 6,35) and a back-shell applied (Fig. 6,36). Correction is effected by successive removal of layers of felt, the application of elastic compression and changes of plaster shell as indicated. The patient is Figure 6,34.

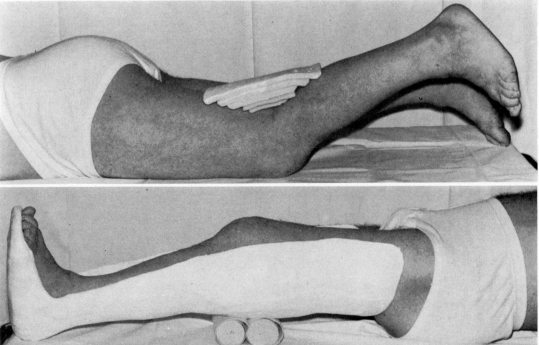

is released to exert an extension force on the joint. In this manner it helps to maintain and increase extension while at the same time limiting excessive flexion and rotation strains (Helfet, 1963).

### Serial Plaster Back-Shells

This method, of universal application in a variety of forms, is the safest and most common means of correction in general use. It is applicable to mild to moderate deformities of relatively recent origin with, say, 25° of flexion in so far as the range of correction to be undertaken is within the range of hingeing motion (Fig. 6,34).

**Technique.** The patient is placed in the prone position and the maximum correction secured. A lightly padded back-shell is applied in a degree or two short of the maximum so that the soft tissues are not under tension and muscle spasm induced. The cast extends from the uppermost aspect of the thigh to the tips of the toes and surrounds three-quarters of the circumference of the limb. It is held in position by a crêpe bandage. It is changed at the end of one week

for one in a greater degree of extension; and so on till the optimum correction is achieved.

The method favoured by the author is to fill the V of the flexion deformity with successive layers of damp cottonwool or, more extravagantly, tapered layers of orthopaedic felt (Fig. 6,35). The back-shell is then applied (Fig. 6,36). To correct the deformity a layer of cottonwool (or felt) is removed at intervals of a few days, the back-shell re-applied and pressure exerted by the firmly applied elastic bandage. By the time the last layer is removed considerable reduction should have been effected; but in any event it will be time to renew the now ill-fitting shell.

### Methods of Traction

Traction, skin or skeletal, fixed or weight, in the Thomas bed-knee splint is applicable to a wide variety of conditions in the lower limb and particularly to the injuries and affections of the knee joint. There is constant reference to its use in this work. In rheumatoid arthritis it is applicable to mild to moderate deformities and at a stage before posterior subluxation has

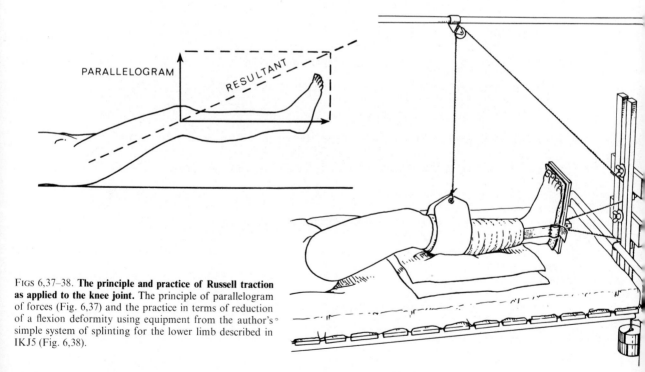

FIGS 6,37–38. **The principle and practice of Russell traction as applied to the knee joint.** The principle of parallelogram of forces (Fig. 6,37) and the practice in terms of reduction of a flexion deformity using equipment from the author's simple system of splinting for the lower limb described in IKJ5 (Fig. 6,38).

occurred. The splint with minimal traction has wide application in the treatment of rheumatoid arthritis as, for example, in the post-operative treatment of synovectomy or posterior release.

The Bohler-Braun-type splint is used with skin or skeletal traction when an extension force is required through the flexed knee in the normal, but injured joint so that the forces can be applied in flexion to relax, for example, the calf muscles. In the disease processes and in rheumatoid arthritis in particular it is used to stretch contracted structures in the early stages of the reduction of a flexion deformity.

**Russell traction.** This is an ingenious form of traction which employs the principle of double pulleys with double ropes so that a single weight exerts double the longitudinal traction. The means whereby it can be employed in conjunction with the system of splinting described is illustrated in Figures 6,37 and 6,38. This method of traction was originally intended for the treatment of fractures of the shaft of the femur. It is applicable to flexion deformity at the knee in so far as it is simple to apply, involves the minimum of apparatus and is readily dis-

mantled and re-applied when periods of intermittent traction are indicated.

**Manipulation : General**

The role of manipulation in the correction of flexion deformities in rheumatoid arthritis is debatable. In general, a less dramatic approach in the form of serial shells is to be preferred as less liable to stimulate unfavourable reaction. There are other circumstances of pathology, for example, poliomyelitis in which manipulation may be indicated. It is important, no matter what the background, that a hinging action is not imposed on a joint in which there is posterior subluxation of the tibia. If in such circumstances there is an indication for manipulation the gliding action must be simulated by pulling the tibial head forward and forcing the femur backwards before hingeing the joint (Fig. 6,40). If this action cannot be effected the application of force will result in dislocation.

A deformity of recent origin or one to which no treatment has been applied or effort made to

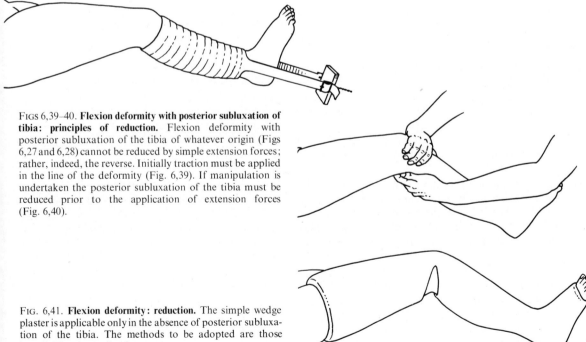

FIGS 6,39–40. **Flexion deformity with posterior subluxation of tibia: principles of reduction.** Flexion deformity with posterior subluxation of the tibia of whatever origin (Figs 6,27 and 6,28) cannot be reduced by simple extension forces; rather, indeed, the reverse. Initially traction must be applied in the line of the deformity (Fig. 6,39). If manipulation is undertaken the posterior subluxation of the tibia must be reduced prior to the application of extension forces (Fig. 6,40).

FIG. 6,41. **Flexion deformity: reduction.** The simple wedge plaster is applicable only in the absence of posterior subluxation of the tibia. The methods to be adopted are those least liable to complication.

maintain function is more likely to react favourably to manipulation than one which has persisted in spite of every effort to the contrary. This is a situation in which posterior release may offer the only prospect of correction.

**Technique.** The amount of force which may be employed cannot be defined: it is a matter of clinical judgement. Where there is deformity to be corrected or motion to be restored function has been deficient in varying degree and possibly as low as zero; and in no pathological background more than rheumatoid arthritis. Decalcification may be extreme with fragility of the cortex and supporting trabeculae. A compression fracture is readily inflicted on the tibial head in particular if force is expended. In such circumstances extreme caution should be exercised in the application of leverage: the femur, the fixed point, should be secured immediately above the joint, the tibia, to be moved, gripped immediately below the joint.

### Wedged Plaster Cast

It will be evident that the simple wedging of a plaster cast exerts a hingeing action only upon the joint and in theory therefore is applicable only within the range of such action (Fig. 6,41). In brief, the technique consists of the application of a plaster cast reaching from as high as possible in the thigh to the roots of the toes in the maximum tolerable degree of correction. It is suitably padded at the bony prominences of the heel, ankle and patella and at points liable to pressure in the corrective process such as the posterior aspects of thigh and calf. When the cast is dry, a day or so later, a transverse cut opposite the centre of rotation in the posterior aspect of the femoral condyles is made which surrounds the posterior two-thirds of the circumference. The cast is then extended to the limit of tolerance and the resulting gap filled with plaster. The wedging is repeated on two or three occasions at intervals of, say, two or three days. The production of local pain indicates the existence of local pressure and demands a change of cast if skin necrosis necessitating abandonment of treatment is to be avoided.

**Posterior subluxation.** There are a variety of turn-buckle devices, competing in ingenuity, which added to the cast aim to simulate the gliding action necessary to reduce posterior subluxation and restore the normal relationship of tibia to femur until the angle is reached at which the joint becomes a hinge. These methods demand skills and standards of supervision rarely available and are in general to be avoided in favour of methods less liable to disastrous complications.

### Skeletal Fixation and Traction

It will be evident that the only biomechanically sound method of reducing a flexion deformity in the presence of marked posterior subluxation must fix the lower end of the femur while traction is applied to the upper end of the tibia in such a direction as to simulate in reverse the gliding motion responsible for the subluxation until such time as, say, $25°$ is attained when hingeing motion can be added to longitudinal traction. Such a method has been developed in the Clinica Primavera el Ortopedia under the direction of Professor Aurelio Perez Teuffer in Mexico City and has been observed in use there. A Steinmann pin is driven through the lower end of the femur and a horseshoe with a rigid bar attached applied to the pin and the bar secured to an overhead beam. The lower end of the femur is thus pushed backwards and rigidly fixed. Traction in the desired direction is applied to a pin driven through the upper end of the tibia (Figs 6,42 and 6,43).

This method, which is applicable to the deformities of poliomyelitis in which similar problems of background subluxation occur, illustrates the principles underlying reduction.

### Operation

In persistent flexion deformity which resists reduction by conservative means or is adjudged not to be amenable to such measures, lengthening division or release of all the posterior soft tissue structures including hamstring tendons, posterior capsule and origins of gastrocnemus may be indicated with the object of enabling the patient, often a child, to walk in a full length caliper. The circumstances in which such radical surgery may be indicated are arthrogryposis, cerebral palsy, meningomyelocele and, of course, poliomyelitis and rheumatoid arthritis.

### Technique: Posterior Release

**Approach from the side.** The technique is based on that of Wilson (1929). The first incision is located on the lateral aspect of the lowest third of the femur and proceeds through fascia lata between flexor and extensor muscles. The lateral popliteal nerve is localised beheath the biceps tendon and freed from the neck of the fibula below to the junction of middle and lowest thirds of the femur above. The tension of fascia lata and biceps is tested. The former is sectioned obliquely if lengthening is contemplated, the latter divided immediately above the head of fibula. The lateral ligament is located and isolated. The periosteum in the distal quarter of the femur is incised longitudinally and erased in continuity with the femoral attachment of the capsule. At this stage a second skin incision is usually necessary on the medial side. It proceeds as on the lateral side between flexor and extensor groups. The vastus medialis is retracted anteriorly to expose the periosteum which is incised longitudinally and stripped in continuity with the capsule. The medial ligament is located and preserved. The forefinger is passed into the popliteal space and any contracted structures limiting extension located. The medial hamstrings are sectioned or lengthened as circumstances demand.

**Direct approach.** If flexion is not extreme the direct approach may be preferred. It is accomplished with the patient in the prone position through a lazy S incision. The operation proceeds, locating and identifying the

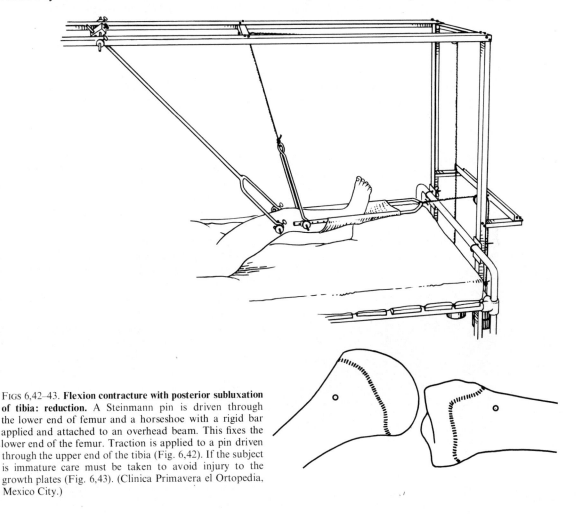

FIGS 6,42–43. **Flexion contracture with posterior subluxation of tibia: reduction.** A Steinmann pin is driven through the lower end of femur and a horseshoe with a rigid bar applied and attached to an overhead beam. This fixes the lower end of the femur. Traction is applied to a pin driven through the upper end of the tibia (Fig. 6,42). If the subject is immature care must be taken to avoid injury to the growth plates (Fig. 6,43). (Clinica Primavera el Ortopedia, Mexico City.)

various tissues involved in the deformity and dividing or lengthening such structures as the circumstances demand.

AFTER-TREATMENT. At the termination of the operation skin traction is applied below the knee and a compression bandage to the joint. The patient is nursed in a Thomas bed-knee splint. Initially the joint is nursed in that degree of flexion which could be attained without tension and gradually extended over the next two weeks or so with the aid of traction. Otherwise treatment is directed towards the eventual aims of operation whether it is a mobile joint under muscular control or less idealistic end result.

## Flexion Deformity: Post-infantile Paralysis

If the lazy S is an attractive approach in which each contracted structure can be identified and sectioned as necessary, its use is not practical in marked deformity, say, 70° or more, in that access is unsatisfactory (Fig. 6,44). In any event at an excessive angle there is considerable risk of breakdown of the skin wound. In such circumstances the approach is of necessity from the lateral side and in the presence of muscle wasting presents no difficulty. The lateral popliteal nerve is identified and retracted. The contracted structures are identified and divided as necessary

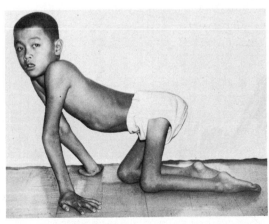

FIG. 6,44. **Poliomyelitis.** Flexion contractures of both knees the result of poliomyelitis showing the means of locomotion. Correction of the deformity by the methods described permits ambulation in the erect posture with the aid of full-length calipers and crutches (courtesy of Prof. P. Balasybramaniam, Kuala Lumpur).

keeping close to the bone deep to the neuro-vascular bundle. In gross deformity complete correction is undesirable and should not be attempted. In this regard, too, it is unnecessary and undesirable to divide or erase the posterior capsule on which the joint may eventually depend for stability. It is not contracted to a degree which will not stretch with traction. If it is found impossible to divide all tight structures from the lateral side a second incision on the medial side may be indicated.

AFTER-TREATMENT. At the termination of the operation detachable skin traction is applied to the leg below the knee and a compression bandage to the joint. The patient is nursed in some form of flexed knee splint or in Russell traction (Figs 6,37 and 6,38) and the joint gradually extended until full extension is attained when the anticipated long leg brace can be fitted.

## LATE, QUIESCENT OR BURNT-OUT RHEUMATOID ARTHRITIS PRESENTING AS PAINFUL PAN-ARTICULAR OSTEOARTHRITIS

The problems of osteoarthritis occurring in burnt-out rheumatoid arthritis differ from those of osteoarthrosis:

**General.** In burnt-out rheumatoid arthritis other joints are usually affected so that the total problem is poly-articular in a patient who has suffered years of ill-health: motivation may be absent. In contradistinction, osteoarthrosis affects one, or at most both, knee joints in a patient otherwise normal, of good morale and with a strong will to recover.

**Local.** In burnt-out rheumatoid arthritis both medial and lateral compartments are affected equally and, in general, without angular deformity (Fig. 6,45). The condition is thus not amenable to the spectacular success which, for a number of reasons, follows correction of angular deformity by osteotomy. In such circumstances total replacement may be the only treatment available.

On the other hand, the problem may at the extreme (Fig. 6,46) be one of angular deformity, a combination of flexion and valgus, possible subluxation, all coupled with lateral rotation of the tibia due to foot deformity. Such circumstances pose considerable problems if pain is to be reduced and function improved.

### ARTHROPLASTY: TOTAL REPLACEMENT

## Historical Note

The first arthroplasty of the knee joint, if not designated as such, was carried out by Fergusson (1856) who excised the damaged joint of a young woman. It is said that five years later she 'could run up stairs or jump off a chair as if she had no disease and no operation'. It is perhaps significant in relation to the author's views on these matters that 'the patella was not removed'. Such a result would be difficult to match more than a hundred years later. Verneuil (1860) is credited with suggesting an interposition membrane to prevent the adjacent bones becoming adherent. In the early years of the twentieth century the operation consisted of the reshaping of the bone ends and the covering of the raw cancellous surfaces with a free graft of fascia lata (Figs 6,47 and 6,48). The underlying principle remains the basis of many forms of arthroplasty. The current interposition membranes, in one form or another, are a combination of stainless steel and plastic.

The evolution of arthroplasty of the knee has been recorded recently (Blundell Jones, 1972) and will not be repeated.

## General Considerations

The natural caution of the Scot, the knowledge that patients are not expendable and that failures may have to be lived with, dictates that the utmost care be exercised in the recommendation and execution of procedures in which complications are common and from which, when they fail, only salvage measures are available. Total replacement of the knee is such an operation. In the present stage of development it is limited to patients with crippling rheumatoid arthritis who will make modest demands of the joint, and patients with bicompartmental or pan-articular osteoarthrosis (Ch. 10), in an older age group, who too, because of age, will make modest demands of the joint. In the current scene only arthrodesis can provide the robust function

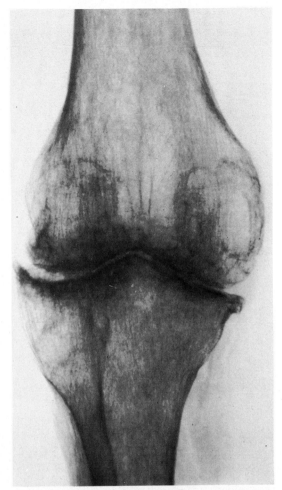

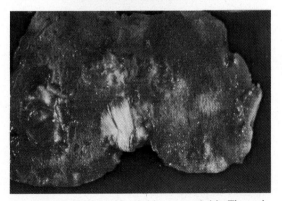

FIGS 6,45–46. **Rheumatoid arthritis: osteoarthritis.** The problems are different from osteoarthrosis. Medial and lateral compartments are equally affected and without angular deformity (Fig. 6,45). In extreme examples destruction of articular cartilage has been complete (Fig. 6,46). In such circumstances total replacement (or arthrodesis) is the only treatment available.

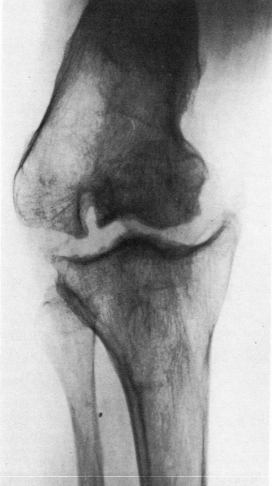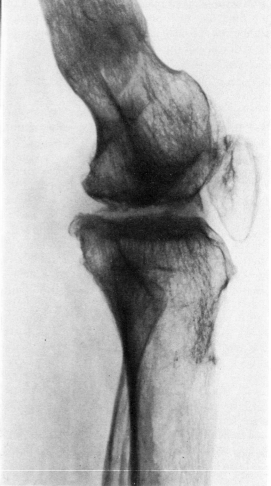

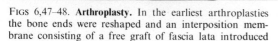

FIGS 6,47–48. **Arthroplasty.** In the earliest arthroplasties the bone ends were reshaped and an interposition membrane consisting of a free graft of fascia lata introduced (Fig. 6,47). In this example an osteotomy of the femur has been performed presumably to correct flexion deformity (Fig. 6,48). See also Figures 5,18 and 5,19.

demanded by the young vigorous patient required to do heavy physical work. But development proceeds apace. Arthrodesis precludes arthroplasty. It, like arthroplasty, should not be lightly undertaken.

## Hemiarthroplasty

This form of replacement is applied to monocompartmental osteoarthrosis (Ch. 10). In patients with limited disability the demands made on the prosthesis are considerable. In any event the coefficients of friction are different on each side of the joint. It is probable also that debris from the prosthetic articulation accelerates wear in the remaining articular cartilage. The author would concur with the view that the indications for this type of replacement must be limited. The problem is resolved either by osteotomy or some form of bicondylar replacement (Insall *et al.*, 1976). In this regard, however, it is of interest that Laskin (1978), in confirming unsatisfactory results in the medial compartment using the Marmor prosthesis, reported the possibility of better results on the lateral side of the joint. This finding is worthy of pursuit in view of the less satisfactory results of osteotomy in lateral compartment osteoarthrosis.

## Indications for Operation

Joints untreatable other than by arthrodesis.

## Contraindications, Relative and Absolute

**1. Cardiovascular, respiratory or renal disease** of a degree implying operational risk.
**2. Peripheral vascular disease.** This includes a previous history of deep vein thrombosis.
**3. Presence of possible source of infection in, say, foot or particularly occult infection in genitourinary tract.**
**4. Neuropathic joint** (Figs 9,37 and 9,38).
**5. Ankylosis** (Fig. 5,15) **or arthrodesis** (Fig. 5,27). A patient, particularly a female, whose knee is ankylosed from rheumatoid arthritis, sepsis or subjected to arthrodesis in youth for tuberculosis, seeks, not unnaturally, a mobile joint. It is essential to appreciate that function in the form of a simple hinge is dependent on muscular action; and if this action has been eliminated by arthrodesis, *and the patella absent or ankylosed to the femur*, the interposition of a hinge between femur and tibia without muscular control is an unphysiological procedure which cannot other than fail. It results in disappointment for patient and deserved loss of reputation for the surgeon. Thus the circumstance in which arthroplasty is most desirable, namely longstanding ankylosis, is just the circumstance in which arthroplasty for technical reasons is contraindicated.

There is a possible solution to this particular problem. It is amputation and provision of an artificial limb. This is the only method of providing a mobile knee joint. It will be clear, however, that the occasions in which such a measure is indicated are rare. In a country with an advanced prosthetic industry and readily available aftercare services, amputation might be indicated in a woman for cosmetic and even social or domestic reasons. To part with a useful limb, even with a rigid knee, and the loss of independence related thereto is a decision not to be lightly undertaken. The patient (D.L., male, aged 31) whose radiographs are illustrated in Figures 5,27 and 5,28, whose knee was arthrodesed at the age of 7 for tuberculosis, when told that arthroplasty was impossible actually sought an artificial limb with which to gain knee flexion. He was, however, of low intelligence and capable only of working as a labourer. He was strongly advised against such measures. There are other situations of manual dexterity or intellectual employment in which contraindications might be less clearly defined.
**6. Previous infection** (Fig. 5,20).
**7. Previous patellectomy.** Extension lag, the commonest cause of failure in major knee surgery, entails absence of quadriceps control and the imposition of unacceptable stresses on the prosthetic replacement. It follows that only methods which retain the patella should be chosen. In other circumstances the necessity to transplant the tibial tubercle in the course of operation should be anticipated.
**8. Presence of scars.** Scarring of skin from previous injury or operation, in particular transverse scars, are a contraindication relative or absolute (Fig. 5,22).
**9. Overweight.**
**10. Absence of motivation.**

In addition, and particularly in regard to the variety of prosthesis to be employed, will be considered: (1) age, (2) weight, (3) occupation, (4) range of motion, (5) degree of flexion contracture, (6) degree of angular deformity, (7) integrity or otherwise of ligaments, (8) degree of decalcification. In rheumatoid arthritis, for example, trabecular bone may not support a surface prosthesis.

## Associated Hip and Foot Deformities

In rheumatoid arthritis in particular it is seldom that a knee presents as an isolated problem. The other knee, one or both hips, to say nothing of foot deformities, confuse the issue and produce problems of management of which examples can be itemised.
1. If both knees are affected and the subject of flexion deformities and it is proposed that both be replaced it is important that the second knee be dealt with before the resumption of weightbearing otherwise the first joint will readopt a flexion deformity.

2. If the opposite, or the hip of the same side, is the site of deformity, the hip should be dealt with before the knee. The importance of considering the mechanics of the limb as a whole in calculating the correction required, as in high tibial osteotomy (Ch. 10), is stressed.

It will be evident that the elimination of a flexion-adduction deformity of the hip with its compensatory valgus angulation at the knee has a beneficial effect on the latter joint to the point of occasionally eliminating the necessity for operation. Furthermore, the elimination of shortening, if the hip involved is on the opposite side, also eliminates the necessity to walk with a flexed-knee gait and the danger of developing a fixed flexion deformity.

There is one biomechanically unrelated reason why hip replacement should precede knee arthroplasty: the physical manoeuvres involved in hip replacement may impose considerable torsional stresses on the knee. This is clearly undesirable after replacement.

When foot deformities accompany knee deformities consideration of treatment by corrective footwear, or operation, should be deferred until knee replacement has been accomplished.

## Biochemical Considerations

The aims of arthroplasty are (1) to eliminate pain; (2) to correct deformity; (3) to resurface destroyed joint surfaces with prosthetic components; (4) to obtain secure fixation; and (5) to achieve static and dynamic stability of the joint. To explain that a variety of designs are available with these aims in view could only be described as a gross understatement. In the current scene no one type has demonstrated overwhelming clinical advantage over all other (Scales, 1976). In such circumstances recommendations, when rapid advances are being made, are hazardous and justified only because decisions about patients with an urgent problem have to be made.

In the multiplicity of implants available can be recognised classifiable varieties:
1. **Simple hinge.** The first replacements consisted of simple hinges (Walldius, 1953; Shiers, 1959) allowing flexion and extension but with total restraint from other movements. The most successful recent models are so designed that the patella is retained to articulate with an upward protrusion of the femoral component. In *theory* a rigid hinge attached to the femur and tibia by long stems, secured within the medullary cavities by cement, creates an unacceptable biomechanical situation. In the knee, as opposed to the hip, there is a check to motion at the limits of extension and flexion. The forces involved at the attachments of the stems of the prosthesis to the shafts of femur and tibia, particularly in the absence of quadriceps control, are considerable. Furthermore, a simple hinge does not simulate the knee joint mechanism with its combination of rotation, rocking and gliding. When the foot is fixed to the ground, for example, the last action of extension is medial rotation of the femur to complete the screw-home movement. There are thus constant torsional forces imposed from the ground in the course of ambulation incapable of being absorbed.

In *practice* such a device is introduced in circumstances of gross degenerative disease with angular deformity and instability and in which the joint would not even merit the description 'simple hinge'. In such conditions the prosthesis achieves the object of relief of pain combined with an improved level of function.

In a recent survey comparing the results of four models of replacement prosthesis by the knee-rating system (Table 7) (Insall *et al.*, 1976) a simple hinge (Guepar) emerged as superior from many standpoints despite the fact that it was used in joints with the most severe involvement and yet equalled any of the other prostheses in the quality of results both in rheumatoid arthritis and in osteoarthrosis. It had also the lowest proportion of failures.

The method of insertion of the Stanmore prosthesis will be described. It has certain advantages:

1. It is technically the simplest device to insert requiring the minimal accessory instrumentation.
2. It can be used in the presence of gross angular deformity. The inbuilt normal valgus angulation reduces errors in the correction of weight-bearing mechanics to a minimum.
3. It is not dependent for stability on correct ligamentous tensioning.

4. It can be used in circumstances of decalcification in which surface replacements must fail.

5. It is an admirable salvage device (Figs 6,67 and 6,68).

On the other hand must be considered:

1. It is no more than a simple hinge with the biomechanical restrictions inherent therein.

2. It is reputed to be complicated by infection more often than less voluminous devices probably as a result of the dead spaces which exist on either side of the prosthesis.

3. It is more difficult to salvage than surface replacements.

**2. Surface or condylar prostheses.** These replacements, in the widest variety, consist of two-, three- or four-piece prostheses which resurface the femoral and tibial condyles. They are unconnected and virtually unconstrained except by the contours of opposing surfaces and the presence of the collateral and sometimes of the cruciate ligaments. In theory they should be less liable to loosening from the imposition of torsional and lateral strains. It will be deduced

that such devices are not to be applied in gross degenerative disease or where instability or deformity is severe.

In the field of surface prostheses has been designed at the Hospital for Special Surgery, New York, a graduated system which covers every eventuality from unicondylar to total condylar replacement (Insall *et al.*, 1976). The relatively simple instrumentation covers all types.

The technique of total condylar replacement will be described in some detail to demonstrate the complexity of these procedures and the accuracy which must be practised if failures due to errors of technique are to be reduced to a minimum.

This type of surface replacement has advantages over the rigid hinge as outlined above:

1. It aims at reproducing the complex movements of the normal knee.

It has inherent disadvantages:

1. The operation is demanding in technical

TABLE 7
Knee-rating scale (Hospital For Special Surgery)

| Pain (30 points) | | Muscle strength (10 points) | |
|---|---|---|---|
| No pain at any time | 30 | Excellent: cannot break the quadriceps | |
| No pain on walking | 15 | power | 10 |
| Mild pain on walking | 10 | Good: can break the quadriceps power | 8 |
| Moderate pain on walking | 5 | Fair: moves through the arc of motion | 4 |
| Severe pain on walking | 0 | Poor: cannot move through the arc of | |
| No pain at rest | 15 | motion | 0 |
| Mild pain at rest | 10 | | |
| Moderate pain at rest | 5 | Flexion deformity (10 points) | |
| Severe pain at rest | 0 | No deformity | 10 |
| | | Less than 5° | 8 |
| Function (22 points) | | 5–10° | 5 |
| Walking and standing unlimited | 12 | More than 10° | 0 |
| Walking distance of 5–10 blocks and | | | |
| standing ability intermittent | | Instability (10 points) | |
| ( $>\frac{1}{2}$ hour) | 10 | None | 10 |
| Walking 1–5 blocks and standing ability | | Mild: 0–5° | 8 |
| up to $\frac{1}{2}$ hour | 8 | Moderate: 5–15° | |
| Walking less than 1 block | 4 | Severe: more than 15° | 0 |
| Cannot walk | 0 | | |
| Climbing stairs | 5 | Subtraction | |
| Climbing stairs with support | 2 | One cane | 1 |
| Transfer activity | 5 | One crutch | 2 |
| Transfer activity with support | 2 | Two crutches | 3 |
| | | Extension lag of 5° | 2 |
| Range of motion (22 points) | | Extension lag of 10° | 3 |
| 1 point for each 8° of arc of motion to | | Extension lag of 15° | 5 |
| a maximum of 18 points | 18 | Each 5° of varus | 1 |
| | | Each 5° of valgus | 1 |

expertise despite the relatively simple accessory instrumentation.

2. It is dependent on the accurate tensioning of the lateral ligaments. Its use may thus be contraindicated in gross deformity.

3. In general surface replacements are contra-indicated in gross decalcification. In this regard, however, this particular replacement distributes the load over a wide area and is less dependent on the support of the weak cancellous tissues of the medial tibial condyle.

**3. Stabilised gliding.** In what has been described as a third generation, an attempt is made to compromise between hinge joints and surface prostheses. They consist of a two-piece surface replacement connected in such a manner that stability is provided while retaining gliding movement and polycentric action.

The technique of insertion of the Sheehan prosthesis will be described.

This type of semiconstrained replacement has advantages over the rigid hinge and un-constrained devices in so far as:

1. It seeks to reproduce a more normal action of the joint.

2. It incorporates a measure of inbuilt stability.

3. The wide distribution of compression forces makes it applicable to decalcification situations rather than certain surface replacements.

The disadvantages include:

1. The instrumentation is extensive, consisting of some 17 items.

2. The necessity for a high degree of operative technical expertise.

3. Dependence on correct tensioning of lateral ligaments. The strength of the central tibial stud and the design of the device in general is not such as to withstand the forces inherent in angular deformity.

4. It is thus unsuitable in gross deformity.

5. The device is voluminous and requires removal of a considerable mass of cancellous tissue both from femur and tibia. Salvage by Stanmore prosthesis is possible but if arthrodesis is required minimal peripheral bone remains for compression contact.

## Choice of Prosthesis

It will be evident, even among the legion of devices in current production, that indications emerge as between say the simple hinge and surface replacements. It is repeated that in the variety of designs available no one type has as yet demonstrated overwhelming clinical advantages. Total knee replacement, if advancing rapidly, must still be regarded as in the experimental stage. The techniques employed in the insertion of many of the models is demanding. There is little margin for error. It will be evident that the advantages of sophisticated design are lost unless location is achieved with precision. If the correction of deformity, possibly in three planes, and the insertion of two components is an exacting operation, the insertion of four components correctly aligned with a margin of error in each of less than 5° and accurately adjusted for tension, is virtually impossible in the average surgeon's hands. In general, therefore, four-component surface replacements are not to be recommended.

## Principles of Operation

There are some basic principles which must be observed in all forms of total replacement arthroplasty.

**Skin incision.** In most early descriptions a lateral parapatellar incision is advised so that skin and capsular incision do not coincide. This incision, however, is vulnerable to slow healing and superficial skin necrosis. In the current scene a vertical mid-line incision is favoured; but which is the best incision has yet to be resolved. The skin incision, however, may be determined by a previous parapatellar incision which may require to be excised to gain access to the joint without leaving a barrier of fibrous tissue to the healing of a new incision. Reference is made to the fact that extensive scarring from a previous injury or operation may constitute a contra-indication to operation. In any event whatever the approach the incision must be of sufficient length to avoid excessive skin traction by, or compression from, retractors in the course of a prolonged operation if superficial necrosis is to be avoided.

**Elimination of angular deformity.** It is essential that the normal biomechanics of the lower limb as a whole be restored that is to say the correct alignment of hip, knee and ankle joints and with the normal 5° to 10° of valgus angulation at the knee.

Varus or valgus deformity may be of bony origin, usually due to a depressed tibial condyle, of ligamentous origin, or both. The correction of fixed varus angulation may require division of the medial capsule from the upper tibia and erasure of the inferior insertion of the medial ligament from the lower tibia. The correction of fixed valgus angulation may require division or lengthening of the iliotibial tract and erasure of the superior attachment of the lateral ligament from the femur. Release of such structures to correct deformity entails exposure of the lateral popliteal nerve if the risk of paralysis is to be reduced to a minimum.

The instrumentation of some varieties of total replacement incorporate devices to ensure correct alignment (see 'Total Condylar Knee Prosthesis' below).

**Lateral release.** It is a common experience where total replacement has entailed the reduction of a long-standing valgus deformity that the patella cannot be restored to the mid-line due to contraction of the lateral expansion. In performing a lateral release it should be remembered that the medial capsule has already been divided in entering the joint. Caution should be exercised in the division of soft tissues lest the blood supply of the patella be endangered.

**Reduction of wear-potential.** It will be evident that the restoration of normal biomechanics will reduce wear-potential due to excessive local stresses on the polyethylene component. The wear rate is greatly accelerated if loose fragments of acrylic cement become detached to form an abrasive agent between the components. It is important, therefore, that towards the termination of any procedure meticulous attention be paid to the removal of any excess of cement from the periphery of the components.

## Practical Considerations

It is proposed that the method of insertion of three different types of prostheses be described. It is not to be interpreted that this constitutes recommendation based on personal experience: each may be improved, or superseded. In any event a surgeon contemplating the insertion of a specific prosthesis would be wise to contact the manufacturer regarding modifications of design and/or of the instrumentation of insertion.

### STANMORE KNEE

The prosthesis is made from vacuum melt/vacuum cast cobalt/chromium-molybdenum alloy which possesses satisfactory mechanical properties in laboratory tests. There is a separate prosthesis for right and left knees. The femoral intramedullary stem is set at 8° to the tibial stem in the coronal plane allowing the hinge to be maintained in a horizontal position when weight-bearing (Fig. 6,49). It is also set anterior to the tibial stem in the sagittal plane so that the long axes of the femur and tibia retain their correct anatomical relationship.

Both femoral and tibial stems are sufficiently long to extend into the medullary cavities ensuring secure fixation to the cortical bone with acrylic cement. The cancellous bone of the adjacent ends of the tibia and femur is left largely undisturbed.

The joint permits more than full anatomical flexion (150°) and has a stop at 2° of hyperextension to ensure that the joint is self-locking when carrying a full load.

The patella is retained. The width of the prosthesis is no more than the average width of the European patella. The soft tissues are therefore protected from rubbing on the replacement during movement and are protected from contact with the metal in a fall or similar direct injury.

The patella articulates throughout with a reciprocally-shaped groove which holds it in the correct anatomical position during movement.

The bearing surfaces are metal on high molecular weight polyethylene.

The axle is positively located and cannot rotate, being held in position with a titanium alloy type 318 circlip (Fig. 6,49). Assembling the joint at operation is therefore simple.

A minimum of special surgical implements are required: a measuring block to ensure that adequate bone has been resected, a trial axle to enable the joint to be assembled and moved through a full range of movement before final fixation, and a patella template to check that the

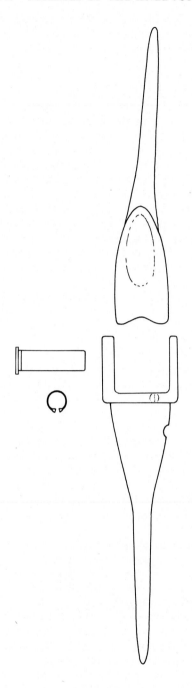

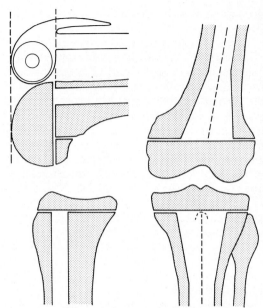

Figs 6,49–53. **Stanmore knee: Technique of insertion.** The frontal view of prosthesis to show femoral component with large flange for patella, tibial component, axle and retaining circlip (Fig. 6,49). At insertion the femoral condyles are resected at right angles anteroposteriorly (Fig. 6,50) and in anatomical valgus angulation of about 10° (Fig. 6,51). The plane of section is determined by placing the femoral component parallel to the femur with its distal surface in the same plane as that of the condyles which are marked at the level of the plateau on the prosthesis (Fig. 6,50). The posterior parts of the femoral condyles are trimmed to allow increased flexion of the artificial joint (Fig. 6,50). The tibia is resected immediately above the tubercle at right angles in both planes (Figs 6,52 and 6,53) (after Lettin *et al.*, 1978).

articular surface of the patella is congruous with the groove on the prosthesis. A special tool is also required to insert the circlip (Wilson, Lettin and Scales, 1974).

**Operative technique.** A skin incision just lateral to the mid-line is favoured. It extends from 7·5 cm (3 in) above the patella to the level of the tibial tubercle. The skin flap is reflected medially to the medial margin of the patella and the joint entered by a medial parapatellar incision through the capsule. This ensures that skin and capsular incision do not coincide. The ability to displace the patella to the lateral side is accomplished by incising the attachment of vastus medialis immediately distal to the muscle fibres. The knee is then flexed to a right-angle.

No more stripping of soft tissues is undertaken than is necessary to expose the femoral condyles. To select the site of resection the stem of the femoral component is aligned with the femoral shaft and kept parallel with the anterior surface. The inferior surface of the component is held in the same plane as the condyles. The femur is then marked at the level of and in the plane of the plateau of the component. The site is approximately 2·8 cm from the apex of the convexity of the condyles. Resection is made at right-angles to the shaft of the femur in the antero-posterior plane and at approximately 10° to the long axis in the lateral plane to allow for the angle at which the femoral component is set to the tibia in order that the hinge is horizontal. Section of the femur is completed by trimming of the posterior cortex of the cut surface in an oblique fashion in order to permit full flexion after insertion of the prosthesis (Figs 6,50 and 6,51). Activity is now transferred to the tibia where stripping of soft tissues is limited to that required for resection immediately above the tubercle. In contradistinction to the femur it is

undertaken at right-angles to the shaft in both antero-posterior and lateral planes (Figs 6,52 and 6,53).

If there is considerable varus (or valgus) angulation the medial (or lateral) tibial condyle may be depressed (Figs 6,54 and 6,55). In such circumstances it is better to resect the head of the tibia first because the depression of the condyle will determine the amount of bone required to be removed. That to be removed from the femoral condyles will be determined accordingly.

It is at this stage that a check is made as to whether sufficient bone has been resected to accommodate the prosthesis. To this end the 'gauge block' is inserted with the limb in extension and under slight distraction. If it is shown that some increase in interval is necessary bone is resected from the femur. Maintaining the angles, and the posterior level, recorded above in the preparation of the medullary cavities sufficient cancellous bone is removed not only to accept the stems of the components but with the addition of the cement. The

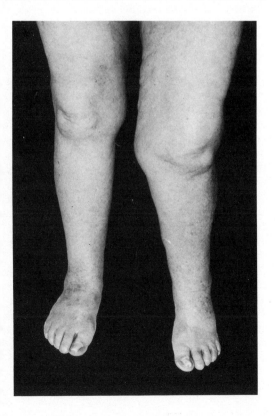
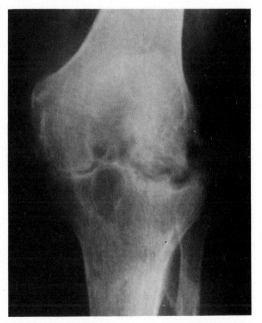

FIGS 6,54–55. **Stanmore knee: technique of insertion.** In angular deformity (Fig. 6,54) if one or other tibial condyle is depressed (Fig. 6,55) it is better to resect the head of the tibia first because the depression will determine the amount of bone to be removed.

cancellous tissue adjacent to the cut surfaces is retained. Fixation of the prosthesis depends on anchoring the stems of the components in the medullary canal of the shaft of femur and tibia rather than in soft cancellous bone. It is at this stage that the articular surface of the patella is examined and checked against the template in order to ensure congruity with the patellar bearing surface of the femoral component. Excision of peripheral osteophytes is usually required. A trial of reduction is then undertaken. The tibial component is inserted first. When both are in place the trial axle is introduced from the medial side. The joint is then put through its full range of movement, say, zero to 100° of flexion in order to ensure that the axis of rotation of the tibial on the femoral component coincides with the axis of rotation of tibia on femur. If, in full flexion, the tibia contacts the femur, the former must be bevelled in the manner described for the femur. It is essential to the success of the technique that this position is noted in order that the components are cemented in the correct position. It will be evident that if the axes do not coincide a stress situation will be created which may result in loosening of one or other or both components.

The stage is now reached for the cementing of the components. To this end venting tubes, linked by Y connector, are introduced into both medullary cavities and mechanical suction maintained. Cement is introduced into both medullary cavities simultaneously, the suction tubes withdrawn and the tibial and femoral stems introduced while the cement is soft. The components are articulated using the trial axle. It is important that the notch on the anterior margin of the tibial plateau is aligned with the tibial tubercle. Bone debris and excess cement is removed by curetting and irrigation. The mechanical aspects are completed by the removal of the trial axle in favour of the permanent device which may be inserted from either side. This axle is retained by a titanium circlip introduced into the retaining groove by the circlip compression instrument.

The operation is completed with the introduction of suction drainage and closure of the subcutaneous tissues and skin with interrupted sutures. A compression bandage is applied and the tourniquet removed.

FIGS 6,56–58. **Total condylar knee.** The prosthesis consists of a cobalt chrome femoral component (Fig. 6,56) and a high-density polyethylene tibial (Fig 6,57) and patellar components (Fig. 6,58).

### TOTAL CONDYLAR KNEE

The prosthesis consists of a cobalt/chrome femoral component and high-density polyethylene tibial and patellar components (Figs 6,56 to 6,58). The femoral component is anatomically shaped when viewed laterally in that the radius of curvature posteriorly is less than the anterior part. Thus, in extension there is conformity with the tibial component, but as flexion progresses rotary and antero-posterior sliding motions are permitted. The femoral component has a grooved flange for the patella. There is available a patellar articular surface replacement should this be required.

The tibial articular surface is cupped to receive the femoral component and stability is further increased by a median intercondylar eminence. Tibial fixation is enhanced by a stout central peg which is shaped to fit against the strong posterior cortex of the tibia.

All components are available in a variety of sizes; the tibial component in a variety of thicknesses.

**Principles of operation.** Insertion of the prosthesis requires excision of the cruciate ligaments. Stability thus depends on the correct tension of the collateral ligaments in both flexion and extension. The level of division of the tibia determines the fit of the prosthesis in flexion. This level is decided with the knee in right-angled flexion so that after insertion the collateral ligaments are taut in this position. The amount of bone removed from the femoral condyles determines the fit in extension. This level is decided with the collateral ligaments under tension so that after insertion they are taut in extension. The shape of the new surfaces provides some measure of inherent stability when weight-bearing in extension. The principal source of stability however depends on the correct tensioning of the soft tissues.

### Instrumentation

Four instruments are required for the accurate placement of the components:

**1. Tibial cutter.** This instrument is in the shape of a cross and has a stem which is inserted into the intramedullary canal of the femur. On the cross arm there are two slots which correspond to the thick and thin tibial components. There is a spike for fixation (Fig. 6,59).

**2. Femoral trimmer.** This instrument consists of a block with anterior and posterior slots also located by an intramedullary stem. Its purpose is to trim the anterior and posterior femoral condyles (Fig. 6,60).

**3. Femoral cutter.** This instrument applies traction on the tibia via a plate which fits on the previously cut surface of the upper tibia. There are two slots which correspond to the thick or thin tibial component previously selected. It has a handle for applying traction. The plate is the exact size of the tibial component and contains a slot corresponding to the fixation peg (Figs 6,61 and 6,62).

**4. Spacer and alignment rod.** The spacer is a block the size of the prosthesis. It is used to determine the fit and orientation of the cuts both in flexion and in extension. An alignment rod is included. There is a clip-on attachment to the plate which corresponds to the dimensions of the prosthesis when the thick tibial component is used (Figs 6,63 and 6,64).

**Operative technique.** A mid-line skin incision centred on the patella is employed. In an individual of average size it will be about 30 cm long. The skin flap is reflected medially to the medial margin of the patella and the joint entered through a parapatellar incision through the capsule. The patella is dislocated laterally, part of the fat pad excised and if necessary a portion of the patellar tendon insertion detached from the tibial tubercle. The periosteum and insertion of the pes anserinus are separated from the flare of the tibia and the deep portion of the medial collateral ligament divided from the margin of the tibia. This provides access to the posterior aspect of the tibia when inserting the tibial component.

The joint is then flexed to a right-angle. A centering hole is made into the intramedullary canal of the femur so that the intramedullary stem of the instrument lies on the posterior cortex of the femur (Fig. 6,59). The insertion of the posterior cruciate ligament into the femur is a guide to proper location. The knee must be flexed to exactly 90° using the longitudinal bar of the instrument as a guide. The cross arm is positioned at right angles to the shaft of the tibia. Orientation is easier if the alignment rod is inserted first into the intramedullary canal of the tibia. When the instrument is correctly positioned it is fixed by driving the spike into the tibia. The alignment rod is then removed and the upper tibia resected through the appropriate slot using a reciprocating saw. The tibial cut should be at right angles to the shaft in both the antero-posterior and lateral planes. The slot selected should remove just enough of the tibia to provide a flat surface.

The femoral trimmer is then inserted and positioned so that it lies transversely across the lower end of the femur using the epicondyles as reference points (Fig. 6,60). Approximately equal amount should be removed from the medial and lateral condyles. The line of the cut should be parallel to the cut made in the tibia. The fixation spikes are driven into the lower femur and bone resected directly through the slots. Care should be taken not to converge the anterior and posterior cuts as this will produce a loose fit.

The removal of the upper tibial fragment is

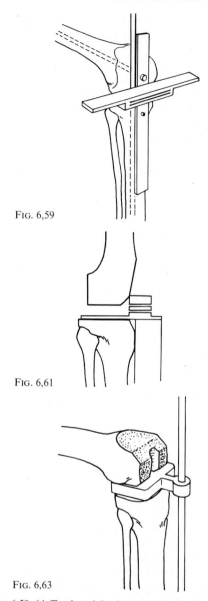

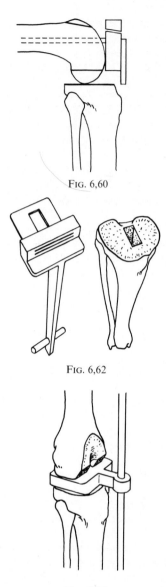

FIG. 6,59

FIG. 6,60

FIG. 6,61

FIG. 6,62

FIG. 6,63

FIG. 6,64

**FIGS 6,59–64. Total condylar knee: instrumentation.**
Fig. 6,59. *The tibial cutter* is the shape of a cross and has a stem which is inserted into the medullary canal of the femur. On the cross arm there are two slots which correspond to the thick and thin components. There is a spike for fixation.

Fig. 6,60. *The femoral trimmer* consists of a block with anterior and posterior slots located by an intramedullary stem. Its purpose is to trim the anterior and posterior femoral condyles.

Figs 6,61 and 6,62. *The femoral cutter* applies traction on the tibia via a plate which fits on the previously cut surface of the tibia. There are two slots which correspond

to the thick or thin tibial component previously selected (Fig. 6,61). It has a handle for applying traction (Fig. 6,62). The plate is the exact size of the tibial component and contains a rectangular slot corresponding to the fixation peg (Fig. 6,62).

Figs 6,63 and 6,64. *The spacer and alignment rod* consists of a block the size of the prosthesis. It is used to determine the fit and orientation of the cuts both in flexion (Fig. 6,63) and extension (Fig. 6,64). It includes an alignment rod. There is a clip-on attachment to the plate which corresponds to the dimension of the prosthesis when the thick component is used (after Insall).

facilitated by dividing the cruciate ligaments the remnants of which are excised.

It is at this stage that the spacer and alignment rod is used to check the fit in flexion (Fig. 6,63).

The knee is then extended and the femoral cutter applied to the cut surface of the tibia and traction applied to tighten the collateral ligaments (Fig. 6,64). The line of resection of the lower femur is marked through the slot with an osteotome. The proximal slot is used when the thick tibial component is selected and the distal slot when the thin component is to be used (Fig. 6,62). The knee is flexed again and the femoral trimmer reinserted. The block is at right angles to the shaft of the femur. The final position of the femoral component should be from zero to 5° of valgus. The cut on the femoral condyles should either parallel the block of the trimmer or diverge slightly to the lateral side. If the previous steps of the operation have been carried out correctly the marking on the femur should be repeated. This step corrects varus or valgus deformity and flexion contracture.

The anterior and posterior surfaces of the femur are bevelled and a slight recess created centrally between the femoral condyles. These cuts accommodate the deep surface of the femoral component.

The articular surface of the patella is removed leaving enough thickness to anchor the patella implant. A central hole is made and deepened as far as the anterior cortex. The edges are undercut with a curette.

The knee is flexed and the position for the tibial stem marked on the upper tibia using the slot on the femoral cutter (Fig. 6,62). The slot is positioned centrally and should point in the same direction as the foot.

It is at this stage that the spacer and alignment rod is used to check the fit in extension. The rod should pass through the centre of the hip joint say 3 cm medial to the anterior superior spine and the centre of the ankle joint (Fig. 6,64).

A trial fit is carried out. The components should be tight in flexion. It should not be possible to dislocate them anteriorly or posteriorly; but up to 1 cm of antero-posterior motion is inherent in the design. The knee is then extended. If stable there should not be more than 5 mm of opening on either side. The patella should lie centrally. If there is a tendency to

lateral subluxation the lateral retinaculum should be divided (see 'Principles of Operation'). The tibial and patellar components are cemented at the same time; the femoral component later. All components are cemented with the joint in flexion. It is in this position that excess cement is most readily removed.

The procedure terminates with the introduction of suction drainage, closure of the soft tissues and the application of a compression bandage.

## SHEEHAN KNEE

The femoral component (Fig. 6,66), made in mirror image for left and right knees, has two separate bearing surfaces with a gap for the stabilising stud of the tibial component. It interlocks between the femoral bearing surfaces engaging an inner radius thus ensuring stability of the joint. The external surface of the femoral component has a curvature simulating that of the normal knee permitting a constantly changing instant centre of rotation. This is achieved by blending two external radii together; and this facilitates manufacture of the prosthesis. The internal femoral radius engages in the groove of the expanded tibial stud. It simulates stability inherent in the cruciate ligaments by preventing anterior or posterior movement, but at the same time permits a combination of sliding and rolling to occur between the surfaces. Collateral ligament stability is also achieved by this mechanism: approximately $2 \times 3°$ of side-to-side rock are permitted in the extended position, increasing to 6° to 7° when the knee is semiflexed.

When the knee is fully extended the tibial stud fits the intercondylar notch of the femoral component (Fig. 6,66) thus preventing axial rotation. In 30° of flexion the condyles show gradual widening of the intercondylar gap to allow approximately 20° of axial rotation when the knee is flexed to a right angle.

The inner femoral radii gradually taper from 50°; and with the knee flexed beyond a right angle there is no direct linkage between the components. If apposition of soft tissues occurs posteriorly by the calf and thigh coming in contact, the tibial component is free to subluxate anteriorly and thus prevent a tensile or distraction force on one or other component.

There is no patellar surface as such on the prosthesis. The patella approaches the bearing surface at approximately 50° of flexion and

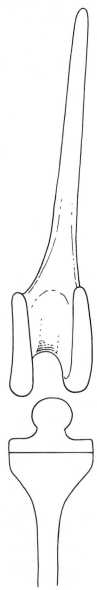

remains in contact with it for the remainder of the range. The transition point where the patella passes from the lower femur on to the prosthesis is very smooth; and beyond 50° of flexion a hemiarthroplasty of the patello-femoral joint has in fact been achieved.

The tibial component, made of high-density polyethylene, has two bearing surfaces and an expanded intercondylar stud shaped like a rugby football when viewed from the side (Fig. 6,65); the required movement and stability are achieved by an accurate selection of radii. The radius of the main weight-bearing surface is 50 mm.

Both components have an intramedullary stem which, especially in soft osteoporotic bone such as is frequently encountered in rheumatoid arthritis, is the ideal method for both fixation and alignment. In addition, the degree of destruction or collapse of the condyles does not influence the final stability of the joint. Flats, so blended with the stem that no points of stress concentration remain, prevent rotation. The stems are long enough to pass well into the cortical region to obviate stress concentration particularly in the lower femur.

**Operative technique.** Through a long, almost-straight medial parapatellar incision the patella is dislocated laterally, care being taken not to damage the insertion of the patellar ligament. The knee is flexed to a right angle and a jig is introduced to outline the area of femur to be removed. This area with its attached cruciate ligaments is removed with an oscillating saw and the lower part of the femur is reamed out. A trial femoral component is inserted and aligned with a tibial jig to allow a centering hole to be drilled in the tibial plateau after any rotational deformity has been corrected. Reaming of the tibial surface is undertaken with the knee in full flexion, and largely through the notch of the femur so that no disturbance of the posterior capsule is made.

The tibial component is inserted first and the tension of the knee is adjusted as necessary by sinking the component further into the tibia. Both components are cemented separately while the knee is held in flexion so that varus or valgus stresses are not applied. The collateral ligaments are thus not put on the stretch while the cement cures.

FIGS 6,65–66. **Sheehan knee: posterior aspect.** The lips of the ellipsoidal tibial stud (Fig. 6,65) engage with the inner bearing channels of the femoral condyles (Fig. 6,66) simulating the stability inherent in the cruciate ligaments in the first 90° of flexion. In full extension the tibial stud (Fig. 6,65) fits the intercondylar notch exactly thus preventing rotation.

The tourniquet is released and haemostasis secured before meticulous closure of the wound in layers with three suction drains—one superficial and two deep. The limb is supported in a compression bandage, the drains are removed after 48 hours and weight-bearing permitted as soon as the patient feels able to stand, usually on the third day after operation (Sheehan, 1978).

## AFTER-TREATMENT: GENERAL

It is prudent to institute dorsi- and plantar flexion exercises of the foot immediately. Quadriceps setting and assisted straight-leg-raising begin as soon as the suction drainage tubes are removed in, say, 48 hours. Weight-bearing with the aid of crutches is encouraged as soon as the immediate effects of operation and the patients inclination permits usually from the fourth day onwards. It is at this time too that flexion exercises, within the confines of the compression bandage, begin. The skin stitches, as has been indicated, are not removed until the third week. If a satisfactory range of flexion has not been achieved by that time a gentle manipulation under general anaesthesia may be indicated.

## COMPLICATIONS

Total replacement of the knee is an operation performed for diseases in an age range in which complications are inevitable. If the contra-indications to operation are observed they can be reduced to a minimum.

## Immediate

### 1. Infection

**Superficial.** Reference has been made to the vulnerability of skin incisions in the area concerned to delayed healing and superficial necrosis. It is the author's practice to defer the removal of sutures until 3 weeks have elapsed rather than the customary 10 days; and to exert caution in the practice of flexion exercises if healing is delayed.

The appropriate antibiotic is administered.
**Deep.** This is the complication most feared. The incidence should be reduced to a minimum if the contraindications to operation, relative and absolute, are observed and the theatre environment and aseptic techniques appropriate to such a vulnerable undertaking. When deep infection occurs, every effort should be made to contain and resolve the infection short of open drainage. A small proportion of cases can be salvaged only by removal of the prosthesis and compression arthrodesis (see 'Arthrodesis') or in the last resort by amputation.

LATERAL POPLITEAL PARALYSIS. Where replacement involves the correction of several valgus and/or flexion deformities operation may be followed by lateral popliteal palsy. The condition is usually temporary and resolves within six months.

## Late: Causes of Failure

**Infection.** For reasons not fully understood, but sometimes of metastatic origin, infection may develop years after the uncomplicated insertion of a prosthesis. The breaking down of a scar for no apparent reason may be the result of the development of sensitivity to materials such as nickel or cobalt.

When infection occurs every effort should be made, as in immediate infection, by the use of antibiotics, continuous closed irrigation, etc., to avoid the necessity for open drainage. In favourable circumstances of an exposed prosthesis healing may sometimes be effected by a plastic procedure in the form of a local rotational skin-flap.

**Loosening of prosthesis.** This late complication is manifest in the onset of pain accompanied by synovial effusion and the development of angular deformity. It is considered that a high proportion of failures so related are due to errors of technique at operation whereby perfection of local alignment, or of the limb as a whole, is not achieved. Other causes include collapse of trabecular bone, stress fracture (Fig. 6,68) and deformation of the tibial component. The precise nature of the pathological process underlying the development of a radiolucent line at the cement-bone interface remains in doubt. There is little doubt however that if it is wider than 2 mm and increasing it is an indication of impending failure.

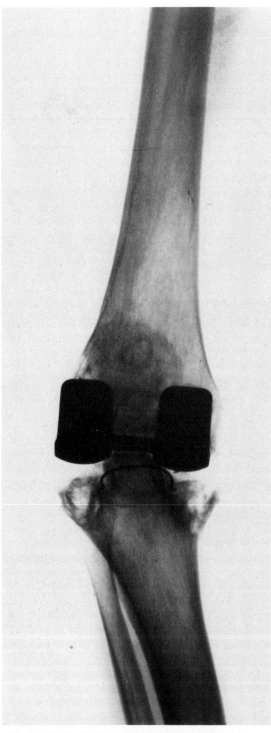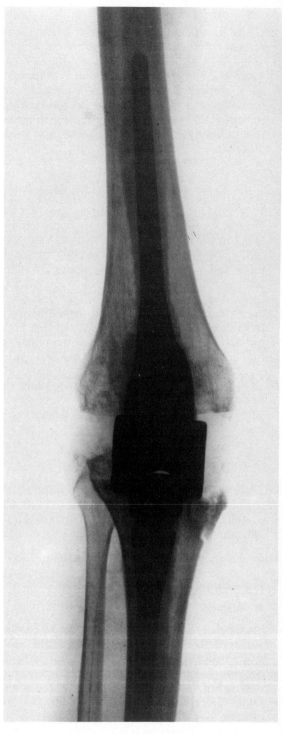

FIGS 6,67–68. **Failed total replacement: treatment.** This geometric replacement performed in North America failed after three years and presented with pain and instability. Note varus angulation with fracture of medial cortex of tibia (Fig. 6,67). At reoperation, when a Stanmore hinge prosthesis was introduced, both components of the original replacement were found to be loose. Note restoration of the normal valgus angulation (Fig. 6,68). (Mrs M.G., aged 79.)

**Wear of prosthesis.** Wear, particularly of the tibial component, may occur in the normal course of events. In the Stanmore knee for example, the polyethylene bush at the axle has been known to wear and to require replacement (Lettin, personal communication). In a majority of cases wear of one or both components or of the patello-femoral joint is of iatrogenic origin: failure to remove exposed cement with resultant production of abrasive debris.

## EVALUATION OF RESULTS

In a situation with so many varieties available and in a rapidly changing scene some method of measurement of efficiency or otherwise is desirable. The knee-rating system of the Hospital for Special Surgery, New York (Insall *et al.*, 1976) has been selected as simple and not too time-consuming in practice. This rating system allots a maximum of 100 points subdivided into 6 categories: pain, function, range of motion, muscle strength, flexion deformity and instability. From the total points scored subtractions are made for use of walking aids, extension lag and varus and valgus deformity. The final total is the knee rating. A rating of 85 or more indicates an excellent result. Knees with a score of 70 to 84 are considered to have obtained a good result. Joints rated between 60 and 69 are considered to have achieved a fair result only. A score of less than 60 is considered to be a failure. It is below the rating achieved by arthrodesis.

## ARTHRODESIS

Arthrodesis is the acceptance of failure of conservative measures, surgical and otherwise. The necessity for the operation has not been common even in a considerable turnover of cases and particularly of the insoluble problems of others. That 241 arthrodeses should have been performed in 35 years could not be judged to be excessive by any standard and in particular when in the majority the underlying pathology was rheumatoid arthritis. It is appropriate therefore that arthrodesis should be considered under this heading.

**Background Note**

It is said that the technique of arthrodesis of the knee joint is a lost art having been superseded by reconstructive measures. On the other hand it has been said also, and with some truth, that the commonest reason for arthrodesis in the current scene is arthroplasty, by which is intended, failed arthroplasty. If the need for arthrodesis for tuberculosis has been virtually eliminated the necessity for arthrodesis in recent years has been increased by the frequency of complications in reconstructive measures and the necessary use, but sometimes misuse, of the corticosteroids.

In this series on which opinions are based, 12 arthrodeses only were added to the total (Table 8) in the six years 1972–78, by six orthopaedic surgeons working in the same hospital. This indicates the infrequency with which the operation is performed in the current scene and thus the difficulty of receiving instruction and of gaining practical experience in the course of training. It is one of the reasons why the operation is, in general, badly done. The operation appears to the uninitiated to be simple of execution, virtually certain in outcome. In other hands the subtleties of performance, and pitfalls, are recognised.

**Other indications for arthrodesis.** If in the past (Table 8), and possibly in the current scene, rheumatoid arthritis remains the most common indication for arthrodesis, there are other disease processes in which it may be indicated:

1. Failed total knee replacement.
2. Tuberculosis.
3. Infective arthritis.
4. Trauma.
5. Paralytic poliomyelitis.
6. Haemophilia.
7. Neuropathic joint.

**Restrictions imposed by arthrodesis.** There is a finality about arthrodesis which demands that the resultant social, domestic and marital repercussions require explanation and discussion, particularly if there is an alternative solution; but not in any detail if there is no alternative. Patients rapidly accommodate to a stiff knee and learn, for example, to ascend stairs two at a time. Ripple rubber or plantation rubber soled shoes increase adhesion and act as shock absorbers.

On the other hand in public transport the leg extends into the aisle of bus or subway train and the patient so disabled receives little consideration from other passengers. There are problems in aircraft and particularly in the use of the toilet. Social activities may be curtailed by the necessity to sit in a seat nearest the aisle in a theatre, cinema or football match. There is difficulty in getting in and out of a car. Inability to activate the controls is overcome with automatic transmission; in other circumstances by hand controls.

**Liability to injury.** The vulnerability of the leg to fracture is increased as a result of arthrodesis (Moore and Smillie, 1959). The risk occurs in the early stages of rehabilitation when a massive single graft is used (Fig. 6,79). With other methods it occurs at a later stage and is related to loss of flexibility in avoiding a hazard.

TABLE 8
Arthrodesis of knee. Reasons for operation. 1942–78

| Diagnosis | Number |
|---|---|
| Rheumatoid arthritis | 100 |
| Tuberculosis | 30 |
| Osteoarthrosis | 61 |
| Infective arthritis | 14 |
| Paralysis | 5 |
| Gunshot wound | 3 |
| Recent fracture | 1 |
| Pigmented villonodular synovitis | 2 |
| Deformity/instability | 16 |
| Neuropathic joint | 1 |
| Not specified | 8 |
| Total | 241 |

**Dissatisfaction with result.** A patient with an intolerable disability from late rheumatoid arthritis is unlikely to complain of a stiff knee when relieved of pain and achieved stability. On the other hand a patient, arthrodesed in childhood, has no memory or interest in the reason; only with the consequent disability.

In a series of 124 patients (Green, Parkes and Stinchfield, 1967) 2 only expressed dissatisfaction, both of whom had the operation performed for tuberculosis in early childhood. In 39 patients in whom fusion was performed for rheumatoid arthritis, 2 were dissatisfied

(Brattstrom and Brattstrom, 1971). This series of 241 cases has not been investigated in this regard. One patient purposefully expressed dissatisfaction. He too had arthrodesis performed for tuberculosis as a child (Figs 5,27 and 5,28).

**Trial of acceptability.** Arthrodesis of the knee joint has a feature not common to many operations that the restrictions imposed can be simulated prior to a decision which is final.

Arthrodesis is an operation of necessity; seldom of choice. In a failed arthroplasty there may be no alternative other than amputation. There are circumstances of quadriceps paralysis, for example, in which the operation is one of choice as an alternative to the wearing of apparatus which may be unacceptable, unobtainable or which imposes an intolerable financial burden.

If the knee is stiff, or virtually stiff, it can be explained that the physical conditions after successful arthrodesis will be the same; and that it is possible to guarantee complete absence of pain. If there remains a useful range of movement but accompanied by pain, as may obtain in quiescent rheumatoid arthritis, or a complete range of painless movement as in paralysis but with instability and the necessity to wear a full-length caliper, a test of acceptability may be advisable in a patient who expresses doubts on her ability to accept the restrictions imposed by a fixed knee. In such circumstances a light plaster cuff is applied to the limb leaving the ankle and foot free. She then returns to her home with instructions to resume her normal domestic and social routine. She reports in an arbitrary period of one to four weeks with her mind made up in the knowledge that the physical circumstances of arthrodesis have been simulated; but that she will not be required to carry a plaster cast for more than four months after operation.

**Bilateral arthrodesis.** The disadvantages of single arthrodesis, for obvious reasons, are less evident in those of short stature. If the patient is tall and requires a bilateral fusion it is recommended that the legs are deliberately shortened with the purpose of decreasing the difficulty of getting up from the sitting position and in reaching the feet.

**Aim at symmetry.** Some attempt should be made to match for contour the arthrodesed knee with the normal side. If there is slight varus then the knee should be arthrodesed in slight varus. This is a relatively simple matter to accomplish by the method described. Figure 6,70 shows the cosmetic result of matching the arthrodesed left knee with the normal side.

**Arthrodesis/amputation.** When both knees have been destroyed in youth or middle-age and the patient required to undertake physical work, an alternative to the restrictions imposed by a bilateral arthrodesis is arthrodesis on one side and amputation at or about the knee on the other. This gives one painless, stable but rigid limb and one in which the knee is artificial but mobile.

## Arthrodesis in Rheumatoid Arthritis

Rheumatoid arthritis, the most common reason for performing arthrodesis (Table 8), imposes biomechanical problems not encountered in other conditions in so far as not only is the opposite knee likely to be involved but all the weight-bearing joints may be affected in some degree. The improved function which results from arthrodesis imposes additional and un-accustomed strains on these joints and the mobile knee in particular is incapable of compensating for shortening, even more so than a normal joint.

Reference has been made elsewhere (Ch. 10) to 'good knee', or 'long leg' arthropathy. In rheumatoid arthritis the opposite knee is most unlikely to be 'good' although it will be 'long' in varying degree. In such circumstances it is important to compensate completely for discrepancy of leg length by the raising of both sole and heel of the shoe to permit the maximum extension possible of the knee and to avoid overloading the forefoot.

The special pre-operative and post-operative measures applicable to rheumatoid arthritis may be summarised (Brattstrom and Brattstrom, 1971):
1. Non-weight-bearing quadriceps exercises for the moveable knee.
2. Compensation for discrepancy of leg length by raising both heel and sole of the shoe.
3. Education of the patient to use the arthrodesed side as the stable standing leg and to use it as much as possible in daily life in order to save the mobile one. An example cited is walking backwards downstairs.
4. Follow-up at six-monthly intervals in order to anticipate the mechanical problems imposed on the other joints by arthrodesis.

## Arthrodesis of Neuropathic Joints

A review of the literature in English (Drennan, Fahey and Maylahn, 1971) revealed that in 144 cases in which arthrodesis had been attempted in neuropathic joints by a variety of methods only 55 per cent were successful. These authors showed evidence that failure or otherwise of fusion, other things being equal, may depend on whether or not a synovectomy is undertaken at the time of operation rather than the method of arthrodesis adopted. It is postulated that fibrosis and thickening of the synovial membrane caused by chronic irritation may create a barrier to the vascular supply of the knee and cause blood to be shunted past the site of fusion.

The same authors point out that the pre-disposition of the Charcot knee to post-operative complications and failure of fusion could in addition be related to the fact that patients suffering from tertiary syphilis are often un-reliable and frequently have impaired balance. Post-operative supervision must be related. accordingly. Unprotected weight-bearing should not be undertaken until there is radiological evidence that fusion is complete; and this may entail the use of a plaster cast for as long as five months.

## Arthrodesis for Failed Arthroplasty

It has been indicated that in the current scene the commonest indication for arthrodesis is failed total arthroplasty (41 examples in 5 years, 1971–76, Brodersen et al., 1977). In the circumstances of infection, presence of cement and wide resection of bone demanded by the original operation, it will be anticipated that fusion is more difficult to achieve than in most other indications. In the series referred to infection, present in 80 per cent of the cases, generally cleared with removal of the prosthesis and primary closure over suction irrigation tubes and systemic antibiotics.

The technique recommended involves the use

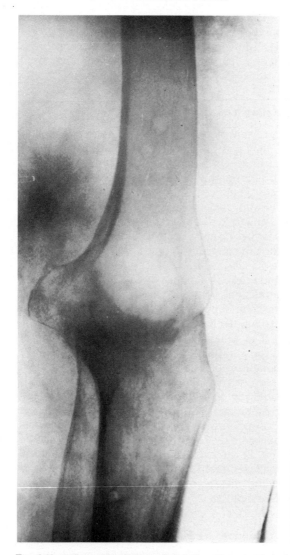

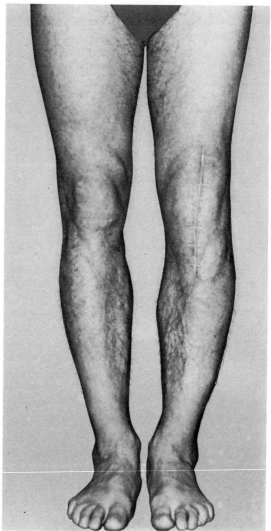

FIG. 6,69. **Arthrodesis: technique of operation.** The technique favoured retains the contours of the femoral and tibial condyles. This enables reduction of angular deformity in either plane to be achieved with the minimum sacrifice of bone while at the same time producing maximum bony contact.

FIG. 6,70. **Arthrodesis: technique of operation.** It is important from the cosmetic viewpoint to match the curves of the normal leg. The technique which retains the contours of the condyles enables this to be accomplished without difficulty.

of compression in the manner to be described. It is to be noted, however, that in a recent series (Hagemann, Woods and Tullos, 1978) a preference is shown for double rather than single pins for exerting compression. The paucity of bone producing inadequate surface contact may necessitate the use of bone grafts. In this regard consideration should be given in suitable cir-

cumstances to gaining access to the medullary cavity of the tibia by the removal of bone grafts which could then be used in crossed fashion after the manner of Brittain (1942) (Fig. 6,72).

### Arthrodesis in Haemophilia

In haemophilia some form of internal fixation

such as crossed screws inserted after the manner of the crossed bone grafts of Brittain (1942) is to be preferred to the compression method. It is undesirable to risk the theoretical danger of haemorrhage and infection inherent in the use of percutaneous pins in the haemophiliac (Houghton and Dickson, 1978).

### Arthrodesis in Childhood

In this series (Table 8) 7 examples only were children under the age of 15 years, 6, in the distant past, for tuberculosis and the seventh for deformity/instability from a suppurative arthritis of infancy producing total destruction of the lateral femoral condyle.

When arthrodesis is required in childhood the compression technique should be avoided as liable to produce growth changes in the presence of open epiphyses. If a means of internal fixation is desirable the single central graft (Hatt, 1940) does not affect growth but should be taken from femur or tibia not closer than 2·5 cm from the epiphyseal plate (Van Gorder and Chen, 1959). The patella should be retained intact or, if diseased, excised; but in no circumstances merely denuded of articular cartilage. It is known that such a patella can fuse to the femur and, closing the growth plate, be responsible for a gross recurvatus deformity (Van Gorder and Chen, 1959). When a progressive flexion deformity develops it is usually due to the fact that arthrodesis has been carried out in some flexion and therefore excessive pressure is applied to the posterior aspects of the growth plates while at the same time pressure is reduced on the anterior aspects. If such angular deformities occur osteotomy may be required when the epiphyses are mature. **Methods available.** There are a variety of techniques and the author has personal experience of some of them. These include simple apposition of the exposed bone ends; apposition of the bone ends supplemented with crossed pins included in a plaster cast (Fig. 6,73); crossed bone grafts (Brittain, 1942) (Fig. 6,72); and single central graft (Hatt, 1940) (Fig. 6,71). There are other methods, particularly of internal fixation. These include intramedullary nail; plate and screws; stainless steel wire sutures; and staples. The means of fixation which receives

the greatest measure of acceptance in the current scene is the compression method of Key (1932) elaborated and developed by Charnley (1948). This is the means of immobilisation practised, with modification of technique as disease processes demand (see below), to the exclusion of others in recent years. It is of interest and practical importance that the technique adopted does not influence in material degree the outcome of operation in terms of success or failure of fusion (Moore and Smillie, 1959; Green *et al.*, 1967); for in the interval of time required when opposed bone ends are sclerosed and union likely to be slow, compression appears to hold advantages. It may be a disadvantage in conditions where the bone ends are rarefied and fragile. Too much importance should not be placed on the time taken for fusion to occur. A patient with a stiff knee is scarcely more inconvenienced with a plaster cuff than without. He is able to walk and sometimes can return to work.

### Technique of Operation

Two assistants are necessary: one operative, one to hold the leg. The operation is performed under tourniquet, the patient supine with a small sandbag beneath the knee. The limb is draped in such a manner that full flexion can be produced without danger to aseptic technique. An anterior mid-line incision is made extending from the upper limits of the suprapatellar pouch to a point below the tibial tubercle. The quadriceps tendon is split in the same line, beginning at the upper extremity of the pouch continuing down over the patella and splitting the patellar tendon to end at the tibial tubercle. The capsule is then erased from the medial and lateral tibial tuberosities. In disease the suprapatellar pouch is dissected out completely; otherwise it is ignored. The patella is excised preserving the coverings in continuity with quadriceps and patellar tendon.

It is at this stage that a decision has to be made as to the means of fixation.
**Compression method.** The technique currently practised, and which commends itself to the author, is the retention of the curves of both femoral and tibial condyles. The joint is fully

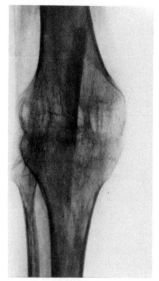

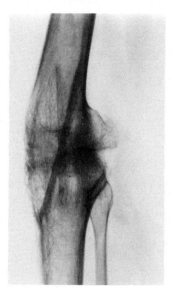

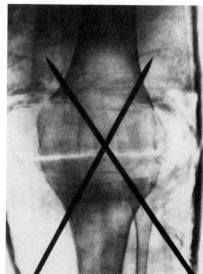

FIG. 6,71          FIG. 6,72          FIG. 6,73

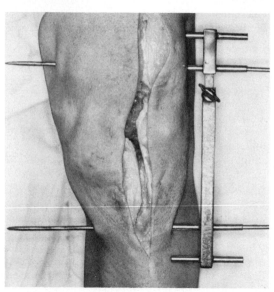

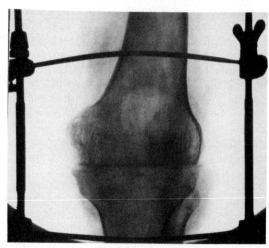

FIG. 6,75

FIG. 6,74

FIGS 6,71–76. **Arthrodesis: methods of internal fixation.** It is possible a variety of methods may be required in solving the problems of arthrodesis posed by failed total replacement. Single massive graft (Hatt) (Fig. 6,71). Crossed grafts (Brittain) (Fig. 6,72). Crossed Steinmann pins (Figs. 6.73) and compression technique (Figs 6,74 to 76). Note use of template to ensure that Steinmann pins are parallel (Fig. 6,74). The action and benefit of compression is seen in Figure 6,75 by comparison with Figure 6,73 in which a space is seen between the opposing bone ends. The location of the incision in Figure 6,76 was determined by the necessity to excise a scar.

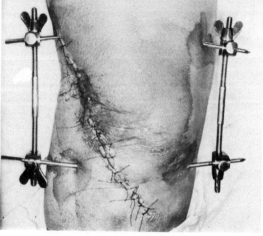

FIG. 6,76

flexed. The femoral articular cartilage is removed down to cancellous bone. The same procedure is followed in the tibia, hollowing out the centres of the condyles but leaving the limiting cortex intact. The opposing surfaces are brought into contact and the necessary adjustments made by deepening the concavity of one or other tibial condyle to correct valgus or varus, lowering the central area as necessary to obtain better contact and by antero-posterior rotation adjusting the joint to the exact degree of flexion required. The method has the advantage of bringing the largest possible areas of bone into contact in natural stability and avoids the necessity of a decision, right or wrong, within 5° and does not reduce unduly the size of the tibial head which sometimes occurs when the twin saws are used.

But alternatively the articular surfaces of the femur and tibia are removed by means of a twin-bladed saw, permitting two parallel cuts to be made which remove both surfaces at the same time, thus ensuring the most perfect apposition. A few degrees of flexion, but no more, is the most desirable position. The proximity of soft tissues does not permit the entire bone to be transversed by the saw, which can be used to only about half the depth and the remainder completed with an osteotome with the joint in maximum flexion.

In either method, before the final adjustment is made and before the pins are inserted, the bone of the opposing tibial and femoral surfaces, particularly any remaining sclerotic areas, is broken up by driving in a small gouge at various points and partially levering out fragments of cancellous tissue in order to increase both the area and the roughness of the opposing surfaces and contribute to vascularisation.

Gravitational forces in the course of healing tend to produce extension or even hyperextension. Immediately before closing the wound it is the practice to insert cancellous bone chips, collected in the course of operation, into the region of the intercondylar notch anteriorly. These chips, by producing a small increase in flexion, are under a compression force when the joint is in extension.

**Application of compression.** No matter whether the 'retention of contour' or 'parallel saw cut' method is used, the insertion of the 4 mm Stein-mann pins is most readily accomplished by means of a template.

The distal Stinmann pin should be introduced first because it is easier to insert a pin at right-angles to the axis of the tibia than to correct for the valgus angle which the femur makes with the tibia if a pin is inserted first into the femur (Charnley, 1953). The template is applied and adjusted so that the femoral pin is in the desired position parallel to the tibial pin (Fig. 6,74).

It is important, from the viewpoint of avoiding post-operative pain and infection, that the pins are inserted without tension on the skin. To this end when the site in the tibia at which the first pin is to be inserted has been selected, the skin incision is closed temporarily using Alliss' tissue forceps. The pin is then introduced. The tissue forceps are released while the site at which the femoral pin is to be inserted is selected and the template applied. The temporary closure of the skin is repeated while the second pin is introduced. With this technique, undesirable tension at points of entrance and exit will not occur (Fig. 6,74).

The clamps are now applied and tightened with the purpose of achieving a load as near 45 kg (100 lb) as possible (Charnley, 1953). In practice a degree of compression is applied which holds the opposing surfaces in firm opposition when the limb is supported by the calf. Suction drainage is introduced and the wound closed.

One of the few disadvantages of this form of arthrodesis is the difficulty which exists in applying a pressure bandage to the joint. In this regard it is important that the pins should be sufficiently long, say 25 cm (10 in) and that the clamps are applied at a distance from the skin sufficient to permit cotton-wool and bandages to be introduced. A posterior plaster shell is applied over the compression bandage to prevent hyperextension.

AFTER-TREATMENT. At the termination of the operation the limb is placed in a half-ring Thomas bed-knee splint. In the adjustment of the slings care is taken that the Steinmann pins cannot contact the metal side-irons of the splint (Fig. 6,77).

Experience has shown that no matter how much care has been taken, considerable post-operative oozing occurs. This need not occasion alarm in the knowledge that no blood has been lost at operation, provided the compression bandage has been applied with the care the situation demands.

The stitches are removed about the fourteenth day and a skin-tight plaster back-shell applied to prevent extension. The patient is returned to bed and the Thomas bed-knee splint reapplied. In the standard treatment compression is maintained until a total of six weeks have elapsed, when the apparatus and pins are removed in favour of a skin-tight walking plaster cast which does not include the foot or ankle.

After-treatment can however vary with age, physique and circumstances of the case. It is possible to make the patient ambulatory at the end of three weeks using a patten and crutches and incorporating the limb including the pins in a skin-tight plaster cast. Weight-bearing is deferred until the pins are removed at the sixth week. In exceptionally favourable circumstances a plaster cast incorporating the pins may be applied at the end of the third week. The pins are withdrawn thereafter and weight-bearing commenced. In all cases the walking cast is retained for a minimum of 12 weeks; and there are circumstances, of osteoarthrosis in particu-

lar, when the cast may require to be retained for a considerably longer time.

If protection is required when the plaster cast is finally removed the corset-caliper (1KJ5, Fig. 11,21) is to be recommended as a temporary measure.

## Means of Internal Function

**Crossed pins.** This is the simplest method. When the bone ends are opposed in acceptable position they are held in position by long Steinmann pins of 4 mm diameter inserted crosswise and entered through the tibia so that they engage the cortex of the femur on the opposite side (Fig. 6,73). The skin is held in the position in which it will be sutured before the pins are entered so that tension is avoided at the points of entry. Suction drainage is introduced before the skin is closed.

AFTER-TREATMENT. The compression bandage, in outer layers of which are incorporated plaster slabs, is applied over and including the pins. The limb is immobilised in a half-ring Thomas bed-knee splint. When the sutures are removed a skin-tight plaster cast is applied including the pins which, if necessary, are cut short. They are removed at the end of six weeks when weight-bearing in the cylinder cast is

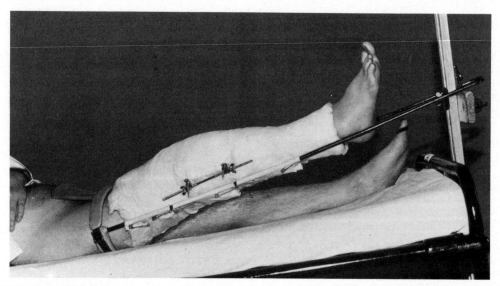

FIG. 6,77. **Compression arthrodesis: after treatment.** In the immediate post-operative phase the patient wearing a compression bandage is nursed in a half-ring Thomas bed-knee splint.

instituted. The cast is retained until union is complete.

**Bone graft.** The graft is cut from the crest and anteromedial aspect of the tibia beginning at a point about 5 cm (2 in) below the upper limit of the shaft and extending distally about 12·5 cm (5 in). A cranked osteotome of about 1·25 cm (½ in) diameter is introduced through the upper part of the bed in the tibia from which the graft was taken and driven upwards into the femur to provide a suitably located track. The massive graft is then driven home. The graft should be regarded as a means of attaining union rather than a method of internal fixation. Stability cannot be expected to depend on the strength of the graft, nor on the cancellous tissue with which it is in contact (Fig. 6,71). Alternatively two grafts are cut and driven across the joint in the form of an X using two cranked osteotomes (Fig. 6,72) (Brittain, 1942).

AFTER-TREATMENT. The employment of a tourniquet precludes the immediate use of a plaster cast, which does not provide elastic pressure. It has therefore been the practice to apply a compression bandage incorporating long plaster slabs, which reach from the groin to the ankle joint, and to immobilise the limb in a half-ring Thomas bed-knee splint as a temporary measure. The only completely satisfactory method of immobilisation for this type of arthrodesis is that provided by a plaster spica which includes both hip and ankle joints. The initial compression dressing should not be retained for longer than a few days, for it rapidly becomes loose and may permit a hyper-extension deformity to occur.

In 8 to 16 weeks, depending on the rapidity of fusion, the spica is discarded in favour of a thigh-length walking plaster of the type which permits ankle movement or a walking caliper incorporating a knee corset (IKJ5, Fig. 11,21). The splint is retained until the arthrodesis is completely consolidated.

### Errors, Omissions and Complications

**Deformity.** In general it can be said that the use of the twin saw is applicable where there is little deformity. In such circumstances broad areas of cancellous bone can be brought into intimate contact.

Where there is a gross deformity it may not be possible to obtain the two flat opposing surfaces produced by the twin saw without a sacrifice of bone, which reduces the area of contact to cortical rather than cancellous tissue with consequent delay in healing and unnecessary shortening in the final result. In these circumstances conservation of tissue is essential and means retaining the normal conformation of the less deformed condyles, rather than attempting to produce flat surfaces.

FLEXION. The extended or nearly extended position should be adopted. Some flexion, as used to be taught, results in difficulty in getting

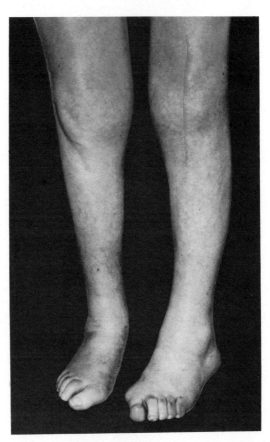

FIG. 6,78. **Arthrodesis of the knee.** It is a serious technical error to arthrodese the knee with the tibia in internal rotation. The error occurs because of failure to appreciate that in extension the tibial tubercle is displaced to the lateral side as in completing the screw-home movement; not opposite to the intercondylar notch. Fusion in internal rotation produces an ugly gait (L.M., female, rheumatoid arthritis, case of J.W.I.).

M

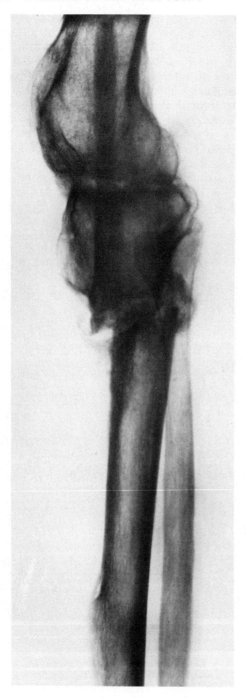

FIG. 6,79. **Arthrodesis: complication.** Stress fracture at top of donor site following use of single central graft.

the heel to the ground, loss of power in the calf and unnecessary shortening.

ROTATION. Care must be taken not to fuse the joint in internal rotation. It is an unsightly deformity and causes difficulty in walking (Fig. 6,78). The error occurs from failure to appreciate the normal relationship of tibia to femur. It is the screw-home movement which determines that the tibial tubercle is lateral to the mid-line of the patellar (trochlear) notch of the femur in extension and not opposite to it. This may not be evident when the patella has been removed.

LATERAL ANGULATION. The consideration, in relation to valgus or varus, is comparison with the other side. The normal 9° of valgus may not always be possible to attain. If a greater degree must be accepted, weight-bearing should be deferred.

**Plaster fixation.** When plaster immobilisation is used in after-treatment the foot should not be incorporated in the cast. If weight-bearing is permitted the foot-piece detracts from the compression stimulus. If the limb is required to be suspended and patten and crutch used, incorporation of the foot has a distracting influence on the arthrodesis site which delays union.

## JUVENILE RHEUMATOID ARTHRITIS: JUVENILE CHRONIC POLYARTHRITIS (STILL'S DISEASE)

**Definition.** Juvenile rheumatoid arthritis, a chronic form of arthritis first described by Cornil in 1864, has protean manifestations. It can begin as a fulminating systemic disease like that described by Still (1897); it can have a poly-articular onset similar to that observed in adult rheumatoid arthritis; or it can present as single-joint disease which may or may not progress to poly-articular arthritis.

### Diagnosis

The condition is rarely mono-articular although the major manifestations affect one knee joint. The clue as to the nature of the pathology may exist in the form of minor swellings, possibly without symptoms, in other joints. The most valid criterion for diagnosis is the persistence of joint involvement of several months duration in a patient who has no other demonstrable disease.

**Involvement of other joints.** If mono-articular onset is not uncommon patients whose disease remains mono-articular are few. But the longer involvement remains mono-articular the less likely are other joints to be affected.

**Sex.** Females predominate in the ratio of 2 to 1.

**Age at onset.** The age at which the disease is manifest varies widely between 18 months and 15 years. It is the impression that the age at onset is unrelated to prognosis.

## Laboratory Tests

**ESR.** If, in general, the sedimentation rate is raised to a degree corresponding to the systemic activity of the disease this does not apply to the mono-articular variety.

**Radiological changes.** It has been indicated elsewhere that radiographs depict bone; not cartilage. It will be evident therefore that when there is narrowing of the joint space and/or erosions of bone destructive changes in the articular cartilage are advanced and thus the prognosis in terms of future function poor; and the earlier the changes occur in the course of the disease the worse the prognosis. Improvement in the appearance of the joint once changes have been observed rarely occurs. In view of the relationship of radiographic appearance to prognosis plates should be taken at, say, intervals of six months. The advent of changes may be an indication for synovectomy (see below).

**Radiology in rheumatoid arthritis.** In relation to the above recommendation it should be appreciated that rheumatoid arthritis is a life-long disease. No patients are subjected to more radiological examinations than those in which the disease arises in childhood. At what stage does further exposure to X-rays become dangerous?

## Treatment

The knee joint problem, unless mono-articular, must be seen against the background of a general disease of unknown origin with a wide variety of manifestation in joints and organs other than joints and of prognosis impossible to estimate in the early stages of the disease. In such circumstances the aim of treatment is the prevention of flexion deformity combined with the maintenance of function.

In the active stage or during an exacerbation, bed-rest combined with splinting on the lines indicated under 'Flexion Deformity: Prevention' are indicated. Active exercise is the only form of therapy likely to be rewarding; and as improvement occurs a balance between rest and exercise must be struck. The nature and prognosis of the disease and the aims of treatment must be explained to the parents. The importance of the prevention of deformity and the maintenance of function by splinting, passive stretching and active exercise is stressed looking forward to such time when, sooner or later, the disease for which there is no dramatic cure, is 'burnt out' (Figs 6,80 to 6,85). The patient attends hospital only until the measures have been mastered by parent and child and performed thereafter in the home three times a day. Physical activities are not otherwise controlled other than by the restrictions imposed by the disease.

Regular medical supervision is essential at intervals related to the activity and progress of the disease.

**Drug therapy.** The only drug recommended is aspirin. It is given in doses of 80 mg/kg body weight per day, usually in divided doses with meals. It is discontinued in children who have been in remission for any considerable period of time, say, six months.

If patients have been receiving steroid therapy before referral it is recommended that withdrawal is completed as soon as practicable in the circumstances of the case.

## Prognosis by Conservative Non-operative Means

In general it can be said from the wide variety of small series reported that some 50 per cent of patients recover, virtually completely, with rational conservative therapy on the lines indicated. In those who recover the only important permanent sequelae may be defects of growth.

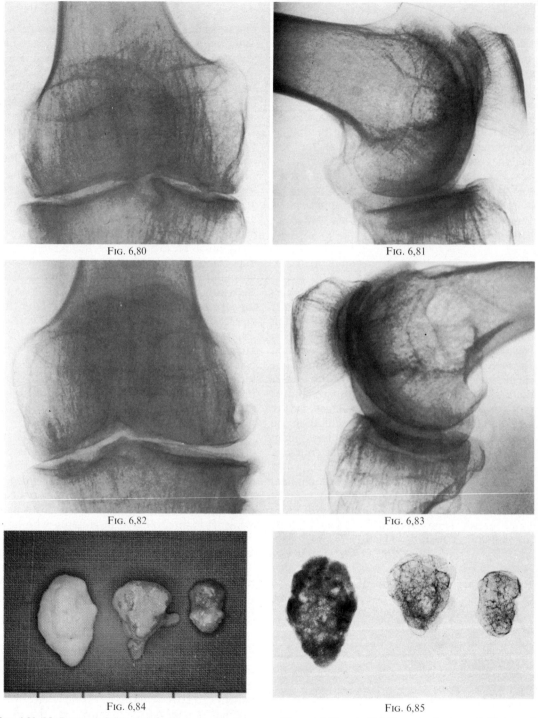

Fig. 6,80

Fig. 6,81

Fig. 6,82

Fig. 6,83

Fig. 6,84

Fig. 6,85

Figs 6,80–85. **Burnt-out Still's disease.** These are the knee joints of a patient (Mrs J. B., aged 40), from which loose bodies (Figs 6,84 and 85) were removed 15 years previously when a bilateral limited debridement was performed. The extension in both knees was complete and there was a full range of flexion. She is symptomless. Debridement can be a useful operation even in the long term (Figs 6,80 to 6,83).

Figures 6,84 and 6,85 illustrate the natural history of loose bodies. The largest was free. The other two had an attachment to synovial membrane. Note quality of articular cartilage in loose body without blood supply; and thinness and erosion of articular cartilage in those with a blood supply. But note also sclerosis of bone in loose body without blood supply, and normal appearance of bone in those with blood supply.

## Indications for Synovectomy

In making a decision regarding the necessity for synovectomy it will be remembered that articular cartilage is thick in children and total destruction is late. This is the reason why many recover excellent function even after years of swelling and thickening of the soft tissues about the joint. Major surgical interference with a joint which is destined to recover spontaneously is clearly undesirable. In such circumstances the ability to recognise the clinical course of the type of disease which is likely to go into remission is important. The timing and even the necessity for synovectomy in juveniles is much more difficult to establish than in the adult (Ansell, 1967).

If criteria for synovectomy must be established those which have evolved from the retrospective study of Eyring, Longert and Bass (1971) are as follows:

1. Persistence of active synovitis for more than 18 months without radiological evidence of destruction and without significant loss of motion, despite adequate conservative measures.
2. Presence of active synovitis with radiological evidence of destruction regardless of the duration of the disease.
3. Presence of active synovitis with significant loss of motion in the face of prolonged conservative therapy.

**Technique.** The operation and after-treatment do not differ in material degree from that described for the adult. A recent review of results McMaster (1972) prefers short lateral and medial parapatellar incisions (Marmor, 1966) as not only less destructive than a single medial parapatellar incision but permits earlier post-operative exercise to be pursued; and this confirms the author's impression. The suprapatellar pouch and as much synovial tissue as possible is removed. The menisci are retained or excised as the situation demands. In the event of excision, which is usually necessary, the manoeuvre described under 'Technique of Operation' permits wide access to the synovial membrane of the posterior compartment.

## Results of Operation

Synovectomy can be a useful procedure in juvenile rheumatoid arthritis capable of arresting or influencing favourably the process of the disease in the majority of cases. In a minority it fails and the knee may become worse. In the series of 30 synovectomies in 27 children reviewed by McMaster (1972) 17 remained symptomless, 6 were adjudged to be slightly better and 7 were worse. It is the general opinion that the best results occur in the mono-articular variety.

**Effect on growth.** It has been suggested that hyperaemia of the synovial membrane in the region of the growth plate is responsible for increased growth; and that valgus angulation is due to asymmetry of vascular supply (Brattstrom, 1963). It appears that synovectomy may be beneficial in this regard in that valgus deformity may correct spontaneously and rate of overgrowth decrease (McMaster, 1972).

# COMPLICATIONS OF RHEUMATOID ARTHRITIS

## 1. IN THE NATURAL COURSE OF THE DISEASE

### Suppurative Arthritis

**Introduction.** Suppurative arthritis is a common and serious complication of chronic rheumatoid arthritis. The diagnostic and therapeutic problems posed were first described by Kellgren *et al.* (1958). The mortality recorded is as high as 35 per cent (Karten, 1969). The most recent reports probably based on early recognition of the complication, but certainly on more effective chemotherapeutic agents, suggest a considerably improved prognosis (Myers, Miller and Pinals, 1969).

**Joint incidence.** The knee is by far the most common joint affected. In a minority of cases more than one joint is involved.

**Organism.** The most common infecting organism is *Staphylococcus aureus,* coagulase positive. Haemolytic streptococcus and a variety of other organisms may be implicated.

**Aetiology.** There is some evidence that infective arthritis after bacteraemia may develop in joints previously damaged by disease other than rheumatoid arthritis (Willkens, Healy and

Decker, 1960). It is significant that Myers *et al.* (1969) during their interest in the matter encountered the complication in systemic lupus erythematosus (3 cases); haemophilia (1 case) and Charcot's arthropathy (1 case). The joint involved was the one previously affected by the basic disease. It has been shown that leucoytes in the synovial fluid in a joint affected by rheumatoid arthritis have diminished activity in phagocytosis of staphylococci; and this may explain the increased susceptibility to infection (Bodel and Hollingsworth, 1966).

The source of infection can seldom be determined with certainty. In 10 of a series of 16 cases (Myers *et al.*, 1969) probable sources were: skin (3); pneumonia (2); surgical wound (2); osteomyelitis (1); urinary tract (1); and intra-articular injection of corticosteroid (4).

## Diagnosis

Suppurative arthritis complicating chronic rheumatoid arthritis is frequently overlooked, the signs and symptoms misinterpreted as activation of the disease (Kellgren *et al.*, 1958). This is presumed to be the explanation of the high mortality. The infected joint is swollen and with increase in local temperature is not dissimilar to rheumatoid arthritis. There is systemic reaction but the pyrexia may be low-grade and intermittent. The fact that the ESR is raised is not helpful. Leucocytosis is moderate or may be absent. The diagnosis, as in so many medical activities, depends on background knowledge of the frequency of the complications leading to the aspiration of purulent fluid from the joint and repeated blood culture.

**Treatment.** Initial treatment differs in no material respect from that applicable to suppurative arthritis arising *de novo* (Ch. 5) and will not be repeated.

**Prognosis.** It is characteristic of suppurative arthritis superimposed on rheumatoid arthritis that the infection is difficult or impossible to eradicate and recurrence is common following discontinuation of antibiotic therapy. In some examples such therapy must be continued virtually on a permanent basis. It will be recognised that infection superimposed on rheumatoid arthritis is frequently the final insult to the damaged articular cartilage leaving

no alternative to the recommendation for arthrodesis.

## LEAKAGE OF SYNOVIAL FLUID: RUPTURE OF POSTERIOR CAPSULE: GIANT SYNOVIAL CYST OF THE CALF

**Pathological anatomy.** Popliteal cysts are a common accompaniment of rheumatoid arthritis if it is only for the reason that rheumatoid arthritis is a common disease and distension of the gastrocnemio-semimembranosus bursa the known accompaniment of pathology within the joint. In rheumatoid arthritis is the added feature that the synovial lining of an existing bursa can be directly affected by the disease. Cysts of the calf as a complication of rheumatoid arthritis are not herniations of the synovial membrane of the knee joint or extensions of previously existing bursa but the result of rupture of the posterior capsule or of a gastrocnemio-semimembranosus bursa: the so-called cysts are not lined with synovial membrane but merely the inflammatory response to the irritation of leakage of pathological synovial fluid from the joint. The reason for rupture of the capsule is not far to seek. It is the site of a degenerative pathological process and as such unable to withstand the pressure created in flexion which has been shown to be as high as 1000 mm of mercury (Palmer, 1970).

## Clinical Features

Leakage of synovial fluid through the posterior capsule as a complication of rheumatoid arthritis, unlike suppuration, is not so much that it is missed as that it is misdiagnosed. It may be difficult to distinguish from deep venous thrombosis.

There are four clinical forms (Myles, 1971):

**Acute.** This may occur in active arthritis and presents with sudden severe pain behind the knee and in the calf. There is erythema, oedema and marked tenderness accompanied by a general systemic reaction. The appearance is that of acute cellulitis and as such not likely to be confused with popliteal vein thrombosis.

**Subacute.** This is the form which most readily simulates deep venous thrombosis. There is gradual onset of pain behind the knee and in the calf, with swelling of the leg; sometimes, at an early stage, with induration, oedema and erythema of the calf. In thrombosis oedema starts at the ankle.

**Chronic: (a) painless oedema.** This form occurs in arthritis of long duration, not necessarily active. Oedema of the legs is common in rheumatoid arthritis. In many examples the precise cause is difficult to determine probably because it is multifactorial in origin. Painless synovial leaks, sometimes associated with cysts of the calf, may be responsible for chronic painless oedema.

**(b) Cyst of the calf.** Cysts, which may assume major proportions sometimes reaching to the ankle, are a well-known feature of chronic rheumatoid arthritis. They may be a source of pain from tension and/or from irritation of the adjacent soft tissues.

### Diagnosis

The establishment of a diagnosis is of most immediate concern in the acute and subacute form. The knowledge that leakage of synovial fluid into the popliteal space and thence downwards is more common than spontaneous deep venous thrombosis is basic to the avoidance of error.

**Arthrography.** Contrast arthrographs may be used to confirm the presence of a leak and are more likely to be of assistance in defining the tract or cyst formation determined by gravity in the subacute and chronic forms than in the acute in which the original extravasation is likely to be diffuse. In any event arthrograms are more of academic interest than for actual assistance in determining a diagnosis which in circumstances of urgency in determining treatment is based on background knowledge of the pathological anatomy of rheumatoid arthritis and a reasonable level of clinical acumen. Nevertheless, arthrograms may be necessary where doubt exists as to the nature of the swelling and to determine the extent of the cyst prior to surgical intervention.

TECHNIQUE. The joint is aspirated under the strictest aseptic precautions and 5 to 20 ml of contrast material injected. The patient then flexes and extends the joint, stands up and takes a few paces. A lateral radiograph then shows the material extravasated diffusely into the calf in acute ruptures or defining the cyst in the chronic variety.

### Treatment

The importance of the complication is the striking similarity of the symptoms and signs to those produced by deep vein thrombosis. The undesirability of unnecessary anticoagulative therapy in the circumstances is evident. A 'deep venous thrombosis' in a patient with rheumatoid arthritis of the knee should be suspect and anticoagulant therapy withheld until the diagnosis of rupture of the posterior capsule has been excluded.

In the acute or subacute forms rest, elevation and compression is required. In a tension situation aspiration may be indicated. It will be recognised that the potential for recurrence is inherent in the basic pathology; and surgical intervention in one form or another may be inevitable.

In active disease local excision in the course of symptomatic surgery is liable to be followed by recurrence in so far as treatment has not been directed to the cause. If rheumatoid arthritis cannot be cured by surgery, subtotal synovectomy, when indicated on general grounds but not otherwise, is likely to be effective. In other circumstances local excision may be indicated.

TECHNIQUE. A long incision is necessary; and that part of it which exposes the upper limits in the popliteal space should be of the lazy S variety and not vertical to avoid a keloid scar. The cyst will be found between gastrocnemius and soleus muscles to which it may be adherent and can be traced upwards to communicate with the knee joint beneath the medial head of gastrocnemius.

### COMPLICATIONS OF TREATMENT

#### 2. IATROGENIC

##### *Corticosteroid Arthropathy*

In the current scene intra-articular corticosteroid injections are in common use in the treatment of rheumatoid and other forms of arthritis. It should be accepted that the effects are palliative and transitory. They have no beneficial therapeutic effect other than temporary relief of symptoms. On the other hand there is an increasing volume of evidence, clinical and experimental, that intra-articular injection of steroids prevents cartilage repair and can inflict serious and permanent damage on the arthritic joint. It is evident that only the obvious disasters are reported. The signs of less severe damage may be difficult to distinguish from the natural course of the original disease. Whether intra-articular steroid therapy has any place in the long term management of a relentless disease such as rheumatoid arthritis or is of value in helping a patient to come to terms with such a disability has always been open to question. 'The case against multiple injections is so strong that the practice should, in our opinion, be discarded, which implies that even a single injection requires strong justification.' (Bentley and Goodfellow, 1969.)

### Varieties

It appears that there are two types of corticosteroid arthropathy: (1) the development in an otherwise normal knee of an area of avascular necrosis bearing such·a resemblance to osteochondritis dissecans as to be known as 'hydrocortisone osteochondritis dissecans' (see Ch. 11). The immunosuppressive regime associated with organ transplants is liable to produce such changes. The situation therefore may be a complication of an operation undertaken for the relief of a lethal disease and differs as such from the arthropathy which occurs after the local or systemic treatment of rheumatoid or other forms of arthritis. No doubt the problems posed by immunotherapy will be solved in the future; and (2) the rapid deterioration and disorganisation of a knee joint already the site of rheumatoid or other form of arthritis and which follows either systemic, or more usually, repeated intra-articular injections of hydrocortisone.

**Clinical features.** In the knee the syndrome produces intermittent episodes of pain and swelling, a feeling of instability and giving-way incidents. Radiographs demonstrate a condition not dissimilar in appearance to osteochondritis

dissecans (Fig. 6,86) or a generalised progressive destructive process.

**Treatment.** Management follows general principles, aspiration, compression, maintenance of extension and quadriceps exercises. A loose body producing symptoms may require to be removed. In no circumstances should repair of the lesion be attempted: it will result in failure.

In extreme examples of a destructive process pain and instability may be such that the patient is unable to stand. In such circumstances arthrodesis may be indicated and has been successfully accomplished (Aichroth *et al.*, 1971).

### Rupture of Patellar Tendon

Spontaneous rupture of the patellar tendon is an accident of some rarity in the young athlete. There is evidence that local injection of hydrocortisone at the junction of patella and patellar tendon for the relief of pain in, for example, jumper's knee (Ch. 2) entails the risk of rupture;

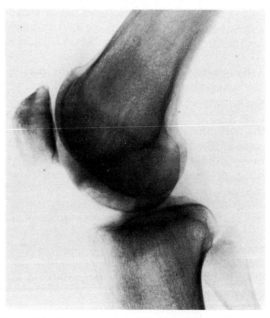

FIG. 6,86. **'Hydrocortisone osteochondritis dissecans'.** A lesion resembling osteochondritis dissecans may develop in the knee of a patient undergoing local or systemic corticosteroid 'therapy'. It is important that the source of the lesion is recognised. Treatment is expectant and may require excision of a separating mass of cartilage and bone. Conservative surgery is contraindicated (see IKJ4, p. 298).

and such has been reported (Ismail, Balakrishnan and Rajakumar, 1969). The risk is greatest if the injection has been administered with the purpose of permitting the athlete to continue his activities. The practice is to be condemned.

Bilateral rupture in patients suffering from systemic lupus erythematosus receiving long-term systemic corticosteroid treatment, from the number of cases reported in the literature, appears to be common.

## REFERENCES

AICHROTH, P., BRANFOOT, A. C., HUSKISSON, E. C. & LOUGHRIDGE, L. W. (1971). Destructive joint changes following kidney transplantation. *Journal of Bone and Joint Surgery,* **53B,** 3, 488.

ANSELL, B. M. (1967). Results of synovectomy in rheumatoid arthritis of the knee. In *Synovectomy and Arthroplasty in Rheumatoid Arthritis,* p. 54. Edited by G. Chapchal. Stuttgart: George Thieme.

BENJAMIN, A. (1969). Double osteotomy for the painful knee in rheumatoid arthritis and osteoarthritis. *Journal of Bone and Joint Surgery,* **51B,** 4, 694.

BENTLEY, G. & GOODFELLOW, J. W. (1969). Rupture of patellar ligament after steroid infiltration. *Journal of Bone and Joint Surgery,* **51B,** 3, 503.

BODEL, P. T. & HOLLINGSWORTH, J. W. (1966). *Journal of Clinical Investigation,* **45,** 580.

BRATTSTROM, M. (1963). Asymmetry of ossification and rate of growth of long bones in children with unilateral juvenile gonarthritis. *Acta rheumatologica scandinavica,* **9,** 102.

BRATTSTROM, H. & M. (1971). Long-term results in knee arthrodesis in rheumatoid arthritis. *Acta rheumatologica scandinavica,* **17,** 86.

*British Medical Journal* (1977). Editorial, **ii,** 717.

BRITTAIN, H. A. (1942). *Architectural Principles in Arthrodesis,* p. 46. Edinburgh: Livingstone.

BRODERSEN, M. P., FITZGERALD, R. H., BREWER, N. S., BRYAN, R. S., PETERSON, L. F. A. & COVENTRY, M. B. (1977). Arthrodesis for failed total knee arthroplasty. *Journal of Bone and Joint Surgery,* **59B,** 506.

CHARNLEY, J. (1948). Positive pressure in arthrodesis of the knee joint. *Journal of Bone and Joint Surgery,* **30B,** 478.

CHARNLEY, J. (1953). *Compression Arthrodesis.* Edinburgh: E. & S. Livingstone.

CORNIL, V. (1864). Mémoire sur des coincidences pathologiques du rhumatisme articulaire chronique. *Mém. Soc. de Biol. (Paris),* **3,** 25.

DICK, W. C., SHENKIN, P., NUKI, G., WHALEY, K. & BUCHANAN, W. W. (1970). Effect of synovectomy on the clearance of radioactive Xenon ($^{133}$Xe) from the knee joint of patients with rheumatoid arthritis. *Journal of Bone and Joint Surgery,* **52B,** 1, 70–76.

DRENNAN, D. B., FAHEY, J. J., MAYLAHN, D. J. (1971). Important factors in achieving arthrodesis of the Charcot knee. *Journal of Bone and Joint Surgery,* **53A,** 6, 1180.

EYRING, E. J., LONGERT, A. & BASS, J. C. (1971). Synovectomy in juvenile rheumatoid arthritis. *Journal of Bone and Joint Surgery,* **53A,** 4, 638.

FERGUSSON, W. (1861). Excision of the knee joint—recovery with a false joint and useful limb. *Medical Times and Hospital Gazette,* **1,** 601.

GREEN, D. P., PARKES, J. C. & STINCHFIELD, F. E. (1967). Arthrodesis of the knee. *Journal of Bone and Joint Surgery,* **49A,** 6, 1065.

HAGEMANN, W. F., WOODS, G. W. & TULLOS, H. S. (1978). Arthrodesis in failed total knee replacement. *Journal of Bone and Joint Surgery,* **60A,** 790.

HATT, R. N. (1940). The central bone graft in joint arthrodesis. *Journal of Bone and Joint Surgery,* **22,** 393.

HELFET, A. J. (1963). *The Management of Internal Derangements of the Knee.* Philadelphia: Lippincott & Co.

HOUGHTON, G. R. & DICKSON, R. A. (1978). Lower limb arthrodesis in haemophilia. *Journal of Bone and Joint Surgery,* **60B,** 387.

INSALL, J. D., CHITRANJAN, S. R., AGLIETTI, P. & SHINE, J. (1976). A comparison of four models of total knee-replacement prostheses. *Journal of Bone and Joint Surgery,* **58A,** 6, 754.

INSALL, J., RANAWAT, C. S., SCOTT, W. N. & WALKER, P. (1976). Total condylar knee replacement. *Clinical Orthopaedics and Related Research,* **120,** 149.

ISMAIL, A. M., BALAKRISHNAN, R., & RAJAKUMAR, M. K. (1969). Rupture of patellar ligament after steroid infiltration. *Journal of Bone and Joint Surgery,* **51B,** 3, 503.

JONES, G. B. (1968). Arthroplasty of the knee by the Walldius prosthesis. *Journal of Bone and Joint Surgery,* **50B,** 3, 505.

JONES, G. B. (1972). *Arthroplasty of the Knee. Modern Trends in Orthopaedics.* London: Butterworths.

KARTEN, I. (1969). *Annals of Internal Medicine,* **70,** 1147.

KELLGREN, J. H., BALL, J., FAIRBROTHER, R. W. & BARNES, K. L. (1958). *British Medical Journal,* **i,** 1147.

KEY, J. A. (1932). Positive pressure in arthrodesis for tuberculosis of the knee joint. *Southern Medical Journal (Nashville),* **25,** 909.

LASKIN, R. S. (1978). Modular total knee-replacement arthroplasty. A review of eighty-nine patients. *Journal of Bone and Joint Surgery,* **58A,** 766.

LETTIN, A. W. F., DELISS, L. J., BLACKBURNE, J. S. & SCALES, J. T. (1978). The Stanmore hinged knee arthroplasty. *Journal of Bone and Joint Surgery,* **60B,** 327.

MACKEEVER, D. C. (1943). The use of cellophane as an interposition membrane in synovectomy. *Journal of Bone and Joint Surgery,* **XXV,** 3, 576.

MCMASTER, M. (1972). Synovectomy of the knee in juvenile rheumatoid arthritis. *Journal of Bone and Joint Surgery,* **54B,** 2, 263.

MARMOR, L. (1966). Synovectomy of the rheumatoid knee. *Clinical Orthopaedics,* **44,** 151.

MIGNON, A. (1900). *Bulletin de la Société de Chirurgie, Paris,* **26,** 1113.

MOORE, F. H. & SMILLIE, I. S. (1959). Arthrodesis of the knee joint. *Clinical Orthopaedics,* **13,** 215.

MUIRDEN, K. D. & MILLS, K. W. (1971). Do lymphocytes protect the rheumatoid joint? *British Medical Journal,* **iv,** 219.

MYERS, A. R., MILLER, L. M. & PINALS, R. S. (1969). Pyarthrosis complicating rheumatoid arthritis. *British Medical Journal,* **ii,** 714.

MYLES, A. B. (1971). Posterior synovial leaks in arthritis of the knee. *Proceedings of the Royal Society of Medicine,* **64,** 262.

PALMER, D. G. (1970). Tendon sheaths, bursae and protrusion cysts in rheumatoid arthritis. Twentieth Annual Meeting of the New Zealand Orthopaedic Association, September 14–18, 1969. *(Journal of Bone and Joint Surgery,* **52B,** 1, 188).

PARADIES, L. H. (1969). Synovectomy of the knee. In *Early Synovectomy in Rheumatoid Arthritis,* p. 129. Proceedings of the Symposium on Early Synovectomy in Rheumatoid Arthritis. Amsterdam, The Netherlands, April 1967. Edited by W. Hijmans, W. D. Paul and H. Herschel. Amsterdam: Excerpta Medica Foundation.

PERRY, J., ANTONELLI, D. & FORD, W. (1975). Analysis of knee-joint forces during flexed-knee stance. *Journal of Bone and Joint Surgery,* **57A,** 7, 961.

SCALES, J. T. (1976). Replacement of the knee joint. *British Medical Journal,* **ii,** 638.

SHEEHAN, J. M. (1978). Arthroplasty of the knee. *Journal of Bone and Joint Surgery,* **60B,** 3, 333.

SHERMAN, M. (1951). The non-specificity of synovial reactions. *Bulletin of the Hospital for Joint Diseases,* **12,** 110.

SHIERS, L. G. P. (1954). Arthroplasty of knee. Preliminary report of a new method. *Journal of Bone and Joint Surgery,* **36B,** 553.

SMILLIE, I. S. (1941). Simple system of splinting for the lower limb. *Lancet,* **ii,** 304.

SPEED, J. S. (1924). *Journal of the American Medical Association,* **83,** 1814.

STILL, G. F. (1897). *Medico-Chirurgical Transactions,* **80,** 47.

STREJECK, J. & POPELKA, S. (1969). Bilateral rupture of the patellar ligaments in systemic lupus erythematosus. *Lancet,* **ii,** 714.

TRICKEY, E. L. (1969). Double osteotomy for the painful knee in rheumatoid arthritis and osteoarthritis. *Journal of Bone and Joint Surgery,* **51B,** 4, 679.

VAN GORDER, G. W. & CHEN, C-M. (1959). The central-graft operation for fusion of tuberculous knees, ankles and elbows. *Journal of Bone and Joint Surgery,* **41A,** 1029.

VERNEUIL, A. (1860). De la création d'une fausse articular par section ou résection partielle de l'os maxillaire inférieur, comme moyen de reméchier à l'ankylose vraie ou fausse de la machoire inférieure. *Archives Générales de Médecine,* 5me Ser., **15,** 174–195, 284–316.

VOLKMANN. (1877). Quoted by Speed (1924).

WALLDIUS, B. (1953). Arthroplasty of the knee using a plastic prosthesis. *Tidskrift I Militär Hälsovärd,* Val. **78.**

WARDLE, E. N. (1964). Osteotomy of the tibia and fibula in the treatment of osteoarthritis of the knee. *Postgraduate Medical Journal,* **40,** 536.

WILLKENS, R. F., HEALY, L. A. & DECKER, J. L. (1960). *Archives of Internal Medicine,* **106,** 354.

WILSON, J. N., LETTIN, A. W. F. & SCALES, J. T. (1974). Twenty years of evolution of the Stanmore hinged total knee replacement. In *Total Knee Replacement.* London & New York: The Institution of Mechanical Engineers.

WILSON, P. D. (1929). Posterior capsulotomy in certain flexion contractures of the knee. *Journal of Bone and Joint Surgery,* **11,** 40.

# 7.   Haemorrhagic Arthropathy

## HAEMARTHROSIS

### Traumatic Haemarthrosis

The commonest cause of haemarthrosis is accidental trauma. It takes the form of an intra-articular fracture, or rupture of soft tissue with a blood supply such as ligament or synovial membrane in the presence of an intact enveloping capsule. The second most common is haemorrhage of iatrogenic origin from operative trauma as a complication of arthrotomy usually for the purpose of meniscectomy.

**Clotting.** There is within major joints a system which preserves the synovial cavity from obliteration after injury. It works by preventing coagulation of blood shed into the joint and by removing rapidly and without organisation any clots which form. At operation it is not uncommon to find small clots in a haemorrhagic effusion; but the majority of the blood remains fluid.

The extent to which blood remains fluid, however, is probably related to the nature and extent of the injury and the influence of the products of injury on coagulation. It is influenced also by rupture of the capsule and the consequent escape of the contents, whether the patient is standing or supine, into the soft tissue of the calf.

**Absorption.** Erythrocytes within the joint cavity escape by passing between the synovial cells and are to be found lying between the cells and in the subsynovial tissues (Key, 1929; Roy and Ghadially, 1967). Others are phagocyted by the synovial cells and are fragmented and converted into unicentric or multicentric whorled membranous bodies and siderosomes.

If blood remains within the joint and is not aspirated as recommended (see below) the haemosiderosis which results is responsible for unnecessary periarticular fibrosis.

**Rapidity of onset.** The outstanding feature of traumatic haemarthrosis and the one which distinguishes it from traumatic synovitis is the rapidity of onset. A haemarthrosis arises within minutes, at least within half an hour of the causative injury, whereas a traumatic synovial effusion does not appear until some hours later. The swelling which takes place in a matter of minutes rather than hours cannot be other than due to the outpouring of blood.

**Pain.** Haemarthrosis is accompanied by considerable pain, probably initially the result of the rapid distension of the capsule and possibly later from irritation of the synovial membrane by the products of the breakdown of red corpuscles.

**Palpation.** If the effusion is tense, palpation is not helpful. In other circumstances a greater sense of resistance may be encountered by the palpating fingers; but the operative factor is probably 'a high index of suspicion' engendered by knowledge of the mode of onset.

**Systemic reaction.** An untreated single-incident traumatic haemarthrosis may produce systemic reaction with rise in temperature, general as well as local, and thus induce the suspicion of infective arthritis.

**Aspiration.** The ultimate confirmation is aspiration which has the additional advantage of constituting an important therapeutic measure.

### Post-operative Haemarthrosis: Clinical Features

In the immediate post-operative phase following arthrotomy, pain of considerable intensity but in any event of a degree greater than to be expected as a reaction to operation, and particularly when accompanied by oedema of the leg distal to the compression bandage, should be regarded with suspicion as indicating the possibility of intra-articular haemorrhage. The situation may occasion alarm in so far as systemic reaction and increase in local temperature raises the possibility of infection.

### TREATMENT

#### Prevention

A large number of knee joint operations, the most common of which is meniscectomy, are performed under tourniquet and depend for haemostasis thereafter on a compression bandage. The fact that haemarthrosis is unusual, but by no means rare, is due to the fact that the synovial tissues divided are peripheral and therefore subject to compression applied from without. Not all areas of synovial membrane however are under compression, for example, that of the posterior compartment and the antero-central aspect of the fat pad. It is the liability to haemorrhage from the latter area which prompted the measures which avoid, in the removal of synovial tags, leaving raw areas within the joint (Ch. 4). It is the author's practice and strong recommendation that the surgeon who performs the operation should apply the compression bandage and not leave this important part of the immediate post-operative treatment to an inexperienced assistant.

In the current regime the joint is rested after arthrotomy under the compression and splintage of the bandage for a matter of four days; and quadriceps exercises in any form, or flexion exercises, are not recommended until this interval has elapsed. On the other hand, dorsi and plantar flexion exercises at the ankle joint are practised assiduously from the start and at least once every waking hour as a prophylactic measure against venous stasis and appear to be effective in so far as deep vein thrombosis is an uncommon complication of meniscectomy.

Haemarthrosis, however, must be accepted to be the occasional complication of arthrotomy, and of meniscectomy in particular. This complication in both aetiology and treatment has been described in IKJ5, and will not be elaborated.

**Suction drainage.** This method at first sight appears to be the solution to the problem of post-operative haemarthrosis. It is employed in the major intra-articular proceedings such as synovectomy; but otherwise, only in the extra-articular procedure of transplantation of tibial tubercle for recurrent subluxation of the patella.

**Meniscectomy.** That the means should exist of preventing the worst of the common post-operative complications has obvious attractions. On the other hand it must be remembered that excision of a meniscus is normally followed by regeneration; and there is evidence that regeneration is important to the prevention of local

osteoarthrosis. Regeneration is dependent on the existence of blood in the wedge-shaped gap which exists between femur and tibia after excision of a meniscus. It is not known to what extent suction drainage influences the presence of blood at this site; and thus the basic material of the replacement fibrous tissue meniscus.

**Anticoagulants.** If meniscectomy is the most common operation performed on the knee joint, and possibly the most common orthopaedic operation, the complication of thrombosis, whether affecting the deep veins of the calf or of a coronary artery, are relatively uncommon. If, however, for one reason or another, anticoagulants are required in the immediate post-operative period the danger of haemarthrosis is considerable.

On one occasion, to which reference is made in IKJ5, but repeated here, pentothal was injected in error into the brachial artery in the course of meniscectomy (J.F., aged 36, professional footballer, meniscectomy number M2566). The arm in question recovered completely. There occurred, however, as a result of the anticoagulant therapy, a haemarthrosis on the second day following operation. It was aspirated and compressed and did not recur in noticeable degree. Convalescence was protracted in spite of the patient's knowledge of quadriceps exercises and what was required of him. The knee never became completely normal although it did reach a stage of recovery which permitted him to return to professional football for a short time. He has been lost to follow-up.

The complication of pulmonary embolus has been a rare complication of meniscectomy in the author's experience. There is no record of the number in 10 000 operations; but it cannot have been large. On two occasions in recent personal experience anticoagulants were given and some haemorrhage into the joint occurred and required aspiration. Recovery, as is usual in haemarthrosis complicating meniscectomy, was delayed; but not to a material degree.

**Sequelae of post-operative haemarthrosis.** The reaction in terms of recovery to post-operative haemarthrosis following meniscectomy varies within wide limits. In a recent example a case, which required aspiration on two occasions, examined five weeks later showed no synovial thickening and admitted to having taken part in athletic activities against advice. On the other hand the impression conveyed by the majority of cases has been unfavourable: recovery has been delayed and examination revealed synovial thickening even at a late date. There remains the strong impression, in this complication of arthrotomy, that recovery is influenced in major degree by aspiration; and that those cases in which aspiration has not been undertaken are the ones in which delay in recovery has been most retarded and with the possibility of future degenerative changes.

## Treatment

**Aspiration.** It is generally recognised, and on a number of counts, that the presence of blood within the synovial cavity, for whatever reason, is undesirable. It should be removed by aspiration using a wide-bore needle as soon as reasonable in the circumstances prevailing. (For technique see Chapter 3.)

## SPONTANEOUS HAEMARTHROSIS

Spontaneous haemarthrosis is defined as the occurrence of bleeding into the joint not initiated by an incident of trauma noticeable to the patient. It is unusual; but it does occur. It is characterised by swelling which takes place rapidly and reaches the stage of distension which creates a tension situation with resultant pain which may be of considerable degree. Causes encountered within the author's experience, not necessarily in order of frequency, include: (1) scurvy; (2) haemangioma; (3) villonodular synovitis; (4) malignant tumour; (5) idiopathic.

### Scurvy: Vitamin C Deficiency

**Background note.** This disease, of great historical interest, is now unusual in adults except under conditions of mass starvation and deprivation, occasionally in alcoholics, extreme diet faddists and in the uncared-for aged often living alone on a diet deficient in vitamin C. In the current scene the manifestations in the knee in the form of haemarthrosis are of such uncommon occurrence as to be liable to misdiagnosis.

**Clinical features.** It is not proposed to recite the textbook features of scurvy. In recent years two cases only of haemarthrosis the result of vitamin C deficiency have been encountered:

The first, an elderly woman of considerable wealth who lived alone, was admitted to a private hospital by her general practitioner and the author summoned on account of the tense swelling of one knee. The diagnosis presented no difficulty (she refused to have the joint aspirated) in the obvious presence of multiple petechial haemorrhages and thereafter the history of a totally inadequate diet.

The second, a middle-aged man also living alone, presented at a consultative clinic as a bilateral effusion. The fact that the effusion was blood was not appreciated at the initial examination. He was admitted to hospital for investigation. The finding, on aspiration, that both joints contained blood was the first suggestion of the possible cause and then only were other stigmata noted.

Both cases responded dramatically to the administration of vitamin C.

### Idiopathic

Occasionally recurrent haemorrhage takes place into the joint without the source being discovered. A case is recalled which had successive haemorrhages into the joint over a matter of six weeks. A point in treatment had been reached where exploration was under consideration when the bleedings ceased and did not recur. Khermosh (1963) reported two young adults who had recurrent haemarthrosis after injury. No cause was found. Eventually synovectomy was performed without the actual source of the bleeding being discovered. The synovium presented an inflammatory non-specific reaction with deposition of haemosiderin. The presence of villi and giant cells pointed to the possible diagnosis of pigmented villonodular synovitis.

Two further examples are quoted:

In the first, the patient, a schoolmaster, presented with a haemarthrosis following a trivial injury. The blood was aspirated, a compression bandage applied and quadriceps exercises instituted. He returned to work after a week. One week later he presented with a further haemarthrosis. Again aspiration, compression and exercises were prescribed. One further haemorrhage occurred before complete immobilisation in a plaster cast was undertaken and maintained for six weeks. No further haemorrhage occurred.

It is probable that the explanation of such a case, in the absence of blood diseases and scurvy which, of course, were eliminated by investigation, lies in the presence of superficial vessels in the synovial membrane readily divided by minimal trauma. The recurrences took place because the area affected was not placed at rest and granulation tissue not permitted to become fibrous tissue, in other words, to heal. It is evident therefore that in the absence of cause sufficient time should elapse for healing to occur before instituting exercise and particularly weight-bearing exercises.

In the second, also a male, a tense haemarthrosis developed while sitting at a table playing cards. There was no history of any previous trouble with the joint. A radiograph taken in the course of routine investigation revealed the presence of multiple loose bodies in the posterior compartment. The explanation in this case was trauma to the synovial membrane by the loose bodies which were subjected to pressure when the knees were crossed as in sitting.

## HAEMOPHILIA A AND B

**Background Note**

König (1892) showed that the recurrent haemarthroses which occur in haemophilia result in progressive destruction of the joint involved.

**Definition.** Haemophilia A is a hereditary bleeding state due to deficiency or total lack of an essential bloodclotting factor called anti-haemophilic globulin (AHG) or factor VIII. The condition is inherited as a sex-linked recessive character and thus mainly affects males. A second disease haemophilia B (Christmas disease), due to deficiency of another essential bloodclotting factor (factor IX) is inherited in the same way as haemophilia A and has the same clinical features. The incidence is about 10 per cent of haemophilia A. It is distinguishable only by laboratory tests.

The clinical features characteristic of these diseases are due to the haemorrhagic consequences. Severely affected patients suffer apparently spontaneous bleeding into muscles and joints which recurs progressively throughout childhood and without specific treatment leads to disablement by the time adolescence is reached. Before 1940 the outlook for the haemophilic patient was poor and the average expectation of life was 16 years; it was thus essentially a disease of childhood (Biggs, 1969).

**Joint incidence.** It is said that one half of all haemophilics bleed into joints and that half of the episodes of haemorrhage into joints affect the knee. The knee is thus the most important single major joint involved in this rare disease, the articular manifestations of which are, in general, polyarticular. It is most often the joint which draws attention to the existence of the condition; the most common joint involved in a polyarticular situation; and the one which provides the major problem of arthrosis in those patients who survive the first years of life.

RIGHT OR LEFT. In young haemophilics there is a tendency to recurrent involvement of one particular joint rather than serial involvement of different joints. In one series (Stuart, Davies and Cumming, 1966) four out of five haemophilics with recurrent haemarthrosis in the knees showed a predilection for activity in the right knee rather than the left. The right knee was involved more often in from 64 per cent to 100 per cent of occasions. This tendency for preference of the left or right side was not noted in other joints.

**Haemarthrosis**

In the haemarthrosis of haemophilia blood remains fluid within the joint and, following lysis of the red cells and degradation of the haemoglobin, is phagocyted by the synovial cells. Much of the iron-containing pigment remains in the surface layer indefinitely; and repeated haemorrhages result in progressively increasing haemosiderosis. The iron content has been found to be as high as 70 per cent of the ash weight of synovial tissue (Rodnan et al.,

1957). The capacity of the articular tissues to remove red cells and the products of their breakdown is said to be little impaired by antecedent haemorrhages (Rodnan, 1962).

## Arthropathy

The aetiology of the arthropathy associated with the repeated haemarthroses of haemophilia is incompletely understood. It is probably, as in so much orthopaedic pathology, multifactorial. The principal damage appears to occur during growth when the immature articular cartilage receives a blood supply from the underlying bone. It is not unlikely that subchondral haemorrhages produce gross degeneration in the form of localised defects and replacement fibrosis in overlying cartilage.

The direct effect of repeated haemorrhage on the synovial membrane is to produce a gross appearance not dissimilar from pigmented villonodular synovitis; and further destruction of articular cartilage may be so related. There are, too, the possible effects of intra-articular pressure, long periods of immobilisation and the vicious circle of degeneration associated with ambulation in incomplete extension.

In relation to the practical aspects of aetiology it is said that initially painless haemarthroses are the principal threat to joint deformity (France and Wolf, 1965) and thus, eventually to the haemophilic arthropathy. In haemophilia, intra-articular haemorrhage, in contradistinction to periarticular or muscle haemorrhage, may be painless. Bleeding into periarticular tissues and/or muscle produces immediate pain and muscle spasm so that the patient is forced to rest and possibly to seek advice. Bleeding into the joint imposes no such restraint. Thus, unless specifically instructed, he continues to move and to weight-bear. In the ensuing weeks the knee, or knees, become swollen, painful and hot, and assume, as would be expected in the circumstances, a position of flexion. There may be a systemic reaction related to a situation whereby continuous or intermittent haemorrhages occur faster than the products can be absorbed. If the haemarthrosis is painful from the onset the opportunity arises of recognition of the cause, and, in the knowledge of the implications, preventative measures in the form of immobilisation in extension, instruction as to how to live with the disease and how to prevent deformity become a practical proposition.

**Radiological features.** In the child the earliest finding is enlargement of the epiphyses by comparison with the normal side and due it is presumed to local hyperaemia. With destruction of articular cartilage comes loss of joint space proceeding to sclerosis of articular margins particularly in the tibia (Fig. 7,3). Subchondral cysts indicate the site of haemorrhages (Fig. 7,1). Subchondral fractures superimposed on the cysts produce the appearance of a gross destructive process (Fig. 7,4).

A radiographic sign frequently recorded and said to be specific to haemophilia is deepening of the intercondylar notch (Fig. 7,3). The rational explanation of this phenomenon is the fixed flexion contracture present so that the antero-posterior projection is to a large extent a tunnel view.

### TREATMENT

The management of haemorrhage into joints, in particular into the knee joint, consists of:
1. Prevention.
2. Treatment of the acute incident.
3. Treatment of the established arthropathy.

## Prevention

The majority of doctors, including orthopaedic surgeons, have little opportunity to gain experience of the treatment of haemophilia. Some do not appreciate the serious implications of haemorrhage into muscles or joints. Haemophilia is a rare disorder and its management highly specialised. In general therefore it is desirable that patients should be treated at hospitals where every facility is available at all times. This, of course, is not always possible. In such circumstances it is most important that the benefits of plasma therapy in haemarthrosis be widely known.

It is not proposed to describe in detail the treatment of haemophilia in the current scene but rather to stress the importance of prevention of haemorrhages into the joint during the vulnerable age range 5 to 20 years, not only in the immediate interest of the patient in terms of suffering and reduction of time lost from school or work, but in the interest of reduction of the irreparable damage which occurs to the most important of the weight-bearing joints.

**Plasma therapy.** One of the many advances in the management of haemophilia in recent years has been the prevention of the deformities associated with repeated haemarthroses particularly in children. This has been achieved principally by the administration of sufficient plasma containing both antihaemophilic globulin (factor VIII, AHG) and Christmas factor (factor IX) within 24–48 hours of the onset of pain and swelling. The development of concentrates of AHG (factor VIII), especially in the form of cryoprecipitate which can be held in store ready for use has simplified the treatment of the 85 per cent of clinical haemophilic patients who are deficient in factor VIII. The influence of treatment on deformity and therefore upon prognosis is seen in the results of an investigation in south-east England (Ali *et al.*, 1967) in which it was demonstrated that boys between the age of five and leaving school whose haemarthroses were untreated with the appropriate factor developed deformities in 1 in every 7 joints affected; whereas those who received timely treatment developed deformities only in 1 in 39 of the joints affected.

In the past the problem of prophylaxis has been the necessity for frequent intravenous drips; and since the veins are the lifeline of the haemophilic patient such treatment was not without inherent risks and was impracticable. Advances in haematology have reached a stage where concentrates of the antihaemophilic factor have reduced the volume of fluid to be given intravenously and the use of the cryoprecipitate preparations brought the volume down to one that can be given by syringe. This has permitted prophylaxis to reach a stage of development where cryoprecipitate, stored in the domestic deep-freeze, is administered in the home by the mother, trained in the technique of intravenous therapy, to the child at the onset of an incident of haemorrhage (Rabiner and Telfer, 1970).

## Treatment of the Acute Incident

**A. Immediate plasma therapy.** One infusion aim-

ing at *in vivo* level of the missing factor to 15–20 per cent of normal is generally adequate. To cover aspiration of the joint, or a deep muscle haematoma, several daily infusions aiming at 40 per cent of normal will probably be required (Dormandy, 1977).

**B. Aspiration.** The evacuation of blood from the joint is at all times desirable; and there must be few exceptions. If controversy existed in the past as to the advisability of aspiration in haemophilia there is no doubt in the current scene that aspiration under cover of plasma therapy is advantageous not only in reduction of the immediate tension situation, which may be such as to endanger the circulation, but also of reducing the long-term liability to arthroplasty.

Aspiration produces immediate relief of pain and early recovery of function and is not to be compared with the previous treatment of allowing slow resolution to occur in the immobilised joint, a process which often extended over many weeks. It does not lead to complications provided it is undertaken under plasma cover. After aspiration the patient is kept at rest in the compression bandage for 24 hours. If there is no recurrence of pain or swelling, and if movement has returned to its previous range, the plasma infusion is stopped and return to weight-bearing permitted. If such progression does not lead to return of pain and swelling he is discharged wearing his compression bandage.

**C. Application of cold.** In bleeding such as occurs in haemophilia, heat is contraindicated, whereas the application of cold is beneficial. While the physiological mechanism of vascular constriction may be obscure, it is known that cold brings about vascular constriction, probably reflexly (Quick, 1970).

**D. Compression/immobilisation.** If aspiration is desirable so is compression not only in the hope of reducing liability to further haemorrhage but in the interests of reduction of pain by immobilisation. If aspiration is undertaken a compression bandage should be applied (Ch. 3). In other circumstances a padded plaster cast supported in a half-ring Thomas bed-knee splint is indicated.

## Intra-articular Fractures

The component bones of the knee joint are the

common site of fractures from relatively minor trauma as a result of limitation of movement, associated osteoporosis and loss of protection from muscle wasting.

**Treatment.** Three principles are involved in the haemostatic management of injury in haemophilia: production of initial haemostasis, maintenance of haemostasis and immobilisation (Kemp and Matthews, 1968). The importance of absolute rest is stressed. Movement incurs the risk of further bleeding at the fracture site or into the adjacent soft tissues. Uncontrolled bleeding at the latter site involves the risk of compression of nerves and vessels. It is for this reason that circumferential unpadded plaster casts are undesirable until haemostasis is complete and swelling is in the course of resolution.

Healing of fractures is characterised by absence of periostal reaction but is not delayed.

## TREATMENT OF ESTABLISHED ARTHROPATHY

**The treatment** requirements of established haemophilic arthropathy are not dissimilar from those of rheumatoid arthritis except in so far as they affect a different sex in a different age range.

In early youth it is a matter of prevention of deformity, in general, on lines indicated above, locally, by instruction in the means whereby extension can be maintained by (a) passive stretching, (b) quadriceps exercises, and (c) the use of plaster night shells.

In the gross flexion deformities in youth the principles of treatment are not dissimilar in application from similar deformities in the more common conditions of poliomyelitis or rheumatoid arthritis (Ch. 6). The method of undoing flexion deformity devised by the author and illustrated in Figure 6,31 and renamed 'reversed dynamic slings' is particularly useful (Stein and Dickson, 1975). The other methods applicable will not be repeated except to emphasise that consideration must be given to the exceptional underlying pathology; and that the utmost care is exercised in the application of forces which in other circumstances are readily tolerated.

In adult life the local practical problem is that of a defect of function manifest in loss of extension and limited flexion (Figs 7,1 to 7,4).

The resultant disability, in a patient conditioned to disability, may not be such as in other circumstances would demand operative action of one kind or another but in the physical circumstances manifest, probably arthrodesis.

## Synovectomy

**Biochemical basis of operation.** The frequency of haemarthroses in the haemophiliac has been ascribed to the low level of thromboplastic activity in normal synovial membrane and joint capsule (Astrup and Sjølin, 1958). and the additive deficiency in plasma thromboplastin formation within the synovial blood vessels may contribute to delayed haemostasis. Sjølin and Astrup (1958) have also demonstrated the presence of a thromboplastin inhibitor in the synovial membrane of a haemophilic, while the persistence of bleeding in joints which are the site of arthropathy may be related to the presence of fibrinolysin activators in granulation tissue.

If repeated haemarthroses occur it is the common experience that even prompt medical and orthopaedic treatment, even in special centres, slows down but cannot prevent the advance of haemophilic arthropathy towards eventual ankylosis. The clinical and histological similarity between haemophilic arthropathy and pigmented villonodular synovitis has prompted a trial of the effect of synovectomy on the control of bleeding and thus on the future function of the joint (Storti et al., 1968). It is claimed from the outcome of 14 synovectomies that: (1) there was no recurrence of bleeding in the knees subjected to synovectomy; that pain and disability disappeared; and that joint function was regained; (2) that bleeding into sites other than the joint subjected to synovectomy have ceased or become rarer and of shorter duration than in the pre-operative period, suggesting that the removal of the synovial tissue might have benefited the patient as a whole; (3) there were no complications. Two hypotheses are offered: (1) that hyperactivity of the enzymatic fibrinogen-fibrinolysin system leads to a persistence of intra-articular bleeding and occurrence of haemorrhage at other sites; (2) that synovectomy, by removing a considerable amount of synovial tissue, which

FIGS 7,1–2

FIGS 7,3–4

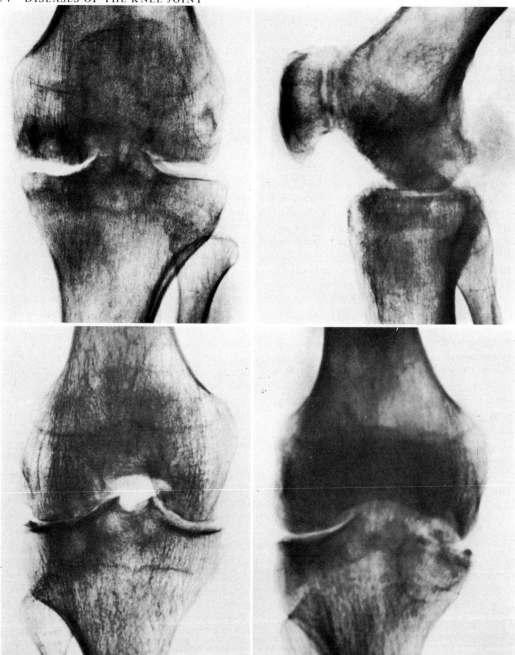

FIGS 7,1–4. **Haemophilic arthropathy.** Figures 7,1 and 7,2 knee joint of G.S., aged 42, to demonstrate destruction of articular cartilage of medial femoral condyle (Fig. 7,1) and particularly in the weight-bearing arc with a bony block to complete extension (Fig. 7,2).

Figure 7,3. In this example the destructive process is less evident. Note equal involvement of medial and lateral compartments with evidence of a healed intra-osseous haemorrhage in the lateral condyle of tibia.

Figure 7,4. In this case an intra-osseous haemorrhage has resulted in destruction of the medial condyle of tibia.

histologically resembles an angioma, eliminates an active source of fibrinolytic tissue activators.

**Indications for operation.** There are circumstances of chronic synovitis similar to rheumatoid arthritis in which the possibility of synovectomy requires to be considered as a means of maintaining function and preventing destruction of the articular surfaces. The hazards of the procedure should be equated against the haematological background of the case, the possibilities for control of bleeding and the potential for improvement of function and prognosis. In general the operation should not be performed below the age of 5 or after the age of 30. (For Technique see Chapter 6.)

## Conservative and Reconstructive Surgery

In centres where haemostatic factors are available in sufficient quantities with the necessarily related technical know-how and laboratory facilities, conservative surgery such as meniscectomy and synovectomy and reconstructive measures such as arthrodesis can be undertaken with indications not dissimilar to those which obtain in other forms of arthritis or osteoarthrosis.

It is necessary to raise the factor VIII or IX to normal levels pre-operatively and to maintain the level above 40 per cent until healing is complete. The pre- and post-infusion levels of the factor in the blood must be checked daily. Since the half disappearance time of factor VIII is usually in the order of 8–12 hours and of factor IX 18 hours, it will be necessary to treat a post-operative case two or three times a day for the first week. A pre-operative check must be made in all cases to ensure that antibodies to factor VIII are not present (Dormandy, 1977).

**Complications.** Haematomata, and sloughing of skin with slow wound healing are complications to be anticipated. When wounds fail to heal by first-intention, slow healing by granulation tissue does not necessarily require continuous cover with a haemostatic agent. The granulation tissue seems to give protection against further serious bleeding (Duthie and Rizza, 1970).

## Haemophilic Arthropathy: Record of a Case

The patient (J.W., a farmer aged 33) when first seen at a hospital at the age of 28, gave a history of intermittent pain in his knee for about 15 years. He stated that in the last 2 to 3 years he had noted that he had loss of full extension. He had been told by various doctors 'that he had cartilage trouble'. Apparently at any time when he visited hospital with incidents in the knee, operative treatment on the so-called torn meniscus had not been carried out as he had been told that his blood-clotting time was abnormally prolonged. He offered the information, however, that when he cut his hands or face he had never noticed any significant abnormality about the time bleeding stopped. On the last occasion he was in hospital following incidents with the knee he had been told that there were loose fragments of cartilage in the joint, but when the question of operative treatment arose it had once again been deferred because of the suspicion of blood dyscrasia.

On investigation in hospital at that time it was found that his only brother had died at the age of four after tonsillectomy. His mother's brothers and his cousins had no abnormality.

Examination showed that in addition to the limited functioning of the knee joint there was restriction of movement in the left shoulder and in the left ankle. When examined there was a large haematoma in the right antecubital fossa, and another in the left leg above the ankle. Thromboplastin generation test was carried out and showed that he had mild haemophilia. No operation was carried out.

He was first seen by the author 5 years later. The purpose of the consultation was to 'seek operation for internal derangement and to remove any loose fragments of articular cartilage or meniscus'.

On examination extension was limited by bony block to 150°. Flexion to a right-angle. There was thus a range of movement of 40° (Fig. 7,7).

His radiographs, Figures 7,5 and 7,6, showed gross changes. When comparison was made between radiographs of five years previously it was evident that rapid deterioration had occurred.

He was advised that subject to consultation with a haematologist operation should be undertaken at an early date. It was pointed out to him that faulty mechanics of walking with his flexed knee was throwing additional strains on his spine, especially in the heavy occupation which he pursued. He would not, however, accept that any harm was occurring; nor that any deterioration had taken place in

the previous five years. He insisted that he was able to work as a farmer, and capable of operating tractors and a combine harvester. He did not wish his knee to be made straight.

In view of the possibility that he would

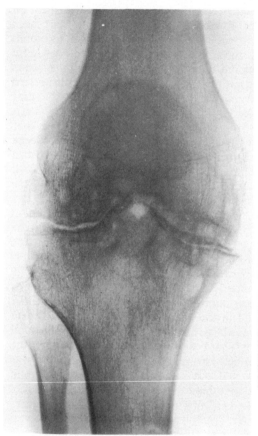

Fig 7,5

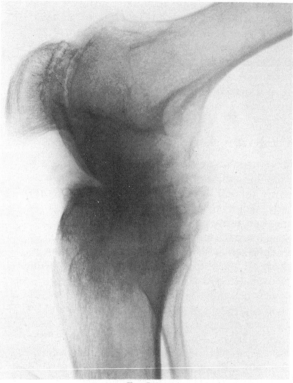

Fig 7,6

Fig 7,7 ▶

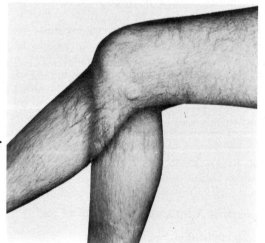

FIGS 7,5–7. **Haemophilic arthropathy.** Left knee demonstrating destruction of the articular cartilage of every compartment (Figs. 7,5 and 7,6). Extension was limited to 145°, flexion to 80° (Fig. 7,7). (J.W., aged 33.)

eventually accept operation the advice of a haematologist was sought. He suggested that if the patient sought arthrodesis an assay of his antihaemophilic globulin (Factor VIII) would be required in order to assess whether his deficiency of that substance was such as likely to be easily corrected by Factor VIII concentrate. It was recommended that if he sought operation reference to a haematology laboratory would be necessary for the purposes outlined.

This patient is known to be of independent character and to have served sentences in jail. He is prepared to accept medical advice only when it suits his preconceived ideas. At the time of writing he has not returned. It is unlikely that he will be seen again until a further incident, mechanical or otherwise, occurs in the joint.

This case is quoted to demonstrate: (1) failure to recognise the nature or importance of the bleeding incidents in youth as is liable to occur in 'mild' haemophilia; (2) the decreasing incidents with age; (3) the establishment of a gross arthrosis with extension limited by a bony block at 150° and with a total range of motion of 40°; and (4) the personality problem common in haemophilics in this case probably related to the appreciation that the condition had been misdiagnosed and mistreated in youth, a situation not conducive to confidence in the medical profession.

## REFERENCES

ALI, A. M., GANDY, R. H., BRITTEN, M. I., DORMANDY, K. M. (1967). *British Medical Journal,* **iii,** 828.

ASTRUP, T. & SJØLIN, K. E. (1958). *Proceedings of the Society for Experimental Biology and Medicine,* **97,** 852.

BIGGS, R. (1969). Haemophilia. *Proceedings of the Royal Society of Medicine,* **62,** 913.

DORMANDY, K. (1977). Haemophilia A and B. *Prescribers' Journal,* **17,** 1, 8.

DUTHIE, R. B. & RIZZA, C. R. (1970). Reconstructive surgery in haemophilia and Christmas disease. *Journal of Bone and Joint Surgery,* **52B,** 4, 772.

FRANCE, W. G. & WOLF, P. (1965). Treatment and prevention of chronic haemorrhagic arthropathy and contractures in haemophilia. *Journal of Bone and Joint Surgery,* **47B,** 247.

KEMP, H. S. & MATTHEWS, J. M. (1968). The management of fractures in haemophilia and Christmas disease. *Journal of Bone and Joint Surgery,* **50B,** 2, 351.

KEY, J. A. (1929). Experimental arthritis. The reaction of joints to mild irritants. *Journal of Bone and Joint Surgery,* **11,** 705.

KHERMOSH, O. (1963). Recurrent haemarthrosis of the knee. *Journal of Bone and Joint Surgery,* **45B,** 806.

KÖNIG, F. (1892). Die Gelenkerkrankungen bei Blutern mit besonderer Berücksichtigung der Diagnose. Sammlung klinischer Vörtage von R. von Volkmann. N. F. Chirurgie, nr. 11, 233.

QUICK, A. J. (1970). Effect of cold on bleeding. *Lancet,* **ii,** 1307.

RABINER, S. F. & TELFER, M. C. (1970). Home transfusion for patients with haemophilia A. *New England Journal of Medicine,* **283,** 1011.

RODNAN, G. P., LEWIS, J., WARREN, J. & BROWEN, T. (1957). Hemophilic arthritis. *Bulletin of Rheumatic Diseass,* **8,** 137.

RODNAN, G. P. (1962). Experimental hemarthrosis: the removal of chromium-51 and iron-59 labelled erythrocytes injected into the knee joint of rabbit and man. *Arthritis and Rheumatism,* **3,** 195.

ROY, S. & GHADIALLY, F. N. (1967). Ultrastructure of synovial membrane in human hemarthrosis. *Journal of Bone and Joint Surgery,* **49-A,** 8, 1636.

SJØLIN, K. E. & ASTRUP, T. (1958). *Danish Medical Bulletin,* **5,** 242.

STEIN, H. & DICKSON, R. A. (1975). Reversed dynamic slings for knee-flexion contractures in the hemophilic. *Journal of Bone and Joint Surgery,* **57A,** 282.

STORTI, E., TRALDI, A:, TOSATTI, E. & DAVOLI, P. G. (1968). Synovectomy for haemophilic haemarthrosis. *Lancet,* **ii,** 572.

STUART, J., DAVIES, S. H. & CUMMING, R. A. (1966). Haemorrhagic episodes in haemophilia. A 5-year prospective study. *British Medical Journal,* **ii,** 1624.

# 8. Angular Deformity: Childhood

## CONGENITAL SUBLUXATION OR DISLOCATION (GENU RECURVATUM CONGENITUM)

The earliest angular deformity of the knee is encountered in the newborn in the form of congenital subluxation or dislocation.

**Background note.** Chatelain, a Swiss physician, is credited with the original description of congenital dislocation of the knee in 1822. Since then a voluminous bibliography has accumulated.

**Incidence.** The condition is rare. In the Newington Children's Hospital, Connecticut, U.S.A., in the 25-year period 1942–67, 16 cases were admitted in comparison with 650 cases of congenital dislocation of the hip (Curtis and Fisher, 1969).

The author's experience is limited to the cases described by D. S. Middleton (1935), with whom he had the privilege to work, and, since then, six examples all associated with the multiple musculo-skeletal deformities of arthrogryposis multiplex congenita (myodystrophia foetalis).

### Aetiology

There are three basic varieties of widely differing origin, degree of deformity and prognosis.

**Mechanical.** This may take the form of malposition *in utero* or a birth injury. The malposition *in utero* postulated is that of the foot locked in the axilla or mandible causing hyperextension of the knee. This position was demonstrated radiologically in one of McFarland's (1929) cases. In regard to birth injury, if this is the description of the pathology, it is said that so-called genu recurvatum is most common following breech delivery.

**Primary embryonic defect.** This type is accompanied by other defects such as spina bifida, cardiac abnormality, hare-lip, etc.; and the knee deformity may be unimportant in the total clinical picture.

**Primary mesenchymal defect.** This is the origin of those cases which are associated with fibrosis of the quadriceps. The muscle changes are said to be similar to those found in arthrogryposus multiplex congenita.

### Pathological Anatomy

Congenital hyperextension of the knee exists in three forms:
1. Simple genu recurvatum (Fig. 8,1);
2. Anterior subluxation (Fig. 8,2); and
3. Anterior dislocation (Fig. 8,3).

It will be evident in such circumstances, and particularly in relationship to the aetiological background, that the pathological anatomy, related to treatment, is important only in frank dislocation. It will be appreciated that wide variation is encountered and that individual experience, in a condition of some rarity, is limited. In these circumstances the pathological anatomy such as may be encountered at operation in complete dislocation is described.

There is (1) anterior displacement of the tibia on the femur; (2) contracture and fibrosis of the quadriceps affecting the lateral elements while the vastus medialis remains unaffected (Curtis and Fisher, 1969). Lateral dislocation of the patella recorded may be so related; or to the existence of valgus deformity; (3) lengthening or absence of the cruciate ligaments. Various theories have been advanced in this regard: such findings are inevitable in complete dislocation; (4) anterior dislocation of the flexor tendons so that they act as extensors (Stern, 1968); (5) absence of vascular or neurological defects.

### Clinical Features

The affected knee is hyperextended with multiple anterior skin creases and a prominent bony swelling in the form of the femoral condyles (Fig. 8,4) with the possible presence of other less obvious deformities such as congenital dislocation of the hip, club foot, etc. which

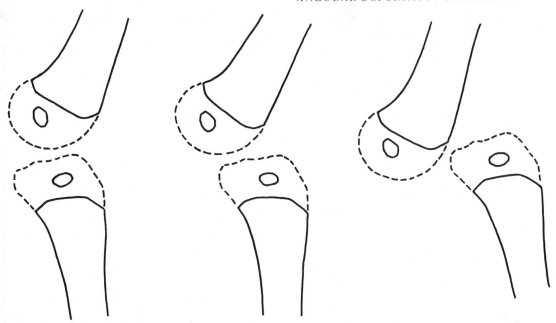

FIGS 8,1–3. **Congenital subluxation/dislocation.** Simple genu recurvatum (Fig. 8,1), anterior subluxation (Fig. 8,2) and anterior dislocation (Fig. 8,3).

might suggest a background of arthrogryposus multiplex congenita. The existence of multiple deformities not only determines treatment but priorities in treatment, the possible necessity for operation and eventual prognosis.

## Treatment

**Conservative.** It is important, as in congenital dislocation of the hip, that treatment is undertaken as soon, in the first few days of life, as practical considerations permit. The aim of treatment is correction of the relationship of tibia to femur; and the ease with which this can be accomplished is related to the degree of displacement. In a simple hyperextension deformity of mechanical origin the tendency for birth injuries to return to normal is active if suitable physical conditions are provided. Gentle traction applied to the quadriceps may permit restoration of the relationship of tibia to femur in extension or slight flexion. In this regard 'gallows' traction, particularly in a portable frame, is useful in that it permits the infant to be nursed at home (Fig. 8,5). The reduction attained is maintained by a plaster cast. Serial casts are then applied

in progressively greater degrees of flexion at, say, two-week intervals until right-angled flexion is achieved. At this stage an ankle strap attached to a pelvic band is used to prevent recurrence (Fig. 8,6). If relapse occurs in deformities which fail to respond to manipulation and plaster and in frank dislocations, operative reduction is indicated.

Recalcitrant cases may be divided into three categories: (1) those in which treatment was protracted, perhaps because the simple con-

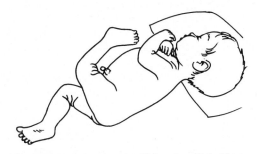

FIG. 8,4. **Congenital subluxation/dislocation: clinical features.** The affected knee is hyperextended with multiple anterior skin creases. There is a prominent bony swelling produced by the femoral condyles in the popliteal space.

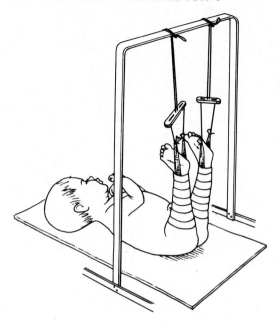

FIG. 8,5. **Congenital subluxation/dislocation: treatment.**
Gallows traction is useful in effecting reduction. It can be incorporated in a portable frame to permit the infant to be nursed at home.

servative measures outlined above were not undertaken sufficiently soon after birth; (2) those in which there is fibrotic replacement of the quadriceps with contracture, possibly a localised form of arthrogryposis multiplex congenita; and (3) those associated with multiple deformities in the generalised form of arthrogryposis multiplex congenita.

In regard to (2): fibrotic replacement of the lateral elements of the quadriceps is associated with adhesion of the patella and quadriceps to the anterior aspect of the femur in the absence of the suprapatellar pouch. It has been pointed out that this situation is easily detected by the simple measure of performing an arthrogram (Laurence, 1967).

**Operative.** The nature and extent of operative measures depends on the circumstances of the case. In general a long incision located towards the lateral side is necessary to gain access to the abnormal quadriceps components. The tendon is lengthened by Z or inverted V-plasty. The capsular incision is then extended laterally on both sides to mobilise and displace backwards the medial and lateral ligaments and the

iliotibial band from their inferior insertions. When this is achieved reduction can usually be affected in flexion. The quadriceps tendon is resutured in the lengthened position with the joint in 30 to 45° of flexion (Figs 2,6 and 2,7).

AFTER-TREATMENT. At the termination of operation a padded plaster cast is applied in the 30 to 45° of flexion. Immobilisation in this position is maintained for six weeks. At the end of this time some freedom is permitted depending on the findings and success of reduction at operation. A night shell in flexion and/or a caliper with a check to extension may be required depending on the age and circumstances of the case. In an older child weight-bearing is deferred for, say, 12 weeks and then only in a caliper preventing hyperextension and incorporating a knock-knee apron. The caliper may require to be worn for several years.

**Prognosis.** In general the prognosis in cases of hyperextension and subluxation of mechanical origin treated immediately after birth by the simple conservative measures described is good. In circumstances of dislocation complicated by other deformities, particularly if operation is unduly deferred, or in arthrogryposis multiplex congenita, it must be guarded and clearly depends on the circumstances of the individual case.

## ARTHROGYPOSIS MULTIPLEX CONGENITA (AMYOPLASIA CONGENITA)

### Treatment

**Flexion.** When angular deformity at the knee is

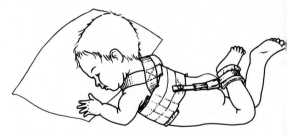

FIG. 8,6. **Congenital subluxation/dislocation: treatment.**
When restoration of the relationship of tibia and femur has been effected an ankle strap attached to a pelvic band is used to prevent recurrence.

TABLE 9

Results of treatment in 28 knees with flexion contracture in
arthrogryposis multiplex congenita.
(Lloyd-Roberts and Lettin)

| Method of treatment | Number of knees | | |
| --- | --- | --- | --- |
| | Lasting improvement | Temporary improvement | No improvement |
| Physiotherapy | 0 | 0 | 0 |
| Manipulation and splinting | 6 | 9 | 0 |
| Posterior release | 9 | 1 | 0 |
| Supracondylar* osteotomy | 4 | 8 | 2 |

*Fourteen osteotomies in twelve knees, two repeated later and six amputated.

one of multiple deformities, flexion contracture is more common than hyperextension in the ratio of 28 to 5 (Lloyd-Roberts and Lettin, 1970). In the course of treatment 15 flexed knees were treated by serial plaster casts, and of these, 6 achieved full and lasting correction. The remaining 9 were improved but subsequently deteriorated and necessitated operation.

SUPRACONDYLAR OSTEOTOMY. This procedure failed if persistent deformity compromised walking or splinting in the young child. They record two disasters from popliteal occlusion necessitating urgent amputation, and two in which stiffness and deformity were such that the problem was solved only by through-knee amputation. In two cases the osteotomy, repeated at the age of 15 years, was followed by lasting improvement. It appears that deformity recurs rapidly after supracondylar osteotomy and, when the operation is repeated, further posterior subluxation of the tibia occurs so that eventually it articulates with the posterior aspect of the femoral condyle.

POSTERIOR CAPSULOTOMY. The most successful operation in correcting deformity without loss of stability, but not in restoring motion, was posterior capsulotomy including division of deforming muscular, tendinous and fascial contractures. The operation is difficult in a young child with marked flexion, distortion of the normal anatomy and much subcutaneous fat. Two incisions medial and lateral are recommended. The plane of capsule is established on both sides avoiding the tendency to search at too proximal a level. A blunt instrument is passed in contact with the capsule

from the medial to the lateral side and the neurovascular bundle isolated and lifted away by a sling of gauze. The posterior capsule can now be divided under direct vision followed by division of tight hamstring tendons and superficial fascia. The structures which now limit extension are nerves and blood vessels. In such circumstances it is prudent to apply a plaster cast with the knee in some flexion, achieving extension gradually in two or three serial plaster casts.

Operation and after-treatment in the manner described achieved correction in 9 cases out of 10; and these have not relapsed (Lloyd-Roberts and Lettin, 1970).

Hyperextension. It is pointed out that hyperextension does not necessarily delay walking. If the knee can be flexed to the neutral position or more, walking calipers can be fitted.

## AFFECTIONS OF THE GROWTH PLATES

The hazards to the epiphyses in chronological order of occurrence and potential for future angular deformity are as follows:

1. **Birth injury.** The earliest affection of the normal knee takes the form of separation of the lower femoral epiphysis sustained in the course of a breech delivery. If displacement is considerable and the related massive callus alarming, in contrast to total separation at later ages, accurate reduction is unnecessary. In the infant there is a strong and persistent trend to restoration of the normal anatomy. The potential for future disability is minimal.

**2. Osteomyelitis and infective arthritis of infancy.** After birth the most serious immediate risk to the epiphyses is infection in the form of osteomyelitis and infective arthritis. The potential for disability in the form of angular deformity is considerable.

**3. Physiological genu varum/tibia vara.** At the walking stage and immediately thereafter the hazards are concerned with the biomechanics of weight-bearing; in the extreme, tibia vara. In addition there is the potential for deformity inherent in avitaminosis and conditions of systemic origin listed in Table 10.

**4. Trauma.** It is probable that the most serious hazard incurred from, say, age 10 to maturity, is trauma in one of two forms (1) single-incident, or (2) microtrauma, in the form of abnormal mechanics, weight-bearing or otherwise.

This work is not primarily concerned with single-incident trauma, but it is, as it must be, concerned with the long-term effects of trauma. The injuries to the epiphyses constitute such a situation.

## MICROTRAUMA: BIOMECHANICS OF ANGULAR DEFORMITY

That the mature knee should be of 'normal' conformation and the limb of normal length depends on the 'physiological' use of the joint; and that no abnormal pressures are applied to the growth plates for any prolonged interval of time especially during a period of rapid growth.

The effect of pressure is to retard growth on the aspect under compression, with relaxation, and possible acceleration of growth, on the opposite side. This has the effect of producing the angular deformity of genu recurvatum, genu valgum or genu varum or a combination of the former with one or other of the latter; and, as has been indicated, the more rapid the period of growth the greater the resultant discrepancy in length and deformity.

The most common example is almost within the 'physiological' category: the effect of the compression forces involved in the mechanics of walking as seen in the wearing of high heels in women. If such heels are worn prior to epiphyseal maturity increased pressure is applied to the anterior aspect of the upper tibial epiphyseal

plate with the result that growth slows down anteriorly, and is possibly accelerated posteriorly producing the slight genu recurvatum which is almost the normal conformation where the use of such footwear exists; indeed there is some evidence that unless high heels are worn at an early age difficulty may be encountered in their use at a later stage.

In the pathological category is the well-known effect of prolonged recumbancy in the supine position in childhood, whether in plaster cast or otherwise, necessitated by such affections as tuberculosis of the hip and resulting in genu recurvatum (Figs 9,1 and 9,2); and the effect of walking thereafter with an adducted hip and the resulting genu valgum. But any condition of the hip or even of the foot which produces abnormal stresses at the knee can have such an effect, for example, slipped upper femoral epiphysis, malunited fracture or even, as has been recorded, the erroneous amputation of the great toe in infancy.

## PHYSIOLOGICAL GENU VARUM AND VALGUM

**Introduction**

Angular deformity in the form of genu varum or valgum is the commonest deformity of childhood with which the clinician is confronted.

The developing child is the centre of parental adoration but of critical evaluation by well-meaning relatives and friends. One of the situations in which he is watched and appraised is when he begins to stand and walk. Abnormalities, imaginary or otherwise, observed in the overall appearance of the child arouse comment and become a source of worry to the parents. Outward bowing of the lower extremities is a cause of particular concern (Holt, Latourette and Watson, 1954).

In the early years of the century almost all cases of bow legs and knock knees were thought to be due to rickets; and there was good reason for the assumption. It is evident now that the diagnosis in a high proportion of cases was incorrect. But, strange as it may appear, the problem still remains and is encountered with perplexing frequency.

**Shape of legs in infancy.** In discussing the aetiology of tibia vara Golding, Bateson and McNeil-Smith (1969) point out that all infants are born with legs which show radiographic varus and this converts at a later date to radiographic valgus. In a survey conducted in Bristol, England (Bateson, 1966) the change from varus to valgus took place at one to one and a half years, about the time an English child is walking. In contrast, in Jamaica the change from varus to valgus takes place one year later. The average Jamaican child walks at less than one year and thus has been weight-bearing with varus deformity for one and a half to two years. The period of time in which there is an increased load on the medial side of the knee is considered to be a factor in the frequency of tibia vara in Jamaica. Such are the mechanical problems of weight-bearing at this stage of development and the factors of race and environment involved in the production of deformity, temporary or permanent.

If in recent years there has been an increase in interest in the extrinsic factors maintaining or exaggerating varus deformity (Fig. 8,7) and of habitual postures contributing to the associated medial torsion of the tibia (Figs 8,16 to 8,18) there remains considerable lack of factual information on the biomechanical problems concerned in the phenomenon of conversion of physiological genu varum to physiological genu valgum. One explanation offered is that children, when they learn to walk, tend to hold their feet wide apart in order to maximise stability. This action increases the compression forces acting on the lateral side of the growth plate with consequent relaxation of compression forces on the medial side. The result is faster growth on the medial side (Salenius and Vankka, 1975).

**Natural history.** Morley (1957) examined 1000 schoolchildren of different ages in regard to the incidence of genu valgum. In the age range 3 to 3½ years 22 per cent had a deformity of 5 cm or more. At 7 years 2 per cent only had a comparable deformity. She concluded that treatment is unnecessary. This course of events is well known to orthopaedic surgeons of experience and is the basis for the statement: 'The condition, if treated, recovers in two years; if untreated, in 24 months.'

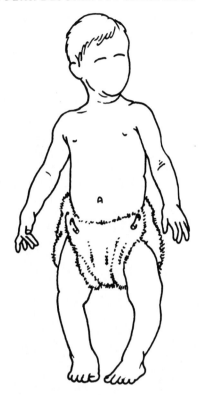

FIG. 8,7. **Genu varum.** If a massive towelling diaper is not the cause of physiological genu varum it is a factor in maintaining and aggravating the deformity when the infant walks.

## Clinical Features

The condition, whether of physiological genu varum (Figs 8,8 and 8,9) or valgum, occurs in children otherwise healthy. Genu valgum is said to be encountered in two distinct types: the overweight but otherwise healthy, vigorous child who has been encouraged to walk too soon; and the thin, undernourished child with poor muscle tone.

**Method of assessment.** The natural history of the condition requires that a standard of improvement or deterioration is established. The interval between the medial malleoli is the obvious yardstick. This is measured with the child standing, the knees straight and in contact. The hand, placed between the malleoli (Fig. 8,10) is an immediately available ruler of some 8 cm. It is a mistake to carry out the measurement in the supine position as is generally recommended.

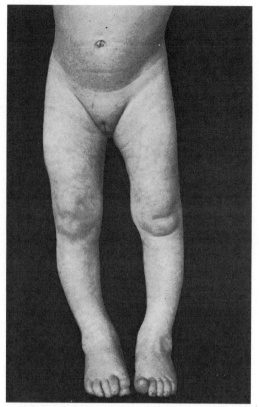

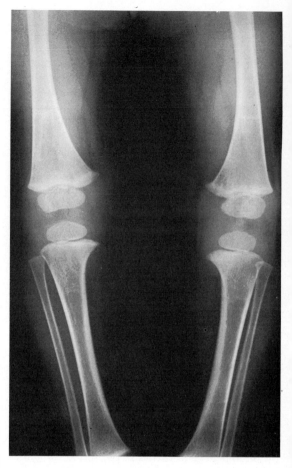

FIGS 8,8–9. **Physiological genu varum.** The gross appearance differs little from the angular deformity of systemic origin (Fig. 8,8) (see Figs 8,29 and 8,34). Typical radiographs show (1) lateral bowing of tibial and femoral shafts; (2) beaking at medial aspects of both femoral and tibial metaphyses; (3) thickening of medial cortex of tibia; and (4) slight tapering of femoral and tibial ossification centres towards the medial side (Fig. 8,9).

This is not the position in which the deformity presents to the mother and her relatives; but in any event is a position resented by the child. The method of assessment, a hand's breadth, is simple, readily applied and appreciated by the mother to whom it is demonstrated. She is informed that deterioration over and above her hand's breadth of, say, 8 cm is possible; but if the interval reaches 10 cm re-examination is essential. The arbitrary interval of 10 cm has been selected as unacceptable socially to all concerned with the child, and, more important, possibly harmful to the development of the joint.

At re-examination an underlying pathological, as opposed to physiological, cause for knock knees should be sought if (1) the distance between the malleolus is excessive, i.e. say 10 cm or more; (2) the deformity is of unequal degree in the two knees; (3) the child is of small stature, and (4) there is family history of bony deformities.

**Radiological examination.** Routine radiographs, in the circumstances of this common diagnosis, are unnecessary. This ancillary examination is undertaken only where doubt exists.

The normal varoid-to-valgoid growth pattern has characteristic appearances. At the genu varum phase there is: (1) lateral bowing of the tibial and femoral shafts; (2) beaking at the medial aspects of both femoral and tibial metaphyses; (3) thickening of the medial cortex of the tibia; (4) femoral and tibial ossification centres taper medially (Fig. 8,9).

At the valgoid phase the patients are older: (1) epiphyseal centres are naturally larger; (2) beaking of the metaphyses on the medial side has been eliminated. It may exist in minimal degree on the lateral side; (3) thickening of the medial cortex may have disappeared. It may exist but in lesser degree on the lateral side; (4) medial tapering of the ossification centres has been eliminated. It may exist in minimal degree towards the lateral side.

It should perhaps be pointed out, as on a previous occasion, that the ossification centre is the only visible portion of the epiphysis. That which is invisible is articular cartilage. The varying shape of the ossification centres is the response to growth phases; not a factor in production (Shopfner and Coin, 1969).

The early stages of tibia vara are difficult to differentiate from physiological genu varum. It is of some importance that in tibia vara changes in the metaphyses affect the tibia only. It is unusual to see abnormalities in the femur (Fig. 8,28).

## Treatment

The attitude to be adopted to the parents of a child considered to be suffering from physiological genu varum or valgum is initially one of explanation and reassurance coupled with advice as may be indicated regarding diet, rest and activity. In the case of the recently walking child with varus the change to valgus is anticipated. In the older child with valgus the method of measuring progress or otherwise is explained and, if the reassurance is accepted, not to return if improvement occurs. If, however, the interval reaches 10 cm to return immediately for re-examination. If reassurance alone is not accepted and active treatment sought, even demanded, it becomes not so much a matter of treating the child as of treating the parents. Nevertheless it is not unprofessional to treat such a case even in the knowledge that it is unnecessary. The young mother may be under pressure from her mother or mother-in-law. Reassurance in such circumstances may not be enough and may lead to the child being taken to

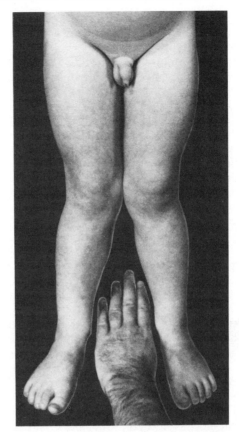

FIG. 8,10. **Physiological genu valgum.** The distance between the medial malleoli is accepted as a measure of the deformity and the hand's breadth a convenient yardstick which can be demonstrated to the parents as indicative of improvement or otherwise. If the interval reaches 10 cm re-examination is indicated.

some unorthodox practitioner with the risks of possible injury but inevitable credit for the natural cure. At worst, the child may be saved from an unnecessary and undesirable operation at the hands of the ignorant or the unethical. In any event the theories propounded regarding the aetiology of tibia vara cast doubt on the wisdom of permitting unlimited weight-bearing over a long period in the presence of an angular deformity. Continuous pressure on one aspect of epiphyseal plates with reduction of pressure on the other may well lead to some permanence of deformity, including rotation, if not necessarily to a condition of such a progressive nature as tibia vara. The use of a mermaid splint (see below), for example, at least ensures that pressure is relaxed on the concave aspect of the angle for a proportion of the 24 hours.

It is important, in a condition which is self-limiting, that treatment prescribed for social reasons, or as a placebo, should not be harmful. It is important also that the mother should be involved and responsible for the treatment of her child.

A wide variety of measures are available of which the following is a selection in current use: **Modification of shoes.** Perhaps the simplest treatment applicable to physiological genu valgum is the application of wedges to the heels or to the soles and heels of lacing shoes. The effect of this popular measure in reducing the deformity is difficult to estimate in a situation which is largely self-limiting. There are those who maintain that the principal function of corrective wedges is to ensure the periodic return of patients for re-examination.

**Manipulation.** In theory, forceful manipulations could damage the epiphyseal plates of femur, or tibia. It is unlikely, in manipulations carried out by the mother, that force would be used of a degree likely to hurt her child; and it is unlikely that force of lesser degree could be harmful.

The mother is shown how, by placing a hand on the inner aspect of the lower end of the femur, to produce a fixed point. Pressure can then be exerted on the upper aspect of the tibia on the outer side to stretch the soft tissues and correct the valgus deformity.

**Mermaid splint.** This night splint, which exists in many forms, has the advantage that it can be applied to varus deformity at, say, two years and to valgus deformity, but in a larger size at, say, four years. The object of the splint is immediately evident. It has the additional merit of involving the mother in the treatment of her child; and at the cost of considerable trouble.

It consists of two light dural gutter splints riveted back-to-back, padded and provided with straps (Fig. 8,11). A splint of suitable size is selected, fitted to the legs, the straps tightened and finally an overall circumferential bandage applied to give the 'mermaid' effect from which the appliance derives its name (Fig. 8,12).

**Adaptation of playthings.** Modification to playthings in common use can at least produce the illusion of remedial therapy in the treatment of

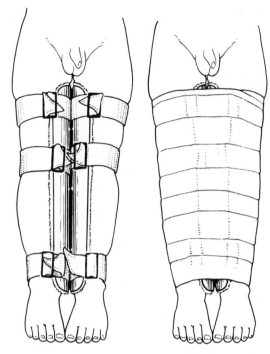

FIGS 8,11–12. **Genu varum/valgus: treatment.** The mermaid splint is applied and straps tightened (Fig. 8,11). It is the overall bandage which gives the splint its name (Fig. 8,12).

genu valgum. If, for example, wooden wedges, base inwards, are bolted to the pedals of a tricycle and the saddle suitably adjusted for height, the effect in use is somewhat similar to wedging of the shoes. A horse on wheels on which the child sits and propels with his feet on the floor can be broadened in the back and adjusted for height so that pressure is exerted on the inner aspect of the knees as the toes reach the ground.

### Operation

It is most important that physiological genu varum, in particular, be recognised for what it is—'physiological'; and that it will correct naturally or convert to valgus. It must be differentiated, and this may be difficult, from tibia vara in particular, and other causes of angular deformity of systemic origin. In no circumstances should operation to correct physiological varus be undertaken no matter

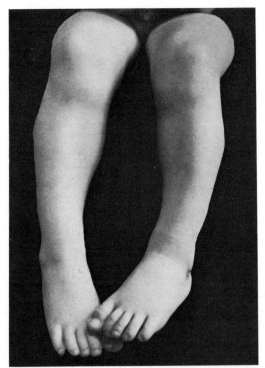

FIG. 8,13. **Medial torsion of tibia.** To determine the site of the torsion the child is seated on the examination couch with the legs dangling towards the floor. In medial torsion located to the tibia the feet look inwards.

Is this the precursor of Figure 8,23?

what the pressures from the parents. The operation will result in a severe valgus deformity. It is a very real trap for the unwary (Golding, Bateson and McNeil-Smith, 1969).

## TORSION

This term is applied to abnormality of the axial relationship of the foot to the thigh. The change may be due to torsion within the femur, rotation at the knee joint or torsion within the tibia or a combination of one and another or all three. It is difficult to isolate the factors concerned, clinically or radiologically.

The methods of measurement applicable to the tibia are clinical, tropometric, which combines the use of a caliper applied to the malleoli with a protractor, and radiological. Experience has shown, however, that while

inspection standing, lying and finally in the sitting position, which isolates the tibia, has the merit of simplicity it is an unreliable means of assessment. A simple mechanical method of measurement is essential for the compilation of records.

**Measurement.** To measure tibial torsion, apparatus has been devised (Wynne-Davies, 1964) whereby a pointer locates the tibial tubercle and a caliper with attached protractor locates the malleoli. In the adult and in the pursuit of the biomechanical basis of bilateral pan-articular osteoarthrosis it has been shown that so-called medial torsion of the tibia is not so much medial torsion as reduction of lateral torsion. Normal lateral torsion in the adult is within the range 15° to 25°. It is probable that torsion outwith this range is abnormal (Figs 8,14 and 8,15).

## MEDIAL TORSION

Children with persistent varus, as opposed to those who in the normal course of events convert to valgus, frequently exhibit an extreme degree of medial tibial torsion which tends to persist after the general alignment of the extremity has been restored to normal. This torsion is more important in terms of appearance, gait and the aetiology of osteoarthrosis in later life than the original varus deformity.

**Clinical assessment.** To locate or confirm medial torsion in the tibia, as opposed to elsewhere in the leg, the child sits on the edge of the examination couch with the feet dangling. In the normal leg the forefoot points straight forward. If there is medial torsion in the tibia the feet will point towards one another (Fig. 8,13).

### Treatment

**Prevention.** There is experimental evidence to show that if continuous torsional load is applied to the growing tibia the primary effect is at the epiphyseal plate (Moreland, 1975). It is said that prevention of medial torsion of the tibia should begin when the newborn infant leaves the hospital. In practice, the opportunity seldom arises until a deformity is noticed. If the opportunity offers advice is proffered on the lines that habitual adoption of a single posture whether at

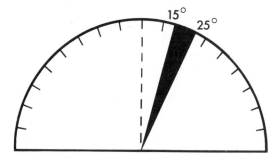

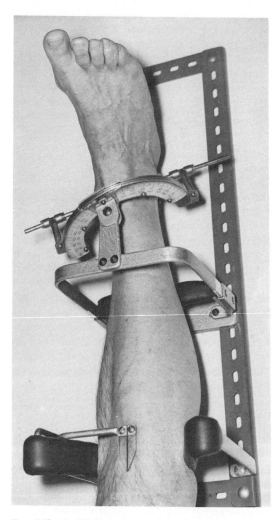

FIGS 8,14–15. **Tibial torsion: method of measurement.** The normal range in the adult is 15° to 25° of lateral torsion (Fig. 8,14). To measure it a pointer locates the tibial tubercle and a caliper with attached protractor locates the malleoli (Fig. 8,15).

sleep or at play is undesirable. If the safest position for the baby is on his stomach he should not be permitted to sleep continuously in the prone-kneeling or extended position (Figs 8,16 and 8,17) but at times in the frog or in the side-sleeping position. If a change from one position to another is encouraged the development of a fixed rotational deformity will not occur. At a later stage habitual sitting postures should be observed. Sitting on the feet (Fig. 8,18) should alternate with sitting in the tailor position (Fig. 8,19): with sitting on the floor with the legs extended; and with sitting on the conventional chair if a postural habit resulting in a rotation deformity is to be prevented.

**Early established deformity.** If habitual sleeping or sitting positions maintained by infants are not necessarily the primary factor there can be little doubt that they contribute to the continuation and aggravation of the deformity. It is usual to find that children with excessive medial rotation are either face or knee-chest sleepers who do so with the feet inverted. Those with knock knee and lateral rotation will be found to be back or face sleepers who do so with their feet in the everted position. Waking habits follow sleeping habits. Knee-chest sleepers tend to sit on their feet (Fig. 8,18); and if this posture has been adopted over any considerable period of time bony prominences and evidence of friction on the skin may be present over the head of the talus and antero-lateral aspect of the calcaneous. The child who sleeps with her feet in lateral rotation tends to sit between her knees (Fig. 8,20). The child who can sit between her knees has certainly been doing so previously.

While it is customary to refer to these postural habits as being responsible for torsional deformities of the tibia, it is inconceivable that the tibia only is influenced. Face sleepers, for example, must exert some torsional force on the femur, although, with the intervening joint, the effect will be less than on the tibia.

If evidence of a habitual deforming posture is present attempts must be made to break the habit by frequent changes of sleeping position and, if possible, by side sleeping. It must be admitted, however, that if fixed sleeping or sitting postures have been established they are difficult to change.

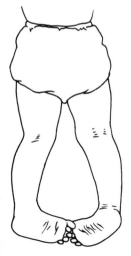 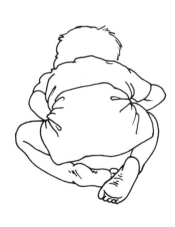 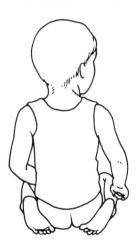

FIGS 8,16–18. **Medial torsion. Faulty sleeping and sitting postures habitually employed are factors in maintaining and increasing medial torsion.** Stomach sleeping in extension (Fig. 8,16); prone-kneeling (Fig. 8,17); and sitting on the feet with the toes turned in (Fig. 8,18).

**Night splints.** The most useful device in countering rotational deformity is a modified Denis Browne splint. Unfortunately the rigid bar of the splint is not readily tolerated after the age of three. In genu varum a long cross bar is used (Fig. 8,21) and the feet gradually rotated laterally to an angle of some 60°. In genu valgum a short cross bar is used and the feet gradually rotated medially some 45°. It is important that the boots fit comfortably and that the rotational force is applied gradually. A method applicable to medial torsion, the more important deformity, is the use of a leather strap between the shoes. The strap is fixed by detachable bolts to the lateral counter and is adjustable for length so that the shorter the distance between the bolts the greater the degree of rotation (Fig. 8,22). The method is readily acceptable to parents and child and has the advantage of permitting movement in every direction with the exception of medial rotation (Kingsbery, 1965).

## ESTABLISHED MEDIAL TORSION

There are, unfortunately, no symptoms, other than the possible psychological or functional handicap, related to medial torsion in adolescence or early adult life. The deformity, if it is recognised as such, is accepted until the onset of symptoms; and then it is too late (Fig. 8,23). The opportunity, possibly the only one, to correct a deformity which inevitably results in osteoarthrosis, by simple conservative means, occurs in early childhood when the parents are concerned with the cosmetic aspects of in-toeing. A further opportunity, but no longer by conservative means, occurs sometimes in the athletically-inclined father's concern for his son's ineptitude at games. Once this stage has passed the only chance is the young man's worry about his appearance.

When such opportunities arise the anxiety of the patient, or his parents, is such that a technically complex, and time-consuming procedure when it entails correction of both varus and internal rotation, is readily accepted. If, from the physician's viewpoint, the operation is regarded as a prophylactic measure, this aspect should not be overstressed: patients seldom appreciate being saved from the disaster they have not experienced.

**Late Established Deformity**

There comes a time when the cortex of the tibia is no longer plastic and malleable and thus no

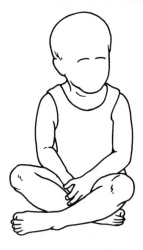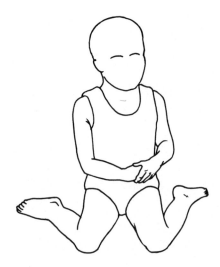

FIGS 8,19–20. **Medial (or lateral) torsion of tibia. Faulty sitting postures habitually employed are factors in maintaining and increasing torsional deformities.** Sitting tailor fashion main- tains medial torsion (Fig. 8,19) whereas sitting between the knees, so-called W sitting, produces lateral torsion (Fig. 8,20).

longer amenable to conservative measures in the form of corrective night splints. Genu valgum may exist with, or without, lateral torsion of the tibia and genu varum exist with, or without, medial torsion. Lateral torsion may exist without valgus and medial torsion without varus. Medial torsion with minimal varus is more common than is generally recognised. It may be the commonest single cause of bilateral osteo-arthrosis in middle-age.

If it is certain that the deformity is established, no longer part of the normal varoid-valgoid sequence and of a degree which merits interference, osteotomy in the supracondylar region of the femur or the infracondylar region of the tibia, or both, may be indicated. Supracondylar osteotomy is more difficult to perform and the correction more difficult to maintain than osteotomy of the tibia. It will be remembered, whether child or adult, that torsion of the tibia cannot be corrected above the tubercle. Osteotomy is usually performed immediately below the tubercle or at the site of maximum deformity. In general, the simpler the procedure the better, keeping in mind, particularly in the female, the desirability of a minimal incisional scar.

**Operative Techniques**

1. The most simple procedure, with no formal

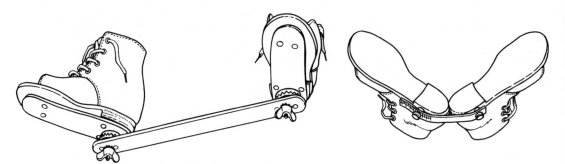

FIGS 8,21–22. **Medial torsion: treatment.** Footplates with a transverse bar are applied to boots which are worn at night. The degree of rotation is adjustable (Fig. 8,21). Alternatively, a strap adjustable for length is attached to the heels of boots and controls rotation (Fig. 8,22).

incision, requires a stab-wound large enough to permit the entry of a bone-awl. A zig-zag line of holes is made across the tibia, the bone fractured, the angulation corrected and a plaster cast applied.

2. If a more precise procedure is indicated an incision some 2 cm long is made over the antero-medial margin of the tibia at the chosen site. The periosteum is incised and elevators passed sub-periosteally round the bone. A zig-zag line of drill holes is made in the tibia and the holes joined with cuts from a narrow-bladed osteotome. This results in an irregular linear osteotomy in which the opposing margins hitch against one another without serious danger of displacement and permitting both angular and rotational deformity to be corrected. Mainten-ance of correction depends on external fixation in the form of a plaster cast.

3. When it is a matter of correcting angular deformity only, and with an intact fibula, no means of maintaining correction may be necessary other than a plaster cast. If, however, both angulation and torsion exist some means of control may be required particularly when osteotomy of the fibula is necessary. The method most favoured is transverse pins passed through the tibia above and below the chosen site for osteotomy and inserted before the bone is divided. The pins provide evidence and control of the correction achieved and are incorporated in the plaster cast.

4. In the older child, the adolescent or the young adult medial torsion and/or varus angulation can be corrected only by a more extensive procedure carried out at the upper end of the tibia avoiding, in the immature subject, the growth plate. At this site the danger of non-union is minimal.

A 'Z' osteotomy with anterior resection of a rectangle of bone permits rotation to be corrected (Fig. 8,25). If resection takes the form of a trapezium, rotation and varus angulation can be corrected. The degree of the angle of the deformity determines the form and size of the trapezium (Fig. 8,26). An osteotomy of the fibula at a lower level and through a minimal incision is required to permit correction (see below). The operation is completed by the use of internal fixation in the form of screws (Fig. 8,27) (Brunelli, 1969).

## Derotation Osteotomy: Complication

**Lateral popliteal nerve paralysis.** The hazards of ischaemia in the limited space of the anterior fascial compartment are well known in the so-called anterior tibial compartment syndrome. It appears that lateral popliteal nerve paralysis is a common complication of derotational osteo-tomy. It is attributed to compression of nerve, vessel and muscle in the anterior compartment. It is recommended that such compression can be avoided if fasciotomy is performed; but better still, and contributing to ease of rotation, the fibula should be osteotomised (Schrock, 1969).

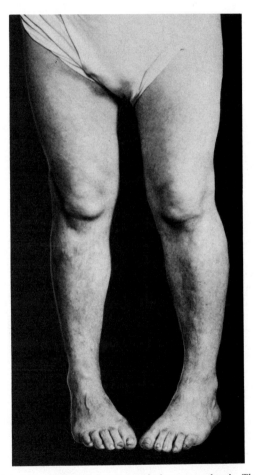

FIG. 8,23. **Medial torsion: pan-articular osteoarthrosis.** The most common single cause of bilateral pan-articular osteo-arthrosis is medial torsion. Figure 8,23 illustrates bilateral pan-articular osteoarthrosis based on medial torsion of the tibia. There is minimal angulation (S.D., male, aged 45). Is Figure 8,13 the precursor of Figure 8,23?

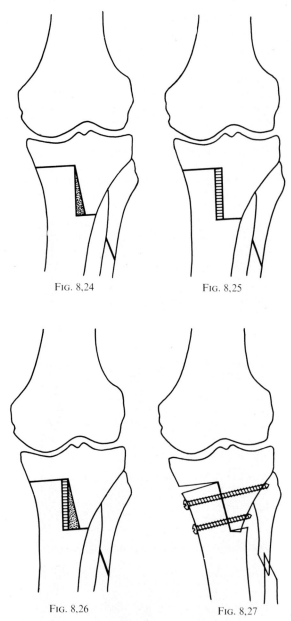

FIG. 8,24  FIG. 8,25

FIG. 8,26  FIG. 8,27

FIGS 8,24–27. **Derotation osteotomy: prophylaxis pan-articular osteoarthrosis.** Z osteotomy below tibial tubercle to correct varus angulation and/or medial rotation of tibia. To correct varus alone a wedge of cortex of calculated angle is resected from the anterior cortex (Fig. 8,24). To correct medial rotation alone the cortex resected is rectangular in shape (Fig. 8,25). To correct both varus angulation and rotation the two are combined (Fig. 8,26). The osteotomy requires subperiosteal division of the distal fibula. Internal fixation is used to stabilise the completed osteotomy of the tibia (Fig. 8,27) (after Brunelli).

# TIBIA VARA (BLOUNT'S DISEASE, OSTEOCHONDROSIS DEFORMANS TIBIAE)

**Background note.** Tibia vara was first reported by Erlacher (1922) and later described in full by Blount (1937) after whom the disorder has been named in recent years. It is suggested, as will be seen, that *tibia vara interna* is the most accurate description (Golding *et al.*, 1969).

**Definition.** The salient features of the condition are the development of a progressive varus deformity at the knee joint of a child accompanied by medial rotation of the tibia. It is generally considered to arise from a disorder of the postero-medial aspect of the upper tibial epiphysis. In early cases it is difficult to distinguish from so-called physiological genu varum (see below). After one or two years the radiological changes in the form of deformity and sclerosis of the metaphysis are characteristic. In the majority of cases both legs are affected.

CLASSIFICATION. Blount described two types: *infantile*, in which the deformity becomes manifest in the first three years of life; and *adolescent*, in which it first becomes evident at about the age of eight.

The infantile variety is the more common, the more severe and the more progressive form.

## Infantile Variety: Aetiology

**Age of walking.** Tibia vara is common in Jamaica and almost unknown in Britain. The average Jamaican child, living in a country district, stands at 5 months and walks at 9 to 10 months. The average child in temperate climates walks at 15 to 18 months. Whether this marked difference is due to clothing, footwear or climate alone, is not known.

All children are born with radiographic varus which later converts to radiographic valgus (Bateson, 1966, 1968). It is clear that Jamaican children walk for longer on physiological genu varum than do English children (Golding *et al.*, 1969). It has been shown that growth on the side of the epiphyseal plate under compression slows down whereas growth on the side under relaxation tends to speed up (Arkin and Katz, 1956). It is thus not unlikely that the basic disorder in tibia vara is nothing more than a simple differential growth in length because of early weight-bearing on a physiological genu varum. Once initiated the static forces involved ensure that the condition is progressive.

**Rotation deformity.** Kessel (1970) has offered an ingenious explanation of the production of the important rotation aspect of the deformity. He points out that the superior and inferior tibio-fibular joints do not lie in the same coronal plane. The superior is posterior to the inferior by a matter of some 6°. This could cause the fibula to act as a camshaft in the event of differential growth between the two bones thus producing rotation in addition to the varus. The tibia grows 5 cm in length from birth to the age of three (Maresh, 1943) and a 5 mm lag in growth of the tibia could in theory produce medial rotation of the tibia by as much as 30°.

## Clinical Features

Tibia vara occurs in otherwise healthy children

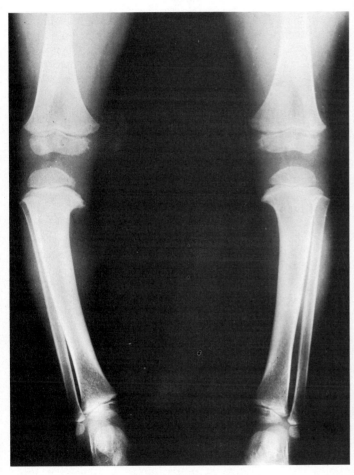
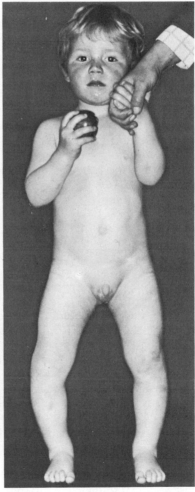

FIGS 8,28–29. **Infantile tibia vara (Blount's disease: osteo-chondrosis deformans tibiae).** Early stage of tibia vara. Note fragmentation of the medial prominence or beak; and that the medial cortex of the tibia is much thicker than the lateral. Note in particular that the condition affects the tibia; not the femur (Fig. 8,28). It is characteristic, as in this case, that the deformity is asymmetrical both clinically and radiologically (Figs 8,28 and 8,29). (S.F., male, aged 3½, case of W.W.)

noted to have excessive genu varum on walking. Usually, but not invariably, the condition is bilateral. In the early stages between, say, 9 and 18 months, it is not possible to distinguish between physiological genu varum of persistent foetal alignment that corrects spontaneously without treatment and the genu varum that progresses to tibia vara. In tibia vara however, over the next few months, a projection or beak develops on the medial aspect of the tibial head where the growth plate is localised subcutaneously. If the disease progresses the beak becomes more prominent to palpation and the varus deformity becomes more obvious. In the established example the varus deformity and the accompanying medial rotation of the tibia are obvious (Fig. 8,29).

## Radiological Features

A range of progressive changes are characteristic of tibia vara. They can be classified into four stages (Golding et al., 1969).

**1. Physiological genu varum.** This condition related to persistent foetal alignment is characterised by:

(a) Medial rotation and varus deformity of the tibia.

(b) Prominence of the medial aspects of the femoral and tibial metaphyses.

(c) Relatively thickened cortex on the medial side of the femoral and tibial shafts.

(d) Irregularity of metaphyseal regions of femur and tibia (Fig. 8,9).

**2. Early stage of tibia vara.** The medial prominence or beak begins to fragment at its medial extremity. The medial cortex of the tibia is much thicker than the lateral. It is unusual to see abnormalities in the distal femur (Fig. 8,28).

**3. Established stage of tibia vara.** The most obvious feature in routine radiographs is that the centre of ossification does not appear in the medial side of the cartilage model. The bony epiphysis appears only in the lateral side; the medial side is almost entirely cartilaginous. The growth plate may widen and disappear medially just proximal to the beak, or split in two. The metaphysis bends medially and runs almost parallel to the proximal end of the medial cortex of the tibia. The epiphyseal cartilage appears to have bent downwards into this depressed area.

**4. Late stage of tibia vara.** The epiphysis is distorted. The secondary centre of ossification has developed and the cartilaginous portion, bent towards the beak, becomes ossified. The growth plate closes laterally, earlier than normal. The wide irregular or split growth plate finally closes in the region of the beak. The lateral radiograph shows that growth posteriorly has been deficient, resulting in a flexion deformity of the tibial plateau on the shaft.

## Differential Diagnosis

It will be evident from the foregoing that the diagnosis in the early stages is difficult, if almost impossible, to differentiate from physiological genu varum especially if the former merges imperceptibly into the latter. At this stage radiological examination is not helpful: marked physiological genu varum shows the same changes in the tibia as tibia vara. In such circumstances it will be evident that care must be taken in a situation which corrects spontaneously and in which the wrong decision, involving osteotomy, results in a valgus deformity of gross proportions. In other circumstances the condition can be mimicked by any disease which involves the epiphyseal plate, such as rickets (Figs 8,33 to 8,38) and metaphyseal dysostosis. It is in such circumstances that radiography is helpful.

## Treatment

**Prevention.** If the theories of aetiology propounded are correct, and the deformity arises from physiological genu varum, it is not unreasonable that weight-bearing activity be reduced, if this is possible, coupled with the use of night splints of the mermaid type (Figs 8,11 and 8,12) or, if internal rotation is marked, splints of the Denis Browne type (Fig. 8,21). It is known that prolonged force can change the shape of a growing bone; but the duration of splintage is more important than the force applied (Golding et al., 1969).

**Operation.** If the theories of aetiology propounded are correct it will be evident that once the condition is established it is progressive and operation in some form is the only measure likely to prove effective; and in this regard the timing of the selected procedure is of major importance.

AGE AT OPERATION. The timing of operation depends on clinical and radiological findings and not on the chronological age of the patient. The correction of an angular deformity cannot be expected to restore normal growth if irreparable damage to the epiphyseal plate has occurred. The danger sign of irreparable damage is distortion and bending of the epiphysis towards the beak.

The timing of operative measures, if the theories of aetiology propounded are correct, will vary from one part of the world to another. In Jamaica the disease begins earlier than elsewhere and osteotomies are performed at age three or four. After this age there is permanent damage to the epiphysis and epiphyseal plate and thus the results of operation are less good. On the other hand, Langenskiold (1952), referring to experience in Finland, advised waiting until the age of eight.

## Operation: Early Stage

**Metaphyseal forage.** Kessel (1969) suggested this possible method of stimulating growth on the medial side of the tibia and has since (1970) described two cases in which the procedure was used with success. The underlying principle is the known fact that overgrowth can be stimulated by injury or disease: Taylor (1963) recorded a genu valgum deformity from stimulation of the proximal tibial metaphysis while the fibula exerted a tethering influence in 72 of the 103 cases he studied. The deformity developed within five months and the degree, as might be expected, depended on the skeletal age.

INDICATION. The simple operation he describes is applicable to definitely established early cases of infantile tibia vara. The results he described suggest that it is worthy of further trial.

TECHNIQUE

'In a few words: I raise a trapdoor of cortex 2 cm × 1 cm on the antero-medial face of the tibia at the proximal end. I remove all the cancellous bone distal to the growth plate, i.e. I try to curette out the whole metaphysis without damaging the growth plate. The

trapdoor is then replaced. The child is fit to go out of hospital the next day.' (Kessel, personal communication, 1970.)

## Operation: Later Stage

**Osteotomy.** Early cases with a definite growth plate abnormality and a small clinical beak may be treated by a dome-shaped osteotomy immediately distal to the tibial tubercle.

TECHNIQUE. The dome which is convex proximally is cut in such a manner that there is a longer curve on the medial side of the proximal fragment of the tibia. This prevents the realigned distal fragment from displacing medially and resulting in a pressure sore with secondary infection of the osteotomy site. The fibula is divided to allow complete correction of the deformity (Fig. 8.30) (Golding et al., 1969).

## Operation: Later Still

**Osteotomy.** Moderately severe late cases with obvious fragmentation of the growth plate on the medial side, a large clinical beak and a thick,

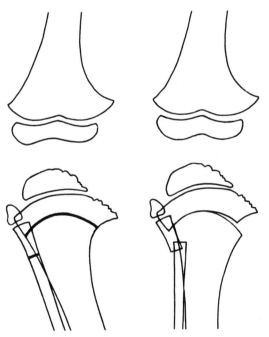

FIG. 8.30. **Tibia vara: treatment.** Early cases may be treated with a dome-shaped osteotomy immediately distal to the tibial tubercle (after Golding et al., 1969).

short medial tibial cortex require a more radical osteotomy; and should usually be over-corrected.

TECHNIQUE. A Steinmann pin is inserted deep to the tibial tubercle and parallel to the knee joint with the patella pointing forwards. A second pin is inserted about mid-shaft, and aligned parallel to the ankle joint with the foot externally rotated about 15°. The angle in two planes between the pins represents the deformity to be corrected. The fibula is approached through a small lateral incision at a point well distal to the lateral popliteal nerve. It is exposed subperiosteally and divided completely. A small section of bone is excised to permit correction (Fig. 8,31). The tibia is exposed subperiosteally through a curved incision distal to the tubercle. An incomplete transverse linear osteotomy is made with a reciprocating saw and completed posteriorly with an osteotome. The pins are now aligned so that the knee and ankle joints are parallel and internal rotation eliminated. A wedge of bone of suitable size is removed from the lateral side of the distal fragment and inserted on the medial side. The osteotomy

should now be stable when the clamps are tightened (Fig. 8,32) (Golding *et al.*, 1969).

*After-treatment.* The pins remain in position for six to eight weeks depending on the age of the patient.

RESULTS. Overcorrection of the deformity with the possible addition of stimulation of the medial aspect of the growth plate, improve, but seldom reverse, the changes which have occurred.

## TIBIA VARA: ADOLESCENT VARIETY

AGE OF PATIENT. This form which is less common than the infantile variety occurs between the age of 8 and 15 years.

AETIOLOGY. It may be secondary to trauma or to osteomyelitis but cases arise in which no cause is apparent.

DISTRIBUTION. This form of the disease is unilateral and does not result in gross deformities.

TREATMENT. It appears that spontaneous re-mission occasionally occurs in the idiopathic

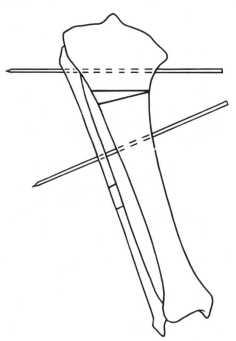

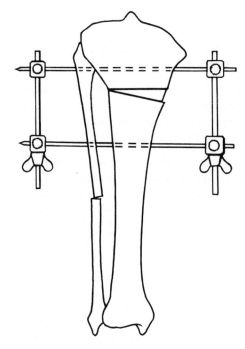

FIGS 8,31–32. **Tibia vara: treatment.** Late cases require linear osteotomy with the transfer of a wedge of bone from the lateral (Fig. 8,31) to the medial side under the control of pins and clamps (Fig. 8,32) (after Golding *et al.*, 1969).

variety of the disease. In the possibility of such circumstances osteotomy should be deferred until growth has ceased (Golding *et al.*, 1969).

## TIBIA VALGA

Hubner (1961) described changes on the lateral side of the tibial head similar to those which occur in Blount's disease. The condition is considerably less common than tibia vara. Several cases have been reported from Jamaica (Bateson, 1966). The disease is characterised by a genu valgum deformity accompanied by marked lateral rotation of the tibia. A palpable beak develops at the lateral extremity of the proximal tibial growth plate. In the radiograph there is thickening of the lateral femoral and tibial diaphysial cortices. The changes in the region of the beak resemble those of tibia vara but are said not to reach the same degree of severity (Golding *et al.*, 1969).

Treatment follows the lines recommended for tibia vara.

## ANGULAR DEFORMITY AS MANIFESTATION OF SYSTEMIC DISEASE

Angular deformity at the knee is the salient clinical feature in infancy and childhood of a number of important conditions of systemic origin and the presenting and often the only complaint of the parents. While physiological bow leg or knock knee is the most likely diagnosis it is important when the slightest doubt exists that the various possibilities listed in Table 10 be considered. The orthopaedic surgeon may be the first clinician offered the opportunity of establishing the diagnosis.

## INFANTILE (NUTRITIONAL) RICKETS (VITAMIN D DEFICIENCY)

**Background note.** The first description of the disease is attributed to Soranus of Ephesus in the first century AD. But it seems probable that it may have been relatively uncommon in the sunny lands which cradled civilisation.

Rickets first became endemic in Britain and continued rampant as a product of the Industrial Revolution into the first quarter of the twentieth century. It was not until the properties of fat-soluble vitamins were appreciated at the end of the First World War that the incidence decreased. By the end of the Second World War, with essential vitamins distributed on a national basis, the disease had virtually disappeared from Great Britain. This happy situation has not been maintained.

In recent years it has been shown that rickets is common amongst immigrant children living in Glasgow (Dunnigan *et al.*, 1962) and London (Benson *et al.*, 1963). But not only immigrants are affected. In the year 1964, 24 children with infantile rickets were seen at the Royal Hospital for Sick Children, Glasgow. From a random selection of 300 children in the age range 6 to

TABLE 10

Differentiation of the radiographic diagnosis of rickets (Pierce, Wallace and Herndon, 1964)

| Diagnosis | Calcium | Phosphorus | Phosphatase | Carbon dioxide | Blood urea nitrogen | Glucose | Amino acids | Comment |
|---|---|---|---|---|---|---|---|---|
| | | | | | | Urine | | |
| Vitamin-D deficiency | N-L | L | H | N | N | Neg. | Pos. | Positive nutritional history |
| Resistant rickets | N-L | L | H | N | N | Neg. | Neg. | Often positive family history |
| Fanconi's syndrome | N-L | L | H | L | N-H | Pos. | Pos. | Often positive family history |
| Renal tubule acidosis | N-L | L | H | L | N-H | Pos.? | Neg.? | Negative family history |
| Chronic renal failure | N-L | H | N-H | L | H | Neg. | Neg. | Renal anomalies usual |
| Hypophosphatasia | N-L | N | L | N | N | Neg. | Neg. | Urine phosphoethanolamine positive |
| Lowe's syndrome | N-L | L-N | H | L | N-H | Pos. | Pos.? | Glaucoma |
| 'Coeliac' rickets, 'hepatic' rickets | N-L | L | H | N | N | Neg. | Neg. | Evidence of steatorrhea or of liver disease |

N = normal;   L = low;   H = high;   ? = equivocal or variably present.

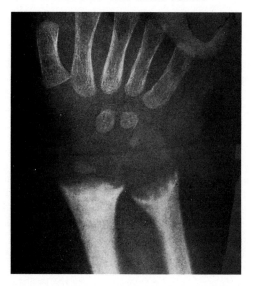

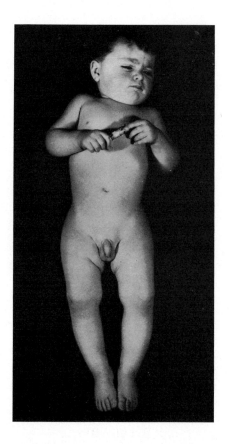

FIGS 8,33–35. **Angular deformity as manifestation of systemic disease: infantile (nutritional) rickets.** The clinical appearance does not differ materially from physiological genu varum (Fig. 8,34). The radiological appearances are characteristic (Fig. 8,35) and confirmed by radiographs of the wrist where the earliest signs are visible (Fig. 8,33).

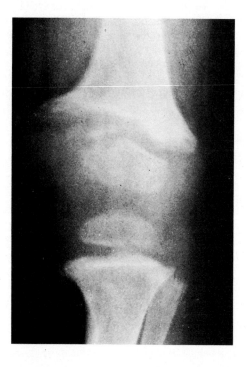

24 months, it was deduced that no less than 1 per cent of white legitimate children of this age in central Glasgow suffered from infantile rickets during the winter 1963–64 (Arneil, McKilligan and Lobo, 1965).

It is known from past experience that immigrant populations tend to suffer from rickets. If the condition is exceptional in the West Indies it is common amongst the infants of those who emigrate to the northern United States. If it is rare in Sicily and Southery Italy, it is common in children of Italians who have emigrated to North America. It is significant that the child illustrated in Figures 8,33 to 8,38 was of Italian origin.

The reappearance of rickets in large industrial cities is largely the result of ignorance. A dietary intake of vitamin D which is adequate on the Indian continent is not sufficient for pigmented individuals transferred to large industrial cities where, as in Glasgow, the hours of sunshine amount to only about 1000 per annum, and

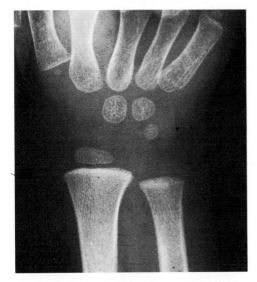

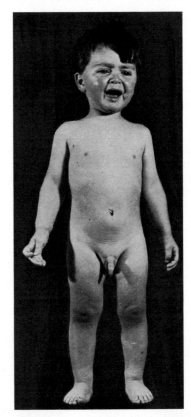

FIGS 8,36–38. **Angular deformity as manifestation of systemic disease: infantile nutritional) rickets.** The clinical appearance of the child eight months after treatment with vitamin D (Fig. 8,37) and the radiographs of knee and wrist taken at that time (Figs 8,38 and 8,36). (A.N., case of J.H.)

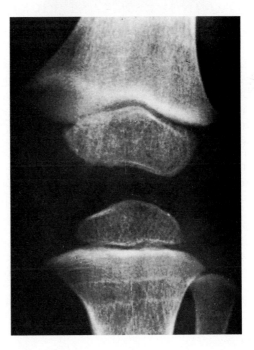

even then limited by high buildings and filtered through industrial smoke. It is clear that clinicians should be alert to the possibility of avitaminosis particularly in the children of immigrants.

## Clinical Features

It has been indicated that the child may be presented as a result of angular deformity and may not, in so far as the appearance of the knees is concerned, differ in material degree from other causes of angular deformity physiological or pathological (Fig. 8,34). The clinician may be alerted by the social background of the child and by other clinical stigmata of nutritional rickets, which need not be listed here, to the necessity for further radiological and biochemical investigations (Table 10).

**Radiological examination.** The earliest stages of rickets are not detectable radiologically. At the stage at which a case is presented as angular deformity of the knee characteristic changes are likely to be present and confirmatory radiographs of the distal ends of the radius and ulna, where the earliest signs are visible, indicated (Figs 8,35 and 8,33).

A wide variety of appearances can be encountered varying with the degree and intensity of the disease. In general the salient features vary between rarefaction and irregularity to total absence of the provisional zones of calcification. The irregular ends of the bones are broad, angled and cupped. The shafts are decalcified and of coarse trabecular pattern.

### Treatment

Recognition of the source of the angulation and the intake of the appropriate dose of vitamin D, with or without splinting, results in correction of the deformity and normal radiographs (Figs 8,36; 8,37 and 8,38).

The reason for the deformity should, if possible, be explained to the parents; in other circumstances social workers should be alerted to the existence of the problem.

## VITAMIN D RESISTANT RICKETS (FAMILIAL OR ESSENTIAL HYPOPHOSPHATAEMIA)

**Definition.** Vitamin D resistant rickets is a specific metabolic disorder, apparently genetically determined, with clinical, radiographic and biochemical characteristics similar to infantile or nutritional rickets, but which progresses to adult life, in spite of antirachitic prophylaxis, and which heals only in response to large doses of vitamin D.

**Biochemistry.** In children the condition is characterised by a very low serum phosphorus, normal or slightly low serum calcium and an elevated alkaline phosphatase.

**Differential diagnosis.** The condition should be distinguished from conditions producing angular deformity in infancy and from other entities with similar clinical and radiological features in particular renal and coeliac rickets from which it is distinguished by the absence of systemic acidosis, renal insufficiency and

malabsorption syndromes (Stamp *et al.*, 1964). See also Table 10.

### Treatment

**Medication.** Vitamin D therapy is urgently indicated in younger children with radiographic rachitic changes and rapidly progressive deformity. Unfortunately the range between essential dosage and overdosage is narrow. The regulation of vitamin D dosage is accomplished by measuring the 24 hour urinary calcium output against the curve of normal excretion; and for such comparison a close estimate of calcium intake is necessary (Stearns, 1964). The matter is one of some complexity and the strictest supervision is necessary if the dangers of hypervitaminosis D are to be avoided. The co-operation of a paediatrician interested in the problem is desirable in the control and management of the therapy.

**Indications for treatment.** There is a wide variety in the manifestations and severity of deformity at the knee joint and elsewhere. In general it is considered desirable to avoid operation in favour of corrective splinting before puberty, if it is only for the reason that recurrence of deformity or the development of a secondary deformity is common (Figs 8,39 to 8,41). There are occasions, however, when angulation is extreme so that the fitting of calipers is impossible. In such cases osteotomies cannot be deferred.

SPLINTING. The type of splinting to be adopted depends on the severity of the case and varies between mermaid splints worn at night and the necessity for full length calipers worn continuously with the exception of periods of non-weight-bearing exercise therapy.

### Operative

**Pre-operative.** When operative treatment in the form of osteotomy is indicated either before or after puberty it is essential that vitamin D therapy is discontinued at least one month before operation lest the child be thrown into acute hypervitaminosis D by the hypercalcinuric effects of bed-rest and immobilisation in plaster casts. In this regard also techniques and methods of fixation, internal and external, should be

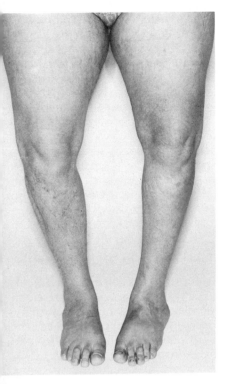
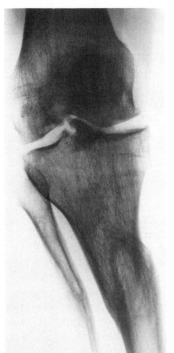
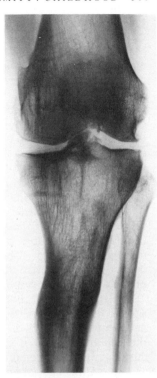

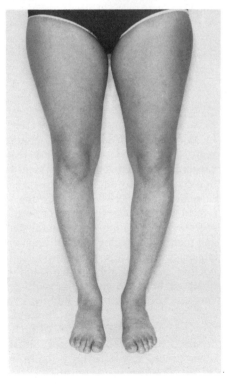

FIGS 8,39–41. **Vitamin D resistant rickets: progression to adult life.** Mother (Dr K.L-W., aged 53, Figs 8,39 and 8,40) and daughter (Mrs M.J., aged 23, Fig. 8,41). It will be seen that in Figure 8,39 in spite of osteotomies recurrence of deformity has taken place with bilateral panarticular osteoarthrosis (Fig. 6,40). The daughter was diagnosed at 15 months and received medication as described. The mother had the impression that the deformity occurred at 10–11 years rather than previously. On the right side there was 8° of varus; 6° of internal torsion. On the left there was 12° of varus and 15° of internal torsion (Fig. 8,41).

chosen which permit the earliest possible return weight-bearing exercise therapy.

**Osteotomy.** The site and type of osteotomy undertaken depends on the location of the deformity and follows the recommendation for similar deformities in childhood and later recommended in this section. The deformities may be such that multiple osteotomies splinted by an intramedullary nail may be necessary to achieve correction in both saggital and coronal planes in terms of medial torsion. In selection of method the desirability of early ambulation should be paramount.

AFTER-TREATMENT. Vitamin D therapy is

reinstituted as soon after operation as the patient can participate in exercise therapy vigorous enough to combat the demineralising effect of inactivity. In the prepubertal child full length calipers are necessary after the osteotomies have healed and, as a rule, to the age of puberty. If puberty has been reached, calipers are required only until the osteotomy site has healed in the knowledge that delayed union is not infrequent following osteotomy in resistant rickets (Pierce, Wallace and Herndon, 1964).

**Prognosis.** If the medical and orthopaedic treatment, conservative and operative, described is important, the hazards of therapy with large doses of vitamin D must be stressed and the danger of cumulative and irreversible renal damage emphasised. There is a wide variation in the clinical severity of the disease and unpredictability in the response to treatment.

The parents of a child with this condition should be warned of the chronic, metabolic nature of the disease; that it must be followed throughout life; that it is especially hazardous during growth for the prevention of deformities and the maintenance of a normal rate of growth; and that recurrence in later years during periods of stress, such as pregnancy and the menopause, in the form of osteomalacia is real (Tapia, Stearns and Ponseti, 1964).

## SCURVY

Separation of epiphyses about the knee are known to occur in scurvy. The separation takes place through the brittle columns of calcified cartilage remote from the epiphyseal vessels and thus recovery without growth disturbance is the rule. Silverman (1970) records the case of a typical separation of the distal femoral epiphysis observed in a 6-month-old infant with clinical and roentgenographic signs of scurvy. One year later, apparent premature union of the central portion of the epiphysis with the shaft was observed and subsequent growth disturbance was recorded when the child was 4 years of age. At 22 years, however, almost complete recovery from the growth disturbance had occurred without compensatory overgrowth of other areas, and with only minor alterations in the configuration of the affected bone.

Apparently, a transitory slowing or arrest of endochondral ossification had taken place in the central portion of the epiphysis and metaphysis with subsequent resumption of normal and accelerated growth, which resulted in restoration of nearly normal dimensions. In such a 'ball-in-socket' epiphysis-shaft junction, closure of the plate may be apparent and not real. Careful serial studies are necessary before considering epiphyseodesis on the healthy side.

These findings are in keeping with the observations made in relation to apparent epiphyseal destruction in infective arthritis in infancy (Ch. 5).

## OTHER CAUSES OF ANGULAR DEFORMITY IN CHILDHOOD

There are a number of less common conditions, mostly genetically determined, which present in childhood or adolescence as angular deformity. It is not proposed that these be catalogued. The following are examples to illustrate the individual problems involved:

### Achondroplasia

The most common complaint of achondroplastic dwarfs is angular deformity in the form of genu varum. The degree of bowing is not necessarily symmetrical. The deformity arises from stretching of the lateral ligament, or originates in the tibia. The femur is not involved (Figs 8.42 and 8.43).

Osteoarthrosis other than of mild degree was not observed in the knees of any adult achondroplastic patient examined (Bailey, 1970).

**Indications for treatment.** The varus deformity of achondroplasia is not accompanied by medial rotation of the tibia. Osteoarthrosis therefore is not inevitable. There is thus no indication for prophylactic measures. Osteotomy may be indicated for cosmetic reasons, or for pain the result of defective weight-bearing mechanics. The osteotomy, since derotation is not involved, can be performed above the tibial tubercle at a site which is particularly broad in the achondroplastic subject. It should be of the opening wedge variety.

CONSERVATIVE MEASURES. In gross ligamentous instability splinting may be indicated.

It should be recognised that the short obese thigh of the achondroplasic dwarf makes the fitting of a caliper difficult in the extreme. In addition the prominent head of fibula, the outcome of varus deformity, renders the lateral popliteal nerve vulnerable to pressure. In such circumstances the forces involved in correction of the angulation by knee-apron secured to the inner iron should be recognised, and the location of straps related accordingly.

## Osteochondrodystrophy (Morquio's Disease)

Angular deformities of considerable degree may occur at an early age and demand correction to preserve function in the joint. It is seldom the simple problem of angulation in one plane but of recurvatus in combination with valgus. When the tibial table slopes downwards and forwards the patella may be located at an excessively low level. In such circumstances the osteotomy should not be deferred until irreversible adaptive changes have occurred in the conformation of the joint. The site of division must not interfere with the growth plate and below the tibial tubercle if the patella is to be raised to a higher level. The osteotomy will be of the opening wedge variety (Fig. 10,56) and require the introduction of wedge-shaped full-thickness iliac grafts; and the possibility of obtaining these from a parent should be considered rather than banked-bone. Staples may be required to maintain stability.

## FLEXION DEFORMITY IN CEREBRAL PALSY

Flexion of the knee is a common deformity in the child with cerebral palsy. It is not proposed that the indications or contraindications for

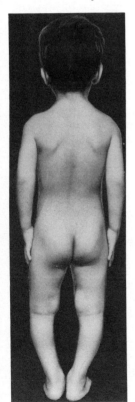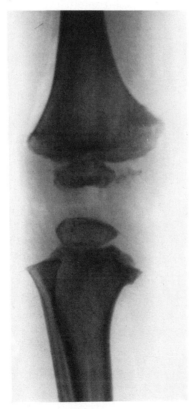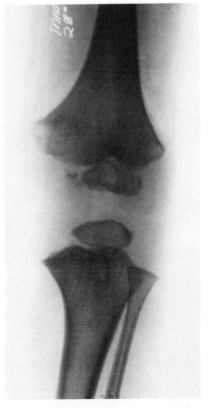

FIGS 8,42–43. **Achondroplasia.** Bowing of the tibiae is not accompanied by rotational deformity and thus osteoarthrosis is not inevitable. Osteotomy may be required on cosmetic grounds (Fig. 8,42). The radiographs show flaring of the metaphysis of the femur and fragmentation of the epiphysis (A.M., aged 5) (Fig. 8,43).

operative treatment be discussed here other than to state that when surgical measures are under consideration the potentialities of the patient and the related outcome of prospective proceedings must be carefully considered. A severely handicapped child with mental retardation lacking in balance to walk will not benefit from the procedures to be described.

The object of operation, if indicated, is improvement of hip extension by balancing the effect of spastic hip flexors, the relief of flexion contracture of the knee and increase in the power of the quadriceps. The deforming elements are overactivity of the spastic hamstring muscles and deficiency of the quadriceps extensor apparatus producing patella alta and an elongated patellar tendon. The procedures available are:

**1. Transfer of the hamstring tendons to the femoral condyles (Eggers, 1952).**
**2. Transfer of the medial hamstrings only.**
**3. Transfer of the hamstring tendons to the femoral condyles combined with advancement of the patellar tendon.**

In reviewing the result of 50 of these procedures in a total of 26 patients (Keats, 1970), it was noted that advancement of the patellar tendon, when indicated, after transference of the hamstrings, produced a striking clinical improvement in 6 of the 7 patients who underwent the operations as a two-stage procedure. In addition, transfer of the medial hamstrings alone and lengthening of the biceps tendon was considered to give good results.

### Transfer of the Hamstring Tendons to the Femoral Condyles

**Technique.** The patient is placed in the prone position and a high tourniquet applied. Two incisions are required. The medial extends from the femoral condyle above to the pes anserinus below. The tendons of semitendinosus, semimembranosus and gracilis are identified and divided about 1 cm from their insertion. The area posterior and immediately proximal to the medial femoral condyle is cleared of soft tissue down to the periosteum. Two separate parallel incisions are made through the periosteum and the intervening tissue elevated. The semitendinosus and gracilis are sutured to the semimembranosus one on either side. The combined tendons are now entered through the tunnel in the periosteum and firmly sutured in position (Fig. 8,44).

The lateral incision, some 10 cm long, exposes the tendon of biceps. The lateral popliteal nerve as it lies beneath the medial edge of the tendon is identified, dissected free, retracted and protected. The tendon is divided immediately above the bifurcation prior to insertion into the fibula. The subperiosteal tunnel proximal to the lateral condyle is made as on the medial side. The

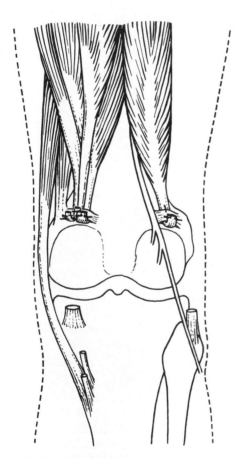

FIG. 8,44. **Flexion deformity in cerebral palsy: treatment. Transfer of hamstring tendons to femoral condyles: Eggers' operation.** Semi-diagrammatic illustration to show transfer of semitendinosus, semimembranosus and gracilis to the medial femoral condyle and biceps to the lateral femoral condyle.

divided tendon is passed through the tunnel and sutured in position.

AFTER-TREATMENT. At the termination of the operation a full-length padded plaster cast is applied with the knee in extension and the foot in dorsiflexion. Windows may be cut at the end of two weeks for removal of the sutures. The cast is retained for about six weeks when exercise therapy and re-education begins. A posterior shell is worn at night until rehabilitation is complete.

## Advancement of Patellar Tendon

**Techniques.** If the epiphysis is open a technique must be adopted which reduces the risk of closure to a minimum (Ch. 2). In other circumstances a bone block may be shifted downwards as in the treatment of patella alta or the bony block carried downwards and to the medial side as in the operative treatment of recurrent subluxation (Ch. 2).

## FLEXION DEFORMITY IN MYELOMENINGOCELE

The neurological state in the lower limbs in myelomeningocele differs from that in cerebral palsy or poliomyelitis. A limb in which there is no voluntary activity may, nevertheless, contain innervated muscles due to the presence of islets of functioning cord which can be shown by the response to electrical stimulation. Such muscles may be capable of causing recurrent deformity. In these circumstances their assessment is essential in planning surgical treatment. In general the correction of deformity by traction or serial plaster casts is contraindicated in the presence of insensitive skin. The aim of operation is to correct the flexion contracture by lengthening or dividing tight posterior structures and to maintain correction by weakening flexor muscles and strengthening the extensor apparatus.

The procedures available are:
1. Flexor tendon lengthening or division.
2. Transfer of flexor tendons to the femoral condyles (Eggers, 1952) just described.
3. Transfer of flexor tendons to patella (Clark, 1956) and described in Chapter 2.
4. Supracondylar osteotomy when soft tissue release is insufficient to correct the deformity.

In the series of 76 children so treated (Abraham, Verinder and Sharrard, 1977) and on which this section is based, there showed ño significant advantage of one procedure over another. If anything the transfer of the flexor tendons to the patella is most effective; supracondylar osteotomy alone the least. Flexor tendon elongation or division or transfer of the flexor tendons to the lower end of the femur appears to be successful only when the power of the quadriceps is at least grade three before operation. Where the quadriceps muscle is paralysed transfer of the flexor tendons to the patella seems to give the best results.

**Indications.** The better the innervation of the quadriceps the more likely it is that any operative procedure which corrects deformity and weakens the power of knee flexion will succeed.

**Contraindications.** The benefits of the correction of flexion deformity can be realised only in patients who have the potential to walk with the aid of long-leg braces. Patients with severe hydrocephalus, or with an intelligence quotient of less than 65, or with upper limb weakness or spasticity, will not be able to do so, and in them flexion deformity should be left uncorrected unless there is a danger of pressure of the heels against a wheelchair.

## CONTROL OF ANGULAR DEFORMITY AND/OR OF LENGTH OF LIMB IN COURSE OF GROWTH

Arrest of growth by epiphysiodesis (Phemister, 1933) is an accepted method of the control of the length of a limb. More recently the application of pressure to the growth plate by staples (Blount and Clarke, 1949) has been used, on one aspect to correct angular deformity, or on both aspects of femoral and/or tibial plates, to control length. In theory removal of the staples is followed by resumption of growth.

These measures should be applied only with caution and with due consideration of the outcome in terms of possible undesirable consequences in the short and long term. If compression is to be applied to both sides of the femoral and tibial plates in an attempt to equalise the length of the legs the certain resumption of growth following removal should not be assumed. In other words stapling should be regarded as a form of epiphysiodesis (Fig. 8,45).

Epiphyseal arrest is considered to be a reliable method of treatment of discrepancy of leg length of 5 to 7·5 centimetres (Green and Anderson, 1970).

### Stapling: To Correct Angular Deformity

Stapling may be used on one aspect of one plate to correct a local angular deformity due to retardation or cessation of growth on the other side (Fig. 8,47). If the indication occurs a short time before anticipated maturity there will be some loss of length. In such circumstances it may be preferable to permit maturity to occur and then to correct angular deformity by an opening-wedge osteotomy above the tibial tubercle. This will at least restore length by the amount the wedge is opened. If used on one side of both femoral and tibial plates for the same purpose an even greater loss of length must be

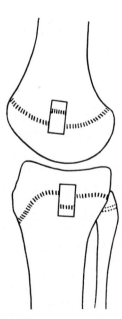

FIG. 8,45. **Epiphysiodesis.** A rectangle of cortex is removed and through the resulting window the growth plate is destroyed by drilling. The rectangular graft is rotated through 180° and re-inserted.

anticipated to say nothing of some possible alteration in the conformation of the joint. In any event, this technique is applicable only at the end of the growing period. The risks inherent in temporary use with the expectation of resumption of growth after withdrawal are too great to be acceptable in the young child.

### Stapling: To Correct Discrepancy of Length

Stapling of the growth plate on one side of an angular deformity in adolescence is very different, in terms of possible harm, to the stapling of both sides of both plates in a normal knee to produce shortening comparable to the abnormal side (Fig. 8,46).

### Epiphysiodesis or Stapling: Technique

**Approach.** The operation is performed in a bloodless field with the knee supported on a wedge-pillow in 30° to 70° of flexion or over the end of the table as for meniscectomy. Radiographic control is essential.

The incision, or incisions, depend on the site and extent of the procedures to be undertaken. The lower femoral growth plate is exposed through an oblique incision 6 to 8 cm in length centred over the plate and sloping downwards and backwards. The proximal tibial plate is exposed through an oblique incision of similar length but sloping downwards and forwards. If exposure of both plates is contemplated the two incisions are joined to form a curved approach convex posteriorly.

The medial aspect of the femoral plate is approached by retracting the vastus medialis anteriorly and the hamstring tendons posteriorly. Flexion reveals the posterior aspect; extension the anterior.

The lateral surface of the femoral plate is exposed by dividing vertically the fascia anterior to the iliotibial band. It is retracted posteriorly and the vastus lateralis anteriorly. Retraction of the soft tissues in flexion, or extension, reveals the posterior, or anterior, aspects of the plate.

To approach the lateral surface of the tibial plate the deep fascia is excised longitudinally anterior to the head of the fibula. To expose the postero-lateral aspect the soft tissues are stripped from the head of the fibula, with due respect for the lateral popliteal nerve, and retracted posteriorly.

Epiphysiodesis aims at destruction of the plate with the object of eliminating further growth. To this end the plate must be exposed. Stapling may aim at the elimination of growth on a temporary basis with resumption when the staples are removed. If this is the aim of operation the growth plate must **not** be exposed. There is thus a difference in the technique to be adopted once the superficial soft tissues have been incised.

**Epiphysiodesis.** The plate is exposed at a point equidistant from the anterior and posterior surfaces by incising the periosteum and erasing it from the bone. A rectangular section of cortex about 2 cm wide, 2 cm thick and about 5 cm in length extending into the epiphysis, but for a greater distance into the metaphysis, is removed. Through the window the plate is destroyed with a small gouge or with a 3 mm drill followed by one of 5 or 6 mm. The resulting space is packed with cancellous bone which may be obtained from the metaphyseal region through the

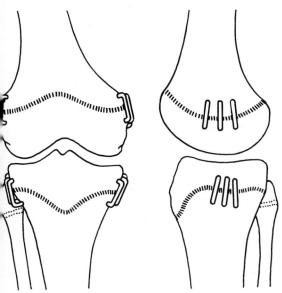

FIG. 8,46. **Epiphyseal stapling for the control of linear growth.** Diagrammatic representation of sites of units of three staples as applied to both femur and tibia. It is prudent to regard such measures as an epiphysiodesis (after Blount and Clarke, 1949).

O*

window from which the graft was taken. The rectangular graft is then rotated through 180° and returned to the bed from which it came (Fig. 8,45).

The procedure is repeated on the opposite side.

AFTER-TREATMENT. At the termination of operation a compression bandage in which are incorporated long plaster slabs is applied. When the stitches are removed a light plaster back-shell or complete cast is applied. Weight-bearing can usually be resumed between the fourth and sixth weeks.

**Stapling.** In each approach dissection proceeds down to, but not through, the periosteum: the epiphyseal plate must not be exposed. The plate may be visible through the periosteum or may be identified by probing with a straight needle. With a needle or needles in position radiographs are taken to confirm the site and curvature. While the plane of the plates is transverse at maturity, when the operation is undertaken the plate of the femur in the antero-posterior view takes the form of a shallow U convex downwards; that of the tibia a shallow U convex upwards (Fig. 8,47).

The staples, usually three in number, are inserted with the cross bars at right angles to the plate as determined by the radiographs. They are driven through the periosteum but are not buried beneath it. Movable soft tissue must not be included. The site of insertion is important. They should be located about the centre of the plate equidistant from the anterior and posterior surfaces. Further radiographs are obtained to make certain that the position is correct before they are finally driven home (Fig. 8,47). If the tibial epiphysis is stapled on the lateral side the anterior third of the head of the fibula may require to be excised to provide access and the entire growth plate eliminated before it is replaced. A small staple is used as the means of internal fixation.

AFTER-TREATMENT. At the termination of operation a compression bandage, in which are incorporated long plaster slabs, is applied. When the stitches are removed at the tenth day a light plaster back-shell or complete cast is used. Weight-bearing may be resumed without support at the end of three weeks and a gradual return to normal activities permitted.

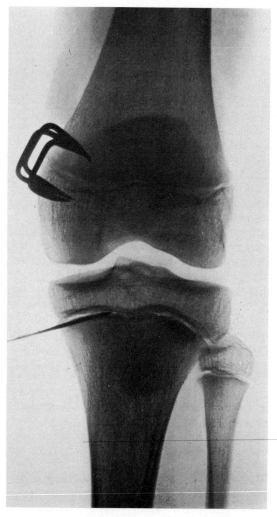

FIG. 8.47. **Angular deformity persisting towards adolescence: treatment.** Epiphyseal stapling may be indicated for the correction of angular deformity persisting towards the approach of maturity. Radiograph taken in the course of operation before femoral staples are driven home and with needle in position to determine exact site of upper tibial epiphysis.

## Epiphysiodesis: Complications

The operation of epiphyseal stapling, while theoretically attractive as a means of correcting discrepancy of leg length, is in such circumstances applied to the 'good' limb. In almost all the reported series there is a high incidence of complications the more serious because they

occur in a previously normal knee. Growth may resume after the staples are removed but this cannot be relied upon in every instance. In such circumstances, as has already been stated, stapling should be considered to be a method of arrest of growth comparable to epiphysiodesis. The hazards of the technique, some of which are irreversible, are such that they are unacceptable except towards the approach of maturity.

### Early

**Fracture or extrusion of staples.** In the early days of the operation numerous examples of fracture, spreading of the limbs or extrusion of the staples were reported. All of these complications have been encountered in the course of the limited experience on which opinions are based. If errors of technique are eliminated, and the importance of the design and quality of the staples recognised, these particular complications can be eliminated. When they occur prompt recognition followed by replacement is indicated.

**Production of unexpected deformity.** It is generally accepted that staples are more easily inserted across the lower femoral growth plate than the upper tibial; and some surgeons for this reason limit their activities to the former site. The staples may fail to influence growth on one aspect while arresting it on the other. A recurvatus, varus or valgus deformity can result. Such complications may occur from errors of technique in placing the staples, to exposure of the plate or to some unknown factor. The deformities, the most common of which is some degree of recurvatus, may necessitate a corrective osteotomy.

**Local cessation of growth.** Exposure of the periphery of the plate at operation may result in local cessation of growth. This will not be of serious importance when staples are inserted near the time of expected closure and with the intention of producing complete arrest of growth. If, however, it occurs in a young child in whom staples are used for temporary arrest with the hope of resumption of growth, the complication can have serious consequences.

**Inaccurate estimation of growth.** Epiphyseal growth estimation charts are based on normal children. Reduction of inequality of leg length after epiphysiodesis usually depends on the growth of an abnormally short limb. In all the series recorded the difficulties of prediction are stressed. Every means of growth estimation must be employed not the least of which is clinical evaluation of the individual patient. The closer the child to maturity the greater the accuracy. In boys over 13 and girls over 12 the predicted correction was accurate (Poirier, 1968).

The follow-up of all patients undergoing epiphysiodesis is essential: an epiphysiodesis on the previously shorter side is occasionally necessary (Green and Anderson, 1970).

## Late

**Laxity of ligaments.** It has been recorded that ligamentous laxity in varying degree was encountered in two-thirds of the cases reviewed some five years after maturity (Poirier, 1968). But bone growth and that of the supporting ligaments are not correlated. If the joint is reduced in size as a result of the use of staples the ligaments may be related to a larger structure.

**Osteoarthrosis.** The author was alerted some 25 years ago when tuberculosis was common to the possibility that epiphysiodesis might be followed by osteoarthrosis:

The patient, a young woman aged 25, had shortening as a result of tuberculous infection necessitating arthrodesis of the knee. A general surgeon had ablated the epiphyses at the lower end of the femur and the upper end of the tibia of the normal leg after the manner of Phemister (1933) in an attempt to reduce the discrepancy between the length of the limbs. No notes were available and it was not known to what extent improvement had been effected. The operation had been carried out efficiently. There was no angular deformity. The point at issue, and the reason why the author was consulted was not the tuberculous joint but the 'normal' knee. The radiographs showed advanced osteoarthrosis, of equal degree in medial and lateral compartments, far beyond what could possibly occur at that age accepting, in the circumstances of arthrodesis, increased wear-and-tear on the normal side (see long-leg arthropathy, Ch. 10). Such gross radiological osteoarthrosis, in the absence of deformity, could not other than be associated with ablation of the epiphyses; and the only explanation offered was that the premature operative closure of the epiphyses had resulted in an abnormal blood supply to the articular cartilage with resulting destruction. This early experience aroused suspicion that epiphyseal ablation, and possibly the stapling operation, as applied to a normal joint, might not be innocent in the long term.

The follow-up to adult life of cases stapled for inequality of leg length or for genu valgum showed a high percentage (18 out of 24 knees) in the latter group with radiological evidence of osteoarthrosis on the side of the stapling (Chen, 1970). This finding, not previously reported, is a further warning that the operation of epiphyseal stapling should not be undertaken without due regard for the possible consequences in both the short and long term.

## REFERENCES

ABRAHAM, E., VERINDER, D. G. R. & SHARRARD, W. J. W. (1977). The treatment of flexion contracture of the knee in myelomeningocele. *Journal of Bone and Joint Surgery*, **59B**, 433.

ARKIN, A. M. & KATZ, J. F. (1956). The effects of pressure on epiphyseal growth. *Journal of Bone and Joint Surgery*, **38A**, 1056.

ARNEIL, G. C., McKILLIGAN, H. R. & LOBO, E. (1965). Malnutrition in Glasgow children. *Scottish Medical Journal*, **10**, 480.

BAILEY, J. A. (1970). Orthopaedic Aspects of achondroplasia. *Journal of Bone and Joint Surgery*, **52A**, 1285.

BATESON, E. M. (1966). Non-rachitic bow leg and knock-knee deformities in young Jamaican children. *British Journal of Radiology*, **39**, 92.

BATESON, E. M. (1968). The relationship between Blount's disease and bow legs. *British Journal of Radiology*, **41**, 107.

BENSON, P. F., STROUD, C. E., MITCHELL, N. J., NICOLAIDES, A. (1963). Rickets in immigrant children in London. *British Medical Journal*, **i**, 1054.

BLOUNT, W. P. (1937). Tibia vara. *Journal of Bone and Joint Surgery*, **19,** 1.

BLOUNT, W. P. & CLARKE, G. R. (1949). Control of bone growth by epiphyseal stapling. *Journal of Bone and Joint Surgery*, **31A,** 464.

BRETT, A. L. (1935). Operative correction of genu recurvatum. *Journal of Bone and Joint Surgery*, **17,** 984.

BRUNELLI, G. (1969). Trapezoidal Z osteotomy in static arthrosis of the knee. *Onzième Congrès International de Cherurgie Orthopédique et de Traumatologie,*Mexico.

CHEN, S. C. (1970). Long-term results of stapling of the knee. *Proceedings of the Royal Society of Medicine*, **63,** 755.

CLARK, J. M. P. (1956). Muscle and tendon transposition in poliomyelitis. In *Modern Trends in Orthopaedics* (Second Series), pp. 116–143. Edited by H. Platt. London: Butterworth.

CURTIS, B. H. & FISHER, R. L. (1969). Congenital hyperextension of the knee. *Journal of Bone and Joint Surgery*, **2,** 255–269.

DUNNIGAN, M. G., PATON, J. P., HEASE, S., McNICOL, G. W., GARDINER, M. D., SMITH, C. M. (1962). Late rickets and osteomalacia in the Pakistani community in Glasgow. *Scottish Medical Journal*, **7,** 159.

EGGERS, G. W. N. (1952). Transplantation of hamstring tendons to femoral condyles in order to improve hip extension and decrease knee flexion in cerebral spastic paralysis. *Journal of Bone and Joint Surgery*, **34A,** 827.

ERLACHER, P. (1922). Deformierende Prozesse der Epiphysengegend bei Kindern. *Archiv für orthopädische und Unfall-Chirurgie*, **20,** 81.

FINDER, J. G. (1964). Congenital hyperextension of the knee. *Journal of Bone and Joint Surgery*, **46B,** 4, 783.

GOLDING, J. S. R., BATESON, E. M., McNEIL-SMITH, G. J. D. (1969). *The Growth Plate and its Disorders*, p. 109. Edited by Mercer Rang. Edinburgh: E. & S. Livingstone.

GREEN, W. T. & ANDERSON, M. (1970). Epiphyseal arrest for unequal leg lengths. *Journal of Bone and Joint Surgery*, **52B,** 776.

HOLT, J. F., LATOURETTE, H. B. & WATSON, E. H. (1954). Physiological bowing of the legs in young children. *Journal of the American Medical Association*, **154,** 390.

HUBNER, L. (1961). Fortscher. *Roentgen*, **94,** 940.

KEATS, S. (1970). *Operative Orthopedics in Cerebral Palsy*. Springfield, Illinois: Thomas.

KESSEL, L. (1969). Quoted in *The Growth Plate and its Disorders*. Edited by Mercer Rang. Edinburgh: E. & S. Livingstone.

KESSEL, L. (1970). Annotations on the etiology and treatment of tibia vara. *Journal of Bone and Joint Surgery*, **52B,** 93.

KINGSBERY, H. C. (1965). *Torsion of the Legs in Young Children*. Read at the Annual Meeting of the Ohio State Orthopaedic Society.

LANGENSKIOLD, A. (1952). Tibia vara. *Acta chirurgica scandinavica*, **103,** 1.

LAURENCE, M. (1967). Genu recurvatum congenitum. *Journal of Bone and Joint Surgery*, **49B,** 1, 121.

LEXER, E. (1931). *Die gesamte Wiederherstellungschirurgie zugleich*, 2 Anfl. Leipzig: Johann Ambrosius Barth.

LLOYD-ROBERTS, G. C. & LETTIN, A. W. F. (1970).

Arthrogryposis multiplex congenita. *Journal of Bone and Joint Surgery*, **52B,** 3, 494.

McFARLAND, B. L. (1929). Congenital dislocation of the knee. *Journal of Bone and Joint Surgery*, **11,** 281.

McFARLAND, B. (1931). Traumatic arrest of epiphyseal growth of the lower end of the tibia. *British Journal of Surgery*, **19,** 78.

MARESH, M. M. (1943). Growth of major long bones in healthy children. *American Journal of Diseases of Children*, **66,** 227.

MIDDLETON, D. S. (1935). The pathology of congenital genu recurvatum. *British Journal of Surgery*, **22,** 696–702.

MORELAND, M. S. (1975). Morphologic effects of torsion applied to growing bone. *Journal of Bone and Joint Surgery*, **57A,** 569.

MORLEY, A. J. M. (1957). Knock-knee in children. *British Medical Journal*, **2,** 976.

PIERCE, D. S., WALLACE, W. M. & HERNDON, C. H. (1964). Long-term treatment of vitamin-D resistant rickets. *Journal of Bone and Joint Surgery*, **46A,** 5, 978.

PHEMISTER, D. B. (1933). Operative arrestment of longitudinal growth of bones in the treatment of deformities. *Journal of Bone and Joint Surgery*, **15,** 1.

POIRIER, H. (1968). Epiphysial stapling and leg equalisation. *Journal of Bone and Joint Surgery*, **50B,** 1, 61.

RANG, M. (1969). *The Growth Plate and its Disorders*. Edinburgh: E. & S. Livingstone.

SALENIUS, P. & VANKKA, E. (1975). The development of the tibiofemoral angle in children. *Journal of Bone and Joint Surgery*, **57A,** 259.

SALTER, R. B. & HARRIS, W. R. (1969). *The Growth Plate and its Disorders*. Edinburgh: E. & S. Livingstone.

SCHROCK, R. D. Jr. (1969). Peroneal nerve palsy following derotation osteotomies for tibial torsion. *Clinical Orthopaedics and Related Research*, **62,** 172.

SHOPFBER, C. E. & COIN, C. G. (1969). Genu varus and valgus in children. *Radiology*, **92,** 723.

SILVERMAN, F. N. (1970). Recovery from epiphyseal invagination: sequel to an unusual complication of scurvy. *Journal of Bone and Joint Surgery*, **52A,** 2, 384–390.

SMILLIE, I. S. & TURNER, M. S. (1979). The influence of tibial torsion on the pathology of the knee joint. *1st Congress of the International Society of the Knee*, April 24–27, Lyon, France.

STAMP, W. G., WHITESIDES, T. E., FIELD, M. H. & SHEER, G. E. (1964). Treatment of vitamin-D resistant rickets. *Journal of Bone and Joint Surgery*, **46A,** 5, 965.

STEARNS, G. (1964). A guide to the adequacy of therapy in resistant rickets due to familial or essential hypophosphatemia. *Journal of Bone and Joint Surgery*, **46A,** 5, 959.

STERN, M. B. (1968). Congenital dislocation of the knee. *Clinical Orthopaedics and Related Research*, **61,** 26, 261–268.

TAPIA, J., STEARNS, G. & PONSETI, I. V. (1964). Vitamin-D resistant rickets. *Journal of Bone and Joint Surgery*, **46A,** 5, 935.

TAYLOR, S. L. (1963). Tibial overgrowth: a cause of genu valgum. *Journal of Bone and Joint Surgery*, **45A,** 659.

WYNNE-DAVIES, R. (1964). Talipes equinovarus. *Journal of Bone and Joint Surgery*, **46B,** 3, 464.

# 9. Angular Deformity: Adult

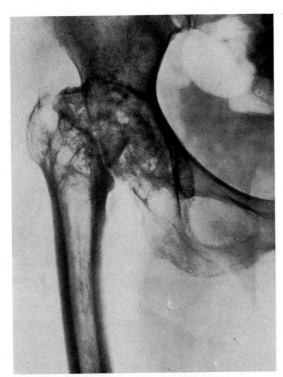

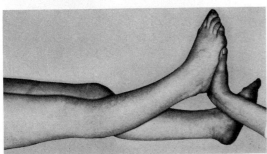

Figs 9,1–2. **Angular deformity of epiphyseal origin.** This patient suffered tuberculosis of the right hip in early childhood (Fig. 9,1). Prolonged immobilisation in the supine position during growth exerted pressure on the anterior aspect of the upper tibial epiphysis and resulted in recurvatus deformity on maturity (Fig. 9,2). Note exaggerated screw-home movement characteristic of genu recurvatum.

Genu recurvatum, valgum or varum of epiphyseal origin is readily corrected by opening-wedge osteotomy. Operation should not be undertaken until hip deformity has been eliminated) Figs 9,3 to 9,7).

## MALFORMATION OF EPIPHYSES

### Tibia

**Aetiology.** A pathological process which over a period of time and particularly a period of rapid growth, exerts pressure on one aspect of the epiphyseal plates about the knee, and thus invariably relaxes pressure on the opposite aspect, is responsible for angular deformity in the mature state. Thus any pathological process which demands recumbency creates such a situation; and in the immediate past tuberculosis of the hip (Figs 9,1 to 9,7) or spine were the obvious examples. Recumbency in the supine position produced genu recurvatum, weight-bearing with adduction deformity of the hip produced genu valgum. There are, however, a multiplicity of other conditions which may be responsible and these include within the experience on which this section is based, major trauma, poliomyelitis, Perthes disease, slipped upper femoral epiphysis, systemic bone disease and even such minor mechanical defects as the loss of a great toe in youth.

In so far as the chronic hip diseases of childhood are most often responsible it is important that deformity of the hip be corrected and the neutral position attained before correction of angular deformity of the knee is considered.

The following are examples:

Case 1. This patient (M.G., female, aged 17) suffered at the age of 9 from a grossly destructive tuberculous infection of the left hip for which she had undergone two unsuccessful extra-articular arthrodesis operations, followed by an intra-articular arthrodesis before bony ankylosis was attained. Finally, at the age of 15 an osteotomy was performed to correct an adduction deformity (Fig. 9,3). The problem, at the age of 17, was the shortening of the limb and the genu valgum (Figs 9,4 and 9,5) made more evident by correction of the hip adduction. When the unsightly deformity of the knee had been

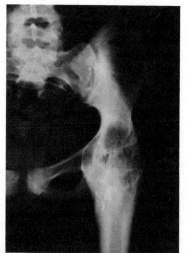

FIG. 9,3

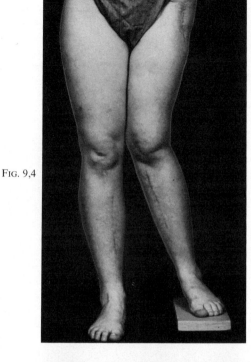

FIG. 9,4

FIG. 9,5

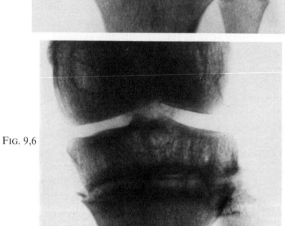

FIG. 9,6

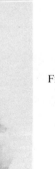

FIG. 9,7

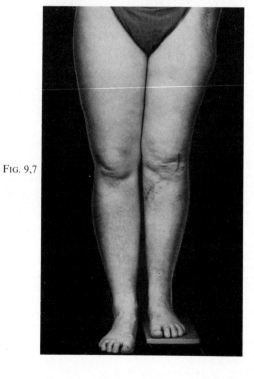

FIGS 9,3–7. Angular deformity of epiphyseal origin. This patient suffered tuberculosis of the left hip at age 9. It was not until age 15 that arthrodesis in neutral position was achieved (Fig. 9,3). At age 17 she presented with valgus angulation and shortening (Figs 9,4 and 9,5). The deformity was corrected by opening-wedge osteotomy within flare of the tibia (Fig. 9,6) with correction of the deformity and reduction of the shortening (Fig. 9,7). (M.G., female, aged 17, see text.)

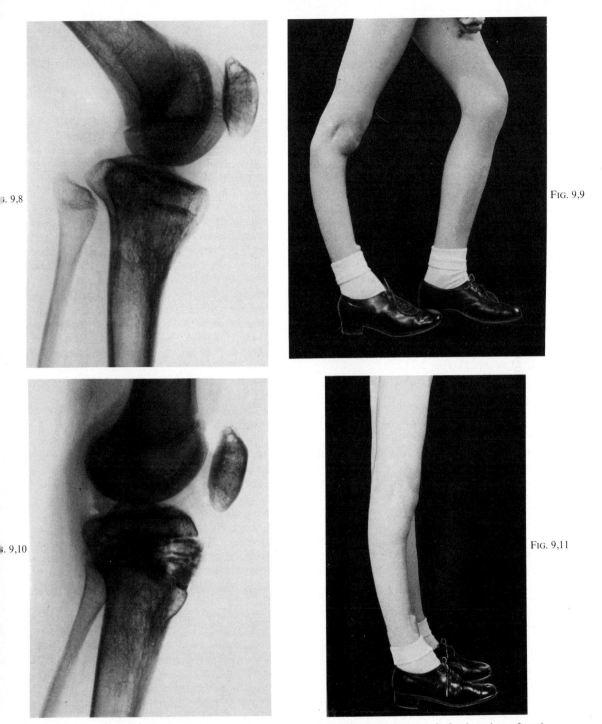

FIG. 9,8

FIG. 9,9

FIG. 9,10

FIG. 9,11

FIGS 9,8–11. **Angular deformity of epiphyseal origin.** Premature closure of the anterior aspect of the upper tibial epiphysis (Fig. 9,8) resulting in a gross recurvatus deformity (Fig. 9,9) was the result of prolonged bed rest in the supine position. The deformity corrected by anterior opening-wedge osteotomy and the insertion of wedge-shaped grafts taken from the iliac crest (Fig. 9,10) and the resulting correction of the deformity (Fig. 9,11). (G.B., female, aged 12, see text.)

corrected (Figs 9,6 and 9,7) she elected to defer the question of equalisation of the leg lengths.

Case 2. The patient (G.B., female) suffered, at the age of 10, an open fracture at the lower end of the tibia in a bomb explosion. There was considerable loss of soft tissue and bone, necessitating a pedicle skin graft and an inlay bone graft at a later date. When her treatment was almost completed she sustained a high supracondylar fracture of the femur in a further accident. Although anatomical reduction was attained in both fractures, she was noted a year later to have acquired a marked genu recurvatum referable to the upper tibial epiphysis (Figs 9,8 and 9,9). It was presumed that the prolonged immobilisation necessitated by the two fractures had produced abnormal stresses which had caused the anterior portion of the epiphysis to close. The deformity was corrected by anterior opening wedge osteotomy (Fig. 9,10) and the result achieved (Fig. 9,11).

## Treatment

Linear osteotomy of the tibial head with correction of angulation by opening-wedge at a site between the tibial tubercle and joint surface is an operation applicable to recurvatus, valgus and varus deformities, and combination of the former with one of the latter, resulting from malformation of the epiphysis occurring in the course of growth. The operation is the basis of the opening- and closing-wedge osteotomies now applied to a variety of conditions and in particular to the angular deformity of osteoarthrosis (Ch. 10).

**Background note.** The original description of the opening-wedge osteotomy in English is attributed to Brett (1935) who recorded a case in which genu recurvatum, the result of poliomyelitis, was corrected by division of the tibia above the level of the tubercle. He stated that the technique used was similar to that suggested by Lexer (1931) with whose work he was not familiar at the time.

TECHNIQUE OF OPERATION. The operation is performed under the control of a tourniquet. The position of choice is right-angled flexion, over the end of the operating-table, as for meniscectomy. The flexed position is favoured in that the posterior capsule and related vessels are relaxed and thus less vulnerable to accidental injury. The relaxation of the collateral ligaments is an aid to the correction of varus or valgus deformity. The incision, which should be made with the joint extended, depends on the angulation to be corrected. A simple varus or valgus deformity can be corrected through a short vertical linear incision on the appropriate side of the patellar tendon. Deformity with a large element of recurvatus requires access on both sides. This can be achieved through a curved transverse incision, the so-called lazy S, which begins on the lateral side of the patella, crosses the mid-line over the tendon and is continued down the antero-medial aspect of the tibia for a short distance (Fig. 9,7). The operation for recurvatus will be described as requiring exposure of both condyles. When the skin flaps have been raised, vertical incisions are made on either side of the tendon and both condyles exposed extracapsulary and subperiosteally. Neither tibial tubercle nor patellar tendon are detached. The osteotomy is performed between the attachment of the tendon and the joint surface behind and within the compass of the tendon. A site is selected about 1 cm below the joint line and parallel to the articular surface. The joint must not be entered. If there is any doubt about orientation, as there may be in the presence of deformity, a guidewire should be inserted in the line of proposed division and radiographs obtained. When the exact direction has been determined fine-bladed osteotomes about 2·5 cm broad are inserted on either side of the patellar tendon and driven backwards as far as but not through the posterior cortex. When the various cuts have been joined a transverse linear osteotomy will have been accomplished. Levers are inserted on either side of the tendon and the upper fragment elevated to correct the angulation by opening-wedge. The correction is maintained by wedge-shaped grafts normally taken from the ilium and inserted in the manner described in detail later in this chapter. In the case of a child, or the wish to avoid scarring, banked-bone or grafts taken from a parent may be considered.

In the majority of cases, particularly if the opposite cortex is intact, the wedge-grafts will be under compression and the osteotomy stable. This should be tested with the joint in extension. If doubt exists staples may be inserted and/or the after-treatment modified accordingly.

(For further details of technique see description of similar procedures performed for other varieties of angular deformity later in this chapter and in Ch. 10.)

*After-treatment.* If the osteotomy is stable and displacement unlikely a compression bandage is applied in the outer layers of the posterior aspect of which are incorporated plaster slabs. The patient is nursed in a half-ring Thomas bed-knee splint. At the end of three weeks, when the stitches are removed, the limb is returned to the bed-knee splint, 1 or 2 kg of traction are applied and active knee flexion encouraged. If stability is in doubt greater caution is observed with an increased interval, say eight weeks, before permitting flexion exercises. Weight-bearing, with the aid of crutches, is not permitted in less than 12 weeks.

**Results of operation.** This is an operation performed in young subjects with a gross disability of form and function. It is the author's experience that results are gratifying in the extreme. There is a dramatic change in the appearance of the limb and, with the patella located at a lower level, marked improvement in power and security. In addition, as a result of the opening-wedge, there is an increase in the length of the limb of 1 to 2 cm (Figs 9,3 to 9,7).

### Genu Valgum

The approach to the lateral aspect of the lateral tibial condyle normally poses problems from the presence of the superior tibio-fibular joint, head of fibula and lateral popliteal nerve. The opening-wedge osteotomy, such as is applicable in this age range, can usually be performed above the flare of the tibia and thus above the tibio-fibular joint (Figs 9,3 to 9,7). The lateral ligament is likely to be lax prior to operation and rendered taut after the introduction of the wedge grafts. If the deformity is gross and the tibio-fibular joint misplaced resection of the head of the fibula may be necessary to gain access to the osteotomy site. This is accomplished in the manner described in Chapter 10.

**Patella: patella baja.** Genu recurvatum is normally associated with patella alta—the genu recurvatum/patella alta complex. Normally there is an advantage, a bonus of osteotomy, that the patella is brought down to a lower level, and, at a greater distance from the centre of rotation, an increase in the power of the quadriceps results. When the recurvatus is the result of anterior poliomyelitis, the quadriceps may have been paralysed during a period of rapid growth. In such circumstances the patella will be located at an abnormally low level. Consideration may require to be given to lengthening of the tendon in order to maintain a reasonable relationship of the patella to the femoral condyles.

### Femur

The extensive curved surfaces of the femoral condyles, opposed to horizontal surfaces of the tibial condyles, ensure a wide distribution of compression forces in the femur and explain the relative absence of angular deformity arising in the femur in the course of growth.

This is fortunate from the viewpoint of operative measures because osteotomy by necessity at a greater distance from the joint surface, and at a greater depth, is less easy to perform and the correction, with a mobile joint immediately inferior, less easy to maintain than osteotomy of the tibia. Nevertheless, if deformity originates in the femur corrective osteotomy must be performed in the femur (Figs 9,12 to 9,15). A variety of procedures are available:

1. The most stable type of simple osteotomy, not involving internal fixation, is performed in the supracondylar region. It should not be performed too close to the joint in order to obtain control of the lower fragment in the post-operative plaster cast.

The femur is approached from the lateral side through the ilio-tibial tract. A short incision is made in the periosteum and elevators inserted one in front and one behind the bone. Multiple drill holes are made in the cortex in the form of a 'V', apex downwards, and the holes joined with cuts from an osteotome. The femur is then fractured and the deformity corrected (Fig. 9,13). It will be appreciated that angulation only, and not rotation, can be corrected by such means. The shape and irregularity of the opposing

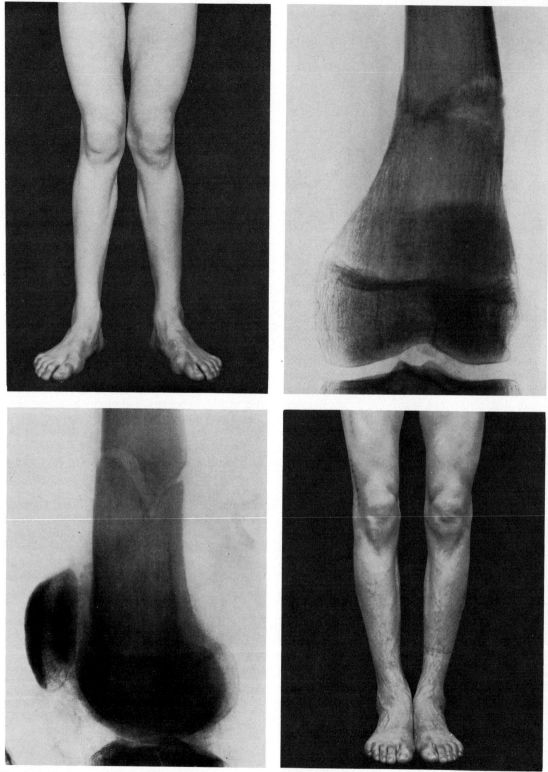

FIGS 9,12–15. **Genu valgum: treatment.** Angular deformity persisting into maturity may demand correction. Genu valgum (Fig. 9,12) treated by supracondylar V osteotomy through multiple drill holes (Fig. 9,13). The correction achieved (Fig. 9,14) and the clinical result six months later (Fig. 9,15) (K.G., male, aged 17, case of J.H.).

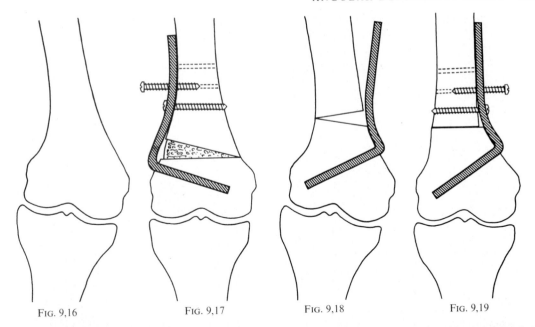

FIG. 9,16          FIG. 9,17          FIG. 9,18          FIG. 9,19

FIGS 9,16–19. **Angular deformity: supracondylar osteotomy.** In the mature subject supracondylar osteotomy demands internal fixation to attain stability particularly if rotation is to be corrected. Opening-wedge osteotomy with the insertion of a wedge-shaped iliac graft restores the length of the limb (Figs 9,16 and 9,17). Closing-wedge osteotomy with removal of a wedge of bone is less difficult to execute (Figs 9,18 and 9,19).

fragments maintain stability in the presence of a post-operative plaster cast in the form of a full-length hip spica including the pelvis and foot.

The cast is retained for a minimum of eight weeks. A longer period may be required in the mature subject (Figs 9,12 to 9,15).

2. If the simple 'V' osteotomy described above is reasonably stable and the correction relatively easy to maintain it has the disadvantage that it does not permit correction of rotational deformity in addition to angulation. If it is necessary to correct rotation before the growth plate has closed, the osteotomy should be performed through a transverse row of drill holes which then permits correction of rotation as well as angulation. It will be evident that accurate control of a situation involving rotation and angulation in two planes is difficult. Control of the upper fragment in so far as rotation is concerned can be achieved by driving a stout Steinmann pin horizontally into the femur in the region of the greater trochanter. The pin permits the degree of rotational correction to be estimated at the time of operation. The pin is incorporated in the padded plaster cast applied at the termination of the operation and which must include the pelvis and foot.

3. In the mature subject the problem of control of the small inferior fragment and the wish to avoid prolonged immobilisation in a plaster cast may determine the use of internal fixation which permits either opening- or closing-wedge osteotomies to be performed (Figs 9,16 to 9,19).

## HERITABLE DISORDERS OF CONNECTIVE TISSUE

Care must be taken to distinguish genu recurvatum of soft tissue origin from that arising in the course of growth in the epiphyses. Generalized laxity of capsular ligaments is a feature of such inherited diseases of connective tissue as Marfan's syndrome, the Ehlers-Danlos syndrome, and osteogenesis imperfecta. In the knee the common resulting angular deformity is recurvatus (Fig. 9,20). Radiographs in such circumstances show the lower end of the femur and upper end of the tibia to be of normal

P·

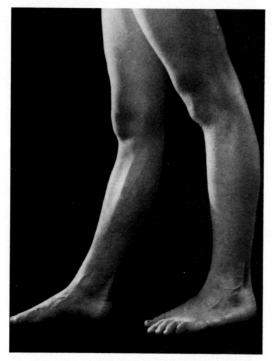
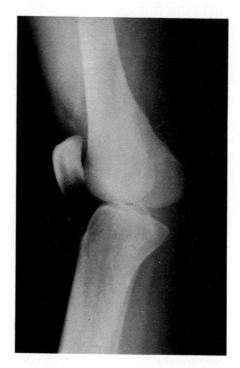

FIGS 9,20–21. **Genu recurvatum not of epiphyseal origin.** There are traps for the unwary in the interpretation of recurvatus deformity. In this example of marked degree (Fig. 9,20), it is seen that the cause is laxity of the posterior capsule (Fig. 9,21), in this case from heritable disease of connective tissue short of the Marfan or Ehlers-Danlos syndromes. There is no deformity of the tibial head and no patella alta (Fig. 9,21).

conformation but in abnormal relationship in the form of a gap posteriorly (Fig. 9,21). An operation on a bone of normal conformation is contraindicated as likely to produce unpredictable mechanical repercussions. In any event if, in the Ehlers-Danlos syndrome, it is decided that surgery is indicated it should be remembered that wound dehiscence is common. The tissues are friable and sutures tend to cut-out. In addition, haemostases may be a problem.

No operation has been practised on deformity arising in a heritable disorder of connective tissue. The only treatment prescribed has been the raising of the heels of the shoes to control hyperextension.

## ANGULAR DEFORMITY OF TRAUMATIC ORIGIN

This volume is concerned with disease as opposed to injury. Osteoarthrosis is, by and large, the result of the trauma of overuse, or wear-and-tear, as opposed to single-incident trauma. Nevertheless, a high proportion of unilateral examples in young adult males with symptoms of pain and/or instability are related to an unrecognised, misdiagnosed or maltreated fracture of the medial or sometimes of both tibial condyles.

Fractures of the medial condyle are relatively uncommon: the inner side of the knee is protected from varus strain by the opposite leg. When fracture occurs it is by some unusual mechanism; and thus may be missed. The common fault is failure to recognise the importance of the injury in terms of end-result and potential for disability by comparison with the much more common fracture of the lateral condyle in which the prognosis, even with considerable displacement, is good. The outcome of injury in the two condyles cannot be compared.

In fractures of both condyles the most common error is failure to maintain reduction in the absence of continuous traction, and of weight-bearing before healing is complete resulting in depression of the medial condyle.

Symptoms of osteoarthrosis as a result of derangement of joint mechanics are not confined to old fractures of the medial condyle but occur after any fracture of the upper third of the tibia which has united with varus angulation (Fig. 9,22) and/or medial rotation (Fig. 9,23). If it is the general rule that osteotomy should be performed at the site of maximum deformity it may be technically easier and safer to alter the weight-bearing alignment within the vascular

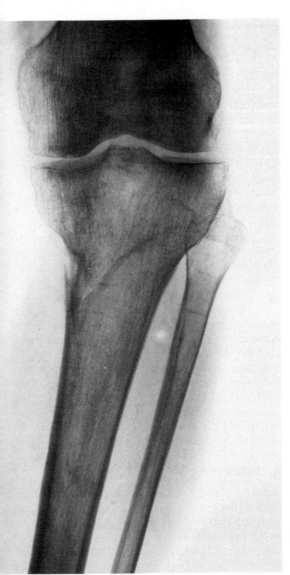

FIG. 9,22. **Angular deformity: adult.** This malunited sub-condylar fracture producing angular deformity of gross degree can be reduced and deformity eliminated by opening-wedge osteotomy within the flare of the tibia.

Minimal downward displacement of the weight-bearing medial condyle interferes with the screw-home movement and particularly with gliding action; and worse, results in overlengthening of the medial ligament with instability comparable to total rupture. Perfect anatomical reduction must be achieved to attain a return of function of acceptable degree.

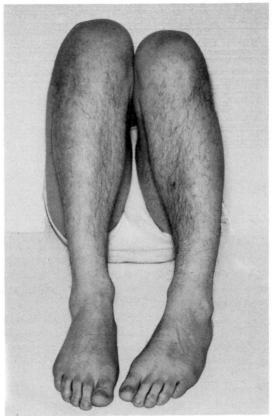

FIG. 9,23. **Angular deformity: adult.** This malunited fracture of the tibia with angular deformity, shortening and gross medial torsion, can be reduced, and in so far as medial torsion is concerned, by derotation osteotomy below the tibial tubercle. In this case the normal leg had 22° of lateral torsion. On the left side it was 3° of lateral torsion. The torsional deformity requiring reduction is therefore more than 20°.

cancellous tissue of the flare of the tibia than at the site of the deformity lower down where the skin may have been damaged in the original injury and the blood supply of the bone suspect.

## Depression of Medial Condyle of Tibia: Clinical Features

There are four principal sources of complaint:
1. **Pain.** The site of pain is the medial compartment and of a type associated with local osteoarthrosis or of a horizontal cleavage lesion of the meniscus.
2. **Instability.** A minimal depression of the medial condyle produces overlengthening of the all-important medial ligament by the extent of the depression at the periphery of the condyle. The instability related to 1 cm of depression is considerable. This may be a contributary factor in the presence of a torn meniscus.
3. **Angular deformity.** The deformity takes the form of varus and is usually of a degree noticeable to the patient by comparison with the normal leg.
4. **Loss of movement.** There is frequently minimal loss of extension in so far as the mechanism of the screw-home movement is deranged. Flexion is frequently limited in gross examples to a right-angle.

## Indications for Treatment

The biomechanical status of the joint as a result of overlengthening of the medial ligament is such that conservative measures in the form of quadriceps redevelopment is likely to be of no more than marginal benefit. The temptation to correct such an apparently local deformity by the insertion of a hemiprosthesis should be resisted. The operation will fail and in the failure create circumstances which cannot be overcome other than by arthrodesis. The situation can be restored only by altering the weight-bearing alignment and in so doing securing a return of the control of the medial ligament.

Restoration of the articular surface will not be followed by an increase in range of motion. Right-angled flexion or thereabouts is compatible with reasonable function and acceptable on social grounds. A lesser range constitutes a contraindication to operation.

## Principles of Treatment

Reconstruction does not aim at isolation of the depressed fragment, which at this stage would be technically impossible, but the raising of the depressed condyle as a whole so that the instability inherent in overlengthening of the medial ligament is restored. The state of the articular surface is not as depicted in the radiographs. A congruous surface of fibrous tissue or fibrocartilage, and related to the residual range of motion, has been established and forms the basis of the restoration.

**Beware scars.** The antero-medial aspect of the tibial head is sparsely covered with skin and, in the male, without subcutaneous fat. If previous operations have been carried out as in fractures there will be a vertical scar or scars. An opening-wedge osteotomy will place the scar under tension and make the skin difficult to close. Experience has shown that healing is slow and it may be prudent not to inspect the wound for removal of the sutures until three weeks have elapsed. If there is a tight vertical, broad or adherent medial scar an opening-wedge osteotomy may be unwise before the scar has been excised and the skin mobilised rather than risk breakdown of the wound and the risk of infection of the joint.

## Technique of Operation

The knee, under the control of a tourniquet, is flexed over the end of the table as for meniscectomy. This position, as opposed to extension, relaxes the posterior capsule and related vessels and reduces the risks should the posterior cortex be penetrated by an osteotome. The joint and medial condyle are approached through a downward extension of the incision used for meniscectomy. This particular operation is the exception to the rule that intra-articular and extra-articular procedures should not be undertaken simultaneously. The exception is condoned on the grounds that the meniscus must be excised. It is usually damaged, but in any event removal is necessary for inspection of the articular surface and in order to obtain the maximum reduction in extension.

The appearance of the articular surface, healed by fibrous tissue, is less alarming than the impression conveyed by the radiograph. The problem is one of angulation downwards, forwards and medially. The deformed condyle is stripped of periosteum on the antero-medial surface proceeding beneath the medial ligament but not further in order to preserve the maximum blood supply. The osteotomy is performed within the flare of the tibia. Even if the fracture has extended downwards into the shaft the osteotomy is performed in the broad area within the flare; and unless this is done there is no bone below to support the wedge-shaped grafts which will be required to maintain reduction. The osteotomy proceeds towards the posterior cortex and then across the mid-line into the lateral condyle. It is important that it be incomplete, that is to say, that the cortex opposite to the point of maximum deformity is not divided. It will be found that by proceeding cautiously a wedge-shaped opening reducing the deformity can be produced by gently levering the articular surface upwards. Some overcorrection is desirable if it can be achieved in so far as some loss of correction can be anticipated from the compression of cancellous tissue. Into this opening are introduced wedge-shaped grafts cut from the whole thickness of the ilium and inserted so that the inner and outer tables accept the compression strain. The spaces between the grafts are filled with cancellous chip (Figs 9,26 to 9,29).

**Iliac grafts: technique.** To obtain the grafts an incision some 10 to 15 cm in length is made over the iliac crest and deepened down to bone. The muscles are stripped from the crest for a distance of some 10 cm and from the inner and outer tables by blunt dissection using an elevator to a depth of about 8 to 10 cm from the crest. Broad-bladed retractors are inserted on either side and three wedge-shaped grafts are cut taking the whole thickness of the crest and both tables. The wedges are of different size. The base of the largest, to be used at the point of maximum correction, will be 2 to 3 cm. The two smaller, one from either side, say 1·5 to 2 cm. A further graft or grafts and/or cancellous tissue are removed if required. Suction drainage is installed and the wound closed (Figs 9,24 and 9,25).

INTRODUCTION OF GRAFTS. A graft of predetermined size is introduced at the site of maximum deformity, anterior, antero-medial or medial as determined by the individual problem.

When the wedge has been inserted at the maximum site of correction the medial ligament and capsule should be taut. It will no longer be possible to gain access to the posterior aspect

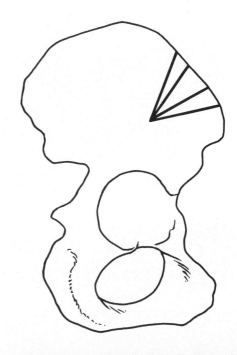

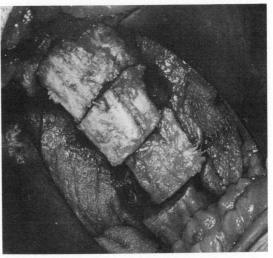

FIGS 9,24–25. **Opening-wedge osteotomy.** Diagrams to show the site and means of obtaining the wedge-shaped grafts from the iliac crest.

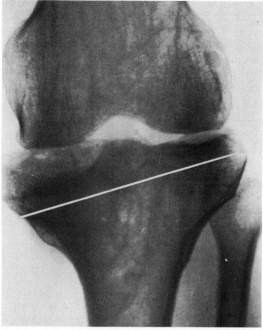

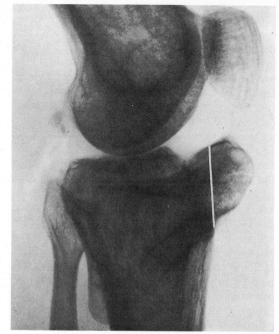

Fig. 9,26

Fig. 9,27

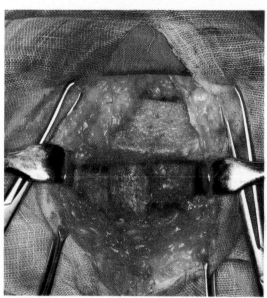

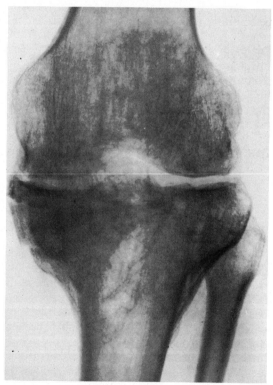

Fig. 9,28

Fig. 9,29

Figs 9,26–29. **Angular deformity of traumatic origin.** Depressed fracture of medial condyle of tibia of six years duration in which a fragment has been extruded anteriorly. The presenting symptoms were instability and loss of extension. The pre-operative radiographs with the direction of the opening wedge (Fig. 9,26). When there is a large anterior projection opening a wedge on the antero-medial aspect brings the projection against the femoral condyle. In such circumstances it is required to be reduced in height and in anterior projection. When this is necessary the bone should be removed prior to the linear osteotomy of the tibial head in so far as when the osteotomy has been performed the upper fragment is unstable, increasing the amount of force required to remove bone and thus increasing the risk of a fracture into the joint (Fig. 9,27). The anterior projection has been reduced in the manner indicated in Figure 9,27, the opening wedge completed and the iliac grafts introduced (Fig. 9,28). The reduction achieved to show site and size of wedge graft (Fig. 9,29). (S. el A., male, aged 56.)

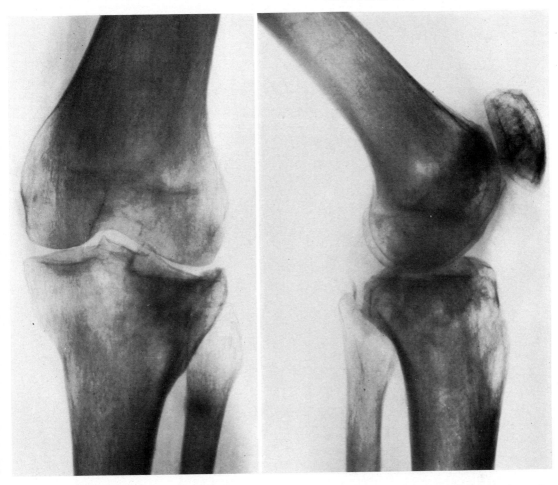

FIGS 9,30–31. **Angular deformity of traumatic origin: timing of operation.** Radiographs of patient who eight months previously sustained a depressed fracture of the lateral condyle of the tibia. It was subjected to operation and internal fixation and the application of a plaster cast four weeks later. The means of internal fixation, of variety unknown, had been removed.

When examined her complaint was of loss of flexion which was limited to 50° and the appearance produced by the 15° valgus angulation.

This deformity can be corrected by opening-wedge osteotomy as described in the text. But note loss of blood supply of central portion of tibial table. Operation, demanded on cosmetic grounds, must be deferred until right-angled flexion has been achieved and until such time as the blood supply has been restored (F.B., female, aged 54, case of L.C.).

of the osteotomy and an unfilled space will exist at the termination of the operation. In anticipation of this situation any small fragments of bone which have become available in the course of operation, or in the preparation of the grafts, should be placed in the space posterior to the ligament before the graft makes access impossible. The resulting reduction should be stable splinted by the patellar tendon and the now taut medial ligament. If stability has not been achieved one or more staples may be inserted which encompass and prevent extrusion of the grafts.

*After-treatment.* At the termination of operation a compression bandage is applied with the knee in a position short of full extension. In the outer layers are incorporated plaster slabs with the purpose of reducing movement to a minimum in

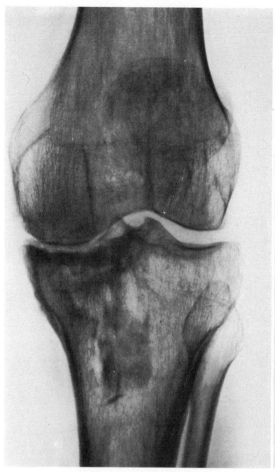 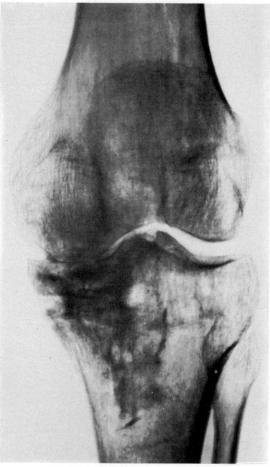

FIGS 9,32–33. **Angular deformity of traumatic origin: timing of operation.** In this case the origin of the mono-compartmental osteoarthrosis with instability and varus angulation was an old fracture of the medial condyle of the tibia which had been subjected to operation and internal fixation in the acute stage and to two further operations, one for the removal of a screw and one for the removal of the medial meniscus. Note aseptic necrosis of areas of bone in the medial condyle (Fig. 9,32).

It is important when a second osteotomy is necessary that the trabecular pattern has returned. To perform an osteotomy in the presence of local increase of density is not only difficult but hazardous. There is a danger of fracture into the joint to say nothing of the possibility of reducing the blood supply still further.

The knee eight months after opening-wedge osteotomy. It was pain free and stability had been restored (Fig. 9,33). (J.R.F., male, aged 42.)

the critical three weeks following operation. At this time the stitches are removed, skin traction applied and the limb placed on the Braun-type splint and active exercise practised against a gently distracting force. Healing of the vascular cancellous tissue of the tibial head can be expected to proceed rapidly, but weight-bearing should not be attempted in less than 12 weeks.

## Results of Operation

Patients in the age range which present with the problems outlined demand a high standard of function. If the results of operation are gratifying in the extreme in relation to the original problems presented they fall short of perfection. The range of flexion for example is not increased. The operation purports to achieve stability with return of confidence and reduction of pain. Perfection of function is unattainable.

**Re-operation.** In an old fracture of the medial condyle, in which the symptom imposed by the depression is instability from overlengthening of the medial ligament, the optimum improvement may not be achieved at the original operation. This is due to the fact that whereas complete stability in extension may be demonstrated at the termination of the operation the stability may not be maintained. This is due to some compression or absorption of cancellous tissue as a result of forces involved. In the young subject with a full range of movement, seeking optimum function, a second operation may be indicated. The timing of a second operation is of importance. In spite of the sense of urgency which such a situation imposes, it should not be undertaken until the bone grafts have disappeared and the normal trabecular pattern of the area is restored. A delay of 6 to 24 months may be necessary (Figs 9,30 to 9,33).

## ANGULAR DEFORMITY: OSTEOTOMY ON COSMETIC GROUNDS

### Indications for Treatment

In the young adult female subject a symptomless varus or valgus deformity, unilateral or bilateral, may be an indication for operation on cosmetic grounds. A cosmetic procedure should not be lightly undertaken. The standard of improvement of appearance anticipated by the patient may fall short of what is physically possible. In any event it should be explained that the operation cannot be accomplished without leaving a scar; and in addition, scars on the iliac crest or crests. In the most successful case it is a matter of exchanging the cosmetic disability of deformity for the cosmetic disability of scars. Furthermore, in the bilateral case, it should be explained that to undergo the first operation is to be committed to the second.

Finally, in an operation performed for cosmetic reasons, as opposed to the more realistic reasons of pain or loss of function, it should be remembered that opening-wedge osteotomy corrects varus; not rotation. The result can thus be disappointing from the cosmetic viewpoint if it has not been recognised that the more important deformity is torsion. The subtlety of the situation in terms of appearance, varus angulation which is obvious, as opposed to rotation which is contributing in major degree to the total effect, may not be obvious in simple mechanical terms to the patient.

In evidence of the occasional necessity for a purely cosmetic operation is cited the following case:

The patient, a female, aged 50, had a relatively minor unilateral valgus deformity of uncertain origin which had existed since youth. In middle age she became so obsessed with the appearance of the leg that she had not left her home for some three years. Such was her state of mind that when her doctor appealed for advice she refused to go to hospital for examination and required to be visited. The purpose of the consultation, to persuade her that she only was aware of the deformity, was unsuccessful. The justification for a major operative procedure, not without risks, did not deter her from demanding correction. In the circumstances the necessity for operation was accepted and achieved, by opening-wedge, the desired objective.

**Motivation.** It is important, in spite of the pressures imposed, that operation is not undertaken for cosmetic reasons without consideration of the possible consequences. It is a sad reflection on human nature, and particularly in this sex and age range, that even greater care in selection must be exercised in a 'free' medical service than in one requiring payment. In the latter circumstance it is unlikely, but not impossible, that such a formidable, time-consuming and expensive procedure is undertaken without the necessary will to recover. In the former, the operation can be too lightly undertaken with the responsibility for the outcome placed on the surgeon.

**Failure of operation.** The hazards which arise are illustrated by the following case:

A young woman, aged 22, was seen who had undergone osteotomies for a bilateral varus deformity. The original surgeon had made every effort to dissuade her from operation but she had become obsessed about the shape

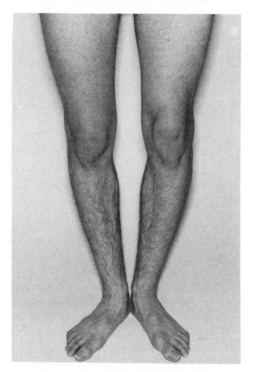

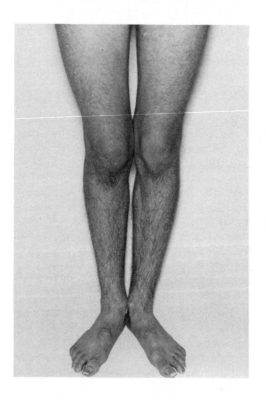

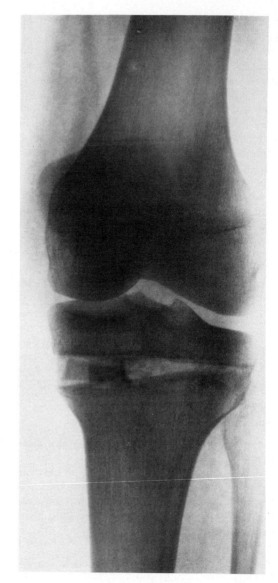

FIGS 9,34–36. **Angular and rotational deformity: opening-wedge osteotomy for cosmetic reasons.** This patient had the unusual combination of 10° varus angulation with lateral torsion of the tibia of 30° (Fig. 9,34). The angular deformity was corrected by bilateral opening-wedge osteotomies above the tibial tubercle (Fig. 9,35) and the result achieved (Fig. 9,36). The lateral torsion was not corrected (R.H., male, aged 17).

of her knees and he was eventually forced to undertake the corrections. Dome-shaped osteotomies were carried out with the desired cosmetic effect on the left side. On the right side however the corrected position had not been maintained in the plaster cast with recurrence of the original deformity. The general effect therefore was worse than that for which the original operation had been undertaken. The purpose of the consultation was to inquire whether a further operation to correct the defect was possible. After a suitable interval (see below) a linear opening-wedge operation was undertaken and was successful in restoring the symmetry of the knees at the cost of somewhat broad scars on both joints and a scar on one iliac crest.

There are three lessons to be learnt from this case:
1. There are hazards in cosmetic operations on both knees which aim at symmetry.
2. The choice of technique must reduce the risks of failure to a minimum. In theory the curved, cup or dome-shaped osteotomy is stable. In the author's view this method is more difficult than linear opening-wedge osteotomy (Figs 9,34 to 9,36) and has the great disadvantage, as far as stability is concerned, that it necessitates division of the opposing cortex.
3. If a second osteotomy is required to obtain further correction, as in this case, or following a fracture, it should not be undertaken until the blood supply of the area has returned to normal and the trabecular pattern is restored.

# NEUROGENIC ARTHROPATHY: CHARCOT JOINTS

**Background note.** It was the French neurologist Charcot (1868) who first described patients with locomotor ataxia who developed chronic painless swelling and instability in the knees and other joints.

## Pathological Anatomy

**Distribution.** The knee is the joint most commonly affected and presents in unilateral or bilateral form.

The loss of proprioceptive muscle sense and insensitivity to pain permits trauma to be inflicted on the opposing articular surfaces in the course of weight-bearing which would not otherwise take place. In time multiple osteoarticular fractures occur with production of loose bodies which may remain free or become embedded in the synovial membrane where there is a blood supply and thus may be responsible for the production of the new bone which is characteristic of the condition. Eventually marked destruction occurs with angular deformity and even dislocation of the bone ends. In gross examples the anterior aspect of the tibial head appears to be shorn off so that the femur is dislocated anteriorly producing shortening, angulation and instability (Figs 9,37 and 9,38).

## Clinical Features

The classical example occurs as a complication of tabes dorsalis. It is still the commonest condition in which Charcot joints are found. It presents as an affection of a single knee, but both knees, the hip, ankle and vertebral joints may be affected simultaneously. The arthropathy is not confined to late cases of untreated syphilis but occurs in a variety of conditions where pain sensation may be deficient, such as meningomyelocele, spinal cord and peripheral nerve injuries, leprosy, yaws and hereditary affections in which there may be insensitivity to pain; and, of course, diabetes. It is common experience that cases are encountered to which a cause can not be ascribed. In the current scene there is a variety attributable to repeated intra-articular injections of the corticosteroids.

The presenting clinical feature in most varieties of arthropathy is pain. In contradistinction, in neurogenic arthropathy the complaint is of loss of function from angular deformity, shortening and instability of a degree which may make even standing erect impossible (Figs 9,37 and 9,38).

## Treatment

The treatment of the neuropathic knee poses problems. The only operation applicable is an arthrodesis; and opinion differs as to the wisdom of undertaking the procedure in view of the frequency of complications and high rate of

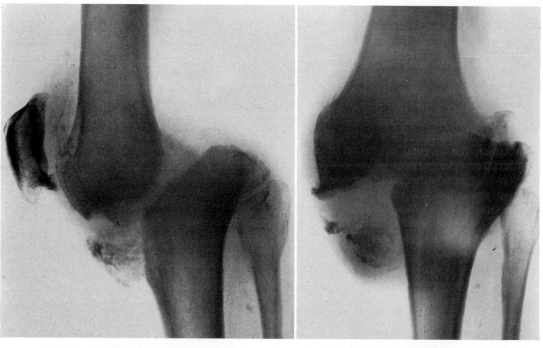

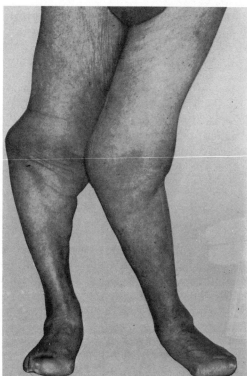

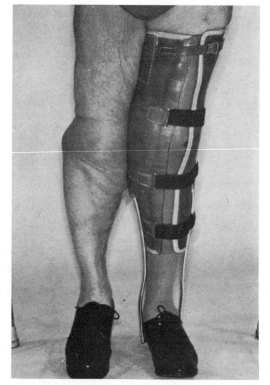

FIGS 9,37–40. **Neurogenic arthropathy:** Charcot joint. In this example, the result of tabes dorsalis from untreated syphilis, there was such gross angulation, shortening and instability that the patient could not stand. It will be seen that the anterior aspect of the head of the tibia is shorn-off permitting the femur to dislocate anteriorly. Note the presence of loose bodies, calcification and ossification (Figs 9,37 and 9,38) (J.L., male, aged 69).

In this bilateral example, the origin of which was not established, a block-leather caliper on the left side enabled ambulation to be maintained with the aid of tripod sticks (Figs 9,39 and 9,40) (case of K.L.G.M.).

failure of fusion. The circumstances of the single successful case recorded in Table 8 are not recalled. A further case is known (not included in Table 8) in which bilateral neuropathic knees fused without difficulty using the compression method. Technical problems relating to arthrodesis are elaborated under 'Arthrodesis', Chapter 6.

The treatment to be undertaken depends on the circumstances of the individual case. In that illustrated in Figures 9.37 and 9.38 for example,

the deformity was gross. The patient had the additional problem of a neuropathic spine and a related drop-foot. Accordingly it was decided that an attempt at arthrodesis should not be undertaken. A full length caliper was prescribed. In a neuropathic joint this appliance may normally take the form of a lacing corset-caliper. In the bilateral example illustrated a block-leather caliper was required in order to provide the necessary rigidity (Figs 9.39 and 9.40).

## REFERENCES

BRETT, A. L. (1935). Operative correction of genu recurvatum, *Journal of Bone and Joint Surgery*, **XVII**, 4, 984.

CHARCOT, J. M. (1868). Sur quelques arthropathies qui paraissent d'ependre d'une lésion du cerveau ou de la moelle épinière. *Arch. Physiol. Norm. Path.*, **1**, 161.

LEXER, E. (1931). *Die gesamte Wiederherstellungschirurgie zugleich*. 2. Aufl. Leipzig: Johann Ambrosius Barth.

# 10.  Angular Deformity: Aged

*'Old age doth in sharp pains abound.'*
Pierre Jean de Beranger (19th century French poet).

## OSTEOARTHROSIS

### Introduction

**Incidence.** The knee is affected by osteoarthrosis more frequently than any other joint. It is the most common condition, in the concept of disease rather than injury, for which advice is sought.

If angular deformity is not an essential feature of osteoarthrosis it is a common finding of widely varying degree in a high proportion of cases. In the circumstances it is thought reasonable to consider the condition under this convenient heading.

### AETIOLOGY OF OSTEOARTHROSIS WITH PARTICULAR REFERENCE TO PREVENTION

### Background Note

**Ultrastructure.** The basic components of articular cartilage are (1) chondrocytes; (2) collagen fibres; and (3) a gel-like ground substance consisting of chondroitin sulphate, keratosulphate, glyco-proteins, salts and water. The scanning electron microscope has enabled a study to be made of the manner in which these components are arranged and the means by which nutrition and lubrication occur. It appears that collagen fibre in the matrix of articular cartilage is disposed at three levels (McColl, 1969):

1. A superficial zone, about 10 per cent of the tissue thickness, consisting of tightly packed parallel bundles of small fibres arranged in such a fashion as to form a protective skin and provide a suitable bearing surface.
2. A mid-zone, about 30 per cent of the depth, consisting of an open meshwork of S-shaped fibres with no definite orientation; and,
3. A deep zone, about 60 per cent of the total thickness, consisting of large, coarse radially orientated fibres which run into the subchondral layer of bone.

It appears that under load the middle zone provides an area of deformability and resilience within the tissue. The fibres gradually become aligned with their long axes at right-angles to the direction of loading or unloading and permitting recovery to take place, the open meshwork gradually returns.

Osteoarthrosic articular cartilage differs from the normal in that it is homogenous. The pattern of the deep zone extends throughout the entire depth and thus there is no response to static compression other than destruction.

**Function of subchondral bone.** Articular cartilage is required to sustain sheer and compression forces. The coefficient of friction is so low that it is unlikely that wear and tear changes occur from simple friction. On the other hand whatever may be the function of synovial fluid it cannot be expected to cushion impact. It is bone which is the longitudinal force attenuator within the musculo-skeletal system. It is bone which spares articular cartilage from impact. But repetitive impulsive loading causes trabecular fractures and the resulting callus formation increases the rigidity of the subchondral bone and renders it less effective as a shock absorber. It is the loss of this protective function which renders articular cartilage liable to destruction (Radin and Paul, 1971; Radin *et al.*, 1972).

**Biochemistry.** The exact biochemical mechanism involved in the development of osteoarthrosis is as yet unknown. In the current scene changes in affected articular cartilage are summarised (Mankin, 1969):

1. Alteration in organic solids:
   (a) Decreased chondroitin sulphate concentration.
   (b) Decreased polysaccharide chain length.
   (c) Altered keratosulphate/chondroitin sulphate ratio.
   (d) Altered distribution of the protein polysaccharide.

2. Changes in metabolic activity:
   (a) Increased D.N.A. synthesis.
   (b) Increased R.N.A. synthesis.
   (c) Increased protein synthesis.
3. Increased enzymatic degradation of protein polysaccharide.
4. Changes in water content and resiliency.
5. Alterations in diffusion.

If this data is speculative it is clear that osteoarthrosic cartilage is not inert and does not lack the capacity to regenerate and repair. If cartilage can provide new cells and can manufacture new matrix there is reason to emphasise the importance of early treatment which may reverse the aetiological factors still unknown and permit repair of the cartilaginous surface.

### General Biomechanical Considerations

**Terminology.** Osteoarthrosis can involve (1) the medial side of the joint to the virtual exclusion of all else; (2) the lateral side to the virtual exclusion of all else; (3) the patello-femoral joint to the exclusion of all else. Various combinations exist: (1) with (2) to the exclusion of (3); (3) to the exclusion of (1) and (2); and (1), (2) and (3) in a degenerative process involving the entire joint.

The knee joint is not divided into 'compartments' as such. Nevertheless, it is customary as a matter of convenience to refer to the 'medial compartment' as indicating the articulation between medial condyle of femur and medial condyle of tibia; and the 'lateral compartment' as indicating the articulation of lateral condyle of femur with lateral condyle of tibia. One or other compartment can be involved in an osteoarthrosic process; and such processes are referred to as **'mono-compartmental'** (Figs 10,1 and 10,2) rather than 'mono-condylar' as constituting a rather more accurate description of the gross pathology. Where the term **'bi-compartmental'** is used it indicates osteoarthrosis involving both compartments of the tibio-femoral joint (Fig. 10,3). The term **'pan-articular'** indicates that the entire tibio-femoral articulation together with the patello-femoral joint are involved (Figs 10,4 to 10,6).

**Primary varus (or valgus).** This is angular deformity usually of socially and functionally acceptable degree present at the termination of growth.

**Secondary varus (or valgus).** This is angular deformity which is the result of degenerative changes in the meniscus or articular cartilage, or both. Secondary varus, or valgus, can for evident biomechanical reasons be superimposed on primary varus, or valgus.

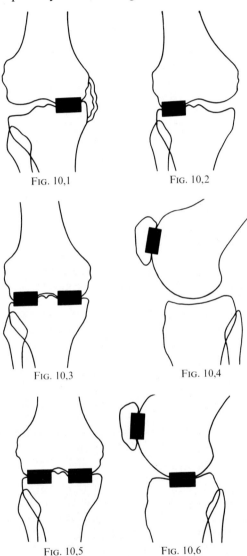

FIG. 10,1    FIG. 10,2

FIG. 10,3    FIG. 10,4

FIG. 10,5    FIG. 10,6

FIGS 10,1–6. **Simple classification of osteoarthrosis of knee.** Figure 10,1. Mono-compartmental (medial). In this variety the secondary varus angulation produces overlengthening of the medial ligament with resultant instability. Figure 10,2. Mono-compartment (lateral). Figure 10,3. Bi-compartmental. Figure 10,4. Patello-femoral. Figures 10,5 and 10,6. Pan-articular. This is the variety which in bilateral form is based on medial torsion.

## Wear and tear

Osteoarthrosis is not, as some would have it, a disease. In the instances when it is, it should be called osteoarthritis. In general it is the result of trauma; not often a single incident, but wear and tear, repeated or microtrauma of mechanical origin in the form of greater compressive forces than the tissues can withstand. It may be a deformity of the hip joint, congenital or acquired, altering the lines of weight-bearing or a fracture entering the joint. It may be no more than overuse, as in professional athletes or physical training instructors. But it is not a disease, for it may be limited to one compartment; in the female, to the patello-femoral joint; in the male, to the medial or lateral compartment or to the tibio-femoral joint as a whole.

But wear and tear is not the only factor concerned. Attention has been directed elsewhere to the anti-complimentary nature of the nutritional requirements of articular cartilage and bone. Any pathological condition, local or general, which increases the blood supply to bone or soft tissue is liable, if maintained, to result in destruction of articular cartilage. Thus conditions, whether of traumatic origin or otherwise, which increase the blood supply to synovial membrane on other than a temporary basis, entail the risk of osteoarthrosis. Examples include 'chronic synovitis', whether of traumatic or idiopathic origin; haemarthrosis from injury or disease (haemophilia); pigmented villonodular synovitis; and, most common of all, other considerations apart, rheumatoid arthritis.

In illustration of the complexity of the mechanical aspects of the problem, reference is made again to the interrelation of the components of the joint. If the first and most common degenerative changes are seen in the menisci, they are not limited for long to the menisci. Destruction of the substance of the medial meniscus brings the opposing condyles into more intimate contact with many possible repercussions such as contact between spine of tibia and medial condyle, compression of fat pad, nipping of synovial fringes and wearing or degeneration of articular cartilage.

The importance of the mechanical factor as such is shown when the condition is limited to one compartment. In a primary varus deformity the weight is borne on the inner side; and the medial compartment is affected. In a valgus deformity the weight is borne on the outer side; and the lateral compartment is affected. That the condition should affect the patello-femoral joint, in the absence of changes in the tibio-femoral joint, provides the best example of all.

**Angular deformity: varus or valgus.** If the middle-aged and elderly of the population in a small industrial city such as Dundee, Scotland, are observed in the street it will be evident that bilateral varus angulation with characteristic gait is common and apparently symptomless. It may be different elsewhere. Valgus angulation of similar degree is considerably less evident possibly because it is less common but possibly also because it is not symptomless and those affected less active; even house-bound. In any event they walk with caution: the waddling gait of varus angulation would place intolerable strain on the medial ligament. The fact that varus angulation, within limits is more readily tolerated than valgus angulation may explain the preponderance of such deformities in some series: valgus angulation imposes a biomechanical situation which is beyond the resources of physician or of physical medicine specialist.

**Varus and valgus.** Occasionally both deformities are present in the same patient. Angulation acquired in youth may in the course of growth require varus adaptation of the opposite knee in order to avoid impingement (Fig. 10,7).

**Patello-femoral joint.** It will be recognised that it is possible to stand erect with the quadriceps relaxed and the patella mobile in every direction provided the knee is in full extension and the screw-home movement completed. But if the joint is flexed, through even a few degrees, the erect position can be maintained only with the quadriceps contracted and the patella pressed hard against the femoral condyles. In women the use of high heels produces such a situation. If the equinus position is adopted before the growth plates close, adaptive changes, resulting in a slight genu recurvatum, occur from increased pressure on the anterior aspect of the plates. But if the use of high heels is deferred to the age of, say, 17, adjustment takes place less readily. If, in addition, the patient is of short stature, walking may be possible only with the knees flexed. This is the mechanical reason why the patello-femoral joint may be worn in women to the exclusion of changes elsewhere in the joint. If chondromalacia of the patella is an entity, in another form it is the precursor of osteoarthrosis of the patello-femoral joint.

## ABNORMALITIES OF BIOMECHANICS WITH TOTAL EFFECT ON JOINT

### Above Knee

Perfection of function in achieving complete

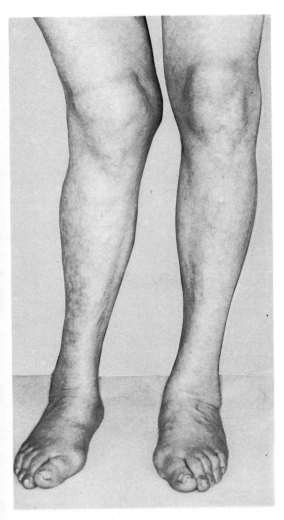

FIG. 10.7. **Angular deformity: valgus and varus.** Right side valgus-angulation, for whatever reason and arising in youth, responsible for a compensatory varus angulation on the left side (M.M.G., female, aged 50).

extension through the screw-home movement is dependent on the normal function of the hip joint. Absence of rotation, inherent in ankylosis, even in the neutral position, leads invariably to generalised osteoarthrosic degeneration.

### 'Coxitis Knee'

This is the name applied to the particular form of osteoarthrosis associated with ankylosis, arthrodesis or indeed any condition of the hip joint in which rotation is severely restricted. It is thus related to fixation of the hip; not to the underlying pathology. But tuberculosis, affecting as it did young people, was once the commonest cause.

**Aetiology.** The condition is attributed to the elimination of the screw-home movement. When the tibia is fixed, that is, when the foot is on the ground, the screw-home movement occurs by medial rotation of the femur. If the hip is ankylosed, the screw-home movement cannot take place. If the position of arthrodesis is imperfect or if ankylosis following disease has occurred in some flexion and adduction, the mechanical stresses on the joint are increased still further.

On a long-term basis absence of the screw-home movement is characterised by: (1) wasting of the vastus medialis, concerned as it is with the screw-home movement; (2) lateral rotation of the tibia, in order to gain stability in extension; (3) abnormal antero-posterior and lateral mobility, from the stresses imposed on a joint in which rotation is impossible; and (4) genu valgum, probably unrelated and due to adduction of the hip.

There is however another important factor in the development of osteoarthrosis other than derangement of the normal mechanics. Tuberculosis of the hip with which the condition was originally associated is a condition of youth necessitating prolonged immobilisation. In any event arthrodesis is notoriously difficult to attain. The effect of prolonged immobilisation on the upper tibial epiphysis is described in Chapter 9. But the articular cartilage of the joint suffers from the absence of movement and associated nutritional deficiency during a time of active growth. The adult articular cartilage is thus vulnerable to degenerative change.

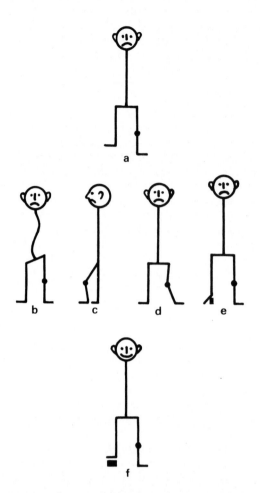

The limited possibilities for treatment, as opposed to prevention, are discussed later.

## Flexed-knee Gait: Good (Long) Leg Arthropathy

If it is impossible to prevent the development of the form of osteoarthrosis known as coxitis knee, there are other forms to which preventative measures are applicable.

It is not uncommon for cases with an arthrodesis of the hip and shortening of the leg uncompensated for by a raise to produce more extreme changes on the 'good' side from walking with a flexed knee than occur in the coxitis knee of the side of the fixed hip (Fig. 10,9).

In inequality of leg length the patient may fail through ignorance, choice or necessity, to compensate for shortening by a raised shoe and

FIG. 10,8. 'Good-leg' or 'long-leg' arthropathy: aetiology.
(a) A short leg, for whatever reason, must be compensated for in some way and the method adopted determines whether or not the patient develops 'good-leg' or 'long-leg' arthropathy.
(b) The classical manner is tilting of the pelvis towards the short side and the production of a scoliosis. This need not necessarily affect the good leg if extension is complete.
(c) and (d) Compensation by flexion of the knee and walking without extension is the commonest single cause of 'good-leg' arthropathy. The superimposition of valgus is a further aggravation.
(e) If the heel is raised and the equinus position adopted, the good knee need not necessarily be affected. Such a method, however, is undesirable in a polyarthritis affecting the peripheral joints.
(f) If the good knee is to be preserved compensation for shortening should consist of raising the sole and heel so that complete extension is utilised in the gait. (After Brattstrom and Brattstrom, 1971.)

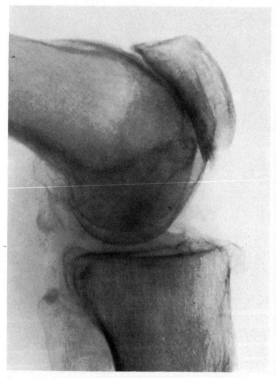

FIG. 10,9. **Good knee arthropathy.** This patient with ankylosis of the right hip in good position had 10·25 cm of shortening but wore a shoe with a raise of only 3·75 cm. Her right knee was symptomless. The left knee the cause of complaint. There is a pan-articular osteoarthrosis but because of walking on a flexed knee all her life the principal changes affect the patello-femoral joint (A.V., female, aged 77).

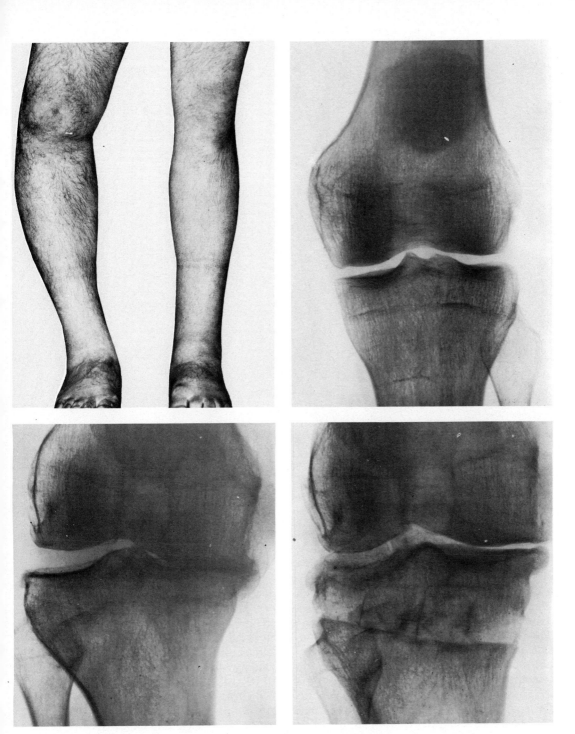

Figs 10,10–13. **Mono-compartmental osteoarthrosis as variety of 'good-leg' arthropathy: angular deformity.** This case illustrates a number of points:

The left leg was paralytic since the age of one when the sciatic nerve was injured in a surgical operation. There was power in the quadriceps only (Fig. 10,10). But note that radiographs of the paralytic leg show no evidence of osteoarthrosis (Fig. 10,11).

The right knee was the site of gross mono-compartmental osteoarthrosis with varus angulation partly from epiphyseal disturbance in the course of growth and partly from later overuse (Figs 10,10 and 10,12).

The deformity was corrected by opening-wedge osteotomy using iliac grafts as described in Chapter 9. Note almost complete correction of deformity (Fig. 10,13) (C.T., male, aged 57).

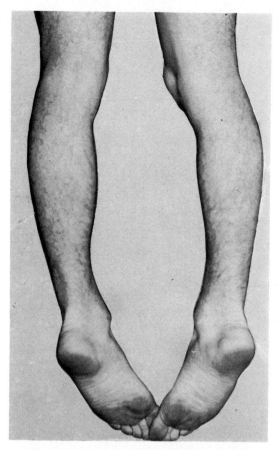 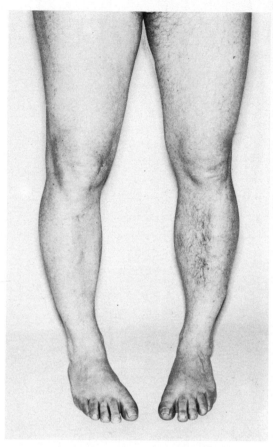

FIGS 10,14–15. **Aetiology of pan-articular osteoarthrosis: medial torsion of tibia.** This patient always slept on his face as a child and when examined at the age of 18 still did so (Fig. 10,14) (A.O., male).

Pan-articular osteoarthrosis in middle age is the invariable outcome of medial torsion (Fig. 10,15). When medial torsion and angular deformity are combined, medial torsion is the more important aetiological factor (J.B., male, aged 62).

walks with the sound knee flexed. The situation is particularly common in women in an effort to avoid the cosmetic defect of a 'surgical' shoe. The patient who adopts this gait for any considerable length of time inevitably and invariably develops a fixed flexion deformity and an osteoarthrosis of the patello-femoral joint and of the articular cartilage of the anterior segment of the femoral condyles. The former is a wear and tear phenomenon due to weight-bearing with the patella pressed hard back against the femoral condyles: the latter occurs because an arc of articular cartilage is not used when complete extension is not used. It thus received limited nutrition from the synovial fluid and undergoes

degeneration. But 'good' leg implies that it is the one which does the work. In addition therefore to the nutrition problem is the factor of hypertrophied muscles with inherent increased wear and tear in the form of longitudinal compression loading of cartilage deficient in nutrition (Figs 10,10 to 10,13).

Prevention, of course, is possible by equalising the lengths of the legs, either by surgical methods, if such are indicated, or, in other circumstances, by raising the height of the shoe of the short leg (Fig. 10,8f).

It is most important to explain to patients the consequences of walking with the knee permanently flexed. (See also Ch. 6.)

**Knee opposing artificial limb.** The good knee in a patient with an amputation develops osteo-arthrosis and it is manifest earlier and in greater degree in above than below knee amputations. The reason is not far to seek: the joint is subject to greater wear and tear in the form of compression forces in getting from the sitting position, ascending stairs and even walking, doing almost the work of both knees. The osteo-arthrosis is usually of pan-articular form; and the degree of involvement of the patello-femoral joint will depend on the degree of flexed-knee gait engendered by the shortness of the opposing artificial limb.

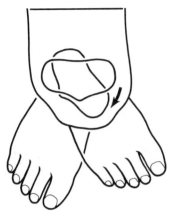

FIG. 10,16. **Aetiology of pan-articular osteoarthrosis: medial torsion of tibia.** Lateral rotation of tibio-femoral and patello-femoral joints is necessary at every step in order that the feet are directed forward rather than medially; and hence the excessive wear.

## BELOW KNEE

### Medial Rotation or Internal Torsion of Tibia.

The role of torsional deformity has been underestimated or passes unrecognised in the aetiology of pan-articular osteoarthrosis (Figs 10,14 and 10,15). Where it is recognised medial rotation of the tibia is usually imputed. But it is not as simple as that. Medial rotation varies in degree as does varus deformity with which it is not necessarily associated. If there is a compound deformity it is the rotation component which takes the greater responsibility for the degenerative changes.

Flexion and extension occur in the sagittal plane. When the tibia is medially rotated, in order to produce a gait in which the feet look directly forward instead of crossing over one another in the act of walking, the tibia must be rotated laterally by the action of the biceps. In combination with this abnormal rotatory action, the very reverse of the screw-home movement, is the possible effect of varus, producing as it does, an abnormal load on the medial condyle of the tibia. The first structure to suffer is the medial meniscus in which a horizontal cleavage lesion is produced; and this in turn is responsible for the progressive degenerative changes in the articular cartilage of the femoral and tibial condyles and the development of bi-compartmental osteoarthrosis. Medial torsion of the tibia seldom occurs in isolation. The possible exception is tibia vara interna (Ch. 8). It is usually a multifactorial situation consisting of medial torsion of femur, rotation at the knee joint and medial torsion of the tibia. If the femur

is involved lateral torsional forces must be exerted on the patello-femoral joint in order that the feet are directed forwards rather than medially. The result is lateral shift of the patella, the development of a patello-femoral osteoarthrosis and, in combination with the changes in the tibio-femoral joint, a pan-articular osteoarthrosis (Fig. 10,17).

### Factors of General Application

**Relationship to muscular development.** There is a relationship between osteoarthrosis and excessive muscle development. Conversely, it is well-known that osteoarthrosis does not develop in the knee joint of a paralytic leg. In the physiological field is the early onset of bilateral osteoarthrosis in the professional soccer player with his highly developed thigh and calf muscles, as opposed to the unaffected joints of the long distance runner. In the pathological field is the osteoarthrosis which develops in the knee related to the hypertrophied thigh which has taken on the function of both thighs in rising from a chair or ascending stairs as occurs opposite an arthrodesis or a full-length caliper.

The knee in paralysis of the quadriceps is subject to abnormal mechanical stresses as, for example, when it is pressed into hyperextension by body-weight to attain stability. It does not

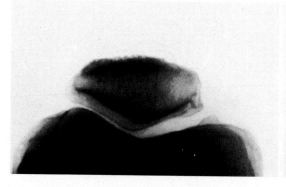 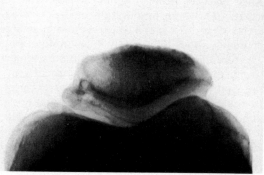

FIG. 10.17. **Pan-articular osteoarthrosis based on medial torsion of tibia.** Lateral displacement of the patellae with degenerative changes in the patello-femoral joints is an early feature of pan-articular osteoarthrosis based on medial torsion and is due to the necessity to exert a lateral torsional force at every step in order to direct the feet in a forward direction rather than medially (H.A.G., male, aged 42).

develop osteoarthrosis (Figs 10.18 and 10.19). But it is not subjected to the compression imposed by hypertrophied quadriceps opposing hypertrophied hamstring and calf muscles as occurs in the professional football player. The longevity of articular cartilage is related to the amount of force it must sustain. The sheer forces acting as in the long distance runner represent but a small percentage of the forces exerted from compression loading. In a multifactorial situation the evidence seems to point to a particularly unfavourable reaction to the excessive compression imposed by hypertrophied musculature just as it is known to react even more unfavourably to excessive compression in the form of impact imposed in the short term.

It appears that in spite of the capacity of the bearing materials of the human knee joint for regeneration, whatever the means of nutrition and lubrication, there is a limit to the acceptance of dynamic compression forces which when exceeded over a period of time lead to osteoarthrosis.

**Relationship to prolonged immobilisation.** It is known that prolonged immobilisation of the knee joint in a plaster cast, as was common in the treatment of tuberculosis of the hip in particular, produced changes in articular cartilage which resulted in osteoarthrosis in later life. The advent of chemotherapy can be expected to reduce the necessity for such measures in the future. There are however other conditions for

which prolonged immobilisation is used in some centres, for example, Perthes disease of the hip and even osteochondritis dissecans of the knee. There is an example of the latter condition quoted in which immobilisation in one form or another was continued for some six years (Ch. 11).

It has been shown experimentally that agitation of the fluid in which cartilage is immersed increases the rate of penetration by as much as fourfold. It can be inferred that the nutrition of cartilage is at least partly dependent on joint movement (Maroudas *et al.*, 1968). Prolonged immobilisation must therefore be detrimental to nutrition.

It is possible that the effect of immobilisation may be greater in the adult, in whom the articular cartilage is entirely dependent on the synovial fluid for nutrition, than in the child in whom the bone cartilage interface appears to be permeable to water and solutes, and evidence that growing cartilage derives a significant part of its nutrition from the underlying bone (McKibbon and Holdsworth, 1966).

**Relationship to obesity.** Overweight can be expected to increase the static and dynamic load on the articular cartilage of weight-bearing joints and has for long been associated with 'osteoarthritis' in the public mind. The bony conformation and related articular cartilage can reasonably be expected to be related to the patient's body-weight and configuration at maturity; and whether his occupation and habits are active or

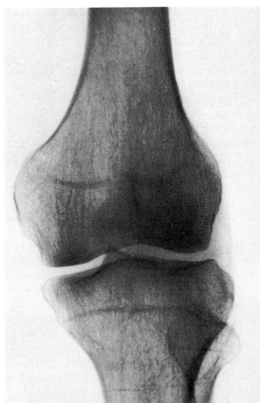
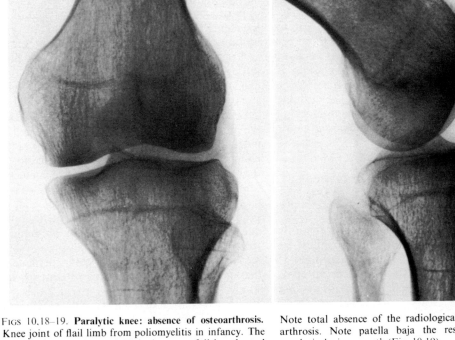

FIGS 10.18–19. **Paralytic knee: absence of osteoarthrosis.** Knee joint of flail limb from poliomyelitis in infancy. The patient (W.F., male, aged 56) had worn a full length steel caliper all his life and worked as a labourer in a factory.

Note total absence of the radiological feature of osteoarthrosis. Note patella baja the result of quadriceps paralysis during growth (Fig. 10.19).

sedentary. It is well-known to the experienced clinician that a sudden change in middle life from a sedentary to an active occupation is associated with the precipitation of 'symptoms' in the knee joints. A sudden increase of weight in middle life produces a similar affect. If such statements are the result of clinical impression a recent review has established a definite relationship between obesity and symptoms in osteoarthrosis (Lawrence, Bremner and Bier, 1966).

**Relationship to varicose veins.** There is an association between lower limb varicosities and osteoarthrosis of the knee joint. The incidence of varicose veins in the general population is 26 per cent (Dodd and Cockett, 1956); in the age range of patients presenting with osteoarthrosis, 22 per cent (Helal, 1965). In a series of osteoarthrosic knees reviewed in respect of varicose

veins, 67 per cent were so affected; and of those with unilateral involvement the varicose veins were either confined to or were worse on the side of the osteoarthrosis. It is of interest, and possible significance in relation to aetiology, that vein disease always predated the symptoms of osteoarthrosis by 3 to 18 years (Helal, 1965). In a recent study of 37 patients with a history of white leg of pregnancy or post-operative deep vein thrombosis with the residual post-thrombotic syndrome in the form of oedema, induration, varicose veins and, in some, ulceration, it has been shown that 23 had osteoarthrosis on the side affected (Phillips, 1972). This is a higher incidence than the 50 per cent in the epidemiological study of the age group concerned (Kellgren and Lawrence, 1957). There is thus a strong suspicion that venous congestion in the lower limb is in some way concerned with the aetiology of osteoarthrosis and more certainly concerned, based on experimental evidence, with the presenting symptom of the established condition, namely, pain.

(See also 'Clinical Features of Osteoarthrosis and Biomechanical Basis of Osteotomy'.)

**Relationship to meniscectomy.** It has been shown experimentally that the ability of the joint to absorb energy may be reduced by up to 80 per cent when both menisci are removed as opposed to 50 per cent when only one meniscus is removed (Krause *et al.*, 1975). This may be one of several explanations why the scars of a double meniscectomy are commonly encountered in bi-compartmental as opposed to pan-articular osteoarthrosis.

### APPEARANCE AND BIOMECHANICAL IMPLICATIONS OF THE AGEING PROCESS

**Incidence.** The knee is the joint most commonly affected. The wearing of joints, manifest as osteoarthrosis, is present in the knee joints of 75 per cent of patients who come to autopsy, whereas only 33 per cent of hip joints are affected (Wright, Dowson and Sellar, 1971).

All mankind suffers the changes of ageing articular cartilage and bone; and at what stage the situation warrants the diagnosis of osteoarthrosis is debatable. One man's ageing joint is another man's osteoarthrosis. To some extent it depends on the threshold for pain: one woman's ache is another woman's agony. The degree of damage or degeneration which may exist in articular cartilage determined at operation but without related symptoms must frequently occasion surprise even in the experienced orthopaedic surgeon.

A considerable familiarity has been accumulated in the course of meniscectomy of the appearance of the ageing knee. If it is possible to distinguish between the ageing and the osteoarthrosic joint it is because observations were made at the stage of degeneration of the substance of the fibrocartilage of the medial meniscus and often before serious injury had been inflicted on the articular cartilage of the medial femoral condyle of a degree which would justify the label of osteoarthrosis.

The following are some of the changes readily demonstrated through the limited exposure required for meniscectomy:

1. The articular cartilage is thin and rigid, yellowish in colour rather than white. It is clearly no longer a 'shock absorber'.

2. The thinness of the articular cartilage of the opposing condyles and the loss of substance in the meniscus inherent in the horizontal cleavage lesion result in loss of joint space so that femur is closer to tibia with the production of so-called settling-down phenomena.

3. Contact between medial eminence of tibial spine may be possible in the 'normal' joint: it depends on the conformation of the spine. When the femur approximates tibia the possibility, indeed, the probability, is increased. It takes the form in the tibia of erosion of the synovium at the attachment of the anterior cruciate ligament. The degree varies. In some examples there is a large area of ligament completely devoid of synovial covering (Fig. 10,20). That the lesion is due to contact with the femur can be demonstrated.

4. There are changes in the articular cartilage of the femoral condyle at the area of contact, the so-called classical site.

5. Approximation of femur to tibia reduces the space available to the fat pad. In consequence the lining synovial membrane is liable to be trapped and results in the presence of ischaemic white fibrous tags which may, or may not, show signs of trapping incidents.

### ABNORMALITIES OF BIOMECHANICS WITH LOCAL EFFECT ON JOINT

#### Angular Deformity

An angular deformity of 10° trebles the load per unit area on the affected tibial condyle (Simonet, Maquet and Marchin, 1963). It is thus evident that minimal abnormalities of alignment carry implications in terms of wear.

In a **primary** varus deformity, that is to say, one existing since maturity, compression forces on the medial side are increased abnormally, and thus this side wears abnormally. Mobility of the meniscus is reduced and the lesion which results is the now well-known horizontal cleavage tear. If the train of symptoms which this lesion produces passes unrecognised and untreated the degenerative process continues to involve the articular cartilage with **secondary** increase of varus from reduction of joint space. If the condition is not too far advanced meniscectomy may still render the patient symptomless and arrest the further progress of degenerative changes. If, however, degenerative changes are excessive, meniscectomy may not reduce symptoms to a tolerable level. It is in such circumstances that an osteotomy to transfer weight-bearing to the unworn lateral compartment may be indicated.

### 'The Torn Meniscus is an Aggressive Agent of Great Power'

The role of the meniscus in the torn state in the aetiology of osteoarthrosis has been underestimated. It is probable that failure to diagnose meniscus tears, longitudinal or horizontal, and effect treatment at an early stage, is the most common single cause of mono-compartmental osteoarthrosis. It is not that meniscectomy is

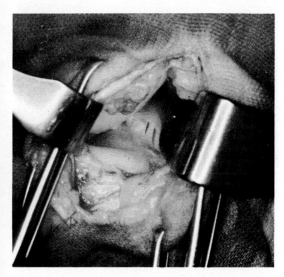

FIG. 10,20. **Age-related changes: 'settling-down' lesion.** The tibial attachment of the anterior cruciate ligament is seen to be devoid of synovial covering as a result of contact with the medial margin of the medial femoral condyle as the joint space is reduced by thinning of meniscus and of opposing cartilaginous surfaces. Two splits are seen in the direction of the bundles of fibres (H.C., male, aged 53).

innocent in terms of future degenerative changes. But the potential for irreparable change is much greater if a damaged meniscus is permitted to interfere with rotation on a permanent basis.

If the longitudinal tear is statistically less common than the horizontal tear it is the more important in potential for osteoarthrosis in so far as it is a lesion sustained in youth and thus the ill-effects manifest at an early age. The horizontal tear occurs at a later age and thus acts for a lesser period of time in a joint subject to lessening physical demands.

It will be clear from observation of the effect of ambulation on the displaced longitudinal tear that articular cartilage is particularly susceptible to break down under longitudinal compression loading, in contrast to a high resistance to wear under the sheer stresses imposed by frictional forces. There is an experimental basis for the phenomena. Repetitive impulsive loading by causing trabecular fractures and callus formation increases the rigidity of the subchondral bone and renders it less effective as a shock absorber. It is the loss of this protective function which renders articular cartilage liable to destruction (Radin *et al.*, 1972).

**Function of the menisci.** It is probable that the principal function of the menisci is to facilitate rotation at the completion of extension; and that other functions ascribed are of secondary importance.

### Effect of Longitudinal Tear

**Nature of lesion.** It is probable that there are no serious effects on articular cartilage until the lesion is complete and displaced to produce the classical 'locked knee' of the young male athlete. The implications of locking have been described in some detail in IKJ5, in brief, rupture of the anterior cruciate ligament and mechanical damage to the medial femoral condyle. It is with the latter lesion that we are concerned in the aetiology of mono-compartmental osteoarthrosis. The initial lesion imposed is a 'split line'. Split lines, the direction of which are constant in any given area of articular cartilage, reflect the arrangement of the collagen fibres. At the weight-bearing site of compression on the medial femoral condyle imposed by the displaced

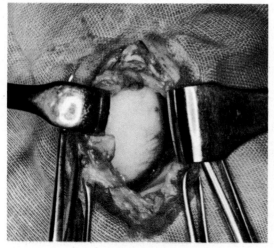

FIG. 10,21

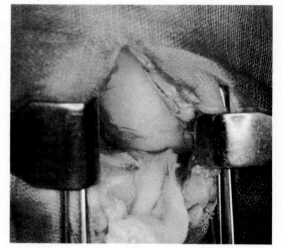

FIG. 10,23

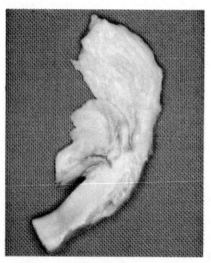

FIG. 10,22

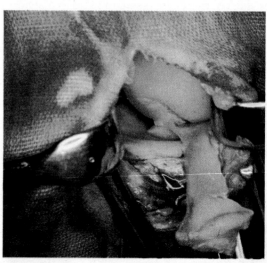

FIG. 10,24

FIGS 10,21–24. **Mono-compartmental osteoarthrosis: aetiology.** Articular cartilage is not designed to sustain impact. These multiple split lines were inflicted on the lateral condyle in a matter of six weeks weight-bearing on a displaced complete longitudinal tear of the meniscus (Fig. 10,21) (S.G., male, aged 17).

Inferior surface horizontal cleavage posterior segment medial meniscus with centrally displaced flap (Fig. 10,22). It is the flap interposed between the condyles which produces loss of complete extension (Figs 10,23 and 10,24). This is the lesion which, undiagnosed and untreated, is responsible for irreversible degenerative changes in the articular cartilage of the opposing condyles of the medial compartment.

Recent lesion of articular cartilage of medial femoral condyle based on split line the result of impact on interposed flap of meniscus (see Fig. 10,22) from horizontal cleavage lesion of posterior segment (Fig. 10,23) (A.H., male, aged 39).

Horizontal cleavage lesion posterior segment medial meniscus with centrally displaced flap (see Fig. 10,22). Note gross lesion inflicted on the articular cartilage of the medial margin of the condyle (Fig. 10,24). 'The torn meniscus is an aggressive agent of great power.'

meniscus, the split line, or lines, are horizontal in direction and vertical in section.

The fate of the single split line once the cause is removed is unknown. Is the pathology progressive? Nor is the fate of multiple split lines (Fig. 10,21), once the cause is removed, known. It seems unlikely that healing occurs. Large areas of chondromalacia and erosions exposing bone are frequently encountered following meniscus lesions in youth. Do they represent a later stage of a pathological progress based on the split line? Here is a subject of long-term clinical research which could be based on the evidence of the arthroscope.

**Patello-femoral joint.** It is not generally appreciated that derangement of the screw-home movement imposed by the displaced longitudinal tear has implications for the patello-femoral joint. The fact that there is a block to rotation alters the distribution of pressure to the trochlear surface of the medial femoral condyle and medial articular surface of the patella with implications for damage in the form of erosion of articular cartilage (Helfet, 1959). To what extent this is responsible for progressive chondromalacia and/or patello-femoral osteo-arthrosis is not known.

### Effect of Horizontal Tear

**Nature of lesion.** The lesion as it effects the meniscus is a degenerative process within the substance of the fibrocartilage presumed to be due to a breakdown in nutrition. The various stages in the development of the pathology have been described in IKJ5.

BIOCHEMISTRY. Analyses of serial horizontal sections of normal menisci show a homogeneous collagen and chondroitin sulphate composition throughout the structure. In the meniscus with a horizontal tear a significant decrease in the collagen/chondroitin sulphate ratio is apparent at the site of the lesion. This decrease is largely attributable to an increased concentration of mucopolysaccharides. It is suggested that this accumulation of mucopolysaccharides, which may be a response to nutritional impairment, alters the physical properties of the central core of the meniscus and perhaps renders it more susceptible to trauma (Peters and Smillie, 1971, 1972). This is a subject of considerable import-

ance not only in meniscus pathology but in the aetiology of osteoarthrosis. It merits further investigation in the fields of ultrastructure and biochemistry.

**Effect on articular cartilage.** In so far as the lesion affects the articular cartilage of the medial femoral condyle (1) the normal, but possibly ageing, articular cartilage of the femoral condyle comes into closer proximity to that of the tibia, where (2) the torn meniscus inflicts friction lesions from its rough surface and compression lesions from the presence of an inferior tag (Fig. 10,22).

Horizontal cleavage does not, in the initial stages at least, involve the convex periphery of the posterior segment but the part immediately internal to it. When the fibrocartilage of this zone is destroyed the femoral condyle sinks into the meniscus just as it does in the congenital disc. The effect of this, apart from bringing the condyles into closer opposition, is to extrude the periphery over the margin of the tibia where, pressing on the tightly applied capsule, it exerts tension on the synovial attachments (Figs 10,25 to 10,28). This is the explanation of the swelling, pain and tenderness on the joint line immediately posterior to the ligament almost pathognomonic of the lesion; and of the sensitivity to pressure of the bedclothes at night which can be explained only on the basis of synovial involvement.

The early lesion inflicted on the tibia is an area of rough granular consistency but not necessarily broken (Fig. 10,29). The early lesions on the femur are more extensive with indented areas, split lines, tags of chondromalacic cartilage to erosions exposing bone (Fig. 10,30). It is clear that these are the changes which in the advanced stage produce the angular deformity described as secondary varus.

It has been possible to follow patients who have had the diagnosis of a horizontal cleavage lesion established but in whom, for one reason or another, operation has not been performed. The commonest reason for declining operation is that the patient has been told that he has 'rheumatism'; and this, to him, is a more acceptable diagnosis than one demanding an operation. Next in order is the intermittent nature of the symptoms. If a patient awaiting operation is requested to report for admission during a quiescent phase, he may fail to come

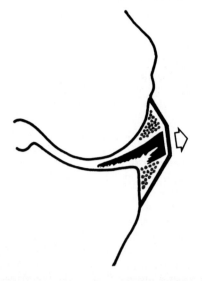

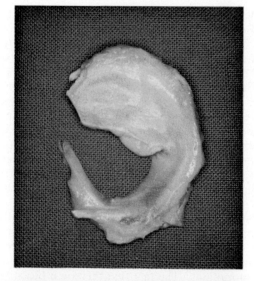

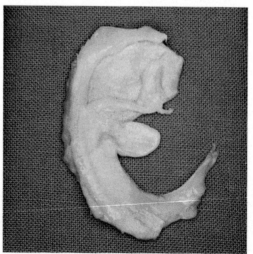

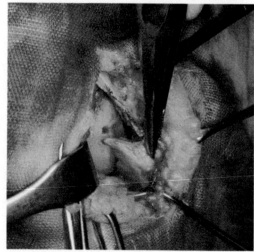

FIGS 10,25–28. **Aetiology of mono-compartmental osteo-arthrosis: Horizontal cleavage of the posterior segment of the medial meniscus. The pathological anatomy explains the related symptom complex.**

Figure 10,25. When the horizontal cleavage lesion occurs the femoral condyle sinks into the meniscus causing it to be extruded medially where it induces tension in the capsule and underlying synovial membrane to explain the swelling, tenderness and pain together with sensitivity to contact with bedclothes (see text).

Figure 10,26. The superior surface of a medial meniscus the site of a horizontal cleavage lesion. Note absence of damage to the surface but note the indentation produced by the femoral condyle.

Figure 10,27. The horizontal cleavage lesion is on the inferior surface with destruction of the substance of the fibro-

cartilage and explains the indentation on the superior surface. It is the sinking of the femoral condyle into the meniscus as in the diagram above (Fig. 10,25).

Figure 10,28. Note at operation that the periphery of the meniscus has been extruded over the margin of the medial tibial condyle.

It will be evident therefore that the alteration to the mechanics of the joint whereby the femoral condyle approaches the tibial condyle by sinking into the meniscus has taken place prior to meniscectomy. This is the reason for the rapid recovery which occurs after operation.

It is the reason also for the loss of joint space in the radiograph and for the onset of mono-compartmental osteoarthrosis if damage is permitted to occur to the articular cartilage prior to meniscectomy.

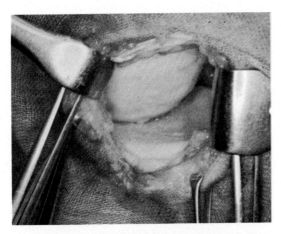

FIG. 10.29. **Mono-compartmental osteoarthrosis: aetiology.** Degenerative changes in articular cartilage. Medial condyles of femur and tibia of patient with meniscus the site of horizontal cleavage lesion of posterior segment of three years duration (W.W., male, age 57).

into hospital. On the return of symptoms, instead of admitting his mistake, he accepts the related pain rather than place himself in the embarrassing position of confessing his error. These are the cases which observed over a period of time, varying between months and years, have provided the evidence of the deleterious effect of an untreated horizontal cleavage lesion on the articular cartilage of the compartment involved.

## Aetiology of Mono-compartmental Osteoarthrosis

**Lateral.** On the lateral side, the less common of the two to be affected but producing the more severe symptoms, factors not common to the medial side obtain. Reference has been made elsewhere (IKJ5) to the frequency with which a local osteoarthrosis may follow the removal of a lateral meniscus particularly in the professional soccer player. Reflection on the pathology encountered suggests an explanation in keeping with the known course of degenerative pathology associated with meniscus tears. It has been stated that the lateral compartment is 'silent'. Gross pathology therein is consistent with minimal symptoms (Fig. 10.30). Moreover, the quadriceps development of the professional soccer player is known to mask gross pathology

while at the same time exerting excessive compression loading. A considerable interval may elapse before the player eventually comes to operation (Fig. 10.31). All this time torn but tough fibrocartilage has been in contact with the less resistant articular cartilage of the femoral condyle on every action of weight-bearing. Hence the degenerative changes of a degree detectable radiologically at such an early age and the formation of reactionary ridges in tibial and femoral condyles possibly accelerated by the removal of the peripheral remnants of the intervening shock absorber.

There is evidence that regeneration following meniscectomy takes a different pattern and is less complete than on the medial side. This is attributed to the intervention of the popliteus tendon, in that a site exists in the arc from which synovial membrane is absent and thus the source of blood clot eventually responsible for the regenerated meniscus of fibrocartilage is deficient. If this is so the absence of a regenerated structure would permit contact between femur

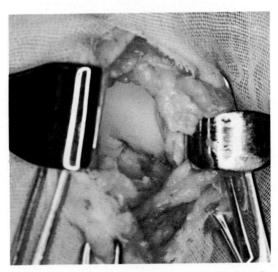

FIG. 10.30. **Mono-compartmental osteoarthrosis (lateral): aetiology.** Appearance of lateral condyle of femur at operation for removal of meniscus the site of a complete transverse tear based on a parrot-beak lesion. Symptoms were minimal and had existed for six weeks only. He played in a first division football game one week previous to operation. (I.J., professional soccer player, aged 23.) The lateral compartment is 'silent' and is responsible for the gross degenerative changes which occur (see Fig. 10.31).

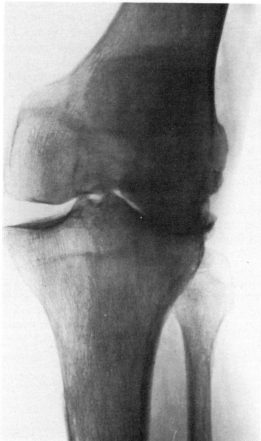
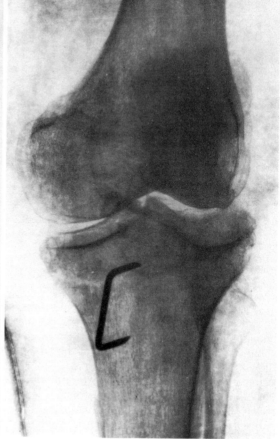

FIGS 10,31–32. **Treatment of mono-compartmental (lateral) osteoarthrosis: closing-wedge.** This mono-compartmental osteoarthrosis affecting the lateral side was related to a torn meniscus operated on 20 years previously but with a 10-year history of symptoms. Weight-bearing radiograph to determine biomechanical status of the joint (Fig. 10,31). Appearance of joint after medial closing-wedge osteotomy correcting valgus deformity and altering weight-bearing alignment (Fig. 10,32) (R.M., male, aged 69).

and tibia with reaction in the form of marginal outgrowths.

## OSTEOARTHROSIS

### Clinical Features: Degenerative Lesions of Medial Meniscus: Horizontal Cleavage

It is evident with the accumulation of experience that lesions of the medial meniscus can be divided into those of **traumatic** and those of **degenerative** origin. The **complete longitudinal tear** is an injury of youth of traumatic origin, if not exclusively so. The **horizontal cleavage** **lesion** of the posterior segment is of degenerative origin, and almost exclusively so.

The aetiology, pathology, clinical features and treatment of the traumatic lesion have been described (IKJ5) as have, if in lesser detail, the more statistically important degenerative lesion. Reference has been made to the influence of traumatic lesions of the medial meniscus in the aetiology of osteoarthrosis. No repetition of the symptoms and signs of the traumatic lesion should be necessary. On the other hand it is proposed, at the risk of some repetition, to reiterate and amplify the clinical features of the degenerative lesion, if it is only for the reason that the train of symptoms and signs, in the absence of a history of trauma, is known to lead to misdiagnosis and mistreatment; as a result, to the initiation of a degenerative process in the articular cartilage of the medial compartment leading to angular deformity and a situation recognised as osteoarthrosis.

It is important that the curious symptom-complex of the horizontal cleavage lesion of the posterior segment of the medial meniscus should be established in the interests of preventative medicine. It will be evident that a lesion of degenerative origin in the fibrocartilage of the meniscus, a structure dependent for nutrition on synovial fluid, cannot heal. The meniscus then inflicts injury to the articular cartilage of the femoral condyle just as the damaged soft bronze of a bearing inflicts damage to the hard steel of the crankshaft. The damage to the articular cartilage is mechanical and is arrested only by mechanical means, namely, excision of the structure interfering with movement at the limit of extension and in particular with the screw-home movement. There is no known method of conservative treatment; in fact, all methods of conservative treatment are to the detriment of the patient in the long term. It is to this end that the features of the symptom-complex are expanded in the context of osteoarthrosis, the condition with which it is usually confused in the early stages when effective treatment is possible.

## History

**Age.** The patient is aged not less than 30. In the last 1500 meniscectomies (8500 to 10000) the average age of males was 50 and that of females 57.

**Sex.** In contradiction to internal derangements relative to the menisci in young women, in whom lesions of the medial meniscus are rare, symptoms are encountered with increasing frequency in the female subject; and in a ratio of not less than 1 case in 5.

**Trauma.** There is no history of injury as such other than of a minor twist in the course of normal activity. The pathology is based on a breakdown of nutrition leading to degeneration of the substance of the fibrocartilage. Minimal trauma, or no trauma at all, is required for the

cleft to occur with the onset of the symptom-complex. But a definite incident placing a shearing stress on the meniscus as, for example, jumping down from a truck with a weight on the shoulders, may be blamed for the onset of symptoms.

**Pain.** The complaint is of local pain. It is not one of general pain in the joint. The pain is accurately located at a point on the joint line immediately posterior to the medial ligament. It is noticeable when sitting in one position for any length of time, as, for example, driving a car. It has the curious feature, almost pathognomonic, that it is present in bed at night. Furthermore, and in the same circumstances, the medial side of the knee is sensitive not only to the other knee touching it but even to contact with the bed-clothes. Some say that sleep is possible only with a pillow between the knees.

The sensitivity of the medial side of the knee to pressure is synovial in origin. An explanation has been offered earlier in the chapter. The pain, turning over in bed, or wakening the patient in the course of sleep, is readily explainable. It is impossible to turn on a soft mattress without flexing the knees. In sleep, this is done without the protection of the quadriceps. It is presumed that contact between damaged structures is transmitted to synovial membrane with consequent pain.

**Insecurity.** There is a feeling of weakness, instability or the tendency to give way. This is particularly noticeable when the necessity to jump down from a height arises. This sensation is explained by the pathological anatomy. The upper surface of the meniscus is no longer attached to the lower. Any shearing stress causes one surface to move on the other with consequent instability.

**Locking.** Loss of last few degrees of extension is a common feature of the established horizontal cleavage lesion. It is not, however, 'locking' in the sense that the complete longitudinal tear produces locking, nor in contradistinction, is there a block to the screw-home movement. Nevertheless, the patient may be aware that extension is incomplete.

The loss of full extension is due to a flap of the posterior segment displaced centrally interposed between the femur and tibia (Figs 10,22 to 10,24). This situation occurs more readily in a joint with age-related changes than in the knee of the young subject. In the ageing knee the opposing surfaces of articular cartilage are thin and rigid and, lacking the depth of articular cartilage of the youthful knee, are prone to loss of extension from the interposition of minimal obstructions.

**Effusion.** The symptom-complex is not characterised by effusion; rather the reverse. The lesion involves avascular fibrocartilage. The meniscus is more rigidly fixed than normal. Even an incident of giving way does not involve stretching of the synovial attachment. There is consequently no effusion.

**Symptoms are intermittent.** It is characteristic of the lesion that the symptoms are intermittent; and the implications of this feature in the development of osteoarthrosis have been described. The intensity of the symptoms depend on whether or not a flap of degenerate fibrocartilage from the undersurface of the meniscus is in its normal place or displaced between the articular surfaces to interfere with rotation.

**Symptoms may be bilateral.** A condition based on degenerative changes can be bilateral just as osteoarthrosis can be bilateral. As in osteoarthrosis, however, symptoms of equal intensity in both knees at the same time are unusual.

### Examination: Horizontal Cleavage Lesion

1. With the patient supine on the couch, test first for full extension using the normal joint as the yardstick. The difference between complete and a few degrees of limitation, such as might be present in a worn joint the site for a horizontal cleavage tear of the medial meniscus with a small displaced tag between the condyles, can be detected only by comparison. (For method see Chapter 1.)

2. With both knees drawn up to a right angle, inspect outline of joint and particularly the medial joint line for swelling (Fig. 1,8). The swelling to be sought is located behind the medial ligament. It is a fullness amounting to loss of outline. It is not readily appreciated without reference to the normal side. It is not evident in extension. Tenderness is accurately located to the same point, the joint line immediately posterior to the ligament. The swelling and tenderness which correspond accurately to the

site of the pain are synovial in origin; and the mechanism of production has been explained. If, of course, considerable extrusion has taken place the convex margin of the meniscus can be palpated as a firm localised tender swelling on the joint line posterior to the ligament (Fig. 10,33).

3. Rotation in flexion with the finger tips on the medial joint line produces a grating sensation and the complaint of pain which the patient recognises as the one with which he has grown familiar (Fig. 10,33).

**Radiological examination.** If compression forces imposed from above act through the centre of the joint subchondral sclerosis of the tibial condyles is of comparable degree and symmetrical in distribution. The earliest radiological signs of incipient mono-compartmental osteoarthrosis are loss of joint space and/or increase of sclerosis. The former is indicative of the development of a horizontal cleavage lesion of the posterior segment of the medial meniscus. The latter, in the absence of loss of joint space, indicative of the presence of abnormal compression forces. Both are present as meniscus

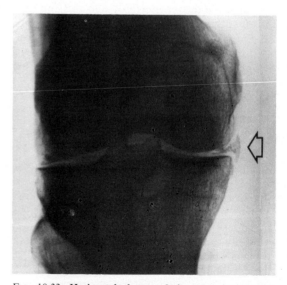

FIG. 10,33. **Horizontal cleavage lesion posterior segment medial meniscus: clinical examination.** If considerable extrusion (Fig. 10,25) has taken place the periphery of the meniscus can be palpated as a tender swelling on the joint line posterior to the ligament. In this example the periphery, the site of calcification, is seen to have been extruded (Fig. 10,33).

degeneration advances with the increase of compression forces inherent in secondary varus angulation.

## Diagnosis

The diagnosis is determined by the precise symptom-complex which has been described. It is the easiest to make of all internal derangements of the knee. There is virtually no condition from which it has to be differentiated. Arthroscopy is superfluous.

## Treatment

Meniscectomy renders the patient symptom-free in spite of radiological changes of marked degree. The important thing is to recognise the source of the symptoms and not subject the patient to some major procedure such as linear osteotomy when in fact a relatively minor procedure is so effective.

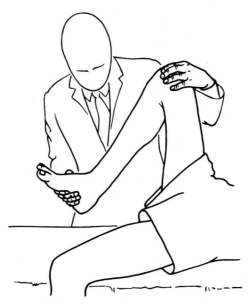

FIG. 10,34. **Horizontal cleavage lesion posterior segment medial meniscus: clinical examination.** Rotation in flexion with the finger tips on the joint line produces a painful grating sensation with which the patient has grown familiar.

### CLINICAL FEATURES: ESTABLISHED OSTEOARTHROSIS

#### Pain

The predominant, often the only symptom, is pain. Three types of pain occur separately or in combination (Helal, 1965).

**1. Muscular.** This is a cramp-like sensation felt in the quadriceps during activity and continuing for a few minutes after exercise. It is the least important of the varieties described. Its existence is elicited by leading questions. The relationship to wasting of the muscle has not been determined.

**2. Capsular.** That pain can be produced by stretching of the capsule is well-established. The circumstances in which this variety is produced is likely to be associated with angular deformity of noticeable degree.

**3. Venous.** This variety takes the form of a dull aching or throbbing pain felt diffusely about the joint, usually worse towards the end of the day and persisting for a while after retiring to bed. In the early stages the pain is felt only when the subject is tired. At a later stage it is aggravated by fatigue. This pain can be reproduced by raising artificially the intramedullary pressure in the tibia (Helal, 1965).

#### Stiffness

Loss of mobility, as opposed to loss of range of motion, is a constant feature of osteoarthrosis as indeed of the ageing joint. The stiffness experienced is probably multifactorial in origin. It is related to decrease of muscle power; to increase of physical resistance in the capsule from alteration in the collagen content with advancing years; to increase in physical resistance within the joint from degenerative changes in the medial meniscus and resulting abrasive injury to opposing articular cartilage; and, finally, to the decrease in the viscosity of synovial fluid which occurs with age.

#### Instability

The complaint of instability is common. When angular deformity takes the form of varus as a result of degeneration of the medial meniscus, articular cartilage and finally depression of the cancellous tissue of the medial condyle of the tibia, the medial ligament does *not* undergo adaptive shortening. There is thus relative overlengthening with consequent instability (Fig. 10,1). This overlengthening can be demonstrated by the examination technique used to test the integrity of the ligament (Fig. 1,2). The manoeuvre, however, is painful in a joint the subject of osteoarthrosis.

### Insecurity: Giving-way

This complaint is common and due to a number of reasons. A joint which lacks complete extension is dependent on a weak quadriceps pressing a worn patella against worn femoral condyles for security. The feeling of insecurity is common and increases with fatigue.

### Loss of Movement

Reduction in the range of movement is seldom a source of complaint. It is generally of more interest to the surgeon than the patient in so far as there is loss of complete extension and frequently of flexion beyond a right angle. Loss of flexion, if not excessive, does not appear to produce social embarrassment in the age range affected but is a source of disability in certain occupations.

### EXAMINATION: ESTABLISHED OSTEOARTHROSIS

1. Observe both limbs standing (Fig. 10,35) and sitting (Fig. 10,36) so that any abnormality of mechanics, which might contribute to abnormal wear and tear, can be detected. Note outline of joint and conformation of limb; compare with the other side (Fig. 10,36).
   In unilateral osteoarthrosis a local reason may be found. If the condition is bilateral a general biomechanical reason is likely to be present; and the most common one a medial torsion deformity.
2. On couch: examine for loss of extension. If present, note degree and estimate cause, soft tissue or bony block.
3. Palpate joint line for tenderness; in particular, that part posterior to the medial ligament with the possibility of a horizontal cleavage lesion of the meniscus in mind.
4. Test range of rotation in varying degrees of flexion until maximum extension is reached; compare with other knee.

5. Palpate margins of condyles. Proliferation of cartilage is evident to the finger tips (Fig. 1,11) long before radiological changes are present in the underlying bone.

In a considerably lesser number of cases the marginal exostoses affect the tibia; and this may occur on either side. The most obvious explanation as to why the tibia should be affected is the relationship to a torn meniscus

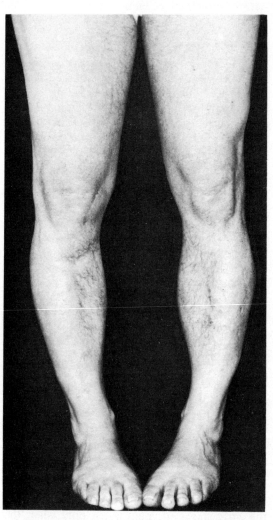

FIG. 10,35. **Varus angulation and medial torsion.** Primary varus and medial torsion. The deformity is increased on the right side (secondary varus) as a result of a degenerative (horizontal cleavage) lesion of the medial meniscus (J.B., male, aged 62).

and/or meniscectomy. It is well-known that changes in the radiographs of the joint follow meniscectomy; and the radiographs of the flat tibial head will show an apparent exostosis, in fact a ridge, much more readily than in the femur. It has been pointed out in describing aetiological factors that proliferative changes appear sooner on the lateral side than on the medial. Nevertheless, there are occasions in which gross degenerative changes have followed medial meniscectomy with pro-liferation of cartilage and bone on the tibia on the medial side. Whether this has been initiated by the longstanding presence of a torn meniscus, known to produce damage to the articular cartilage, or whether it is related to the absence of a regenerated meniscus follow-ing meniscectomy, is difficult to determine.

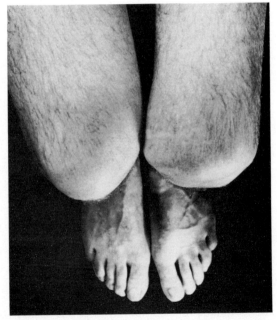

FIG. 10.36. **Unilateral pan-articular osteoarthrosis: clinical features.** When the condition is advanced it will be seen that the joint viewed from above shows broadening of the femoral condyles but, in particular, that the patella has sunk into the femoral groove. These appearances are due to destruction of articular cartilage in the opposing surfaces of all elements of the joint. This is a stage at which con-servative surgery is unlikely to be of avail. This joint has reached the stage when only arthrodesis is likely to be helpful in the absence of any total replacement likely to stand up to the demands of a young adult male (T.W., age 36, motor mechanic, case of W.W.).

6. Note degree of muscle wasting and estimate state of patello-femoral joint. Note range of active and passive movements and reaction, in terms of pain, to passive movements.

7. In consideration of different treatment requirements, determine, in conjunction with outcome of radiological examination (see below), whether the condition is mono-compartmental, bi-compartmental or pan-articular.

### Radiological Examination

There are subtleties and apparent contradictions in osteoarthrosis, of the knee joint in particular, which are not evident except to the experienced. Radiographs depict bone; not cartilage. By the time osteoarthrosis is a radiological entity, the pathology, as it concerns articular cartilage, is far advanced. Radiological changes in the bony outline of the joint bear little relationship to the severity of the symptoms and are not, as has been indicated, a guide to treatment.

If there is angular deformity and/or loss of extension further radiographs are required:

1. A weight-bearing as opposed to a supine antero-posterior view determines the local mechanical situation. It does not, however, convey sufficient information about the mechani-cal status of the limb as a whole which must be estimated with accuracy if an osteotomy is con-templated (see below).

2. If osteotomy is under consideration antero-posterior radiographs under stress, obtained in the same manner as for examination of the medial ligament, are of value in estimating the state of the articular cartilage in the lateral compartment (Fig. 1,2).

When the joint is 'closed' on the medial side it is 'opened' on the lateral side; and for obvious mechanical reasons the opening is exaggerated. The existence of a wide space on the lateral side cannot necessarily be interpreted as indicating that the articular cartilage is intact. The exist-ence of a reasonable space under compression carries with it the implication that the articular cartilage is not unduly worn.

3. A weight-bearing lateral view in maximum extension, if possible, with the quadriceps

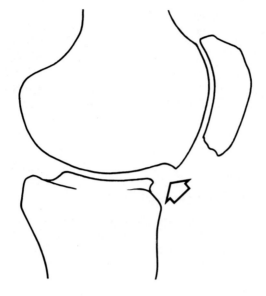

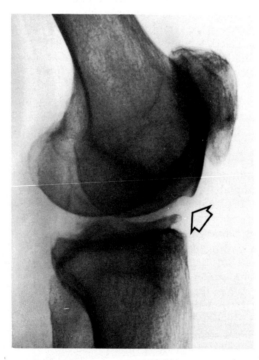

Figs 10,37–38. **Osteoarthrosis: bony block to extension.** At the anterior limit of the weight-bearing arc is a step which in contact with an outgrowth from the tibial head constitutes a positive block to extension. Clinical and radiological examination is directed to the existence of such a block in so far as it is a contraindication to the pursuance of passive stretching (Ch. 6) and maybe an indication for debridement.

contracted is desirable (Figs 1,17 to 1,19). This projection indicates the level of the patella in relation to the femoral condyles and the state of the patello-femoral joint but, more important, establishes whether or not outgrowths of femur and tibia are in contact to constitute a bony block to extension. Such information is of value in estimating the possible outcome of debridement in terms of increase of extension.

In limited extension the salient feature of the lateral view of the tibial element of the tibio-femoral joint is a prominence in the upper end of the tibia near the anterior margin. This prominence rises vertically from the tibial head, is narrow at the base and flattens superiorly so that in the lateral view it is triangular in shape. The mechanism of production of this protuberance is not immediately evident. The shape, however, can be explained on the grounds that bone growing in this region, subjected to pressure from above in weight-bearing, becomes flattened. This explains why it is wider superiorly than inferiorly; and its triangular section.

In the femoral element there is a distinct step in the condyle where the arc of weight-bearing meets the arc of contact with the patella (Figs 10,37 and 10,38). It can be demonstrated radiologically that contact between the prominences occurs at the limit of extension.

**Whole-limb weight-bearing radiograph.** If operative treatment by osteotomy (or total replacement) is contemplated a whole-limb weight-bearing radiograph is essential to assess the tibio-femoral angle and calculate the degree of correction required. Ideally the radiograph is produced on a single plate (Fig. 10,40). If the equipment necessary to produce such a plate is not available a full scale drawing is reproduced from separate plates of hip, knee and ankle superimposed and correlated by means of marks on an opaque vertical ruler. In this way the axis of the femur is superimposed on the axis of the tibia and the tibio-femoral angle measured (Fig. 10,41). If as a result of ligamentous instability a wide gap exists on one side of the joint this must be taken into account in the preparation of the pre-operative drawing to avoid overcorrection. To this end a further tracing is made in which the gap is closed. The tibio-femoral angle is then measured on the second drawing (Maquet, 1976).

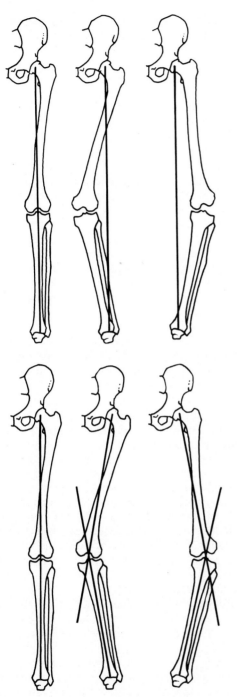

FIG. 10,39. **Biomechanics of mono-compartmental osteo-arthrosis.** In the normal knee a line drawn from the centre of the head of the femur to the mid-point of the body of the talus passes through the intercondylar notch. In osteo-arthrosis affecting the lateral compartment the axis of weight-bearing is displaced to the lateral side. When the medial compartment is affected the axis is displaced to the medial side.

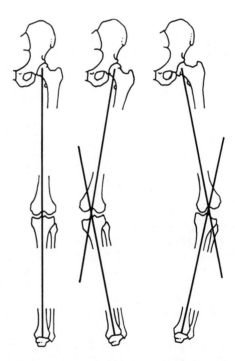

FIG. 10,40. **Biomechanics of mono-compartmental osteo-arthrosis.** The tibio-femoral angle is the angle made by a line joining the centre of the head of the femur to the intercondylar notch with a line joining the mid-point of the body of the talus to the interval between the tibial spines.

FIG. 10,41. **Mono-compartmental osteoarthrosis: treatment by tibial head osteotomy.** To calculate the angle of correction required, the so-called tibio-femoral angle, a whole-limb standing antero-posterior radiograph is required. If the necessary equipment is not available three separate weight-bearing plates centred over femoral head, knee joint and body of talus are taken with a grid placed in front of the cassettes so that the films can be aligned in the correct relationship.

## TREATMENT: CONSERVATIVE NON-OPERATIVE

It is said, but not with complete accuracy, that of the joints prone to osteoarthrosis only the knee reacts to conservative measures. But patients do not seek advice because of sudden deterioration in the pathological process. It is because of the development of a flexion deformity. Once the capacity for extension is lost, the erect position can be maintained only with the quadriceps contracted and the patella pressed hard against the femoral condyles. When the articular cartilage of the patello-femoral joint is worn, as it often is in women, a minor degree of flexion is sufficient to precipate symptoms.

To reduce pain and produce a dramatic improvement of function all that is necessary is to secure a return of full extension by passive means accompanied by active redevelopment of the quadriceps. Unless changes are marked so that a mechanical block to movement is present, it is exceptional for such measures, adequately enforced, to fail to provide relief.

**Passive stretching.** Two methods of increasing extension which do not require special equipment are available to the ambulatory out-patient:

1. The simplest, and all that is necessary in the majority of cases, is passive stretching applied by the patient to her own knee. She sits on the edge of a chair with the leg extended, the heel on the floor. Passive stretching is produced by the pressure of the hand on the anterior aspect of the joint (Fig. 6,29). This measure, practised hourly in combination with quadriceps exercises, by a co-operative patient who has had the method and the reason for it explained to her is most effective.

2. The patient sits in a chair with the heel resting on another chair of similar height. A loop of bandage is placed over the knee and a weight suspended from it so that a passive stretching force is exerted. The size of the weight and the time for which it is applied on each successive occasion depends on the toleration of the patient and the extent of the changes in the patello-femoral joint (Fig. 6,30).

The further conservative methods of increasing extension are applicable more to rheumatoid arthritis and other conditions of soft tissue origin than osteoarthrosis and are described in Chapter 6. It requires to be repeated that it is useless, and discouraging for the patient, to pursue indefinitely passive stretching methods applicable to soft tissue contraction when in fact there is a bony block to extension.

**Rest.** Immobilisation, whether in plaster or otherwise, has no place in treatment. Rest, but not from non-weight-bearing quadriceps exercises, is justifiable only in a crisis and abandoned when the emergency has passed. Nevertheless, rest, if it is defined as reduction of weight-bearing activity, may be essential to the reduction of symptoms; and, sometimes, all that is necessary. The patient is required to 'live within the capacity of his knee joints'.

A joint the subject of degenerative changes is vulnerable to exercise stress or strain. The physical training instructor is advised to modify his activities; the teacher of ballet-dancing her methods and hours of work.

At a lower level of human endeavour as in the labourer, the problem, never simple, may be insoluble by conservative means; and possibly insoluble by any means.

**Reduction of weight.** The relationship of obesity to the symptoms of osteoarthrosis, if not to the cause, has been proved. Reduction of weight is mandatory for effective conservative treatment and may be essential in anticipation of operative action. Acceptance of this advice, proof of which is not far to seek, is an indication of motivation.

**Re-education in gait.** Reference has been made to the gait adopted in varus deformity; and to the possible reason for it. Re-education in walking whereby a greater range of flexion is used can be expected to improve the nutrition of articular cartilage with resulting benefits both in the short and long term.

**Use of walking-stick: limping.** Both the use of a stick and limping reduce the load acting on the affected knee. Both diminish the moment of the force eccentrically exerted by the mass of the body on the affected joint. The stick acts by transmitting a part of the force directly to the ground. The muscular forces necessary for balancing the remaining part are therefore reduced and the magnitude of the resultant force acting on the joint is decreased. Limping shortens the lever arm of the force exerted by the mass of the body by shifting the centre of gravity towards the loaded knee. As a result equilibrium is ensured by a smaller muscular force. The compression force acting on the knee is therefore reduced (Maquet, 1976).

**Injection therapy.** In the present stage of knowledge there is no substance available for injection into the osteoarthrosic knee joint which can be proved to be therapeutically effective. Miller, White and Norton (1958) showed that injections of hydrocortisone were no more effective than similar injections of normal saline. Both produced subjective and objective improvement but no better than was observed after ingenious injections of nothing whatsoever.

If this controlled trial has not received the recognition it deserves it is because there is a large vested interest in the injection of joints; and the fact that such injections are therapeutically ineffective should be widely known and accepted no matter how inconvenient. Osteoarthrosics, like rheumatoid arthritics, are placebo receptive.

HYDROCORTISONE. The use of intra-articular injections of hydrocortisone, a common though perhaps ill-considered practice, must be mentioned only to be discounted (Helfet, 1969).

There is no evidence that hydrocortisone has any beneficial effect in the treatment of osteoarthrosis; rather, indeed, the reverse. Even a single injection can precipitate a disaster. It has no place in treatment.

ARTIFICIAL LUBRICANT. There is evidence that the lubrication mechanism is impaired in osteoarthrosic joints. In such circumstances it might be expected that, whatever the cause of the degeneration, improved lubrication would prove beneficial. The criteria which have been suggested for an artificial lubricant are that it should behave in friction tests and on scanning electron microscopy like hyaluronic acid-protein complex. It should resist thermal, mechanical and oxidative degradation. It should be tolerable within the joint cavity and be retained there. It should be cheap and easy to produce (Wright *et al.*, 1971).

The successful use of silicone fluid as an artificial lubricant in osteoarthrosis has been reported (Helal and Karadi, 1968) but the results have not been confirmed (Wright *et al.*, 1971). It is not to be expected that an artificial lubricant

would be effective in the gross bony incongruity of advanced osteoarthrosis but more likely to be beneficial in burnt-out rheumatoid arthritis where bony contours are often preserved (Helal, 1971). Clearly the matter of an artificial lubricant is one worthy of further pursuit.

## TREATMENT: OPERATIVE

A variety of operative measures are available for the treatment of osteoarthrosis: meniscectomy; debridement; osteotomy; arthroplasty; arthrodesis.

### Meniscectomy

**Biomechanical basis of operation.** The return of function coupled with the relief of symptoms is exceptionally rapid following the excision of a meniscus the site of a horizontal cleavage lesion from the medial compartment even when osteoarthrosic change is in an advanced state. This statement has occasioned surprise bordering on disbelief. It is factual and was acquired in the hard school of experience. The reason on mature consideration is not far to seek: in the young subject there is an upset of joint mechanics as a consequence of a displaced complete longitudinal tear and a further temporary upset of mechanics, if of a different variety, following meniscectomy. In the ageing joint, the manifestation of thinning of articular cartilage and the 'settling-down' lesions and particularly those related to degeneration of the substance of the fibrocartilage have taken place gradually over the preceding months or years. Excision of a meniscus the subject of an advancing horizontal cleavage lesion from between the worn condyles merely removes an obstruction to motion and particularly to the rotatory movement at the termination of extension as the joint is 'screwed home'. The resulting benefit is dramatic in effect.

TECHNIQUE OF MENISCECTOMY. It is not proposed to repeat here the technical details of meniscectomy which have been described in full elsewhere (IKJ5) including the means whereby the difficulties occasioned by the reduction of the space available for manoeuvre in the ageing joint can be overcome. Nor is it proposed to repeat the pre-operative or post-operative care which does not differ in material degree from the measures applicable to the young subject.

## Debridement

**Biomechanical basis for operation.** The irregular osteocartilaginous excrescences, referred to as marginal exostoses, which in widely varying degree are a feature of the pathological process of osteoarthrosis, tend to occur in areas without opposing contact and are not of themselves a source of symptoms. The fact that the margin of the condyle is seen to be raised in the course of operation, for, say, the removal of a degenerate meniscus, is not an indication for interference. Indeed, to do so is meddlesome and to be discouraged as likely to delay recovery without commensurate compensatory benefit in the long term. Nevertheless, marginal exostoses can be a source of symptoms on a number of counts:

1. MECHANICAL OBSTRUCTION TO JOINT MOVEMENT. If the appearance of osteo-cartilaginous excrescences suggest mechanical interference with movement, occurring as they do beyond points of direct contact, it is seldom so. They probably arise on the anterior aspect of the tibio-femoral joint, however, from the stimulus of contact and as such may be responsible for a slow progressive decrease in extension.

It will be clear, however, that if in angular deformity the axis of weight-bearing is changed by osteotomy, the level of the patella will be raised, or lowered, but in any event the track in the groove changed. This may bring opposing excrescences into contact with the precipitation of symptoms. There are circumstances when this advent must be anticipated.

2. MECHANICAL INTERFERENCE WITH SOFT TISSUE MOVEMENT. Local interference with the free movement of opposing synovial membrane is of common occurrence and is a source of pain, a catching sensation and of recurrent effusion. It takes two forms: (a) the trapping of a fringe of synovial membrane by opposing marginal exostoses at either side of the tibio-femoral joint or between patella and exostoses at the patello-femoral joint, or (b)

the production, by the friction of contact in movement, of a hypertrophic area of synovial membrane which may in time become pedunculated. It is the source of a catching sensation, recurrent small effusions, local pain, swelling and tenderness.

3. FRACTURE. Marginal exostoses are mushroom-shaped or pedunculated in section. They are located superficially on the exposed margin of the femoral condyles or lateral aspect of patella. They are liable to fracture from trivial direct injury particularly in subjects with sparse soft tissue covering.

4. DIRECT PRESSURE ON SOFT TISSUE. Occasionally marginal exostoses are so large as to produce direct pressure from within the overlying soft tissues when angular deformity is corrected by high tibial osteotomy (Figs 10,42 and 10,43).

5. DEBRIDEMENT COMBINED WITH HIGH TIBIAL OSTEOTOMY. In regard to the above it is of interest and importance that MacIntosh and Welsh (1977) have reported favourable results from the combination of debridement with high tibial osteotomy performed at the same operation (see below).

## Form of Operation

**'Joint debridement': background note.** The operation as originally described by Magnuson (1941) consisted, in brief, of excision of all degenerate cartilage from the articular surfaces of femur, tibia and patella down to bare bone through a wide exposure. The totality of the attack was stressed. 'The success of the procedure depends on the complete removal of all mechanical irritants from the joints. No half-way procedure will give satisfactory results.' The author has witnessed the execution of even more extreme measures: to the original operation was added subtotal synovectomy, patellectomy and the introduction of two hemi-prostheses. The operation even as originally described, has fallen into disrepute. It is a radical procedure often wrongly applied in unsuitable cases. In any event the basic problem is not, as has been shown, marginal excrescences which are not necessarily offensive. It is an attack on effects leaving the biomechanical and biophysical causes untouched.

## Operation

The possibilities inherent in the procedure, for the reasons recorded above, have not been exploited. The operation, when indicated, should have an objective capable of definition; and when so employed can result in a dramatic improvement of function. There are two forms: **limited debridement** and **local debridement.** The former is applied to the medial femoral condyle or the lateral femoral condyle occasionally to both condyles but seldom to both at the same time. The latter, as the name implies, is applied to a local situation such as may occur in the lateral compartment following meniscectomy whereby marginal ridges may be responsible for symptoms of synovial irritation.

**Technique of limited debridement.** The operation is conducted as for meniscectomy under tourniquet and with the knee flexed over the end of the table. Varus angulation is much the more common deformity and the approach to the medial side is described. The incision is as for meniscectomy. Through it the condyle is inspected and, as far as is possible exerting lateral rotation on the tibia, the posterior segment of the meniscus. In the majority of cases the meniscus is the site of degenerative changes based on the horizontal cleavage lesion and is excised. If it is proposed to proceed to debridement the incision is extended in a curve upwards and medially to the fibres of vastus medialis but not beyond (Fig. 11,22). Retraction of the medial flap provides adequate access for the purpose of the exercise. The joint is flexed and extended to determine the nature and extent of the marginal exostoses, the cause of limitation of extension and the prospects of increase, however slight, by the removal of osteo-cartilaginous excrescences. Some improvement is usually possible unless degenerative changes are extreme. The exostosic rim is removed with a sharp fine-bladed osteotome if possible in one sweep to preserve the normal contour of the condyle (Figs 10,44 and 10,45): and not piece-meal. This can be accomplished by starting anteriorly in extension and proceding in a posterior direction with one assistant retracting while another gradually flexes the joint. The rim of exostoses overhangs the synovial membrane on the medial side, being, as it were, pedunculated. In removing it the osteotome is

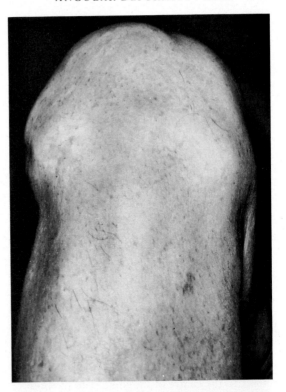

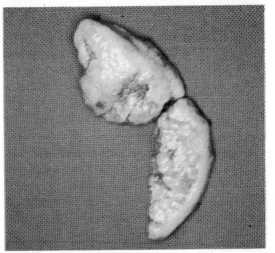

FIGS 10,42–43. **Debridement: indications.** Occasionally the cartilagenous exostoses on the periphery of the affected compartment are so large and the skin cover so poor that correction of the deformity by closing-wedge osteotomy would produce tension in the overlying skin. In such circumstances limited debridement in this example of the lateral compartment is performed three to six weeks prior to the osteotomy, the interval depending on the progress of return of flexion.

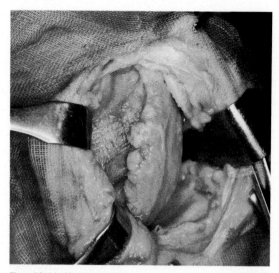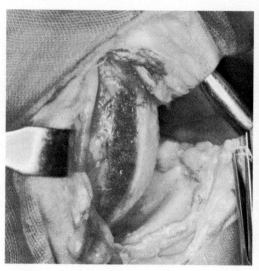

FIGS 10,44-45. **Osteoarthrosis: treatment. Limited debridement.** In mono-compartmental osteoarthrosis debridement of the medial femoral condyle may be indicated to eliminate local symptoms, possibly to increase extension or in anticipation of osteotomy of the tibial head. Appearance of marginal exostosis before (Fig. 10, 44) and after (Fig. 10,45) debridement (J.B., male, aged 62).

placed at a slight angle to the medial aspect of the condyle, that is to say the anterior edge is closer to the centre of the joint. The purpose of angling the osteotome is to make a clean cut on the intact articular cartilage avoiding damage to the synovial membrane as it underlies the overhanging exostoses and, at the same time, reducing the area of exposed cancellous tissue to a minimum.

When the local procedure on the medial femoral condyle is completed retractors should be inserted and an attempt made to inspect and determine the state of the lateral condyle in anticipation of the possibility of the necessity for osteotomy and transfer of weight-bearing to that side.

**Lateral compartment.** The reaction on the lateral side of the joint to degenerative changes in the lateral compartment is more obvious and the marginal exostoses tend to be larger than on the medial side.

At operation it may be found, in contradistinction to the medial side, that the meniscus is absent. It is difficult in these circumstances to distinguish cause from effect; but in view of the finding after lateral meniscectomy it is to be presumed that the lateral meniscus, probably the site of a parrot-beak tear, is destroyed with resulting stimulus to the growth of the massive marginal exostoses.

If the circumstances exist whereby there is doubt as to whether a sizeable portion of posterior segment remains, but in any event to permit inspection of the entire lateral compartment, the hip is rotated laterally and the knee flexed to a right-angle so that the lateral aspect of the ankle comes to lie on the suprapatellar aspect of the other knee. In this position the joint is in maximum varus strain in maximum lateral rotation. In such circumstances a wide gap exists between femur and tibia permitting visualisation of the entire lateral compartment through the limited exposure employed.

**Resurfacing.** The co-efficient of friction imposed by sclerotic subchondral bone is high. There are theoretical attractions in some method of resurfacing exposed areas. Pridie (1959) with this objective in view advocated the perforation of the eburnated areas with multiple drill holes. The advent of a blood supply might reasonably be expected to result in resurfacing by fibrous tissue, at best, by fibrocartilage.

Exposed areas of sclerotic bone widely varying in extent are a common finding in arthrotomy for almost any reason and almost invariable in joints for which debridement is indicated (Figs

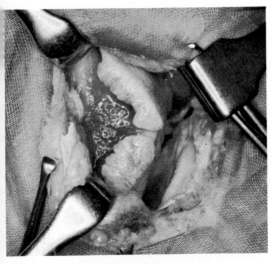

FIG. 10,46

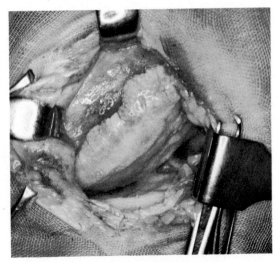

FIG. 10,47

10,46, 10,47 and 10,48). Such areas, other than in extreme examples, are consistent with function of acceptable degree, often indeed, symptomless. Reference will be made later to 'symptomatic surgery.' Reference has been made here and elsewhere to 'meddlesome surgery' (IKJ5, p. 162). It is important not to transform 'limited debridement' into a major procedure.

Drilling of extensive areas of the medial condyle has been practised using a hand gouge, such as is advocated in the surgery of osteo-chondritis dissecans, and producing a regular pattern of closely adjacent holes. Alternatively, and easier of execution, is a criss-cross pattern of right-angled opposing osteotomy cuts inflicted by an appropriately sized fine-bladed osteotome at intervals of, say, 6 mm.

It is not known to what extent such measures influenced the outcome of operation. Nor is it known to what extent the local objective is achieved. In the present state of knowledge and experience this is not a procedure which can be recommended without reserve. It is however worthy of pursuit; and to this end arthroscopic examination might reveal not only the immediate effect of operation but the wearing quality of the surfacing so produced.

CLOSURE OF CAPSULE. It is common practice that whereas limited exposures are made with the knee in right-angled flexion, the incision is

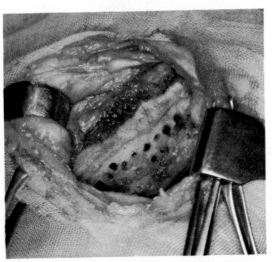

FIG. 10,48

FIGS 10,46–48. **Mono-compartmental osteoarthrosis: treatment. Debridement and 're-surfacing'.**
Figure 10,46. Medial aspect medial femoral condyle to show the massive exostoses, the angle constituting the block to full extension and the injected adjacent synovial membrane.
Figure 10,47. The exposed eburnated bone.
Figure 10,48. Debridement has been carried out and the exostoses excised. Multiple drill holes have been inserted in the exposed bone with the purpose of re-surfacing with fibrous tissue.

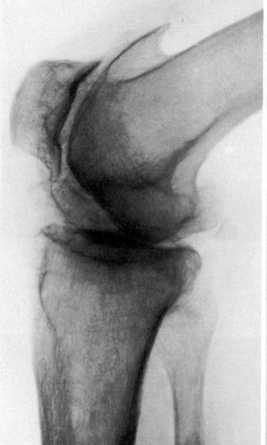
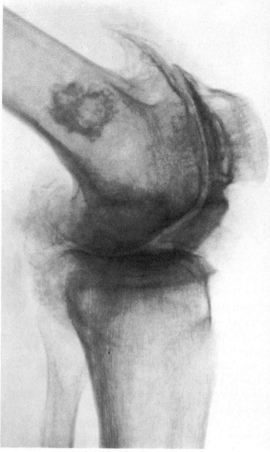

FIG. 10,49. **Osteoarthrosis: treatment.** Function in osteoarthrosis is not necessarily related to radiological findings. Decisions regarding operative treatment should not be so related. These are the radiographs of a schoolteacher on full-time duty who was capable of walking 'for exercise' and of 'Scottish country dancing'. Her reason for seeking advice: 'slight stiffness after sitting for any prolonged length of time'. (A.H., female, aged 55.)

Note marked flattening of the weight-bearing arc and presence of so-called bone island.

closed with the joint in extension. This is not a matter of serious moment. It seems reasonable however, that if the capsule is opened in flexion it should be closed in flexion. In such circumstances it is relaxed in extension, the position in which the compression bandage is applied. It means also that the scar does not require to be stretched in the course of regaining flexion and thus the return of flexion is accelerated. It will be evident that such matters are of little importance in, for example, meniscectomy in the youthful subject in which full flexion is achieved rapidly in any event. It is however a different matter in debridement for osteoarthrosis in which flexion may be limited prior to operation and a return or increase of movement achieved only with considerable effort.

AFTER-TREATMENT. The immediate after-treatment need not differ materially from that prescribed for meniscectomy: in brief, a compression bandage, quadriceps exercises from the fourth day and a return to weight-bearing on the tenth to fourteenth day. If treatment differs from meniscectomy in youth it is in the necessity to pay attention to the return of flexion by deliberate non-weight-bearing flexion exercises

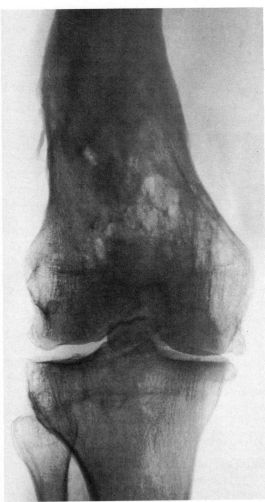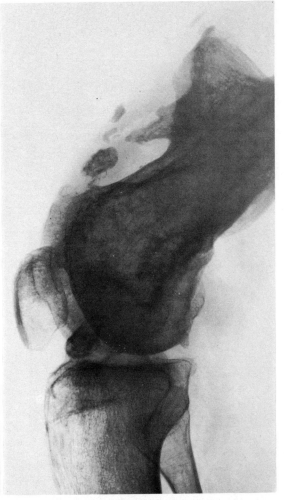

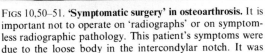

FIGS 10,50–51. **'Symptomatic surgery' in osteoarthrosis.** It is important not to operate on 'radiographs' or on symptomless radiographic pathology. This patient's symptoms were due to the loose body in the intercondylar notch. It was growing in size and from time to time it rotated and locked the joint. It was removed through a 5 cm incision. No other action is necessary or desirable (F.F., male, aged 50).

within the confines of the compression bandage starting on the fourth day. The objective of the operation, increase of extension, must not be forgotten. Any improvement achieved can be maintained only by regular passive stretching and quadriceps exercises on a permanent basis.

**Technique of local debridement.** The minimal incision is located over the offending ridge or ridges. The necessity for removal has usually occurred on the lateral side of the joint and in such circumstances the sites of lateral ligament, tendon of popliteus and lateral popliteal nerve are avoided. When the joint line and opposing ridges are located the absence of a regenerated meniscus is apparent. The local pathology, producing the necessity for operation, is noted to be active from the pink appearance of the cartilage determined by the vascularity of the underlying bone and the injection of adjacent synovial membrane.

The ridges are excised with a sharp fine-bladed osteotome.

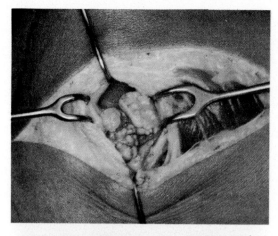

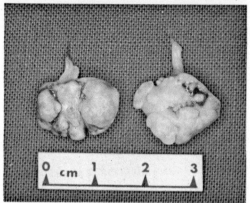

FIGS 10,52–53. **Symptomatic surgery in osteoarthrosis.** These lobulated loose bodies arose from fractures of marginal exostoses and were located immediately superior to the medial margin of the medial condyle of the femur. The muscle exposed is vastus medialis (Fig. 10,52).

The bone element of the loose bodies has retained a blood supply through the pedicles of synovial membrane (Fig. 10,53).

**Result of operation.** The immediate result of operation is the relief of symptoms. But the result may not be maintained. The fact that marginal surfaces denuded of articular cartilage are in contact without intervening regenerated meniscus would suggest that recurrence of the ridges and of the symptoms is likely. Experience is limited to professional football players who had previously suffered a lateral meniscectomy. In two examples the operation has had to be repeated after an interval of two years. Such operations cannot be repeated indefinitely; and

the probable eventual outcome is osteoarthrosis affecting the entire lateral compartment with angular deformity necessitating osteotomy.

Local debridement, for one reason or another, at sites not involved in weight-bearing have a better prognosis in the long term (Figs 6,80 to 6,85).

## Symptomatic Surgery

Many patients come to terms with a disability; even in the knee joint. The most grotesque radiographs may relate to a symptomless joint and are consistent with reasonable function (Fig. 10,49). When such patients develop symptoms it is important not to be influenced by the radiographs. The patient with limited flexion may fail to clear an obstruction with his foot and develop an effusion which will rapidly subside with compression. The patient whose radiographs are reproduced in Figures 10,50 and 10,51 had local symptoms related to the loose body which was growing in size. It was removed through a limited incision with immediate relief. The fracture of an exostosis (Figs 10,42 and 10,53) or the development of symptoms from local irritation of synovial membrane demand similar local surgery; but no more.

## Osteotomy of Tibia

**Historical note.** Osteotomy of the tibia performed simply to correct deformity of the knee was first described by Volkmann (1875) at about the same time as Lister and MacEwan (1878) described supracondylar osteotomy.

Osteotomy of the tibia combined with division of the fibula has been practised in Liverpool since 1928 (Wardle, 1964). At that time the common deformities of the adult knee were the result of childhood rickets. The surgeons who practised it were aware that correction of deformity in adult life by femoral osteotomy, so successful in children, invited the rapid onset of pain and degenerative changes in the knee joint. They gave the reason that correction of deformity above the joint altered the inclination of the axis of movement to the line of weight-bearing in the leg as a whole; and whereas the growing child could adapt the adult could not. Osteotomy below the joint made no such alteration. It corrects deformity by the production of an equal and opposite deformity below the original one leaving the axis of movement of the knee joint at the same inclination to the weight-bearing line of the limb. The application of this procedure to the treatment of osteoarthrosis of the knee is credited to Steindler (1940).

The location of the osteotomy to a site immediately distal to the articular surface of the tibia is ascribed to the author (IKJ1, 1946) (Wardle, 1964). Acknowledgement is made here that the opening-wedge osteotomy so located is based on the procedure of Brett (1935).

**Biomechanical basis of operation.** An angular deformity of 10° trebles the load per unit area on the affected tibial condyle (Simonet *et al.*, 1963). It is established that in angular deformity, usually varus, based on degenerative changes in the medial compartment, the articular cartilage in the opposite lateral compartment may be relatively unaffected, even at a late stage (Fig. 10,54). Alteration of alignment transferring weight to the normal side could in such circumstances be expected to reduce the compression forces on the concave side and at the same time reduce the traction forces on the capsule on the convex side.

There is evidence, with massive documentation (Bouillet and Van Gaver, 1961; Gariepy, 1961; Jackson and Waugh, 1961; Wardle, 1962; Coventry, 1965, 1973, to mention but a few) that osteotomy in one form or another results in reduction or abolition of pain in osteoarthrosis; and that reduction of pain is not entirely due to correction of angular deformity.

**Alteration in pattern of circulation.** It has been known for many years that the success of osteotomy in the relief of pain in osteoarthrosis of the hip joint was not dependent on alteration of mechanics by displacement but on division of the bone (Nissen, 1963). It has been observed in elderly patients in whom osteotomy of the tibia was performed without a tourniquet that division of the bone is associated with the outpouring of dark venous blood from the medullary cavity. This suggested that the relief of intramedullary venous pressure might be associated with the relief of pain (Wardle, 1964). This matter has been pursued experimentally (Helal, 1965) with convincing evidence of venous sinusoidal engorgement in the tibia subjacent to

an osteoarthrosic knee. It appears therefore that in order to relieve pain it is necessary to open the medullary cavity of the tibia distal to the joint. To maintain the relief of pain it is necessary to create a barrier across the medullary cavity isolating the proximal part from any connection with the main venous outflow from the shaft of the bone as a whole. Osteotomy produces this block naturally by bone as in the healing of any fracture (Wardle, 1964).

'LUCKY BREAKS'. It had been known to experienced orthopaedic surgeons for many years that patients with burnt-out rheumatoid arthritis with a fixed flexion deformity at the knee who sustained a supracondylar fracture of the fragile femur in a fall achieved greater relief of pain in the joint than could be explained by correction of the deformity. It seems strange, in the current scene, that this observation was not capitalised at an earlier date.

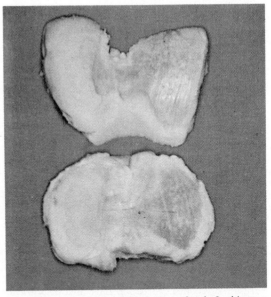

FIG. 10,54. **Mono-compartmental osteoarthrosis.** In this gross example the articular cartilage of the lateral compartment is normal in appearance. The biomechanical basis of the success of opening- or closing-wedge osteotomy in the treatment of mono-compartmental osteoarthrosis with angular deformity depends on the transfer of weight-bearing from the worn to the unworn compartment of the joint.

Note lesion in femoral condyle on the lateral side. This is a common finding and is due to impingement of lateral eminence of tibial spine, the result of loss of joint space.

*Stimulation of chondroblastic activity.* The nutritional demands of articular cartilage and bone are anti-complimentary. Alteration in the circulation pattern by osteotomy may reduce the blood supply of the subchondral bone and provide the stimulus to replacement or to repair by fibrous tissue.

### OPERATION OF OSTEOTOMY

If osteotomy of the head of the tibia is an accepted method of treatment of osteoarthrosis the methods which have been devised for its execution vie with one another in ingenuity and complexity.

It is important that an operation of universal application in patients of an age group likely to require it should be simple in concept, of short duration and that methods of fixation, internal or external, limit the possibility of complications.

The operation as practiced by the author takes one of two forms:
1. **Linear opening-wedge osteotomy.**
2. **Linear closing-wedge osteotomy (Gariepy, 1961).**

### FORM OF OSTEOTOMY: MERITS AND DEMERITS OF OPENING-WEDGE AND CLOSING-WEDGE TYPES AS APPLIED TO VARUS ANGULATION

*Opening-Wedge Osteotomy on Medial Side*

**Advantages**

1. It restores the original anatomy, the length of the leg and the relationship of patella to femoral condyles (Figs 10,55 and 10,56).
2. Absolute accuracy of division is not essential.
3. It is performed entirely within the broad parallel-sided vascular tibial flare and within the compass of the medial ligament and patellar tendon. The stabilising function of the medial ligament is thus restored.
4. The site and degree of correction can be controlled by size of wedge grafts inserted.
5. Fracture of opposite cortex is unnecessary and indeed is to be avoided.
6. Stability is maintained by grafts under com-

pression and by the medial and patellar ligaments. No post-operative splinting is necessary other than by compression bandage incorporating plaster slabs.

7. It is a vascular site, there is minimum interference with blood supply, and with the grafts under compression there is rapid healing.

8. In the absence of the necessity for plaster immobilisation no difficulty is encountered in securing a full return of flexion.

**Disadvantages**

1. The necessity to secure whole thickness wedge-shaped bone grafts from the ilium. This is a procedure with a reputation as a source of pain greater than that incurred at the knee. It is reduced in considerable degree in the current scene by the use of suction drainage.
2. The theoretical risk in older age groups to popliteal vessels by the opening of a wedge.

*Closing-wedge Osteotomy on Lateral Side*

**Advantages**

1. No additional procedure to obtain bone graft is necessary.
2. There is no theoretical risk to vessels or nerves.

**Disadvantages**

1. Operative access to the lateral aspect of tibial head because of presence of fibula and lateral popliteal nerve is more difficult than to the medial aspect.
2. It does not restore the original anatomy, shortens the leg and lowers the relationship of patella to femoral condyles (Figs 10,57 and 10,58).
3. Absolute accuracy is essential to secure closure of wedge.
4. Fracture of opposite cortex is necessary to close the wedge. Furthermore, the closing wedge, excising as it does bone, if it is not performed within the flare of the tibia must terminate with areas of different section in contact not under compression and with resultant fixation problems. Internal fixation in the form of staples, or external fixation in the form of compression, may be necessary.

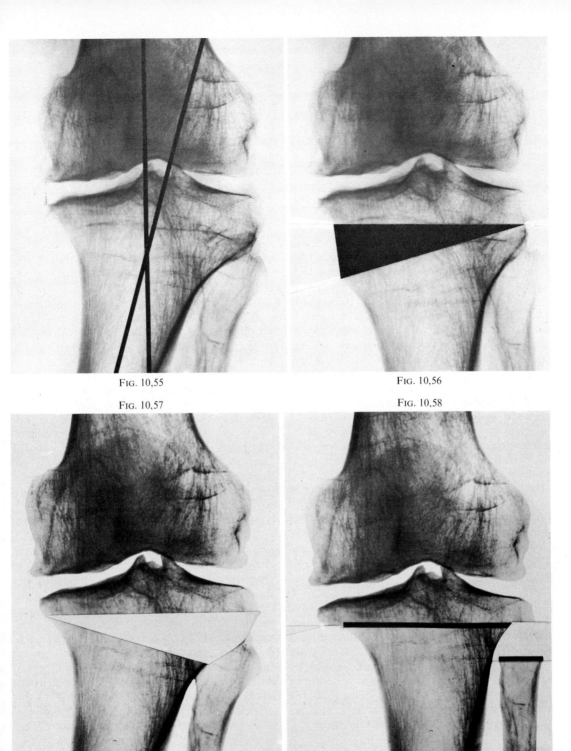

FIGS 10,55–58. **Angular deformity: treatment. Opening-wedge or closing-wedge osteotomy.**
Figure 10,55. Weight-bearing radiograph to show tibio-femoral angle. See also Figures 10,39 to 10,41.
Figure 10,56. Opening-wedge osteotomy on the medial side to restore weight-bearing alignment.

Figure 10,57. Closing-wedge osteotomy on the lateral side to show size of wedge to be removed.
Figure 10,58. Closing-wedge osteotomy after wedge has been removed. The merits and demerits of opening-wedge as opposed to closing-wedge osteotomy are discussed in the text. (Semi-diagrammatic.)

5. For reasons implied in (4) above healing may be delayed.

6. If external fixation and compression is used the theoretical advantage of early movement is offset by an increase in post-operative complications.

7. If plaster fixation is employed, as is the common practice, difficulty is encountered in securing a return of flexion. Manipulation under general anaesthesia may be required.

**Choice.** The more common deformity is varus and thus the problem is one of a choice between an opening-wedge on the medial aspect of the tibial head and a closing-wedge on the lateral aspect.

In general the opening-wedge will be chosen in the younger patient with the highest demands in terms of function whereas the closing-wedge is applicable in less ideal circumstances and the more likely to be chosen in the older age groups.

In valgus deformity in the elderly, as opposed to the adolescent or young adult, it is probable that the opening-wedge method will not be selected on account of possible hazards to circulation or to lateral popliteal nerve (Figs 10, 71 to 10,74). If in the course of operation it is thought that such a risk has arisen the limb should be nursed on the flexed-knee splint and gradually extended until such time as the stitches are removed when the walking cast can be applied.

### Indications and Contraindications to Osteotomy

**Peripheral vascular disease: intermittent claudication.** Linear osteotomy is required most often in the age range which suffers from peripheral vascular disease. Care should be taken especially if an opening-wedge osteotomy is contemplated that tension is not applied to the vessels, either centrally or peripherally, so that a circulatory crisis is precipitated in the foot.

**Medial torsion.** A contraindication to operation in the middle-aged or later may be the existence of considerable medial torsion in addition to varus angulation. Reference has been made to the deleterious effect of medial torsion of the

tibia on the joint. Linear osteotomy above the tibial tubercle can correct varus angulation but cannot correct rotation.

If rotation is to be corrected it must be done in youth before there are irreversible changes in the joint. A method whereby both varus and internal rotation can be corrected has been described (Ch. 8). It will be appreciated that to correct both deformities at once the operation must be performed below the level of the tibial tubercle.

**Flexion deformity.** A fixed flexion deformity of more than 20° is a contraindication to osteotomy of the tibia (Jackson, Waugh and Green, 1969). There may thus be a case for attempting to improve extension by debridement in the first instance.

A fixed flexion deformity greater than 20° may require osteotomy of the femur to be considered with attendant technical difficulty of operation, necessary for prolonged immobilisation and complications.

**Multiple procedures.** The operation should not be performed in combination with any other procedure, intra-articular or extra-articular. The single exception to this rule is recorded in Chapter 9. If an intra-articular operation in the form of meniscectomy, or meniscectomy and debridement, is indicated it should be done previously and the optimum recovery secured before proceeding to osteotomy.

**Symptomless radiographs.** It is a serious error of judgement to operate on symptomless radiographs no matter how extreme in appearance.

**Deformity.** The standard of function in this age group is low. A degree of deformity, particularly varus angulation, which seems alarming to the orthopaedic surgeon is acceptable to the patient provided it is relatively symptomless. It is important not to operate on deformity as such. It is for this reason that such sources of symptoms as the horizontal cleavage lesion of the posterior segment of the medial meniscus should be considered. Elimination of this mechanical interference with function may be all that is necessary; and may avoid more radical measures such as debridement or tibial osteotomy.

### Linear Opening-wedge Osteotomy

This operation has particular application in

angular deformity of adolescents and adults to the exclusion of other forms.

## Angular Deformity: Varus

**Technique.** The knee, under the control of a tourniquet, is flexed over the end of the table as for meniscectomy. It is important that the joint hangs clear so that the posterior vessels and nerve are relaxed and out of danger. A 6 cm vertical incision is made from just above the joint line downwards on the antero-medial aspect of the flare of the tibia. The joint is not entered. The incision is carried through the periosteum and curved elevators inserted sub-periosteally under the medial ligament and patellar tendon. The site of osteotomy is selected, a guide wire inserted and an antero-posterior radiograph obtained. The osteotomy is accomplished with fine osteotomes or reciprocating saw. Care is taken not to divide the cortex on the lateral side. Considerable correction can be achieved without fracture.

In ideal circumstances the correction will be of moderate degree and within the confines of the medial ligament. Where a greater degree is required the medial ligament under tension will be found to limit correction and will require to be released. This is accomplished by determination of the limit of the inferior insertion which is then erased with a periosteal elevator or by a knife blade passed between ligament and bone. This action will be found to permit wide angulation at the osteotomy site.

Bone grafts of the required angle are obtained from the iliac crest in the manner described in Chapter 9. The one depicting the required correction is inserted opposite the medial ligament but, in any event, at the same site if the ligament requires to be lengthened as above.

AFTER-TREATMENT. At the termination a compression bandage is applied in the outer layers of which are incorporated plaster slabs with the purpose of restricting movement which might fracture the intact lateral cortex. In theory, provided the opposite knee is within the bounds of normality, weight-bearing can be resumed on patten and crutches and flexion exercises within the confines of the bandage practised as soon as suction drainage from the iliac crest has ceased and the patient overcome the immediate effects of the operation. In any event it should be recognised that the blood supply in the area of the incision is poor: removal of the skin sutures should be deferred for three weeks. With the ability to practise non-weight-bearing exercises from the start flexion should be regained rapidly. Partial weight-bearing with the aid of crutches can be undertaken about the eighth week. Full weight-bearing is resumed at the twelfth week.

## Linear Closing-wedge Osteotomy

SITE. The wedge is resected at or about the flare of the tibia. A closing-wedge osteotomy can, however, contrary to current practice, be performed within the flare, and has, at this site, the advantage of opposing surfaces of similar diameter. In addition, at this level resection of the head of the fibula is unnecessary to gain access from the lateral side. On the other hand more accuracy of location is necessary. The upper fragment is close to the joint line and therefore thin, so much so that it incurs the liability of fracture into the joint when the wedge is closed. To overcome this hazard care must be taken to remove any obstruction to closure from the osteotomy site and to fracture the cortex on the opposite side manually by opening the wedge before finally closing it (Figs 10,59 and 10,60).

If closing-wedge osteotomy within the flare entails the risk of fracture into the joint, osteotomy immediately below the flare (Fig. 10,61) entails the risk of injury to the anterior tibial artery (Jackson and Waugh, 1974). They point out that the artery passes forward below the lower part of the superior tibio-fibular joint (Fig. 10,62) and above the upper edge of the interosseous membrane. This narrow opening is usually at the level of the lower border of the tibial tubercle and the artery is in danger when the operation is performed at this level. It might be divided or compressed by instruments, stretched or compressed when the wedge is closed.

## Angular Deformity: Varus

**Technique.** The limb is exsanguinated and flexed over the end of the table, hanging clear, as for meniscectomy. It is particularly important that right-angled flexion be adopted; and that the posterior vessels and nerves are relaxed and out of danger. The skin incision may be horizontal below the joint line extending from about the tibial tubercle anteriorly to the head of the fibula posteriorly; or a vertical incision between patellar tendon and fibula may be used.

The proximal extremities of the dorsiflexor muscles of the foot are erased subperiosteally and the flare of the tibia located. The operation is performed as close to the joint as possible within the compass of the patellar tendon. If a large wedge is to be removed it may be necessary to erase the uppermost, but only the uppermost, fibres of the attachment to the tibial tubercle. The sensitivity of the lateral popliteal nerve is well-known. It should not be exposed, handled or retracted. The operation can be performed

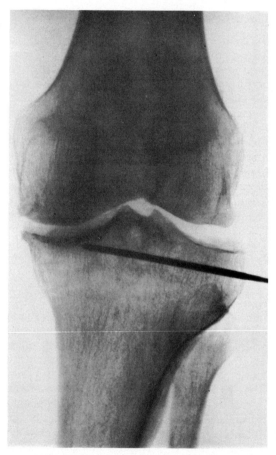

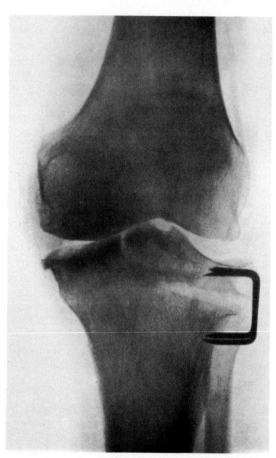

FIG. 10,59. **Closing (or opening) wedge osteotomy of tibial head: technique.** If in doubt as to orientation a guide wire should be inserted and a radiograph taken. The higher within the flare of the tibia the proposed osteotomy the more important is accuracy lest the joint be entered or intra-articular fracture produced. Note that in this case the guide wire is too high. Note the sclerosis of the bone on the side of the joint under compression. It is at or about the point of the guide wire that an intra-articular fracture is liable to occur on closing the wedge (see text).

FIG. 10,60. **Mono-compartmental (medial) osteoarthrosis: closing-wedge osteotomy: error of technique.** It will be seen that a fracture has occurred through the sclerotic sub-chondral bone of the medial condyle probably due to the fact that the osteotomy did not extend far enough to the medial side before closing the wedge. The osteotomy has been performed within the flare of the tibia and without resection of the head of the fibula. The closer the closing-wedge, as opposed to the opening-wedge, osteotomy to the joint line the greater is the danger of this error. It is in this regard that the use of a guide wire is advocated (Fig. 10,59).

without resection of the head of the fibula; but it may be easier to do so. To this end it is exposed subperiosteally from the anterior aspect, the biceps tendon and lateral ligament erased, an elevator passed round the lateral side and sufficient of the head resected to gain access to the tibia. Elevators are then passed round the tibia and the wedge, of predetermined angle, delineated. It is clearly undesirable to produce a fracture entering the joint.

The superior first cut should be 1 to 2 cm below and parallel to the tibial joint surface. The inferior second cut is angled to meet it about the opposite cortex. If there is any question of the exact location of the superior cut, a Steinmann pin is entered and a radiograph obtained (Fig. 10,59). The osteotomy, performed with fine broad-bladed osteotomes, is taken as far as, but not through, the opposing cortex. Force is required to close the wedge with fracture of the opposite cortex; and this is accomplished if necessary by prising open the gap before closing it. But care must be exercised that the fracture occurs at the opposing cortex and not vertically into the joint; and the closer the osteotomy to the joint the greater is the danger. The reason for the hazard is that the bone on the side under compression is sclerosic, whereas the bone on the side under relaxation is osteoporosic. In attempting to close the wedge the rigid bone of the medial condyle is liable to fracture. In this regard too it is important that the cortex be divided anteriorly and posteriorly and that cancellous tissue at the apex of the wedge medially be removed before the gap is closed.

If a flexion deformity still remains it can be corrected by making the wedge appropriately wider anteriorly. In doing so discretion should be exercised in how much flexion to correct in so far as the more bone removed anteriorly between the attachment of patellar tendon and joint line the more relaxed will the tendon become, thus, not only will the mechanics of the patello-femoral joint be altered, but some loss of control of extension may occur.

OVERCORRECTION. In varus angulation Maquet (1976) recommends overcorrection, empirically determined but of 2° to 4°, on the grounds that correcting the deformity to what was 'normal' for that particular patient merely

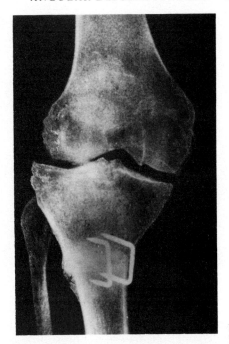

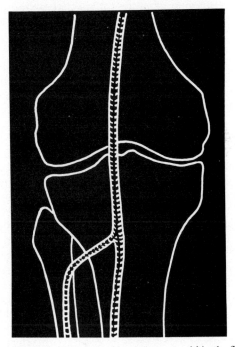

FIGS 10,61–62. If closing-wedge osteotomy within the flare entails the risk of fracture into the joint (Fig. 10,60) osteotomy immediately below the flare (Fig. 10,61) entails the risk of injury to the anterior tibial artery (Fig. 10,62).

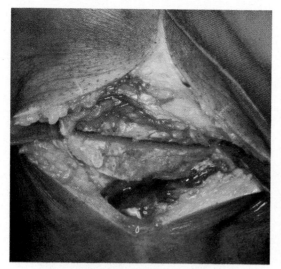

FIG. 10,63

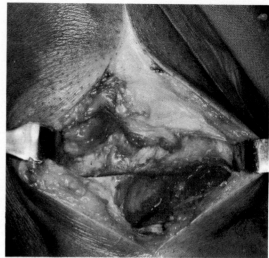

FIG. 10,64

reproduces the mechanical conditions which determined the onset and development of the mono-compartmental osteoarthrosis in the first place. Furthermore it is said to compensate for deficiency of power in the lateral muscles biceps femoris and tensor fascia femoris. It has not been the author's practice to purposefully overcorrect a deformity. The tendency regretfully has been to undercorrect. The exception has been in the opening wedge osteotomy when it has been anticipated that some of the correction will be lost by the collapse of cancellous tissue.

### Angular Deformity: Valgus

**Technique.** A short vertical incision over the anteromedial surface of the tibia immediately below the joint line is favoured. The periosteum is erased from the tibia. The patellar tendon is cleared from the anterior aspect and if necessary the uppermost fibres of insertion are erased from the bone. A medially-based wedge of bone of predetermined angle is removed in a manner similar to that just described. The apex of the wedge should lie above the proximal tibio-fibular joint so that osteotomy of the fibula is unnecessary (Figs 10,63 to 10,65).

INTERNAL FIXATION. In general some form of internal fixation is desirable by staples, one near the head of the fibula posteriorly, and one near the tibial tubercle anteriorly. If a discrepancy in

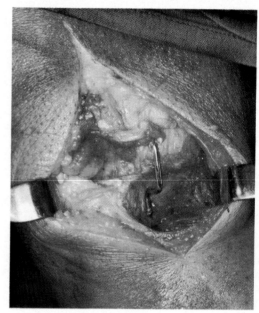

FIG. 10,65

FIGS 10,63–65. **Closing-wedge osteotomy: technique.** The operation can be performed through a limited vertical incision and virtually within the flare of the tibia. A wedge of predetermined angle is outlined and removed (Fig. 10,63) and the resulting wedge-shaped interval closed (Fig. 10,64). Internal fixation in the form of one or more staples may be used. If there is discrepancy in the opposing surfaces a stepped staple (Coventry) may be indicated (Fig. 10,65).

diameter exists between the opposing surfaces staples of the 'stepped' variety (Coventry, 1965) are employed (Fig. 10,65).

If the head of the fibula has been resected the operation is completed by resuture of the lateral ligament and biceps tendon, if necessary, through drill holes.

**After-treatment.** At the termination of either operation a compression bandage is applied incorporating posterior plaster slabs. The limb is placed in a Thomas half-ring bed-knee splint and the end of the bed elevated. On the following day the patient is allowed to stand by the bedside with the aid of crutches. When the stitches are removed at the twelfth day a cylinder cast, not including the foot, is applied with the joint in extension and full weight-bearing permitted with the aid of crutches (Fig. 10,66). Hourly straight-leg raising which increases compression at the osteotomy are practised from the start. At the end of six weeks the cast is removed and mobilising exercises begun.

EXTERNAL FIXATION. The use of transfixation pins, single (Gariepy, 1964), or double (Devas, 1969; Jackson, Waugh and Green, 1969), and compression clamps in theory stabilise the site in the closing-wedge osteotomy, but increase the risk of complications such as pin-track infection, thrombosis and peroneal nerve paralysis particularly in the age range and conformation of joint likely to require this operation. External fixation has not been used by the author. Nevertheless, it is in common use and, indeed, must be used if the dome-shaped osteotomy is employed to be certain of maintaining correction (Figs 10,67 and 10,68). In other circumstances the principal advantage is that mobility of the osteoarthrosic joint can be maintained in the immediate post-operative period and, of course, plaster fixation is unnecessary.

If single pins are to be used the upper is inserted, for reasons which will be evident, from the lateral side not too far posteriorly and parallel to the tibial joint line. The lower is inserted below the osteotomy site at the angle of the wedge to be removed so that, at the termination of the operation both pins are parallel (Fig. 10,69). The double pins are employed not only to permit mobility to be retained but to enable walking with the aid of crutches within a few days of operation (Fig.

10,70). Devas describes the technique of insertion as follows:

'The wedge having been taken the first pin is driven through the tibial plateau above the osteotomy, a small lateral incision having been made over the site of the insertion, which should be approximately at the junction of the middle and anterior third of the tibial plateau and halfway between the joint line and the osteotomy. The pin is driven through until it appears on the medial side. The skin is cut over the point of the pin which is driven through about another 3 to 4 cm. The first osteotomy clamp is placed over the outer aspect of the first pin usually using the centre of the anterior three holes. The connecting bar

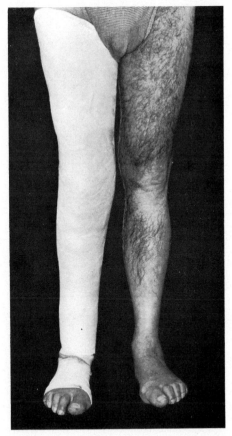

FIG. 10,66. **Closing-wedge osteotomy: after-treatment.** Weight-bearing is resumed as soon as possible in a cylinder plaster cast (J.S., male, aged 68).

is put through from the upper end and the lower clamp placed on the connecting bar and used as a guide for the first pin to be inserted through the tibial shaft, which is done in a manner similar to the first pin. It is important to keep the osteotomy closed at this stage so that the pins will be parallel when the connecting bars are tightened. The second pin through the shaft is then inserted. It is

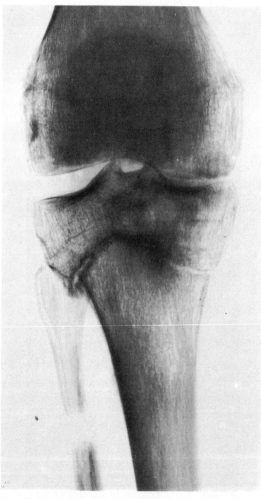

FIG. 10,67. **Angular deformity: operation.** Mono-compartmental (medial) osteoarthrosis treated by dome-shaped osteotomy with the purpose of transferring weight to the normal lateral compartment of the joint. Immobilisation in a plaster cast did not maintain correction and no alteration in the weight-bearing mechanics resulted. The patient however declared that his pain had been alleviated.

important to insert the pins in this order because any error is magnified if the two proximal pins are inserted before both the distal pins. Finally the posterior pin is inserted through the tibial plateau, again using the clamp as a guide. The points of the pins are adjusted so that they do not show outside the clamps when the fixing screws are tightened.

There should be a small gap between the clamps and the skin to avoid soreness. The whole apparatus is then tightened and absolute rigidity of the osteotomy is achieved. The skin only is closed. A light dressing is applied over the wound and pins and the whole enclosed in a crêpe bandage. No attempt is made to pass the crêpe bandage between the connecting bars and the skin. Within a few days the crêpe bandage and wool may be removed and a lighter dressing applied. The patients are allowed to walk as soon as they wish. The pins are usually removed at the end of four weeks.'

## Linear Osteotomy without Displacement

If the relief of pain from osteotomy is the result of alteration of circulatory pattern, particularly in the form of reduction of intramedullary venous pressure, Benjamin (1969) has carried the matter to its logical conclusion by recommending osteotomy of both tibia and femur, not necessarily including correction of angular deformity, for the treatment of both osteoarthrosis and rheumatoid arthritis (see Ch. 6). Experience to date is limited to linear division of the tibia in cases involving the entire tibio-femoral joint without angular deformity when the problem appeared to concern the tibia rather than the femur, in which conservative measures had been exhausted and little hope for relief offered other than by arthrodesis. Double osteotomy has not been practised. The limited experience of simple linear osteotomy of the tibia is not sufficient on which to base an opinion. In an independent assessment of Benjamin's results Trickey (1969) stated, 'The operation has resulted in relief of pain and increase in function in many knees which had no deformity. When a deformity did exist before operation recurrence did not appear to influence the result.' (Fig. 10,67.) In such circumstances the procedure, in single or double form, is worthy of trial in the osteoarthrosis affecting both compartments, coxitis knee, burnt-out rheumatoid arthritis and like problems at present without solution.

**Technique of operation.** 'The tibial osteotomy is through cancellous bone above the tibial tubercle, to ensure rapid union. The femoral osteotomy is done from inside the knee joint, firstly because the cancellous bone at this site seldom fails to unite, and secondly because intra-articular adhesions may be overcome more easily than the muscle adhesions that may follow more proximal osteotomy.

'With the patient supine and the limb exsanguinated by a tourniquet, the knee is exposed through a long medial parapatellar incision. The capsule is incised in the line of the skin incision and the patellar ligament is defined. The knee is flexed, and bone levers are inserted subperiosteally round the lower end of the femur inside the joint; the patella dislocates as these are moved into place. Bone levers are similarly placed round the condyles of the tibia: the knee flexion is essential to

relax the popliteal neurovascular bundle and care is taken that at all times the bone levers are close to bone. The femoral osteotomy is intra-articular, just distal to the upper border of the articular cartilage. The tibial osteotomy is not more than 2·5 cm distal to the joint. Osteotomy of the fibula is unnecessary. If there is flexion, varus or valgus deformity it is corrected by manipulation at both osteotomy sites. After release of the tourniquet the capsule and skin are sutured. A well-padded plaster of Paris cylinder is applied from groin to malleoli and correction of the deformity is maintained by manual moulding as the plaster sets. The position is checked by radiography.

'POST-OPERATIVE CARE. The patient is encouraged to get up on the first or second day after operation, using crutches if necessary but putting full weight on the limb. Five weeks after operation the patient is readmitted to hospital and the plaster is removed. Full weight-bearing is allowed immediately. Mobilisation of the knee is allowed at the patient's own speed, physiotherapy and

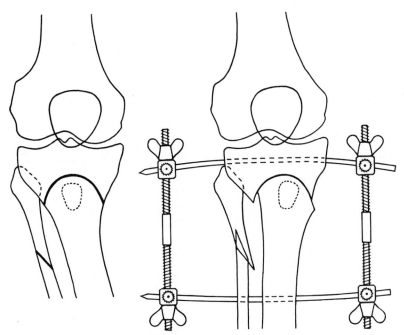

FIG. 10,68. **Angular deformity: operation.** If, for whatever reason, angular deformity is corrected by dome-shaped osteotomy, plaster cast immobilisation alone cannot be guaranteed to maintain correction. Transfixion pins, incorporated in plaster, or with compression clamps are necessary.

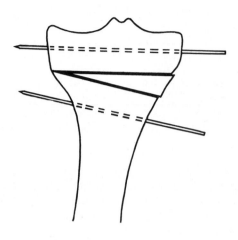 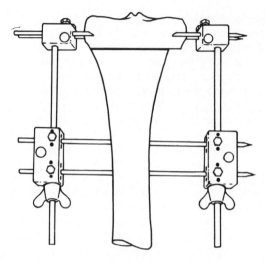

FIGS 10,69–70. **Mono-compartmental osteoarthrosis: Closing-wedge osteotomy.** Method of fixation with single transverse pins (Fig. 10,69) or with double transverse horizontal pins through the upper fragment and double transverse vertical pins through the lower fragment and with compression clamp (Fig. 10,70). (After Devas.)

manipulation being given only if required after 6 to 12 months. In more recent cases, not included in this series, the knee has been gently manipulated to 90° under anaesthesia, after removal of the plaster, with more rapid mobilisation.'

### Results of Osteotomy

This operation in its various forms has achieved a considerable reputation for the relief of symptoms in osteoarthrosis during the short number of years in which it has been practised.

It will be evident that the best results are likely to occur when there is, in fact, an angular deformity capable of correction and with weight-bearing transferred to the relatively normal side of the joint (Figs 10,71 to 10,74). If degenerative changes affect both compartments, as is the rule in burnt-out rheumatoid arthritis, but in some cases of osteoarthrosis, no advantage can result from correction of the weight-bearing mechanics and the only benefit is that of alteration in the pattern of circulation such as is assumed to occur following simple osteotomy without displacement.

**Immediate.** Wardle (1964), who performed the first operation of his series of 35 cases in 1941, recorded that all patients reported complete relief of their pain, in particular of their intractable night pain, within a few days of operation and there has been no recurrence. Twenty-seven of these patients had recovered the minimum range of 90° of active flexion in the knee joint by six months from the time of operation, many of them at three months. A considerable proportion had achieved a full range although movement was limited before operation. At an interval of two years the disappearance of synovial thickening is a striking feature and crepitus is markedly diminished. Later, radiological changes occur in the proximal part of the tibia. Normal bone architecture and density reappear and cysts disappear.

**Late.** In the patients re-examined more than five years from the time of operation certain phenomena have been consistently observed. Clinically there is a striking reduction in soft-tissue synovial swelling. Radiologically the architecture of the tibial bone proximal to the site of the osteotomy tends to return to normal and joint space increases.

### Arthroplasty

In the present state of development, arthroplasty is limited to joints with bicompartmental and

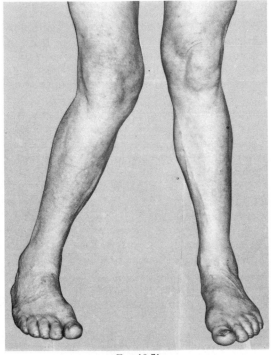

FIG. 10,71

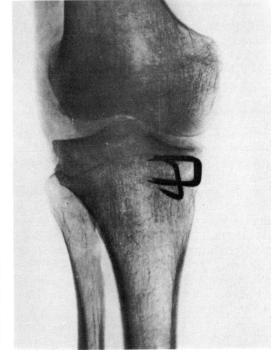

FIG. 10,73

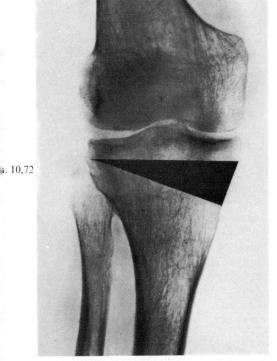

ɪ. 10,72

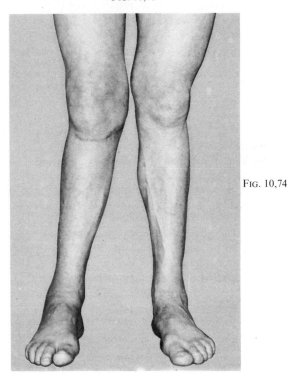

FIG. 10,74

FIGS 10,71–74. **Angular deformity: valgus. Medial closing-wedge osteotomy.** The deformity is bilateral but the right side is much worse than the left which was symptomless (Fig. 10,71). Radiograph outlining of the wedge of bone which was removed (Fig. 10,72). The wedge has been removed with such accuracy that the line of osteotomy cannot be seen. Three staples have been used for internal fixation (Fig. 10,73). The deformity was not corrected completely in an attempt to match the left side (Fig. 10,74). The transverse incision is undesirable and not to be recommended (A.M., male, aged 59).

pan-articular disease untreatable other than by arthrodesis. Patients selected are of an age which will make modest demands of the replacement. (For various techniques see Chapter 6.)

## Arthrodesis

In spite of the frequency with which osteo-arthrosis is encountered, even in gross form, arthrodesis should seldom be indicated (Table 8) other than for failed arthroplasty.

In the young adult male, however, with advanced changes involving the entire tibio-femoral joint, or with gross distortion of the anatomy the result of trauma, who has no skills and depends for his livelihood on manual work, there may be no practical alternative to arthrodesis. Unfortunately the very fact of arthrodesis limits the physical work available to him.

SPECIAL CIRCUMSTANCES OF
TREATMENT

### Coxitis Knee

It will be evident that if mechanical stresses imposed from above can be reduced, and if the age of the patient is such as to make corrective osteotomy a reasonable procedure, the altered mechanics will have a favourable effect on the function of the knee provided secondary changes in that joint are not too far advanced. The initial approach to the problem therefore should, as ever, be the removal, or at least the reduction, of the cause (Bouillet and Delchef, 1968). An adduction deformity of the hip in early life is invariably compensated for by angular deformity at the knee in the form of valgus. If any considerable adduction at the hip is corrected the effect on the distal genu valgum must be considered if the end result in terms of total disability is not to be increased rather than reduced. In other words there are circum-stances in the young subject in which reduction of a hip deformity must be followed, preferably in the course of healing, by correction of the secondary deformity at the knee if the optimal result is to be obtained. The problem of

treatment of which no immediate solution is forthcoming is the coxitis knee in the form of osteoarthrosis affecting medial and lateral com-partments of the tibio-femoral joint in equal degree in the absence of angular deformity of the hip or of angular deformity at the knee. Whether simple division of the head of the tibia and femur without displacement as advocated for the reduction of pain in osteoarthrosis (Benjamin, 1969) would be beneficial in such circumstances has yet to be proved.

The problem as it confronts a patient is a serious one: the impossible combination in terms of function of a fixed hip with a fixed knee. In early cases, if the possibility of a horizontal cleavage lesion of the posterior segment of the medial meniscus can be eliminated, treatment consists of simple measures to preserve full extension combined with quadriceps exercises. When the optimum improvement has been achieved the importance of maintenance exercises on a permanent basis is stressed.

**Conservative surgery.** If a degenerative meniscus lesion is present meniscectomy is indicated in the interests of preserving the articular cartilage of the medial compartment. If meniscectomy is under consideration the question of debride-ment of the medial margin of the medial femoral condyle may arise if a bony block to extension exists or with symptoms related thereto. Finally, in the realms of conservative surgery, is the possible necessity for linear osteotomy of the tibial head. But it may be performed only on the basis of alteration of circulation. Angular deformity cannot be corrected in the presence of a fixed hip.

In any operative measure the difficulties of regaining flexion in the presence of a stiff hip should be remembered. The method of auto-assisted exercises illustrated in Figure 6,15 is applicable in such circumstances.

**Radical surgery.** If conservative measures fail to preserve function at a tolerable level of symptoms radical surgery may be indicated. It is evident that arthrodesis is not to be con-templated in the presence of ankylosis of the hip. Two possibilities remain: (1) arthroplasty; and whether this measure is applicable depends on the age and sex of the patient and the demands likely to be made of the limb: and (2) amputation, at or about the knee. This measure is less radical than might appear in a social climate which accepts amputation and can provide an artificial limb of advanced design and essential service requirements.

## Pan-articular Osteoarthrosis

In osteoarthrosis affecting both compartments the situation is comparable, but by no means the same, to that of osteoarthritis the result of burnt-out rheumatoid arthritis. It is different in so far as a patient of different sex and age range is involved. The patient is usually male and in the third or fourth decade, concerned with the necessity to earn a living and support a family, active and in an occupation with physical, as opposed to sedentary, demands. In women, it is the teachers of such activities as ballet dancing or tennis constantly involved, hour after hour throughout the day, who are affected rather than those they teach. In such circumstances it is important that any local source of symptoms such as a remnant of meniscus or loose body be eliminated. The presence or absence of a flexion deformity is noted and in the former situation the possibility of increase of extension by passive means estimated. If indicated appropriate measures are applied. In all situations the reason and importance of quadriceps development is stressed and the means whereby this can be achieved explained. It is noticeable in male physical training instructors in whom such a situation is common but who are familiar with the problems involved, how much improvement can be achieved and maintained over a large number of years by such methods. There remains the uneducated underprivileged labourer who has suffered symptoms for years, who cannot hold down a job, has had a vast number of passive methods of treatment applied without improvement, is cynical about the ability of the profession to help him and, as a result, is no longer motivated. The selection of treatment in such circumstances is difficult in the extreme. The dramatic results from the removal of a degenerate meniscus with the possibility of debridement of the medial condyle are not applicable. There is no angular deformity and no relatively normal side available on which to transfer weight by wedge osteotomy. What possibilities remain? Osteotomy of the tibial

head and of the femur without displacement can expect improvement only as a result of alteration of the circulation pattern. It is a possibility to be considered and in a limited experience has produced apparent subjective improvement but without proof of lasting relief. Arthroplasty in the form of total replacement is not applicable in this sex or age group in the current scene but may provide the solution in the future. There maybe no alternative to arthrodesis. In such circumstances it is important that the necessity is not anticipated. Arthrodesis is appreciated only when the patient recognises the inevitable. In any event caution in this irreversible decision should be exercised. Pan-articular osteoarthrosis based on abnormal tibial torsion is bilateral although rarely symmetrical in degree of development. That the second knee might demand similar treatment should be anticipated.

## Selection of Operation

In the treatment of osteoarthrosis of whatever origin it is important that the likely outcome of any proposed procedure is anticipated taking all the circumstances of each individual patient into consideration. In the early stages of the mono-compartmental variety before degeneration of the articular cartilage is advanced or more than the minimal angular deformity present *meniscectomy* may suffice. At a more advanced stage meniscectomy may be combined with *debridement* and *resurfacing*. If angular deformity of any considerable degree is present it will be necessary to decide whether *osteotomy* alone is indicated; whether it should be preceded by meniscectomy, debridement and resurfacing; or whether it should be combined with meniscectomy, debridement and resurfacing at a single operation. It should at all times be appreciated that once patellectomy has been performed, and the objective not achieved, salvage procedures available are virtually reduced to arthrodesis.

It should be appreciated too that simple linear osteotomy without displacement can have no effect other than alteration of the circulation pattern. Linear osteotomy, opening or closing a wedge, has the same effect on circulation but has the advantage of altering the alignment of the joint with transfer of weight-bearing to the comparatively normal side. The opening of a wedge will be accepted to locate the patella at a lower level; closing of a wedge will be accepted to locate the patella at a higher level. There is corresponding theoretical increase or decrease of quadriceps power. These theoretical considerations however take no account of the condition of the patello-femoral joint, nor of the existence of exostoses often of major proportions on the margins of the femoral condyles. Alteration of the weight-bearing alignment at the tibio-femoral joint in such circumstances can precipitate symptoms of major degree in the patello-femoral joint.

In osteoarthrosis of moderate degree such considerations should be paramount. It is the author's practice in such circumstances to undertake a limited debridement of the medial femoral condyle coupled, if necessary, with the excision of a degenerate meniscus as a preliminary procedure to possible osteotomy at a later date. This simple procedure, permitting a return to weight-bearing within 14 days, has been so successful in the elimination of symptoms in the patients selected as to appear worthy of consideration prior to any major osteotomy procedure in this age group. A high proportion of patients find the second operation to be unnecessary. If it is, the surgeon can proceed in the knowledge that correction of the angular deformity will not precipitate symptoms in the patello-femoral joint.

The greatest care must be exercised in the selection of operation when the osteoarthrosis is of advanced degree, whether of the common wear and tear variety or superimposed on burnt-out rheumatoid arthritis. This applies in particular to the more radical measures using metal implants whether in the form of hemi-arthroplasty or total arthroplasty. These operations will normally be performed for the relief of pain. If performed for the purpose of enabling the patient to live a more active life, they will fail. The cynical assertion that arthroplasty 'permits the patient to get from his chair to the bar' has a basis in fact. Such operations must not be performed in patients likely to make demands of the knee. It is in osteoarthrosis rather than burnt-out rheumatoid arthritis that such demands are likely and the risk of failure

great. The demands of the rheumatoid arthritic patient are likely to be minimal and the standard of result which is acceptable is low.

In the treatment of osteoarthrosis removal of a degenerate meniscus, debridement and osteotomy can be successive steps. There is a 'finality' in arthroplasty which does not appeal to the cautious surgeon. A failed arthroplasty, hemi- or total, allows three possibilities only: another arthroplasty, arthrodesis or amputation. Failure begets failure. When a succession of failures is followed by an outstanding success the operation responsible is likely to be arthrodesis.

**Patellectomy in osteoarthrosis.** Quadriceps weakness or insufficiency is a constant, and contributing feature of painful degenerative disease of a degree which merits operative action.

Patellectomy is an irrevocable step which, no matter what the arguments for or against in any given situation, always decreases the power of the quadriceps still further. The indications for patellectomy are few. If it must be performed it should be for a single local specific reason, i.e. painful patello-femoral osteoarthrosis (as opposed to tibio-femoral osteoarthrosis) which has failed to react to conservative surgery. In no circumstance should it form part of a widespread surgical attack on the joint or in combination with other procedures. In any event the loss of the patella virtually precludes total knee replacement. The most successful patterns in current practice retain the patella (see case reported later).

### Selection of Treatment: Assessment of Individual Problem

To select the appropriate treatment in any given case the physician must ask himself, and answer, a number of questions:

1. Are the patient's symptoms, in spite of angular deformity and radiological changes, due to a degenerative lesion of the medial meniscus?

It is probable that the most common single error in the selection of treatment is pursuance of conservative measures in one form or another when in fact there is a horizontal cleavage lesion in the posterior segment of the medial meniscus producing mechanical interference with movement and progressive degeneration in related articular cartilage. No improvement will occur until the abnormal meniscus has been excised. Considerable evidence has been accumulated that many cases to which the diagnosis of osteoarthrosis has been justifiably applied are rendered symptomless by no more than meniscectomy. The clear-cut symptom complex characteristic of this local lesion has been described in detail. That simple meniscectomy can be surprisingly rewarding in unpromising circumstances is illustrated by the following example:

The patient, J.F., male, aged 54, a clerk by occupation, had sustained a fractured shaft of femur in youth which had united with medial rotation deformity.

The immediate problem was one of monocompartmental osteoarthrosis with varus angulation. There were, superimposed, obvious signs and symptoms of a horizontal cleavage lesion. The question which arose was whether an osteotomy of the tibial head was necessary. In view of the meniscus lesion, meniscectomy was decided to be necessary as a preliminary procedure and consider later the necessity for osteotomy.

At operation the meniscus lesion was confirmed and the offending structure removed. The medial condyle of the femur had a worn track adjacent to the tibial spine and thought to be caused by it. Adjacent was a strip of relatively unworn articular cartilage. Medial to it was a track corresponding to the site of the meniscus. At the anterior extremity of this track were cartilagenous excrescences. It could be demonstrated that in extension there was contact between femur and tibia.

The condition of the medial compartment was not one in which a favourable outcome was anticipated. The patient returned to weight-bearing and to his home on the fourteenth day. He was instructed to continue with his hourly quadriceps and mobilising exercise therapy and to return for reassessment when the supervising physiotherapist considered he had obtained the optimum improvement. This situation was considered to be achieved at the end of 12 weeks from operation. At this time he declared himself to be completely free of pain. Even the stiffness,

he said, had disappeared. He did not consider any further treatment to be necessary.

2. When (1) has been eliminated, what are the prospects of improvement by conservative non-operative means?

Conservative measures in the form of passive stretching to increase extension and quadriceps redevelopment is the treatment applicable to the majority of cases and may require to be continued on a permanent basis. The most dramatic improvement occurs in the presence of a flexion deformity due to contracture of soft tissue accompanied by quadriceps wasting, the least dramatic in the presence of a bony block to extension and precluding muscular redevelopment. If in doubt as to the necessity or otherwise for surgery it is prudent to pursue conservative measures in the form of exercise therapy even for many months. If with the passage of time it becomes evident that more radical measures are necessary the knowledge of exercise requirements will reduce in material degree the duration of convalescence.

3. If the presence of a bony block to extension and/or the presence of marginal excrescences are such as to preclude improvement by conservative means. In such circumstances is the patient a candidate for limited debridement?

The answer to this question is likely to be based on the individual experience of the physician and estimate of the motivation of the patient. The operation as described does not preclude further surgical measures and indeed may be required prior to further surgical measures. In any event it entails minimal hospitalisation and weight-bearing can be resumed within 14 days.

It has been the author's practice, when both debridement and tibial head osteotomy are required, to perform the operations at separate sessions following the rule that in general intra-articular and extra-articular operations should not be combined. The rule, however, is not a rigid one. MacIntosh and Welsh (1977) have reported a series of 135 knees in which debridement and closing-wedge osteotomy were combined. In the 116 knees in which follow-up was possible at an average of 5·4 years, 81·9 per cent had maintained a good or satisfactory result.

It will be evident that the combination of these procedures at a single operation poses problems of maintaining mobility of the joint. Transfixion pins combined with compression clamps (Figs 10,69 and 10,70) are required for the immobilisation of the osteotomy and to permit manipulation of the joint if right-angled flexion has not been achieved by the tenth post-operative day.

4. Is the osteoarthrosis local, largely confined to one or other compartment, and accompanied by angular deformity so that mechanical benefit will result from opening- or closing-wedge osteotomy? In answering this question he will be aware of the reputation this operation has acquired for reduction of pain and improvement of function.

In pan-articular osteoarthrosis based on medial torsion of the tibia one deformity, and likely to be varus, may predominate. In such circumstances care must be exercised not to misinterpret the situation as mono-compartmental osteoarthrosis.

5. Is the osteoarthrosis more general, bi-compartmental involving the entire tibio-femoral joint, so that no mechanical benefit can accrue from opening- or closing-wedge osteotomy? Is it pan-articular based on a torsional deformity so that the patello-femoral joint is involved? If so, can the source of symptoms be located? Is simple linear osteotomy without angulation justifiable on the basis of alteration of circulation pattern and consequent possible reduction of pain? These are difficult questions to answer in the present state of knowledge and experience. It may be asked in gross examples, has the patient anything to lose?

6. Has this knee reached a stage when only replacement arthroplasty or arthrodesis is worth considering? In spite of the rapid advancement in total replacement the greatest care must be exercised in recommending such operations in pan-articular osteoarthrosis in the relatively young male subjects in which it is likely to be encountered in bilateral form when based on medial torsion of the tibiae. In the elderly, making limited demands on the knee, less caution is necessary (Figs 10,75 to 10,78).

Arthrodesis is the ultimate acceptance of failure. It can no longer be regarded as the operation of choice even in the young subject in view of the advance in the techniques of arthroplasty. There are occasional circumstances of gross unilateral osteoarthrosis in the young male manual worker in which there is no reasonable alternative.

## Motivation

In a lifetime of experience the occasional patient, usually but not always a woman, is encountered who has no serious intention of parting with a chronic knee disability despite her protests. She has a long history with a multiplicity of operations largely unsuccessful and variety of conflicting medical opinions to recall. Her life rotates, to use an inappropriate phrase, about her defective knee joint. It is the constant topic of conversation and centre of attention. She uses elbow crutches bearing little weight on the joint. Pain, despite constant reference to it, is not the problem. The stiff knee which might solve her immediate physical problems is not likely to be more than a nine days' wonder.

It is difficult not to be sympathetic to such patients particularly when it is evident that the disability is in part iatrogenic in origin. It is equally important to recognise that a final solution is unacceptable.

## Report of a Case

The record which follows is an example of a succession of errors of diagnosis, judgement and treatment:

The patient (H.M., female, aged 58) wrote, and the following is a translation of her letter:

'The trouble with my left knee began 40 years ago when I had a skiing accident. In the accident the patella dislocated and the medial meniscus was torn. At operation the medial meniscus was excised and the capsule of the joint plicated on the medial side. In the following year, I tore the lateral meniscus. It also was removed. After the second operation I had no serious trouble for many years. It was about 10 years later that a loose body appeared. The doctor I consulted believed that it occurred as a result of the dislocating patella. A third operation was performed at which the loose body was removed and the

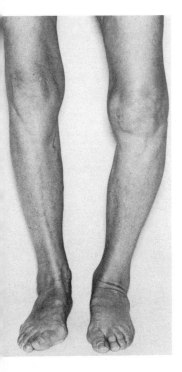

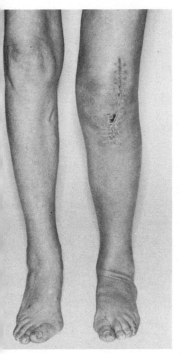

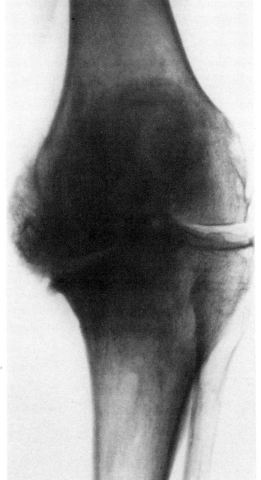

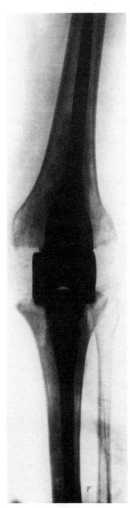

FIGS 10,75–78. **Gross pan-articular osteoarthrosis: treatment by total replacement.**

Figure 10,75. In gross pan-articular osteoarthrosis the fact that one deformity predominates should not be misinterpreted as indicating mono-compartmental disease.

Figure 10,76. Antero-posterior radiograph indicates compression of the medial condyle of the tibia and explains the complaint of instability.

Figure 10,77. Treatment by total replacement with Stanmore hinge. Note reproduction of normal valgus angulation.

Figure 10,78. Clinical result to show reproduction of normal valgus angulation.

patellar tendon transplanted. I made a slow recovery after this operation, but again I had little trouble for many years. During this time I had frequent spa treatment, performed exercises and remained fairly well.

Five years ago I emigrated to the country where I now live. Spa treatment was not available. The climate and my increasing age were probably additional causes for the worsening condition of my knee. Arthritis developed and walking and standing became increasingly difficult.

One year ago I went to England and underwent the operation of MacIntosh arthroplasty. Two hemiprostheses were inserted, one into either side of the joint (Figs 10,79 and 10,80). Initially I made good progress and regained over 90° of flexion. After four months however the prosthesis on the outer side seemed to slip and I developed an effusion. From that moment I made no further progress. I had been using a cane but had to go back to two crutches which

I am using at the moment of writing. There seem to be two major problems. When the outer prosthesis slipped the whole lower leg slipped sideways. It is unstable in a sideways direction. If I push it inward with my hand, it jumps back towards the outer side, about 2 cm.

I have been informed that fixation of the prosthesis with cement is possible. But I would like to know what can be done about the instability of the leg. Unfortunately [patient's word] at the arthroplasty operation, the patella was removed. I cannot lift the leg straight, only flexed. I lack some 40° of extension.

In my opinion the prosthesis on the inner side fits perfectly, I don't feel that I have a foreign body there. But the prosthesis on the outer side hurts when I put weight on it, standing and walking. If I stand for a while, I cannot get the joint to move. I have to manipulate it carefully before I can take the next step.

Another serious problem is the alignment of

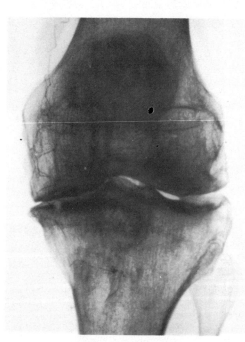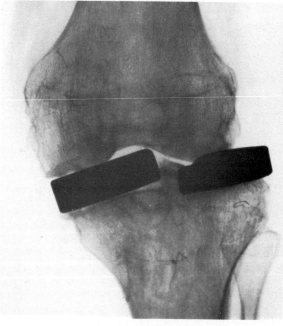

Figs 10,79–80. **Osteoarthrosis: mono-compartmental, bi-compartmental or pan-articular: treatment.** The introduction of hemiprotheses, coupled with excision of the patella, has no place in treatment even of the pan-articular variety and leaves no alternative to arthrodesis (H.M., female, aged 58).

the leg below the knee. It is not of natural conformation.

Everyone in the country in which I live tells me to undergo arthrodesis. I cannot accept this verdict. Is there any other solution to regain stability?'

On examination one month later: examination contributed little information additional to that given in her history. The salient feature was the extension lag amounting to some 30°. There was prominence of the lateral condyle of the tibia and it was possible by pressure on the prominence to move the entire tibia towards the medial side. This abnormal instability could not be controlled by contraction of the quadriceps. There was, however, no soft tissue swelling nor effusion. The joint could be moved passively without pain to the fully extended position; the final 30°, as indicated above, were not under voluntary control.

This case is quoted as an example of the erroneous use of the MacIntosh's hemiarthroplasty technique in osteoarthrosis, to say nothing of the additional error of patellectomy which would make failure inevitable even in a patient demanding a lower standard of function. The problems posed by such errors of judgement are almost without solution.

What salvage procedures are open to such a patient? The longstanding instability and the loss of the patella prejudice any hope of success for revision hemiarthroplasty or total replacement. There remain three possibilities: (1) the permanent use of a caliper splint; (2) arthrodesis; and (3) if the patient will not accept a stiff knee and is unprejudiced against a mutilating operation, ablation at or above the knee joint.

## Angular Deformity: Frail Elderly

There remains to be considered what treatment is available in angular deformity of the elderly, a problem encountered with increasing frequency in an ageing population at a stage when the methods of conservative and operative treatment which have been described are no longer applicable and with contraindications to operation in the form of total replacement. The problem is usually that of a moderate angular deformity, frequently valgus, unilateral or bilateral, which with increasing age and overweight coupled with decreasing muscle power, has passed the critical angle with totally disabling instability accompanied by pain. At this stage, and with an attitude of realism, no treatment is available other than some form of brace or long leg caliper (Figs 10,81 to 10,84).

**Jones knock-knee brace.** If the Jones walking knock-knee brace is no longer used in the treatment of genu valgum in childhood, in modern form it has a place in treatment of the angular deformity in the elderly with painful instability and in whom for one reason or another operation is contraindicated.

The brace is indicated in bilateral cases in particular in which the inner uprights of conventional calipers come in contact as the patient propels one leg past the other. There are the additional advantages in that the brace is simpler, lighter and more easily applied than the standard appliance.

PRESCRIPTION. The correction of the deformity depends on the traditional three point pressure system of maintenance of alignment: pressure is exerted at the greater trochanter and lateral malleolus with the opposing force at the medial condyle of the femur.

The brace consists of a single lateral upright bar of duralumin capable of flexion at the knee by a ring-lock joint. It extends as high as is acceptable towards the greater trochanter and is secured to the thigh with a cuff-top attached with conventional straps and buckles; not a Velcro fastening. A cuff band similarly secured is provided below the knee. The lateral upright is attached to the heel of the shoe with a simple round socket and prevented from extrusion by a medial strap. The third point of pressure corrects the deformity and takes the form of a leather knock-knee apron braced to the lateral upright by straps and buckles; not a Velcro fastening (Fig. 10,84).

**Walking caliper.** In certain gross examples deformity and instability is such that the knock-knee brace described above is not sufficient to

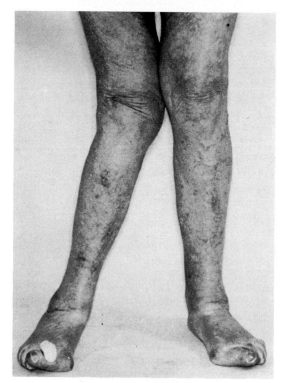

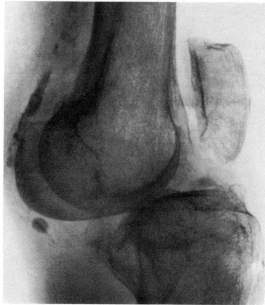

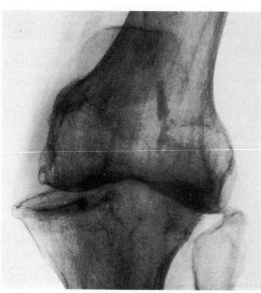

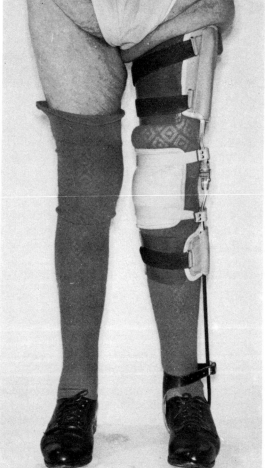

Figs 10,81–84. **Angular deformity: frail elderly.** Gross left-sided osteoarthrosis with symptoms of pain and gross instability (Fig. 10,81). Weight-bearing radiographs showing subluxation. There was calcification of femoral artery (Figs 10,82 and 10,83). This case could be treated by total replacement in the form of Stanmore prosthesis as in Figures 10,75 to 10,78 in the absence of contraindications to operation.

Jones walking knock-knee brace, no longer in use for the original purpose of treatment, corrected the deformity and gave the patient stability (Fig. 10,84) (C.G., female, aged 82).

This brace is particularly useful when the valgus deformity is bi-lateral in that there are no inner uprights to impinge against one another as in the normal full length caliper.

maintain stability and a full-length caliper which may require to incorporate a corset at the knee is necessary. This heavier more cumbersome apparatus is not readily tolerated and walking for the reasons given above is difficult. If one knee is reasonably stable, consideration should be given to the possibility of using a caliper on one side and a knock-knee brace on the other.

## REFERENCES

BENJAMIN, A. (1969). Double osteotomy for the painful knee in rheumatoid arthritis and osteoarthrosis. *Journal of Bone and Joint Surgery*, **51B**, 4, 694.

BOUILLET, R. & VAN GAVER, P. (1961). L'arthrose du genou: étude pathogenique et treatment. *Acta Orthopaedica Belgica*, **27**, 8–187.

BOUILLET, R. & DELCHEF, J. (1968). L'arthrose du genou, conséquence éloignée de l'ankylose de la hanche, étude de 40 cas. *Acta orthopaedica belgica*, **34**, 947–968.

BRATTSTROM, H. & M. (1971). Long-term results in knee arthrodesis in rheumatoid arthritis. *Acta Rheumatica Scandinavica*, **17**, 86–93.

BRETT, A. L. (1935). Operative correction of genu recurvatum. *Journal of Bone and Joint Surgery*, **17**, 4, 984.

COVENTRY, M. B. (1965). Osteotomy of the upper portion of the tibia for degenerative arthritis of the knee. *Journal of Bone and Joint Surgery*, **47A**, 984.

COVENTRY, M. B. (1973). Osteotomy about the knee for degenerative and rheumatoid arthritis. *Journal of Bone and Joint Surgery*, **55A**, 23.

DEVAS, M. B. (1969). High tibial osteotomy for arthritis of the knee. *Journal of Bone and Joint Surgery*, **51B**, 95.

DODD, H. & COCKETT, F. B. (1956). *Varicose Veins and the Pathology and Surgery of the Veins of the Lower Limb*. Edinburgh: E. & S. Livingstone.

GARIEPY, R. (1961). *Correction du genou fléchi dans l'arthrite*. Huitième Congrès Internationale de Chirurgie Orthopédique, 884–886, New York 4–9 September, 1960. Bruxelles: Imprimerie des Sciences.

GARIEPY, R. (1964). Genu varum treated by high tibial osteotomy. *Journal of Bone and Joint Surgery*, **46B**, 783.

HELAL, B. (1965). The pain in primary osteoarthritis of the knee. *Postgraduate Medical Journal*, **41**, 172.

HELAL, B. & KARADI, B. S. (1968). *Annals of Physical Medicine*, **9**, 334.

HELAL, B. (1971). Silicone for osteoarthritic joints. *British Medical Journal*, ii, 654.

HELFET, A. J. (1959). Mechanism of derangements of the medial semilunar cartilage and their management. *Journal of Bone and Joint Surgery*, **41B**, 319.

HELFET, A. J. (1969). Osteoarthritis of the hip and knee. In *Recent Advances in Orthopaedics*. Edited by A. Graham Apley. London: J. & A. Churchill.

JACKSON, J. P. & WAUGH, W. (1961). Tibial osteotomy for osteoarthritis of the knee. *Journal of Bone and Joint Surgery*, **43B**, 746.

JACKSON, J. P. & WAUGH, W. (1974). The techniques and complications of upper tibial osteotomy. *Journal of Bone and Joint Surgery*, **56B**, 236.

JACKSON, J. P., WAUGH, W. & GREEN, J. P. (1969). High tibial osteotomy for osteoarthritis of the knee. *Journal of Bone and Joint Surgery*, **51B**, 88.

KELLGREN, J. H. & LAWRENCE, J. S. (1957). *Annals of the Rheumatic Diseases*, **16**, 494.

KRAUSE, W., POPE, M. H., JOHNSON, R., WEINSTEIN, A. & WILDER, D. (1975). Mechanical changes in the knee post-meniscectomy. *Journal of Bone and Joint Surgery*, **57A**, 570.

LAWRENCE, J. S., BREMNER, J. M. & BIER, F. (1966). *Annals of the Rheumatic Diseases*, **25**, 1.

MCCOLL, J. (1969). Proceedings of the 35th Meeting of the Biological Engineering Society.

MACINTOSH, D. L. & WELSH, P. (1977). Joint debridement—a complement to high tibial osteotomy in the treatment of degenerative arthritis of the knee. *Journal of Bone and Joint Surgery*, **59A**, 1094.

MCKIBBIN, B. & HOLDSWORTH, F. W. (1966). The nutrition of immature joint cartilage in the lamb. *Journal of Bone and Joint Surgery*, **48B**, 793.

MAGNUSON, P. B. (1941). Joint débridement. *Surgery, Gynecology and Obstetrics*, **73**, 1.

MANKIN, H. (1969). Symposium: early degenerative arthritis of the knee. *Journal of Bone and Joint Surgery*, **51A**, 1027.

MAQUET, P. G. J. (1976). *Biomechanics of the Knee*. Berlin, Heidelberg, New York: Springer-Verlag.

MAROUDAS, A., BULLOUGH, P., SWANSON, S. A. V. & FREEMAN, M. A. R. (1968). The permeability of articular cartilage. *Journal of Bone and Joint Surgery*, **50B**, 1, 166.

MILLER, J. H., WHITE, J. & NORTON, T. H. (1958). The value of intra-articular injections in osteoarthritis of the knee. *Journal of Bone and Joint Surgery*, **40B**, 636.

NISSEN, K. I. (1963). The arrest of early primary osteoarthritis of the hip by osteotomy. *Proceedings of the Royal Society of Medicine*, **56**, 1051–1060.

PETERS, T. J. & SMILLIE, I. S. (1971). Studies on chemical composition of menisci from the human knee-joint. *Proceedings of the Royal Society of Medicine*, **64**, 15.

PETERS, T. J. & SMILLIE, I. S. (1972). Studies on the chemical composition of the menisci of the knee joint with special reference to the horizontal cleavage lesion. *Clinical Orthopaedics and Related Research*, **86**, 245.

PHILLIPS, R. S. (1972). Venous pathology in osteoarthritis of the knee. *Journal of the Royal College of Surgeons of Edinburgh*, **17**, 195.

PRIDIE, K. H. (1959). A method of resurfacing osteoarthritic knee joints. Report of paper presented at meeting of British Orthopaedic Association, Torquay. *Journal of Bone and Joint Surgery*, **41B**, 618.

RADIN, E. L. & PAUL, I. L. (1971). Importance of bone in sparing articular cartilage from impact. *Clinical Orthopaedics*, **78**, 342.

RADIN, E. L., PARKER, H. G., STEINBERG, R. S., PUGH, J. W., PAUL, I. L. & ROSE, R. M. (1972). A possible etiological pathway for idiopathic osteoarthritis. *Journal of Bone and Joint Surgery,* **54A,** 6, 1333.

SIMONET, J., MAQUET, P. & DE MARCHIN, P. (1963). Considerations biomécaniques sur l'arthrose du genou. 2. Étude de forces. Osteotomies. *Revue du Rhumatism,* **30,** 777–778.

SMILLIE, I. S. (1974). The biomechanical basis of osteoarthrosis of the knee. Conference on Total Knee Replacement, The Institution of Mechanical Engineers, London.

STEINDLER, A. (1940). *Orthopaedic Operations.* Springfield, Illinois: Charles C. Thomas.

TRICKEY, E. L. (1969). Double osteotomy for painful knee in rheumatoid arthritis and osteoarthritis. *Journal of Bone and Joint Surgery,* **51B,** 4, 697.

WARDLE, E. N. (1962). Osteotomy of the tibia and fibula. *Surgery, Gynecology and Obstetrics,* **115,** 61.

WARDLE, E. N. (1964). Osteotomy of the tibia and fibula in the treatment of chronic osteoarthritis of the knee. *Postgraduate Medical Journal,* **40,** 536.

WRIGHT, V., DOWSON, D. & SELLER, P. C. (1971). *Modern Trends in Rheumatology,* pp. 2, 21. London: Butterworth.

WRIGHT, V., HASLOCK, D. I., DOWSON, D., SELLER, P. C. & REEVES, B. (1971). Evaluation of silicone as an artificial lubricant in osteoarthrotic joints. *British Medical Journal,* **ii,** 370.

# 11. Loose Bodies: Osteochondritis Dissecans and Conditions of Like Radiological Appearance

**Joint incidence.** The knee is the joint by far the most frequently affected.

## Classification

The occurrence of a variety of loose bodies has been recognised since the original arthrotomy of the knee by Ambroise Paré in 1558.

They can be classified as to material content, normal or pathological:

### 1. Fibrin

**Traumatic** as a result of haemarthrosis.
**Pathological** as a result of chronic synovitis; at one extreme, the massive fibrin clot of rheumatoid arthritis, at the other, the melon seed bodies of tuberculous arthritis.

### 2. Fibrous Tissue

**Traumatic** as a result of haemorrhage into a synovial villus.
**Pathological** in any variety of chronic arthritis.

### 3. Fibrocartilage

**Traumatic** as a result of lesions of the menisci.
**Pathological** as a result of degenerative lesions of the meniscus.

### 4. Articular Cartilage

**Traumatic** as the uncommon result of the application of tangential force.
**Pathological** in grossly destructive disease processes.

### 5. Osteocartilagenous

**Traumatic** as in tangential osteochondral fractures.
**Pathological** as in osteochondritis dissecans and conditions of like appearance such as osteonecrosis and hydrocortisone arthropathy. The fractured osteophytes of osteoarthrosis, the sequestra of infective arthritis and neuropathic arthropathy, and synovial osteochondromatosis are other examples.

### 6. Miscellaneous

**Traumatic** as in introduced foreign bodies.
**Pathological** as in tumours, simple or malignant.

This classification has the merit of academic convenience. It is evident in so far as the knee joint is concerned that the majority of examples are but a minor manifestation of a major disease. The loose bodies derived from the articular surfaces of the otherwise normal joint as the result of single-incident trauma or of the ill-defined pathological process, osteochondritis dissecans, are of major importance. In the remainder treatment is the treatment of the causative pathology. In some circumstances, osteoarthrosis being the outstanding example, removal of an osteocartilagenous loose body may be required in the course of symptomatic treatment.

## OSTEOCHONDRITIS DISSECANS

There is one common and important variety of loose body to which measures can be applied not only to prevent separation into the synovial cavity but to restore the articular surface from which it would separate; in gross examples, the prevention of the osteoarthrosis which otherwise ensues. The variety is that which arises from the mysterious condition, **osteochondritis dissecans.**

The opportunity is taken of considering conditions of like radiological appearance and the problems so related.

**Historical note.** Certain knee joints of skeletons dated about A.D. 900 located in the Castle Museum at Norwich, England, show lesions at the classical site in the medial femoral condyle and the centre of the lateral femoral condyle which have the appearance of a pathological basis of osteochondritis dissecans (Figs 11,1 and 11,2) (Wells, 1962). It is probable that the loose body removed by Ambroise Paré in 1558 had the same origin.

## AETIOLOGY AND PATHOLOGY

**Radiology and pathological anatomy: limitations of radiology.** Osteochondritis dissecans is a condition determined by radiological examination. In an investigation into the cause and nature of the disease reference must be made to radiographs. It is characteristic of the condition in general that the many stages in the pathological anatomy which exist before the last isthmus of articular cartilage gives way and the loose body

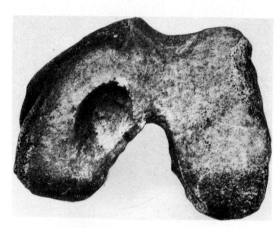

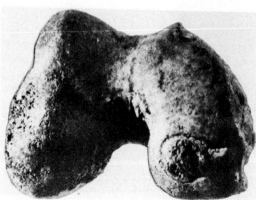

FIGS 11,1–2. **Osteochondritis dissecans?** Knee joints circa A.D. 900 from the Castle Museum, Norwich, England, showing lesion at medial margin of medial femoral condyle (Fig. 11,1) and centre of lateral femoral condyle (Fig. 11,2) both established sites for the development of osteochondritis dissecans (reproduced by courtesy of Dr Calvin Wells).

is cast into the joint are represented by not dissimilar radiological appearances. *The confusion in definition, aetiology, pathology and treatment which exists throughout the voluminous literature devoted to the study of the subject, is based on the fallacy of describing pathological anatomy in terms of radiographic appearances.* In the radiographs of an osteochondritis dissecans-like lesion it will be accepted that the zone of sclerosis can be interpreted in terms of ischaemia. But what of the zone of rarefaction? It could be true rarefaction of bone, but uncalcified cartilage, fibrous tissue and, most important of all, an actual space, all have a similar appearance. It is little wonder so much conflict of opinion on almost every aspect of the disease exists.

It is clear from the variety of appearances in radiographs, particularly of the knee joint at the period under consideration, that the borderline between the normal and the abnormal is narrow. Is the appearance of a small separate ossific centre normal? But a joint showing such a centre or centres does not necessarily proceed to osteochondritis dissecans.

**Differential diagnosis.** The following is a list of conditions said to produce radiological features with some similarity to osteochondritis dissecans:

Anomalies of ossification
Tangential osteochondral fractures
Osteonecrosis
Hydrocortisone arthropathy
Sickle-cell anaemia
Caisson disease
Gaucher's disease
Haemophilia
Systemic lupus erythmatosis
Gout
Chronic alcoholism
Pancreatitis
Sarcoidosis
Wilson's disease

The list is of academic interest. Four are of practical importance: **anomalies of ossification; osteochondral fractures; spontaneous osteonecrosis, and hydrocortisone osteochondritis dissecans.**

The remainder are either a minor manifestation of a major disease and thus unlikely to lead to error, or occur in, for example, caisson disease or chronic alcoholism and affect the hip and not the knee.

In so far as osteochondritis dissecans is concerned it is clear that the condition encountered in a boy of 15 is not the same, despite the radiological appearances, as that which affects the knee joint of an adult for the first time at the age of 25 or more. Equally certain it is that the condition seen in the medial and lateral femoral condyles of one or both knees at the age of 10 is not the same as the lesion of similar appearance seen in the adult (Smillie, 1960).

The radiological lesions of similar appearance are: at the age of, say, 10 an anomaly of ossification, at the age of, say, 15 juvenile osteochondritis dissecans and arising for the first time in the adult, adult osteochondritis dissecans.

## Anomalies of Ossification

**Ossification of lower femoral epiphysis.** The frequency with which irregularities of ossification in various forms are encountered at the periphery of the epiphysis of the femur, is a feature of the radiology of the knee joint in children. Interest in the subject was stimulated by the description by Ribbing (1937) of radiological changes resembling osteochondritis dissecans in the joints of several members of a family suffering from a condition which he named 'hereditary multiple epiphyseal disturbance'. In the course of investigation an osteochondritis dissecans-like lesion was noted to develop in the lower femoral epiphysis of one of the family from an apparent accessory centre of ossification. In a subsequent study (Ribbing, 1944) of some 400 children, aged 1 to 10 years, equally divided as regards sex, 29 per cent of the boys were found to exhibit accessory centres in the lower femoral epiphyses and were affected three to four times more often than girls. The irregularities were seen earlier and disappeared earlier in girls who were seldom affected after 4 years of age. In boys the changes remained to about 10 years of age.

In an attempt to determine the frequency and form of irregular ossification Caffey et al. (1958) obtained radiographs in the form of anteroposterior, lateral and tunnel (Holmblad, 1937) projections of the knees of 147 children between

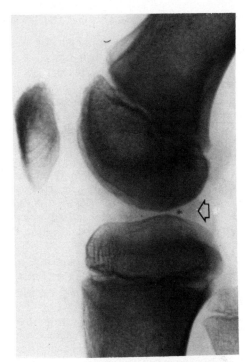

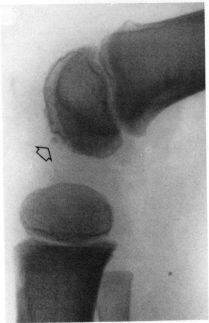

FIGS 11,3–4. **Anomalies of ossification.** Knee joint of boy aged 9 showing irregularity and separate centre of ossification outside the roughened outline of the main mass (Type I) (Fig. 11,3). There is an independent island of bone within the indentation (Type III) (Fig. 11,4). (J.S., aged 5, a younger brother of R.S., aged 12, and A.S., aged 14, see text).

S

the ages of 3 and 13 all known to be free of clinical abnormality in the knee joints.

To assess the findings the irregularities were divided into three groups. The classification is arbitrary; more than one type can be found in the same joint. It is recorded and will be used as it forms some basis for reference and comparison.

*Type I.* There are varying degrees of roughening of the margins and occasionally small foci of calcification immediately beyond the roughened edge of the main centre (Figs 11,3 and 11,5).

*Type II.* There are larger localised marginal irregularities in the form of indentations (Fig. 11,5).

*Type III.* There are marginal irregularities of the same type as Type II except that an independent island of bone is seen within the indentation (Fig. 11,4).

The outstanding feature of the investigation was the finding that marginal irregularities of the epiphyses were more common than those of regular outline. They were present in 66 per cent of the boys and 44 per cent of the girls. In 44 per cent of the total both femoral condyles were affected. The lateral condyle only was involved in 44 per cent; the medial condyle only in 12 per cent. The changes seen were frequently bilateral but were not always symmetrical.

**Nature of anomalies of ossification.** The studies quoted differ in their findings and, in any event, without some standard of irregularity, if such were possible, are not strictly comparable. If any general conclusion can be drawn it would appear that irregularities of ossification, of Type I at least, are a normal variant in the first half of the first decade. Such irregularities are not confined to the knee but appear to be most common in the knee. It is the joint most subject to trauma, minor and otherwise, in childhood and as a result most frequently demands radiological examination. The likely explanation however is the size of the epiphysis of the femur and the rapidity of growth at this site. The zones of proliferating cartilage and provisional calcification are considerably deeper than in a slowly growing epiphysis. It seems evident that when growth is extremely rapid, as it is at the lower end of the femur, the orderly process of cartilage proliferation and provisional calcification can appear outside the radiographic image of the main mass of calcified cartilage during periods of active growth. When the invading osteoblasts replace the provisionally calcified cartilage by bone trabeculae the regular outline is re-established. It is probably a matter of the adjustment

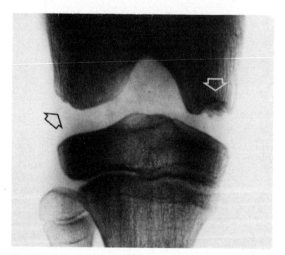

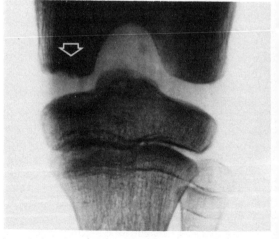

Figs 11,5–6. **Anomalies of ossification.** Knee joints of boy aged 11 showing asymmetrical anomalies Types I, II and III. Right: anomaly in the medial condyle in the form of indentation enclosing island of bone separate from main mass (Type III). Anomaly in lateral condyle in form of irregularity of outline (Type I) (Fig. 11,5). Left: anomaly in the medial condyle in the form of indentation surrounded by band of increased density (Type II). Lateral condyle appears normal (Fig. 11,6).

of blood supply to the needs of bone growth. If this explanation is correct, it seems not unlikely that the transition from smooth to irregular outline could be repeated during periods of accelerated growth.

If an acceptable explanation has been offered of the radiographic appearances of irregularities of ossification which could be classified as Type I, the explanation of the radiographic appearances of Types II and III is less easy. The difference between the two may be merely a matter of degree, or even of the age at which the radiograph was taken. Type II must be presumed to represent a localised segment within the epiphysis in which provisional calcification is retarded. How this occurs is a matter for conjecture. But the fact that the defect is surrounded by a zone of increased density suggests a possible local deficiency of blood supply. On this basis Type III represents a focus of ossification within the area of the defect but separate from the main mass. In the series studied by Caffey *et al.* (1958), Type II and III defects were present in 30 per cent of all male and 17 per cent of all female children.

### JUVENILE OSTEOCHONDRITIS DISSECANS

Juvenile osteochondritis dissecans is the variety which is encountered towards the middle of the second decade and which probably originates in an anomaly of ossification.

But every case of osteochondritis dissecans occurring at this period does not of necessity arise from such a cause. The agents which produce the adult varieties operate at all ages.

#### Relationship to Anomalies of Ossification

In the search for the elusive factors in the aetiology of juvenile osteochondritis dissecans the theory of an association with anomalies of ossification is not new. It was probably Troell (1914) who first suggested the possibility of a superficial accessory nucleus at the epiphysis of the medial femoral condyle as a cause. There are numerous references in the literature to the all-embracing doctrine of Lehmann (1922) of the constitutionally weak epiphysis. Reference has been made already to Ribbing's (1937) observation of osteo-

chondritis dissecans-like lesions developing in the condition he named hereditary multiple epiphyseal disturbance. Lacroix (1941) has stated that the histological structure of loose bodies indicates an irregularity of ossification.

In the course of this series the transition from what was considered to be an anomaly of ossification to what was considered to be juvenile osteochondritis dissecans was observed on many occasions. The evidence is not based on radiological findings, which indicate the change of status only at a late stage, but on consideration of the clinical features of the cases and direct observation of the pathological anatomy in the course of operative treatment. It is proposed to develop the theories and record the observations on which the association is based.

*The common site of anomalies of ossification in childhood, namely, the centre of medial femoral condyle, corresponds to the classical site for osteochondritis dissecans in maturity.* Ribbing (1944), in the course of the investigation referred to, demonstrated that if the sites of accessory nuclei of ossification in the child are projected on to the adult femur, those centres situated most superficially, that is to say those occurring latest in the first half of the second decade, are nearest to the classical site (Figs 11,7 and 11,8). It will be shown later that this site can be demonstrated to be vulnerable to trauma. Thus anomalies of ossification arising later, or persisting, are those most liable to transition to the pathological state. This corresponds to the phenomenon frequently observed, but unproved statistically, that anomalies of ossification in the lateral, as opposed to the medial condyle, tend to disappear spontaneously.

*The transition from anomaly of ossification to pathological process is due to interruption of blood supply.* Anomalies of ossification, no matter what view is held of their relationship to normal, usually disappear spontaneously; but not always. What determines the transition from a variant of ossification to a pathological process is the point at issue. The advent of an accessory nucleus of ossification is determined by the presence of a blood supply, but separated from the adjacent cancellous bone of the epiphysis by hyaline cartilage, it must be precarious. In addition, the very production of accessory centres of ossification is probably an expression of a pro-

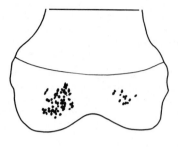

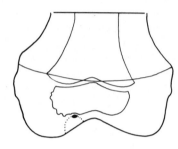

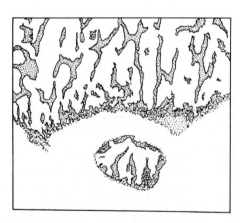

FIGS 11,7–9. **Aetiology of osteochondritis dissecans: relationship of anomalies of ossification.** Diagrammatic representation of sites of accessory nuclei of ossification in children (Fig. 11,7). Outline of femoral epiphysis of child projected on to lower end of femur in adult showing accessory nucleus of ossification in child as lesion at classical site in adult (Fig. 11,8). Photomicrograph of accessory nucleus such as seen in Figs 11,7 and 11,8. The theory is that trauma applied to such a nucleus cuts off the blood supply with transition to osteochondritis dissecans (Fig. 11,9). (Redrawn from Ribbing.)

cess of exceptionally rapid growth; as such they are vulnerable.

Attention has been directed to the fallacy of the interpretation of radiographs in terms of pathological anatomy and the erroneous conclusions which have been drawn as a result. Nevertheless, from what is known of the nature of such conditions as Perthes' disease, Keinböck's disease and even of avascular necrosis of the head of the femur following fracture, the basic pathology of certain anomalies of ossification at the precursor stage, as determined by the appearance of the radiographs, clearly involves a local alteration in the blood supply of epiphyseal bone. The rapid return to radiological normal which follows the simple procedure of drilling the area favours this view.

It appears that in some way the blood supply to the accessory nucleus has been interrupted. The closer the nucleus comes to the surface or towards the classical site as age advances to maturity, the greater will be the vulnerability to injury. It is no longer cushioned by a thick layer of flexible cartilage which disperses the effects of weight-bearing. But when the nucleus approaches the surface it is the very flexibility of cartilage which determines the transition to the pathological process. Movement within the cartilaginous layer between accessory nucleus and parent epiphysis interrupts the blood supply to the ossicle (Fig. 11,9).

It appears therefore that the relationship of anomalies of ossification to osteochondritis dissecans is simply that anomalies of ossification are a manifestation of local deficiency of blood supply in epiphyseal bone occurring at the end of the first decade. They are most common at the lower femoral epiphysis if it is only for the reason that the knee, of all joints, is the one most affected by trauma and, from the viewpoint of blood supply, is the joint with the largest mass of bone distal to an epiphyseal plate. It is a 'pressure' epiphysis not only by reason of the attachment of the powerful quadriceps to the head of the tibia, but from the simple direct pressure of body weight. If by chance the bone affected by the temporary vascular deficiency is subjected to constantly repeated trauma, a fracture, probably of the nature of a fatigue fracture, takes place.

It is possible, from the pattern of symptoms

and from the findings at operation, to draw certain inferences regarding the nature of the later developments. We know that the early changes are reversible and that spontaneous healing occurs. We know also that certain cases, for reasons which will be described, proceed to what we choose to call osteochondritis dissecans. We know that symptomless cases, kept under observation in the hope of spontaneous healing, can suddenly develop giving-way incidents indicating instability of a weight-bearing area. It can be assumed that the change can be due only to the development of the fracture or cleavage lesion in the surface layers of the bone.

*Trauma is the factor in the localisation of the lesion.* It is not unlikely that once an anomaly of ossification and the vascular changes implied, have affected the bone of a femoral condyle, the constantly repeated trauma inflicted by the action of walking is liable to produce a fatigue fracture. Thus the original lesion turns into osteochondritis dissecans with all the possibilities of the eventual separation of loose bodies into the joint. But the liability of an anomaly of ossification to turn into osteochondritis dissecans probably depends on the vulnerability of the site affected. It is greater in the medial than in the lateral condyle; greatest of all at the classical site. But the fact that the lesion occurs at the classical site does not mean that spontaneous healing will not occur, or that it must invariably proceed to osteochondritis dissecans with the separation of loose bodies. As in osteochondritis dissecans arising *de novo,* it probably depends on the anatomical conformation of the particular knee joint and the trauma to which the classical site is subjected. The influence, for healing or progression to osteochondritis dissecans, of the attachment of the posterior cruciate ligament, is unknown.

## Relationship to Disturbances of Bone Growth

'They are either too short or too tall.'

Enchondral dysostosis constitutes the most frequent hereditary disease of the skeletal system in man (Mau, 1958). Dysostotic cartilage ossification in the epiphyses according to Mau is characterised by (1) late appearance of centres of ossification; (2) delayed skeletal maturation particularly of the dissociated variety, i.e. de-

layed maturation in the presence of normal maturation; (3) relatively small size of epiphyseal centres; (4) epiphyses wider and flatter than normal; and with all skeletal proportions changed in this direction the patient is of short stature; (5) tendency to formation of accessory centres of ossification and multipolar ossification.

A dysostotic growth disturbance was in evidence in wide variation of degree among the juvenile cases of the series. In particular was short stature as above. The impression has been gained of recent years, regrettably undocumented, that abnormally tall youths too are vulnerable. The significance of the observation, if true, is not immediately evident except in so far as two families in which two brothers were affected were all abnormally tall. That two different types of stature are involved has not escaped notice (Stougaard, 1964).

An example of the dysostotic constitution in easily recognisable form with disturbance of metaphyseal longitudinal growth as well as disturbance of growth of the epiphyseal centres is quoted:

The patient (D.W., male, aged 19) was of short, broad stature. His height was 5 ft 1 in (154 cm). His legs were short by comparison with his trunk. Both knees showed recurvatus deformity in considerable degree indicating the presence of a mechanical factor (Figs 11,10 and 11,11). The osteochondritis dissecans lesions, instead of location at the classical site, were situated in the centre of the medial femoral condyles of both knees. The reason for admission to hospital was mechanical incidents due to the presence of several large loose bodies in the right knee.

Not all bilateral examples have such conspicuous epiphyseal or metaphyseal growth disturbances. In many unilateral cases the constitutional factor may be even less easy to recognise. The less common varieties affecting multiple joints and the variety affecting families are the most outstanding examples of the constitutional aspect of enchondral dysostosis as it affects osteochondritis dissecans.

**Sex incidence.** In 200 patients investigated were 42 females. When these were subdivided by variety, 16 were classified as juvenile and 26 as

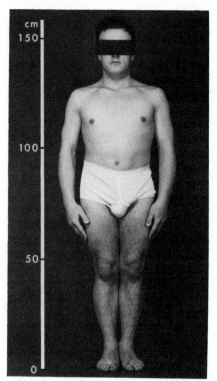

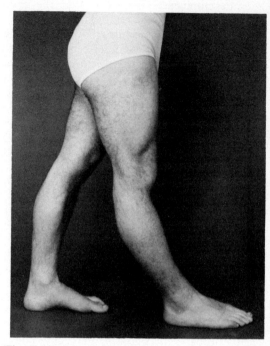

FIGS 11,10–11. **Dysostotic factor in osteochondritis dissecans.** 'They are either too short or too tall.' Stature (154 cm) and physique of patient with bilateral symmetrical lesions at classical site from which loose bodies had separated

(Fig. 11,10). Lateral view to demonstrate biomechanical aspect of aetiology in the form of recurvatus deformity (Fig. 11,11). (D.W., male, aged 19.)

adult. Anomalies of ossification 'normally' disappear in the female knee about 5 years of age; in the male, at about 10 years. This alone, apart altogether from the influence of external or internal trauma, would explain the rarity of the juvenile variety in the female. In addition, the impression, for what it is worth, was gained that the manifestations of the dysostotic constitution are less obvious in the female subject.

The special circumstances which may determine the onset of the adult variety in the female subject are considered later.

**Familial variety.** That osteochondritis of the knee joint can exist in several members of a family is firmly established by numerous references in the literature. Bernstein (1925) recorded two sisters and a brother; Wagoner and Cohn (1931) two families, father, son and paternal uncle, and two brothers; Novotny (1952) two brothers; Gardiner (1955) two brothers and a

sister; Pick (1955) mother and three daughters; Tobin (1957) father, two sons and a daughter; Smith (1960) three brothers; Stougaard (1961) nine cases involving elbow and knee in three generations of a family; Stougaard (1964) ten cases involving elbow and knee in the second and third generations of a family; Hanley, McKusick and Barranco (1967) two brothers. In the present series on which opinions are based, six families were encountered in which more than one member is known to have been affected. They include two brothers on five occasions and a father and son. It is recognised that the record may be incomplete in that families were not investigated except when more than one member was presented. The following is a particularly interesting example:

The father, a doctor, presented the first of the patients (R.S., aged 12) when his right knee became swollen. A radiograph demonstrated a lesion in the centre of the medial femoral condyle. The left knee showed the same condition at a more advanced stage. Both were considered to have progressed from anomalies of ossification to the established lesion. Both lesions were confirmed at operation to be osteochondritis dissecans and treated by 'drilling'. The eldest son (A.S., aged 14), with a massive lesion in the medial femoral condyle of the right knee was then presented. No osteochondritis dissecans lesion was seen in the left knee, but he was noted to have an anomaly of the patella consisting of multipolar ossification with one large fragment and at least two smaller ones at the usual site at the supralateral margin. In addition, he had a well marked Sinding Larsen-Johansson traction epiphysitis at the lower pole. On the right side, that in which the medial femoral condyle was affected, he showed an Osgood-Schlatter traction epiphysitis of the upper tibial epiphysis.

There were three more children in this family, a daughter and two sons. The daughter (E.S.) was first seen at age 16 when she sustained an injury to a knee. Radiographs of both knees were examined in detail in view of the family history, but no abnormality was detected.

The fourth son (A.S.) was first seen at 10 years of age. He had symmetrical anomalies of ossification in both femoral condyles of both knees. He was last seen aged 17 when the radiographs could be regarded as normal.

The youngest son (J.S.) was first seen aged 7 when he showed anomalies of ossification of marked degree in both femoral condyles of both knees, one of which lesions was reported by a radiologist as 'osteochondritis dissecans'. One year later the lesions were even more marked and with multipolar ossification of the patellae. He was last seen aged 13 when the anomalies were still detectable but thought to be in the course of disappearing (Fig. 11,4).

The several possibilities to be considered when osteochondritis dissecans occurs in two or more members of one family are (1) a tendency exists for anomalies of ossification in joints and thus the tendency to develop osteochondritis dissecans in the knee joint, (2) there is a dysostotic constitutional background. This may be the explanation where the members affected are of abnormally short or abnormally tall stature. Familial osteochondritis dissecans of this variety may be the result of selective inbreeding. The dysostotic male tends to select as his mate an even more dysostotic female, (3) the families concerned suffer from a form of hereditary multiple epiphyseal disturbance and (4) joints of a particular conformation are liable to osteochondritis dissecans and certain members of a family may have joints of similar anatomical form.

**Variety affecting multiple joints.** Osteochondritis dissecans affecting both knees is a common finding. There are references to bilateral loose bodies in the earliest literature. In 200 patients investigated in this series 37 (18·5 per cent) are known to have had bilateral lesions. This may be an under-estimation of the incidence in so far as the second knee was not investigated in the majority of cases from which a loose body was removed.

The lesions may be more or less symmetrical but are not necessarily so. The medial condyle may be affected on one side and the lateral on the other; the medial condyle on one side and the patella and medial condyle on the other; the patella on one side and the patella and medial condyle on the other. Two or more different joints may be involved, for example in this series, a knee and a hip on the same side. Such findings eliminate trauma as other than one possible factor in the aetiology.

### Adult Osteochondritis Dissecans

If trauma is accepted, as it must be, to play some part in the production of all types of osteochondritis dissecans lesion, it can be said to play the major part in the adult variety.

Constitutional factors exerting direct influence on growing bone are not in evidence and affect the situation only in so far as they may have determined the final form of the joint.

**Evidence implicating trauma.** If ischaemia is the basic pathology in juvenile osteochondritis dissecans, it is implicated also in the adult variety; but not in the same way. In juvenile osteochondritis dissecans trauma is superimposed on ischaemic bone to produce the lesion. In the adult, endogenous trauma produces the isch-aemia, and continuing, produces the lesion.

Constantly repeated minor traumata have a deleterious effect on the blood supply of bone. The example frequently quoted, and cited here as evidence, is that of Kienböck's disease of the carpal navicular as a result of the use of pneumatic tools. Constant impingement between tibial spine and femoral condyle, head of radius and capitellum, talus and tibia has the same effect; and upon the ischaemic bone is then superimposed the fatigue fracture to produce the lesion which finally results in the discharge of a loose body into the joint.

In the production of the lesion it is necessary to distinguish between the stress fracture which occurs in living bone, capable of reacting, but which has failed to react in time to the stress placed upon it (March fracture) and a fatigue fracture occurring in ischaemic or dead bone unable, like an inert metal, to react. That dead bone does in fact sustain fatigue fractures in a similar manner to metal has been demonstrated experimentally (Walmsley and Smith, 1956).

ENDOGENOUS MECHANICAL FACTOR. In the engineering industry, in the course of assembly of component parts, is what is known as 'tolerances'. This, in non-technical terms, can be described as the limit of size in, say, thousandths of an inch, on the plus or minus side of normal, which is acceptable if the machine in production is to run smoothly. It is said that the chance misfortune of the fitting together of a working part at the limit of tolerance on the plus side, with one at the limit of tolerance on the minus side, results in a unit which lacks the smooth running characteristics which exemplify the normal. If the premise is accepted that adult osteochondritis dissecans is neither a disease nor an anomaly of growth but due to abnormal contact between the component parts of a joint, then something akin to the tolerances of engineering must operate in human joints, otherwise the condition under consideration would be widespread.

That tolerances are an important factor in the vulnerability of joints is widely accepted if not recognised as such. In the hip joint, to take the best example, too shallow an acetabulum predisposes to the development of a wear and tear arthritis, but too deep an acetabulum pre-disposes to exactly the same thing. There is a certain depth which is 'normal' and there are limits on either side of normal; but the joint must be neither too shallow nor too deep.

The delicate balance in the relationship between the components of certain joints can be altered in the course of growth as in the production of recurvatus deformity (Fig. 11,11), or in the course of wear and tear or ageing. Thus the liability of a joint of particular anatomical type to develop the lesion may be decided by the occupation pursued, or in the recreational field, to cite an example, be influenced by the decision to indulge in games of football or in games of chess.

**Medial eminence of tibial spine: contact with medial condyle.** That the medial eminence of tibial spine can inflict a single-incident fracture on the medial condyle of the femur at the classical site is established beyond doubt. Such a fracture in the acute state is described and illustrated in IKJ5, Chapter 10. Conversely, a fracture may be inflicted on the tibial spine; and this too has been illustrated.

Evidence of repeated contact, as opposed to acute fracture, is much more forthcoming and is a common radiological finding particularly in the ageing knee. It takes the form of:

1. SCLEROSIS. The inference to be drawn from increase of density of the medial eminence of the spine is that of repeated contact, or microtrauma, over a long period of time.

2. FLATTENING. Unmistakable evidence of this degree is most frequently encountered where instability is known to exist or where ageing articular cartilage and menisci have brought femur and tibia into closer contact. Both medial and lateral eminence may be affected.

3. FRACTURE. A fracture of the tip of the medial eminence can occur only by contact. It is to be distinguished from the traction lesion which is a form of rupture of the anterior cruciate ligament and which involves the entire tibial spine.


## CLINICAL FEATURES AND TREATMENT

### ANOMALIES OF OSSIFICATION

In a volume which purports to be practical it is

recognised that the major problem in the diagnosis of osteochondritis dissecans in early youth is an anomaly of ossification. Failure to distinguish between the two has confused the literature of the past particularly in regard to treatment. If an anomaly of ossification is not recognised for what it is, it can be claimed, as has occurred, that osteochondritis dissecans can heal spontaneously (Green and Banks, 1953) or by whatever treatment has been applied, usually immobilisation.

## Clinical Features

The problem presents in two forms: (1) a child, usually a boy, is radiographed in the course of investigation after a fall on the knee, and the abnormality noted (Figs 11,3 to 11,6); (2) a child, usually a boy, complains of vague pain in the knee and is, as a consequence, radiographed and the anomaly revealed. In the former circumstance, and with regard to age and sex, the anomaly can be ignored. It is likely to be an incidental finding which will disappear with the passage of time. It is in the latter situation that difficulty arises with the natural assumption that the symptoms are related to the radiological finding. Is it incidental? Is the condition juvenile osteochondritis dissecans? In general, and in the first instance, the age and sex may be helpful.

## Treatment

Observation is the treatment of choice in the hope that the lesion will disappear with growth and the passage of time. In general, and if it is possible to formulate guide lines in a situation which varies so widely in pattern, 'lesions' presenting in a girl over the age of 5 and in a boy over the age of 10 should be suspect and subject to regular clinical and radiological review. But bone age in relation to chronological age may be plus or minus 5 and thus towards the limit of 'normality' is a girl aged 10 or boy aged 15.

There is a symptom which should be sought, but not by leading question, as denoting the possible transition to osteochondritis dissecans. It is persistent incidents of *insecurity* or *giving-way*. The situation is interpreted as indicating the loss of connection between a weight-bearing area of articular cartilage and the underlying bone and thus the circumstance known to exist in established osteochondritis dissecans.

That the diagnosis and management in the 10 to 15 age group poses problems is epitomised in the record of a case:

The patient (M.S., male, aged 12), a pupil in a private residential school (Public School in Britain), had complained of vague pain in the right knee and in consequence was radiographed. The antero-posterior plate showed a

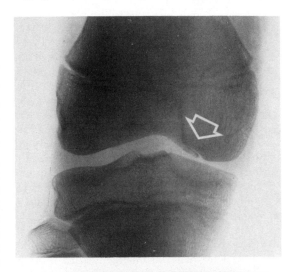

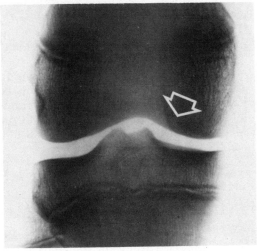

Figs 11,12–13. **Anomaly of ossification: treatment.** This patient presented with a 'lesion' at the classical site which was adjudged to be an anomaly of ossification (Fig. 11,12). A year later the 'lesion' has disappeared (Fig. 11,13). (M.S., male, aged 12, see text.)

'lesion' at the classical site in the medial femoral condyle. The radiologist reported it to be osteochondritis dissecans and recommended that an orthopaedic surgeon be consulted. He confirmed the diagnosis and recommended arthrotomy with the purpose of removing the potential loose body. The father, alarmed at the prospect of an operation at such an early age, sought the advice of a general surgeon who was a personal friend. He suggested that the author's opinion be sought. When seen, three months from the date of the original radiographs, further plates were advised. The antero-postero view showed a discrete oval-shaped bony focus not depressed below the outline of the condyle. There was minimal sclerosis of the base of the crater (Fig. 11,12). When compared with the original radiographs the outline seemed less distinct. The opinion was ventured that the 'lesion' was most probably an anomaly of ossification. In any event, it was pointed out, the boy was within the age-range for anomalies of ossification. In such circumstances he could reasonably be kept under observation without restriction of physical activities.

He was reviewed radiologically at regular intervals. At 3 months the radiographs showed no material change. At 15 months the joint became radiologically normal. It is not known exactly when the final incorporation of the bony focus took place; but it must have been prior to his 13th birthday (Fig. 11,13).

Five years later a proud mother wrote to say that she thought the author would be interested to know that he would be representing his college at the Public Schools Athletic Meeting in London in the 100 metres, hurdles and the shot-putt.

## TANGENTIAL OSTEOCHONDRAL FRACTURES

It is desirable that a distinction should be drawn between tangential osteochondral fractures the result of single-incident trauma and osteochondritis dissecans. The fractures occur at sites at which as the description implies, a tangential force, exogenous or endogenous, can be applied. Such sites are well established and invariably involve the margin of the bone. This feature does not apply to osteochondritis dissecans. There is however a notable exception. It occurs at the classical site.

**Lesion at classical site.** This is the one example to which special reference is necessary if it is only for the reason that it is located at the classical site. It is due to a single incident of trauma from impingement by the medial eminence of the tibial spine. The fracture in the acute state has been observed on a number of occasions. Reference is made to it in IKJ5, Chapter 10. The lesion is important in that it is the outstanding example of the difficulty which exists in differentiating single-incident trauma from repeated microtrauma in the aetiology of the lesion occurring at the classical site *when the pathology is of long standing*. There are implications in terms of treatment (see later).

## SPONTANEOUS OSTEONECROSIS: 'OSTEOCHONDRITIS DISSECANS' OF THE ELDERLY

In recent years an attempt has been made to identify a radiological osteochondritis dissecans-like lesion in the weight-bearing area of the medial femoral condyle occurring in patients over the age of 60 as spontaneous osteonecrosis. The lesion was originally described as a variety of the adult form of osteochondritis dissecans (Smillie, 1960). There are, however, clinical, radiological and other features which may establish the lesion as one of separate if of undefined origin despite the radiological appearances.

**Aetiology.** The precise cause, like that of juvenile osteochondritis dissecans, is unknown. A certain similarity of site, namely the centre of the condyle rather than the margin, will be recognised in osteonecrosis as in osteochondritis dissecans lesions, particularly of the lateral condyle, associated with trauma inflicted by an underlying torn meniscus. The presence of a horizontal cleavage lesion with a displaced flap of meniscus has been a common finding in the author's experience. If the concept of repeated microtrauma is accepted in the aetiology of adult osteochondritis dissecans it would appear to be one factor in the production of osteonecrosis in the elderly.

### Clinical Features

**Age.** The average age of the onset of symptoms was 67 in Muheim and Bohne's (1970) series of 51 patients. Three patients only were younger than 60.

**Sex.** The patients are predominantly female. In the same series of 51 patients 38 were women. It is significant that the two cases illustrated here (Figs 11,14 and 11,15) were both female.

**Pain.** The salient feature of the history is the spontaneous and sudden onset of intense pain at the medial condyle of the femur so much so that the majority of patients recall not only the day but what they were doing at the time (Ahlback, Bauer and Bohne, 1968). The pain decreases in intensity from severe to moderate. In particular it is present when weight-bearing and in bed at night.

**Clinical examination.** There is tenderness to deep pressure over the medial femoral condyle with pain at the limit of forced flexion. There is sometimes a small synovial effusion.

**Radiological examination.** The earliest change is flattening of the articular cartilage of the medial femoral condyle (Ahlback *et al.*, 1968). Later an osteochondritis dissecans-like lesion develops in the weight-bearing area consisting of a zone of translucency surrounded by a halo of sclerosis with (Fig. 11,14) or without (Fig. 11,15) a nidus of dead subchondral bone.

**Scintimetry.** Strontium-85 scintimetry (Bauer, 1968; Bauer and Smith, 1969) shows extremely high values elevated 5 to 15 times over the medial femoral condyle as compared to a symmetrical location in the normal knee (Ahlback *et al.*, 1968).

### Treatment

If the lesion is small the patient can be treated expectantly using simple analgesics for the con-

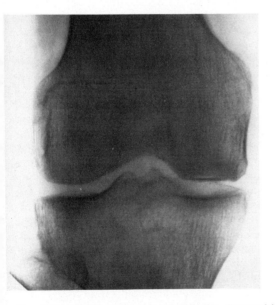 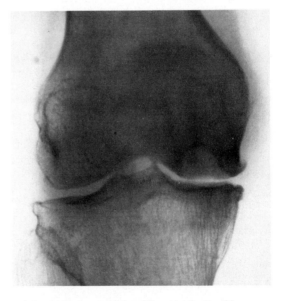

FIGS 11,14–15. **Osteonecrosis: 'osteochondritis dissecans' in the elderly.** The lesion occurs in the centre of the medial femoral condyle. In such circumstances, as in juvenile osteochondritis dissecans, it is the author's experience that there is frequently an underlying meniscus lesion. In this case (M.R., female, aged 73) there was a horizontal cleavage lesion with a centrally displaced flap of fibrocartilage interposed between the condyles (Fig. 11,14). In this case (W.McN., female, aged 86) there was a large osteolytic lesion surrounded by a halo of sclerosis with loss of joint space and other evidence of mono-compartmental osteoarthrosis. No operative action was taken in the absence of serious symptoms (Fig. 11,15).

trol of pain and crutches to reduce the effect of weight-bearing in the hope that healing may occur. If there is clinical and radiological evidence that an osteocartilaginous loose body is separating arthrotomy with removal of the loose body is required. In the age range and circumstances in which this lesion is encountered idealistic measures in the form of repair of the articular surface no longer obtain. If the lesion is large and ill-defined the rapid development of mono-compartmental osteoarthrosis is inevitable. In such circumstances the transfer of weight-bearing forces to the lateral compartment by closing-wedge osteotomy (Ch. 10) should be considered and might require to be combined with arthrotomy on the lines indicated above.

## CORTISONE OSTEOCHONDRITIS DISSECANS

It has been established, but for reasons by no means clear, that patients undergoing corticosteroid therapy either orally or intra-articularly, may develop an osteochondritis dissecans-like lesion in the knee. Such patients are usually past middle age; and the possibility of a background of such therapy should be considered when a patient in this unlikely age group develops a massive osteochondritis dissecans lesion in the medial femoral condyle. It is of particular importance that the nature of the lesion be recognised in view of the progressive nature of the pathological process even after cessation of corticosteroid therapy.

**Incidence.** The condition is not uncommon from the number of cases referred to the author for opinion, the majority of which had received systemic corticosteroids for one reason or another over a period of time. It is of serious significance, however, that two of the cases encountered with previously normal radiographs, the details of one of which is recorded below, received but a *single* injection into the joint.

The true incidence of pathological processes of iatrogenic origin is difficult to determine.

The patient (R.P., male aged 62) was first seen eight months after a minor direct injury when he fell on his knee. The radiograph taken at the time and reviewed later, showed no abnormality of the bone element of the medial femoral condyle. Two weeks later, on continuation of swelling, the patient received a hydrocortisone injection into the joint. There followed one month of immobilisation in a plaster cast.

With the further passage of time and the failure to improve, the advice of another orthopaedic surgeon was sought. It was at this stage that the radiograph showed a large osteochondritis dissecans-like lesion (Fig. 11,16) and the patient was referred to the author. The symptoms were pain, swelling and instability. In view of the size of the defect it was decided that conservative surgery should be undertaken. At operation the outstanding features were the size of the lesion and the presence of a fold of redundant articular cartilage at the anterior extremity due to absorption of the underlying bone. The crater was prepared in the manner to be described and a vascular cancellous bed achieved without difficulty. There was a thin layer of bone on the undersurface of the loose articular cartilage. In such circumstances, together with the favourable technical progress of the operation a favourable outcome was anticipated.

Three months later the radiograph was disappointing in so far as sclerosis appeared to have returned to the base of the crater and the bone element of the separated fragment had become more dense. At operation to remove the means of internal fixation, the articular cartilage was soft and was not fixed to the underlying bone. It was hoped that with a further period without weight-bearing healing might still be achieved. One year from the original operation the radiological appearance had not improved and bore a close resemblance to cases previously recorded (Helfet, 1963). At the third operation the cartilage was detached over about one-third of the total area of the condyle. There was no evidence of healing (Fig. 11,17). The loose articular cartilage was removed. When this patient was first seen the history of corticosteroid therapy was known. But it was not anticipated that a single injection could be responsible for the total failure of reparative measures in a lesion which, in the

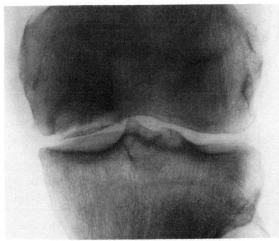 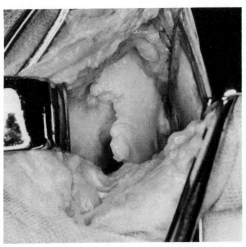

FIGS 11,16–17. **Cortisone osteochondritis dissecans.** Large osteochondritis dissecans-like lesion in medial femoral condyle (Fig. 11,16). Appearance at final operation showing total absence of healing (Fig. 11,17) (see text).

ordinary circumstances of osteochondritis dissecans or osteochondral fracture, would be expected to heal.

The purpose of this record is to direct attention to the importance of recognition of this lesion in the current scene; and the appreciation that it is not one amenable to operative repair. Since this initial humiliating experience a number of patients have been encountered, all osteoarthrosic with radiological osteochondritis dissecans-like lesions and who had received multiple hydrocortisone injections. In such a background it may be difficult to decide whether the lesion is 'hydrocortisone osteochondritis dissecans' or so-called 'osteonecrosis' which might have arisen in the natural course of events in the age range concerned.

### Treatment

The case recorded indicates that repair of a lesion occurring in a background of hydrocortisone therapy should not be contemplated. Subsequent experience indicates that an expectant and symptomatic approach should be adopted. It is possible, as in osteonecrosis, that symptoms could be related to the local lesion. In this situation excision of the separated area of bone and articular cartilage may be indicated (see also 'Complications of Rheumatoid Arthritis', Ch. 6).

### ESTABLISHED OSTEOCHONDRITIS DISSECANS

#### Clinical Features

The classical situation is one of a teenaged male with complaint of symptoms in a knee unrelated to an athletic injury. The complaints are general and vague in the extreme. They consist of pain and giving way incidents. There may be small recurrent effusions so related. The cause may be suspected by the experienced. But it is not a clinical entity; rather a radiological diagnosis. It will be evident, however, that possibilities cover a wide age-range, from at the extreme, say, five in the female child, to osteonecrosis or osteochondritis dissecans of the elderly. It is essentially a diagnosis radiologically determined; and this is the reason why a wide range of radiologically similar conditions is appended at the beginning of the chapter.

**Giving-way.** Instability under stress is perhaps the most characteristic and interesting of the symptoms and yet one of the most confusing in that it suggests a meniscus lesion. It is clearly due to the fact that a weight-bearing area of articular cartilage is unsupported by bone. It may occur even when the lesion is in the classical situation and apparently non-weight-bearing. This may be due to contact by the tibial spine with the area on the lateral aspect of the femoral condyle which is now loose.

**Gait.** Wilson (1967) called attention to the fact that children with osteochondritis dissecans adopt a gait with the tibia in lateral rotation. This gait is employed to prevent contact between the medial eminence of the tibial spine and the classical site. It is confirmed that this sign may be present in the established and particularly the advanced lesion.

If a gait involving lateral rotation of the tibia is adopted to prevent contact between tibial spine and the loose fragments, conversely passive medial rotation of the tibia at 150° extension may induce pain.

**Arthroscopy.** This method of examination has no useful place in the diagnosis or planning of treatment: it has been indicated that bone pathology, as indicated by radiographs, bears no relationship to the visual cartilaginous lesion. On the other hand the arthroscope has a contribution to make in assessing the healing of articular cartilage in cases in which re-operation is unnecessary in the absence of means of internal fixation. In this regard the advent and development of the operating arthroscope raises the possibility of the removal of the nails used for internal fixation without the necessity for arthrotomy at the same time permitting inspection of the restored articular surface. In this regard it is of interest that Jackson and Dandy (1976) record that nails have been inserted in loose osteochondral fragments and later removed under direct vision.

**Treatment**

*'No treatment is better than the wrong treatment'.*
**Immobilisation.** There is no evidence that immobilisation as such has any beneficial influence on healing in established osteochondritis dissecans; rather the reverse in so far as the welfare of the knee joint is concerned. There is evidence that cases recorded in the literature to have healed spontaneously or with immobilisation were unrecognised anomalies of ossification the large majority of which would have disappeared in the normal course of events.

In orthopaedic surgery there are circumstances when no treatment is better than the wrong treatment; and the immobilisation of *established* osteochondritis dissecans in plaster cast or long-leg caliper for an indeterminate period of time with no prospect of healing is an outstanding example.

Reference has been made elsewhere in this work to the deleterious effect of prolonged immobilisation on the growing joint. Figures 11,18 and 11,19 depict the knees of a young man (I.G., aged 30) who, at the age of 12 suffered from osteochondritis dissecans for which he was treated for a period of 6 years in a walking caliper splint. It will be evident that this treatment not only failed to cure the condition but the long period of immobilisation, with the additional factor of pressure of a knee-apron on the patello-femoral joint, has produced degenerative changes which are only too evident in the radiographs. Prolonged immobilisation not only does not cure osteochondritis dissecans but produces irreversible and irreparable changes in the joint. No treatment, with the eventual separation of a loose body, is accompanied by lesser degenerative changes (Figs 11,20 and 11,21).

Immobilisation has no place in treatment other than as a short term post-operative measure (see below).

**Operation**

**Pre-operative considerations.** It is characteristic of established osteochondritis dissecans that the radiological features bear little apparent relationship to the operative findings. The inexperienced, faced with a gross radiological defect, are surprised when there is no obvious lesion of the articular cartilage. It should be stated, however, that it is almost invariably possible to locate the lesion either visually from loss of the normal contour of the articulate surface, or by palpation in the existence of an area unsupported from above by cancellous bone.

**The loose body has separated.** It was once the

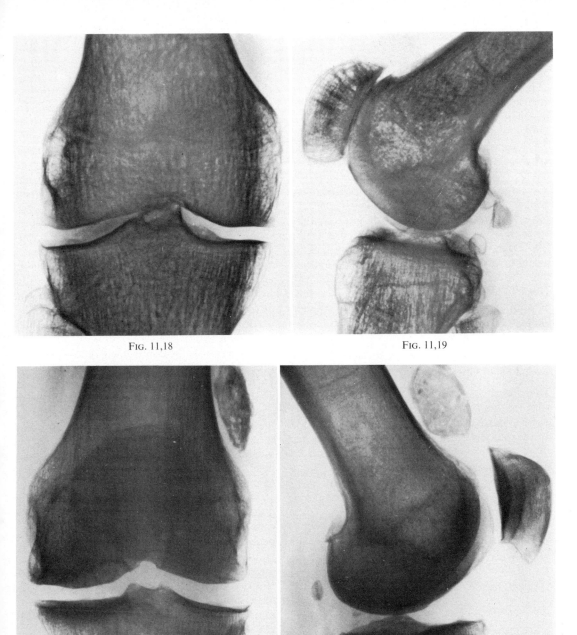

FIG. 11,18

FIG. 11,19

FIG. 11,20

FIG. 11,21

FIGS 11,18–21. **Osteochondritis dissecans: no treatment is better than the wrong treatment**. This is the joint of a patient who at the age of 12 suffered from osteochondritis dissecans at the classical site and was treated for 6 years in a long-leg walking caliper splint. There are generalised degenerative changes throughout the joint (Fig. 11,18). But note in particular the degenerative changes in the patello-femoral joint the result of the pressure of the knee apron (Fig. 11,19). Note presence of loose bodies; but not to be confused with fabella (I.G., male, aged 30, case of C.S.C.).

If the established condition is untreated, sooner or later a loose body separates into the joint. If the lesion is massive as in this bilateral example generalised osteoarthrosis is the inevitable outcome at an early age. But note condition of patello-femoral joint (Fig. 11,21) by comparison with Figure 11,19, Fig. 11,21 is much the better joint. (S.S., male, aged 32.) Note location of loose body to the lateral side of the suprapatellar pouch.

custom to discard any free, loose body. It will be evident that the size of the loose body in terms of the cartilaginous element cannot be determined by the normal routine radiographs. In general, the larger the bone element the larger the cartilaginous element. In any event the larger the loose body the larger the defect in the articular surface and the greater the necessity for repair.

A large loose body is likely to be located in the crater; in the suprapatellar pouch; in the posterior compartment; or in the intercondylar fossa. It is fortunate that the larger it is the less it is likely to have been involved in locking incidents and the less, therefore, the likelihood that the articular surface has been damaged. The smaller loose body, if it has been involved in trapping incidents, may have received such damage to the articular cartilage as to make repair unrewarding.

### Technique of Operation

The operation is performed under tourniquet with the knee flexed over the end of the table as for meniscectomy. The incision is that used for the removal of the medial or lateral meniscus

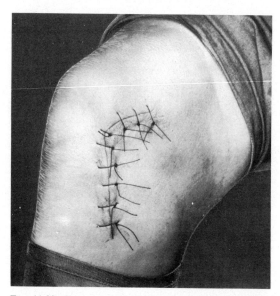

FIG. 11,22. **Osteochondritis dissecans: treatment. 'Drilling' from the side.** To gain access to the side of the condyle above the articular cartilage the incision 'as for meniscectomy' is enlarged in direction upwards and backwards.

depending on the condyle involved, extended upwards and backwards (Fig. 11,22) if necessary but respecting the infrapatellar branch of the saphenous nerve on the medial side. The non-destructive nature of the approach is stressed. Parapatellar incisions which lay the joint widely open are unnecessary and undesirable. The conservative procedures to be described are justified only if the exposure employed is innocent in terms of permanent impairment of function. The use of the retractors described in IKJ5, Chapter 7, together with the special instruments described in IKJ5, Chapter 10, is recommended. Division of the anterior or antero-central attachments of either meniscus is to be avoided. Experience has shown that fixation of the anterior horn by fibrous tissue in the healing process leads to loss of mobility of the meniscus as a whole and a consequent local tear.

Inspection of the condyle will determine what procedure to adopt.

**1. The articular surface is intact.** If no abnormality is apparent, or the site indicated by a raised area surrounded by a shallow gutter, or there is a shallow groove, depression or a flat area, the simple 'drilling' procedure will be indicated in so far as no major operative insult need be inflicted on the all-important articular cartilage.

The first step is accurate localisation of the lesion. To this end inspection, related to the radiographic findings, may be all that is necessary. Flattening of articular cartilage may be evident, or an area imperfectly supported by underlying bone detected by the palpating finger. If no indication of the site exists, or if the indications are indefinite, radiographs with markers of Kirschner wire should be secured to avoid the possibility of error.

APPROACH FROM THE SIDE. In an operation which aims at perfection it is undesirable to inflict even minor injury to the articular cartilage. In the 'drilling' of sclerotic bone beneath an unbroken cartilagenous surface the question of approaching the lesion from the side rather than by direct attack should be considered.

If, after inspection, it is decided to approach from the side, the skin incision is extended upwards about 2·5 cm (1 in) and angled backwards (Fig. 11,22). The underlying tissues and capsule

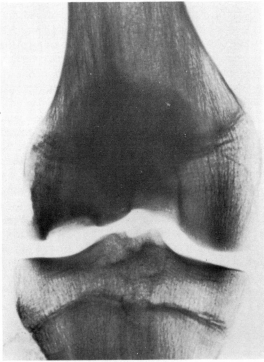

FIG. 11,23.

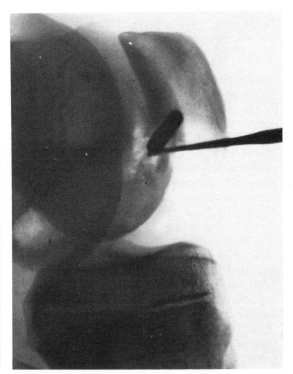

FIG. 11,25.

FIG. 11,24.

FIG. 11,26.

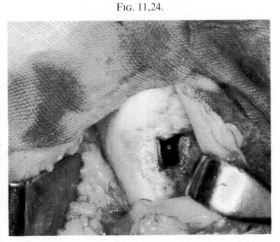

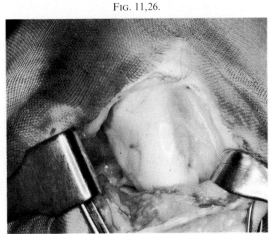

FIGS 11,23–26. **Osteochondritis dissecans: treatment. 'Drilling' from the side.** The side of the condyle affected is exposed by extending the incision as for meniscectomy slightly upwards and backwards (Fig. 11,22). A window is made behind the articular surface. In the current technique the rectangle of bone so produced retains a hinge of synovial membrane on the superior aspect (Fig. 11,24).

If doubt exists as to the exact site of the lesion a lateral radiograph with a marker in position is taken (Fig. 11,25). If a large area of the condyle is depressed but the articular cartilage unbroken (Fig. 11,26) it can be packed up from above with cancellous tissue entered through the window.

are divided until the inferior limit of vastus medialis is encountered. Retraction of the curved flap gives adequate exposure of the condyle posterior to the articular surface.

A window, about 7 mm ($\frac{1}{3}$ in) square, is cut behind the rolled articular margin on the medial aspect of the medial condyle, or the lateral aspect of the lateral condyle, exactly opposite to the lesion (Fig. 11,24). The window is cut in such a manner that the superior synovial attachment is preserved in the form of a hinge. The fragment and attached synovium are then retracted in a superior direction. To gain access some cancellous tissue is removed immediately deep to the opening and preserved. The sclerotic bone of the lesion is then broken up with the point of a fine gouge (Fig. 11,27) entered from the side. In some cases when the gouge touches the hard bony nucleus the sensation is transmitted both to the surgeon and to the assistant holding the retractors; but in any event the difference between normal and abnormal tissue is readily detected. Medial and lateral rotation of the hip bring a wide arc of bone within the compass of the point of the gouge. In other circumstances it is important to be in a position to confirm that the lesion has been entered and sclerotic bone broken up. If doubt exists a radiograph with the gouge or other marker in position is essential (Fig. 11,25). If the articular surface is depressed or unsupported as the result of absorption of underlying bone additional cancellous tissue is readily obtained from the femoral condyle adjacent to the window and packed in to raise the surface to the required level (Fig. 11,26).

At the termination of the operation the block of bone is replaced in the window and driven inwards until it locks in position still retaining the synovial attachment.

If there is a criticism of this procedure it is the tendency to some degree of post-operative haemarthrosis; and aspiration has been required on a number of occasions. There can be no doubt that the compression bandage exerts pressure on the surface concerned; but some

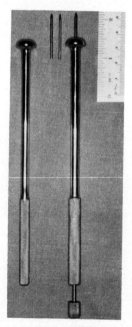

Fig. 11,28. **Osteochondritis dissecans: treatment.** Instruments for internal fixation consist of nail-gun, nails and nail punch. The extruded portion of the trochar of the nail-gun indicates the length of nail yet to be driven. The nails are 25 to 30 mm long and of a diameter of 1·5 mm. They have no heads, but a deep groove is cut at the extreme proximal end to facilitate extraction (see Figs 11,30, 11,31, 11,35 and 11,36 which show use of nails in internal fixation).

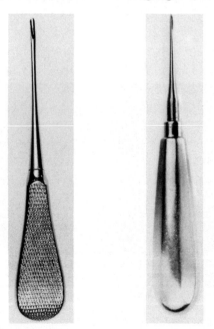

Fig. 11,27. **Osteochondritis dissecans: treatment. 'Drilling'.** Fine hand gouges used in 'drilling' from the side and in the preparation of the crater and bone element of the fragment.

oozing from the vascular bone involved is inevitable. It is hoped that the modifications of technique whereby the plug of bone retains a synovial hinge may reduce this complication.

**2. The loose body is free or virtually free.** In these circumstances a decision must be made whether adequate preparation of crater and bone element of fragment is possible, leaving a hinge of articular cartilage or posterior cruciate ligament intact, or whether preparation is possible only after removal of the loose body from the crater. The choice will depend on local conditions, and particularly on the size and density of the bone element, access to which may be possible only outwith the joint. Radical measures are more certain of success even if they entail the eventual use of internal fixation.

**3. The loose body is quite free.** In these circumstances it is removed for preparation outside the joint. The crater is prepared by excising any fibrous tissue that may line the margins and by 'drilling' the base. In the latter measure the sclerotic bone will be found to be harder than expected and time will be saved by the use of a hand-gouge (Fig. 11,27) or the fine-pointed gouge and mallet illustrated in IKJ5, Chapter 10. If the loose body is free the facility with which it can be replaced is not unnaturally related to the interval between displacement and operation. Preparation of the proliferated margins and of a large dense bone element must take place outside the joint. If on return the fragment sinks too deeply into the crater the level can be adjusted by digging bone outwards from the base or supplementing with autogenous cancellous tissue. The direction in which the nail is inserted is determined to a large extent by the position of the lesion and by the access available. It cannot always be driven at right angles to the surface. A second nail may be necessary if the fragment is large or adjustment of the levels difficult. If the base of the crater has been thoroughly prepared the nail must be driven some distance into the femur before gaining a hold. In general, nails of at least 2·5 cm are necessary (Figs 11,28 to 11,36).

PREPARATION OF THE FRAGMENT OUTSIDE THE JOINT. When the fragment is free, or attached only by a stalk of posterior cruciate ligament or other soft tissue, it is best removed from the joint in order to permit the dense bony element to be drilled or otherwise prepared for revascularisation. There are certain attractions in retaining the isthmus of soft tissue as it enables the loose body to be returned to the crater in a predetermined position. But experience has shown that the breaking up of a dense bony mass is so important that direct access, only possible outside the joint, is essential to ensure the maximum opportunity for revascularisation. Further, if it is true that the attachment of the posterior cruciate ligament to the fragment is at least one of the factors responsible for the failure of healing, then it is not unreasonable that the fragment be freed completely. Thus detachment may not be as radical a move as might first appear.

ORIENTATION. If the fragment is to be prepared outside the joint and particularly if it is not of distinctive outline, for example, almost circular, it is important to have some method of marking so that it is returned to the cavity in the exact position in which it was originally located. To this end, the dental probe, used to manoeuvre the fragment, is inserted at the periphery and the femoral condyle similarly marked. Thus, when the prepared fragment is replaced on the prepared vascular bed, no difficulty or orientation will arise.

In removing the fragment from the joint it should be recalled that synovial fluid is slippy and articular cartilage the slippiest substance known (Charnley, 1955). In these circumstances the greatest care is necessary to prevent escape to the floor either in transit or during preparation. To prepare the bone element, the fragment is placed articular surface downward on a smooth towel moistened with saline. It is held down with forefinger and thumb and the surface broken up with a hand gouge. It is then returned to the crater and aligned with the surrounding articular cartilage. A point is selected suitable for the driving of the nail and a puncture made in the articular cartilage with a straight probe. The fragment is then removed from the joint and the probe driven on through the articular cartilage and bone in the predetermined direction. The nail, entered in the nail gun, is now gently driven through the articular cartilage and bone until the point appears on the deep surface. The fragment, with the nail and nail gun attached, is then returned

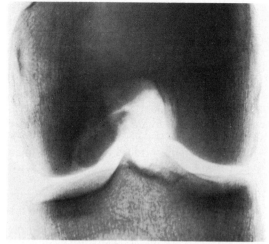

FIG. 11,29.

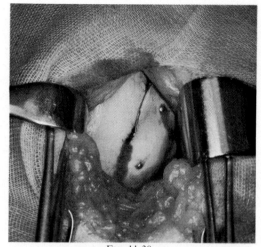

FIG. 11,30.

FIG. 11,31.

FIG. 11,32.

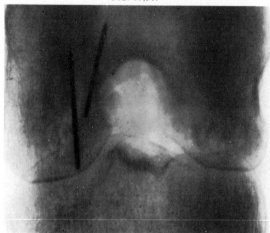

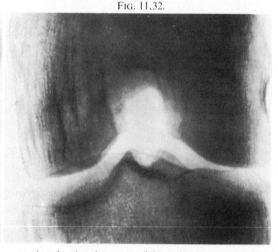

FIGS 11,29–32. **Osteochondritis dissecans: treatment.** Large lesion at the classical site of the medial femoral condyle depicted by tunnel view (Fig. 11,29). The visual appearance at the completion of operation (Fig. 11,30). The appearance four months later and immediately prior to removal of the nails (Fig. 11,31). The appearance one year from the date of operation showing the return of the trabecular pattern (Fig. 11,32) (P.H., male, aged 16).

The tunnel views produce dramatic radiographs. They are not helpful in localisation but may be useful in estimating healing.

to the crater where it will be found that the nail gun enables the position to be controlled without difficulty. When the cartilagenous surfaces are adjusted to the required level the nail is driven home (Figs 11,30 and 11,35).

If towards the termination of the operation the fragment is not lying in perfect position but extruded in flexion, the effect of extension should be observed. It is not unusual to find that when the joint is fully extended the fragment is under compression and fits accurately in position. If such circumstances exist the patient should be nursed for the first two weeks in full extension and at the time when the stitches are removed a plaster cast applied in complete extension. The cast should be retained without weight-bearing for, say, 10 weeks.

NECESSITY FOR COMPRESSION. If there is a large bone component in the potential loose body the curve of the articular cartilage is

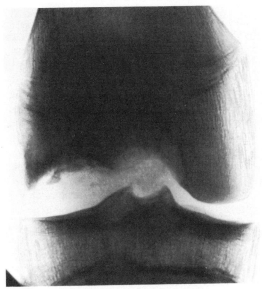

FIG. 11,33.

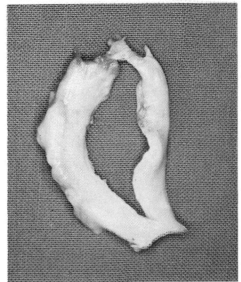

FIG. 11,34.

FIG. 11,35.

FIG. 11,36.

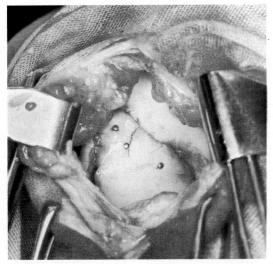

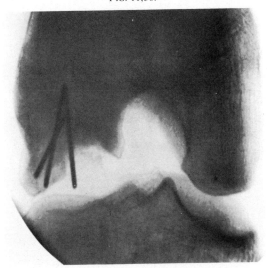

FIGS 11,33–36. **Osteochondritis dissecans of lateral femoral condyle.** Underlying this massive lesion (Fig. 11,33) as is a common finding was a displaced longitudinal tear of the lateral meniscus (Fig. 11,34). Note that lateral margin of condyle is not involved (Fig. 11,33). Appearance at completion of conservative surgery (Fig. 11,35). Post-operative tunnel view to show extent of lesion and provide yardstick for future comparison. Note nails entered at different angles (Fig. 11,36).

preserved (Fig. 11,37). If there is a 'sanding' only of bone the curve of the cartilage is lost as a result of weight-bearing and the profile consequently flat (Fig. 11,38).

The nails described are ideal when the surface involved is small, or in circumstances in which congruity can be achieved without tension. If, however, a large area of flat articular cartilage has to be applied to a curved surface some method of compression is essential. This can be achieved only with screw fixation.

The technique to be adopted takes cognisance of one of the reasons why screws were abandoned in the first place, namely inability to

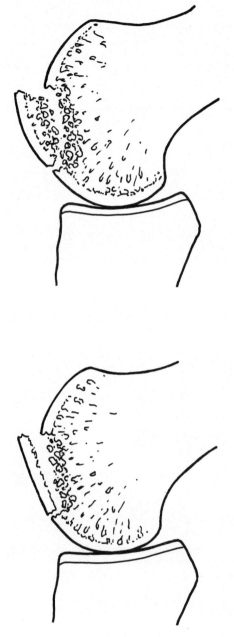

FIGS 11,37–38. **Osteochondritis dissecans: treatment.** If the bone element of the fragment is large, the overlying articular cartilage retains the curve of the condyle (Fig. 11,37). If the bone element of the fragment is minimal, a mere sanding, although the circumstances are favourable to healing the articular cartilage has become flat and if it is to be replaced in the form of a curve nails may be insufficient and compression in the form of a lag-screw is required (Fig. 11,38).

adjust adjacent surfaces after insertion. This problem has been overcome by securing congruity of surfaces by the use of the nails in the normal manner, and, accepting the necessity for compression, inserting one or more lag-screws as the situation demands. When these have been inserted, and the tension adjusted, the nails used as temporary fixation are withdrawn.

**4. The fragment is small or the lesion irreparable.** It is not intended to convey the impression that every lesion should be repaired when this is technically possible. A small area of the articular surface need not be repaired; and indeed it is probably undesirable to do so. There is evidence that small lesions are not necessarily the precursors of mono-compartmental osteoarthrosis. Furthermore, a lesion clearly the result of impingement by a high medial eminence of tibial spine can be expected to recur and should not be repaired.

Nor is it reasonable to repair a defect in the presence of advanced degenerative changes such as may be encountered in the adult or in the so-called osteonecrosis of the elderly. Finally, there is the situation in which repair would be desirable, but because of the multiplicity of fragments or the degenerate state of the articular cartilage, is impossible or unreasonable. In such circumstances the separating fragment or the loose bodies are discarded.

TREATMENT OF THE CRATER. Opinion is divided on what measures, if any, should be applied to the residual crater.

Several possibilities arise:

1. No action is taken other than to trim the margins of the vertical walls of the cavity on the theoretical basis that the opposing condyle glides over the defect without evident incongruity.

2. The cartilaginous margins of the defect are bevelled with the purpose of leaving a shallow cavity. It is probable that this technique is unwise as leaving an area of incongruity greater than would obtain in (1) or (3).

3. The base of the crater is drilled to produce a blood supply which will result in the eventual filling of the cavity with fibrous tissue or fibrocartilage and the elimination of the defect.

The opportunities for the re-exploration of joints so treated is minimal. There is no evidence favouring one technique. In recent years the author, but for no good reason, has favoured leaving, if possible, vertical walls in the crater (Fig. 11,50). In other circumstances and in the presence of degenerative changes the margins of the defect have been bevelled.

This is one more situation in which arthroscopic examination at widely spaced intervals might produce evidence in favour of a particular technique.

BONE-CARTILAGE GRAFTS. Reference has been made previously (IKJ4) to the possibility of repair of extensive defects by bone-cartilage grafts. In transplanting articular cartilage, however, orientation may be important in that the area affected must be stressed to the forces likely to be encountered. Reference has been made elsewhere to the fact that split lines are constant in direction for any given site on the joint surface and is related to the internal structure of the cartilage. This would seem to preclude the transplantation of articular cartilage from one site to another as has been anticipated could be done and has been done (J. L. Bado, 1956, personal communication; C. Lima, 1968, personal communication and Palazzi, 1977). To be successful the articular cartilage transplanted in osteochondritis dissecans would have to be of a structure similar to the area of the defect or it will not withstand the forces likely to be encountered.

### After-treatment

**Radiographs.** It is important that after any operation which aims at the revascularisation of sclerotic bone post-operative antero-posterior and lateral radiographs are obtained before the limb is incorporated in a plaster cast.

In estimating the progress of healing it is not a matter of comparing the original lesion, prior to operation, with one, say, three months later. It is a matter of comparing the immediate post-operative radiograph with one some three months later. The sclerotic bone of the crater and the sclerotic bone of the fragment are altered in appearance, as they should be, by the drilling process, and this is why post-operative radiographs of good quality are essential if a reasonable comparison is to be made.

**Immobilisation.** Experience has shown, after much experimentation with liberal regimes, that the after-treatment most likely to result in healing of the lesion in the age range most commonly involved is immobilisation in a non-weight-bearing plaster cast. Moreover it is the only means whereby compression can be exerted on the anterior aspect of the lesion without the necessity for internal fixation.

The initial regime is that applied after meniscectomy with quadriceps exercises beginning on the fourth day and retention of the original compression bandage until removal of the stitches on the tenth day. It is at this time that a cylinder, but non-weight-bearing, plaster cast is applied. If absorbable sutures have been employed in the skin and in the absence of haemarthrosis or other swelling, the cast can be applied on the fourth day. Ambulation without weight-bearing is permitted using a patten and crutches. In 8 to 12 weeks, depending on the estimate of healing time, the cast is removed and mobilising exercises begun with the purpose of regaining a range of flexion, a right-angle or more, which will permit the removal of the means of internal fixation if such has been employed.

Hourly quadriceps exercises are practised throughout the period of immobilisation and thereafter in conjunction with flexion exercises.

**Bilateral lesions.** In bilateral examples, whether of the medial or lateral condyle, the pathology is never of the same degree. The common finding is that on one side it is advanced to the state at which the loose body has separated while on the other, which may have been symptomless, the articular cartilage is intact. In such cases it can be assumed that the pathology on the less developed side will advance with the passage of time to a state comparable with the side of the gross changes.

The technique to be adopted in such circumstances is to operate on the side of the advanced pathology, and, immediately thereafter, say within one to two weeks, on the second side. This sequence is necessary because it would be unreasonable to operate on the advanced side and expect the patient to become ambulatory carrying his entire weight on an abnormal knee.

When both knees have been subjected to operation at the same time the only possible solution to the resumption of ambulation is the use of

TABLE 11

Experience of operative treatment of osteochondritis dissecans of the knee joint (1940–78)

| Method | Number of lesions |
|---|---|
| Drilling | 100 |
| Drilling and internal fixation | 110 |
| Removal of meniscus; immobilisation, etc. | 14 |
| Loose body removed | 299 |
| Total | 523 |

bilateral patten-ended calipers with or without the use of cylinder casts depending upon the extent to which the patient can be relied upon to follow instructions. The very young readily accept such calipers and even discard their crutches. The method has been applied with success even in young adults. In this regard it should be remembered that footwear should be regarded as nothing more than coverings for the feet. They should be as light as possible so as not to induce traction or other mechanical influence on the knee joint (Fig. 11,39).

**Removal of means of internal fixation.** A criticism which has been levelled at the use of stainless steel nails as a means of internal fixation has been the necessity for removal; and a second operation undesirable *per se* and on economic grounds. It is maintained that the second operation is advantageous to the patient, and to the surgeon in that it provides positive evidence, visual and, if necessary, palpable, that the lesion has healed (Fig. 11,62). It is repeated that radiographs depict bone; and not cartilage. Cases have been encountered in which the radiographs indicated a more favourable situation than in fact obtained.

In recent years failure of healing, evident at exploration rather than radiographically, has not only underlined the desirability of the situation whereby the means of internal fixation is removed, but demonstrated the cause of the failure. The lessons learnt have necessitated some revision of the technique to be employed in certain circumstances; and these advances have been incorporated in the text.

The advent of the operating arthroscope has eliminated some of the criticisms of this form of internal fixation. It is not difficult to design instruments to enter and grip the groove in the nail head. Such instruments in expert hands could extract the nails without the necessity for a second 'open' operation. The successful extraction of nails has been recorded (Jackson and Dandy, 1976).

**Technique.** If internal fixation has been used the nail is removed when the requisite degree of mobility has been attained by active means. The forcible flexion of a stiff knee under anaes-

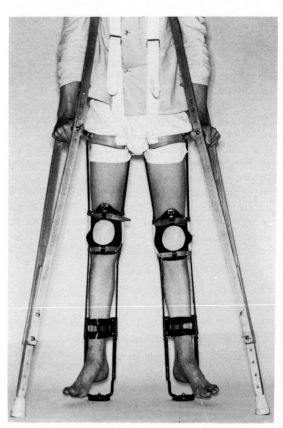

FIG. 11,39. **Bilateral lesions: after-treatment of operations.** In unilateral examples ambulation can be resumed with a patten on the sound side and crutches. If there are lesions in both knees ambulation requires the use of patten-ended calipers which can be applied over cylinder casts if compression by hyperextension is required or if the patient cannot be trusted to comply with instructions. Shoes, if worn, should be of the lightest possible variety in order not to exert a distracting influence on the joints.

Note stature of patient. 'They are either too short or too tall'.

thesia in order to gain access to the site is liable to provoke undesirable reaction and delay recovery.

The scar of the original incision is excised. The access required is minimal. The anterior and antero-central attachments of the meniscus should not be disturbed. The nail is extracted by hooking the point of the fine gouge into the groove on the neck (IKJ5, Fig. 10,3), using the special 'tack-lifter' extractor (IKJ5, Fig. 10,7) or using a pair of suitably-pointed dental forceps (IKJ5, Fig. 10,7). The deep fixation of the affected area is then tested with the saline-moistened gloved forefinger. The further treatment, and particularly the decision as to when to permit weight-bearing, depends on the assessment of the degree of healing determined by radiographs and the visual and digital evidence at operation in relation to the degree of recovery of the quadriceps. In general, the regime normally applied to the meniscus operation has been employed and a return to weight-bearing permitted about the fourteenth day.

**Do the nails require to be removed?** The criticism of metal as a form of internal fixation is the apparent need for a second operation to effect removal. On the other hand internal fixation in the form described inflicts the minimal damage to the articular surface and is known to provoke no reaction four months from the date of insertion. The exploratory operation, with the visual evidence of healing it provides, has attractions for the surgeon and advantages for the patient. But does the nail require to be removed? With increasing experience of this method of internal fixation it was considered at one time that the groove might provide a means of retention as well as of extraction. It was thought probable that in a nail driven flush with articular cartilage fibrous tissue would fill the space and provide permanent fixation. But nails in the femoral condyles are subjected to exceptional gravitational and centrifugal forces (Figs 11,40 to 11,43).

A nail so deeply embedded that it could not be found except at the expense of damage to the virtually perfect articular surface was later extruded to be located in the synovial pouch below the joint line on the lateral side (Fig. 11,42). J. D. Mineiro (1968, personal communication) experienced a case in which a nail was extruded, passed through the posterior capsule to be located in the soft tissues of the popliteal space from which it was removed only with difficulty (Fig. 11,43). It would seem expedient, as was originally intended, to make the extraction of what has been shown to be an innocuous means of internal fixation the occasion for estimating the results of treatment and determining the prognosis.

Nevertheless, it is accepted that there are arguments in favour of a nail which in favourable circumstances could be left *in situ* on the assurance that it would not work long and migrate. Such a nail is in the course of development (Cameron, Piliar and Macnab, 1974). It is based on the nail of the author's design into one side of which is inlaid a porous vitallium strip. It has been shown experimentally that bone grows into the pores of the metal and that such pins have no tendency to migrate and thus would not require to be removed.

### RESULTS OF TREATMENT

It will be evident (Table 11) that a considerable experience has been accumulated over more than three decades of the methods of treatment described. In the Table the figure for removal of loose bodies is high; and abnormally so for two reasons: in the earlier years and before the various techniques for repair had been developed, loose bodies were excised when repair might have been effected; and indeed it was the massive defects which resulted which provided the stimulus to the development of conservative surgery. Moreover, not all the loose bodies which have been removed can be said with certainty to have arisen from an osteochondritis dissecans lesion. Some for example may have been the result of osteochondral fractures.

### Causes of Failure

If the techniques described result in the restoration of the articular surface in a very high proportion of cases there has been the occasional failure. The possible causes have been analysed in the hope of elimination.

**Drilling.** If drilling from the side avoids direct assault on intact articular cartilage (Figs 11,44 to 11,47) it has the disadvantage that approach

T

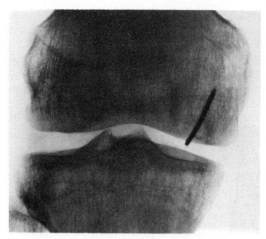

FIG. 11,40

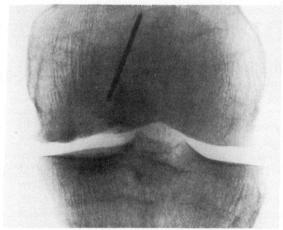

FIG. 11,41

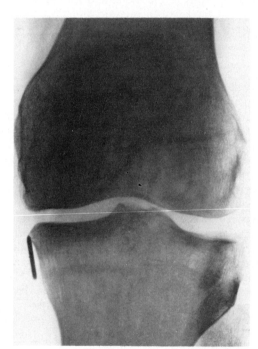

FIG. 11,42

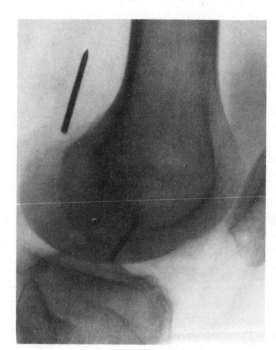

FIG. 11,43

FIGS 11,40–43. **Osteochondritis dissecans: treatment.** If at operation the nail is bent (Fig. 11,40) or otherwise cannot be removed without damage to the articular cartilage one course of action is to drive it deeper into the bone so that the risk of dislodgment is minimised. In this example (Fig. 11,41) the patient is known to have walked after the original repair. It is assumed that the nail head was driven beneath the articular surface by the pressure of weight-bearing. Weight-bearing following operation usually results in failure of healing. This case, undeservedly, healed. He was followed for 18 months. The nail had not moved (F.McG., male, aged 31). In normal circumstances nails should be removed. This one, left *in situ* because of inaccessibility, was later removed from the synovial pouch below the joint line on the lateral side (Fig. 11,42). This one was extruded passed through the posterior capsule and was located in the popliteal space (Fig. 11,43). (Case of the late Prof. J. D., Mineiro, Lisbon.)

to the sclerotic nidus of bone is less direct. It is undoubtedly more difficult to be certain that the bone elements of the particular potential loose body has been completely and systematically perforated. Cases have been encountered in which the bone element has been reduced in size radiologically; but not eliminated. This appears to suggest that part has attained a blood supply, but part, as a result of faulty technique, has not been in a favourable state to attain a blood supply. There are other possibilities to account for failure. In recent years, and in an attempt to avoid the consequences of immobilisation in plaster, a liberal attitude has been adopted to recovery using a patten on the sound leg and crutches with free movement, with the exception of weight-bearing, on the operated knee. It is possible that the responsibilities so related are not acceptable in the age range to which the drilling operation applies. Furthermore, the freedom of movement means that the posterior cruciate ligament can exert influence on immobility of the fragment; and, moreover, contact by medial eminence of tibial spine as an aetiological factor has not been eliminated (Figs 11,48 to 11,51).

It is possible, therefore, that the attitude to retaining mobility was overdone to the extent of responsibility for failure. If there has been a lesson to be learnt from recent failures it is that if in doubt as to the reliability of the young patient, plaster immobilisation should be prescribed in the knowledge that three to four months of immobility is likely to be less damaging in the long term than failure of healing. This is the reason for the current recommendation of plaster immobilisation.

### Repair and Internal Fixation

**1. Inadequate preparation of the crater and/or of the bone element of the fragment.** In the earlier years of the series the occasional failure was traced to inadequate preparation of both crater and bone element of the separating fragment. Examples of failure so related have been demonstrated from other sources, in criticism of the technique, in which it was obvious from the sclerosis evident in post-operative radiographs that conditions favourable to healing had not been provided. It is less than useless to bring the dead bone of the fragment into contact with the dead bone of the crater no matter what the means of internal fixation, nail or screw, and to expect healing to occur. It is positively harmful for the opportunity for healing has been lost.

**2. Unstable replacement.** It is a simple matter to attain stability of reduction of a small fragment; but in the majority of cases in which conservative surgery is indicated the fragment is a large one and part of a curved surface; in particular because the separated fragment is flat and the surface to which it is to be applied curved. In such circumstances it is not unusual after preparation of the base of the crater and of the bony element of the fragment, to find in the course of replacement that whereas congruity of opposing margins can be obtained at one aspect of the crater, the fragment tends to spring out on the opposite side. It may be a simple matter by altering the contour of the cancellous tissue below the fragment to overcome this difficulty. In other circumstances complete stability may be impossible to achieve. In this regard there is little doubt that the smooth headless nails described are not helpful in achieving fixation even when two or three are used at an angle to one another rather than parallel when a flat area of cartilage is applied to a curved surface.

The case which revealed this problem (J.B., male, age 17,) at whose second operation it was anticipated with confidence that the joint surface would be restored, showed one side of the defect to be healed and congruous, the other to have sprung out of the crater leaving the nails behind. The articular cartilage was so seriously damaged by motion that it had to be removed. At removal it was evident that the congruous side had healed by bony union. It was recalled later that at the original operation difficulty had been encountered in keeping that aspect in position. It had been a matter of moulding a flat area of cartilage to a curved surface (Figs 11,37 and 11,38); and the means of internal fixation had been inadequate.

**3. Failure to recognise osteochondral fracture.** It will be appreciated that if the lesion treated is an old osteochondral fracture from single or repeated incidents contact with the medial eminence of the tibial spine rather than 'osteochondritis dissecans' as such, failure is inevitable in the long term: the mechanical aetiological factor remains. In retrospect this is thought to have been the cause of a few failures or partial failures as in the case illustrated in Figures 11,48 to 11,51. The treatment in such circumstances is excision of the unhealed fragment.

**4. Weight-bearing.** Evidence has been accumu-

lated that if instructions have been disregarded and weight-bearing undertaken the lesion fails to heal.

**5. Incomplete immobilisation.** In theory immobilisation in a plaster cast is unnecessary and undesirable. In pursuit of the ideal there

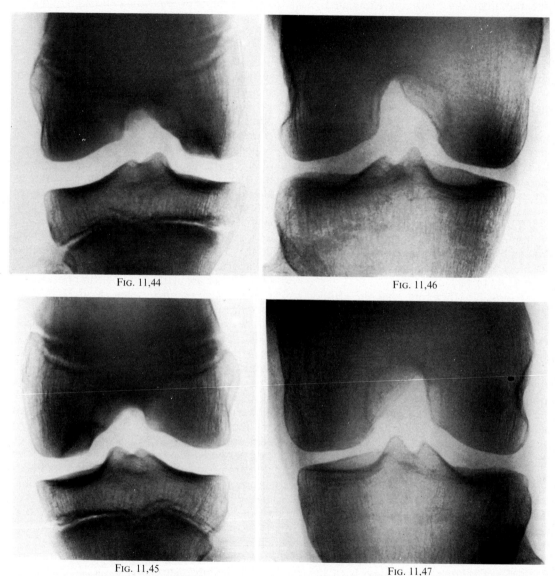

FIG. 11,44

FIG. 11,46

FIG. 11,45

FIG. 11,47

FIGS 11,44–47. **Osteochondritis dissecans: treatment. Long term results of drilling operation.** This bilateral symmetrical example at the classical site was subjected to the drilling operation approaching from the side. The lesion on the femoral condyle consisted of flattening of the articular cartilage. The surface was unbroken (Figs 11,44 and 11,45).

The patient reported 15 years later with some other complaint. The bilateral characteristically shaped scars (Fig. 11,22) were noted on his knees and radiographs obtained. No abnormality could be detected. He regarded his knees as normal (Figs 11,46 and 11,47) (W.S., male, aged 15).

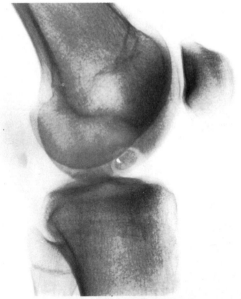

FIG. 11,48

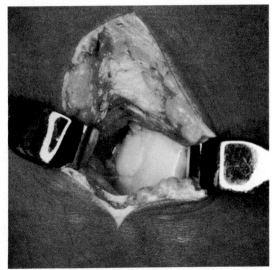

FIG. 11,49

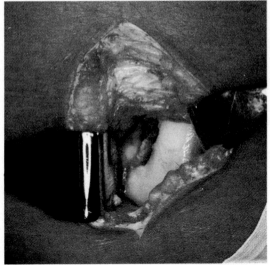

FIG. 11,50

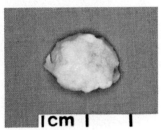

FIG. 11,51

was a time when casts were not employed and the joint exercised freely but without weight-bearing. But certain unexpected failures occurred either from movement, unauthorised weight-bearing, or both. There is strong evidence, it is repeated, that cases in which weight-bearing has taken place do not heal. This is the reason for the current recommendation of after-treatment by non-weight-bearing plaster cast.

FIGS 11,48–51. **Osteochondritis dissecans: treatment. Failure of drilling operation: excision of fragment.** This patient (S.S., female) was subjected to the drilling operation from the side at the age of 15. Four years later she developed symptoms and it was evident from the radiograph that there remained a small nidus of necrotic bone (Fig. 11,48). At operation it was seen that the articular cartilage involved was only about one quarter of the area of four years previously (Fig. 11,49). It was decided, and in view of the evidence of contact between the medial eminence of tibial spine and classical site, that this was the probable cause of failure of healing. The mobile articular cartilage and the necrotic bone were excised leaving a crater with vertical sides (Fig. 11,50). The area of articular cartilage was about 1·5 cm square. The necrotic bone much smaller (Fig. 11,51). Note evidence of blood supply in base of crater (Fig. 11,50) and at margins of necrotic bone (Fig. 11,51) suggesting that this is an osteochondral fracture. If this case is technically capable of repair it is pointless if the cause is contact with the tibial spine.

## OSTEOCHONDRITIS DISSECANS OF LATERAL CONDYLE OF TIBIA

**Historical note.** If osteochondritis dissecans of the lateral condyle of the tibia has proved uncommon in the experience of this series, it is of interest that Wells (1974) had described and illustrated such a lesion in an Anglo-Saxon skeleton circa A.D. 900 (Fig. 11,52). The site and size of the lesion corresponds closely to the

description of the operative findings of the case recorded below (Fig. 11,53).

### Clinical Features

Radiological osteochondritis dissecans in the lateral condyle of the tibia, unilateral or bilateral, appears to be associated, like osteochondritis dissecans of the patella, with lesions elsewhere in the joint. In one case, for example,

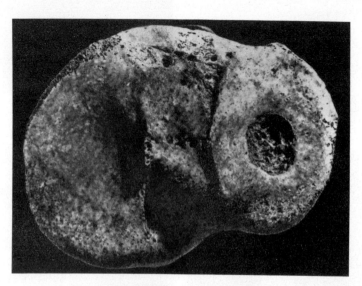

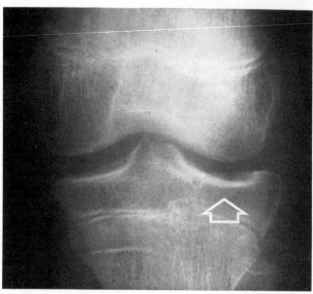

FIGS 11,52–53. **Osteochondritis dissecans of lateral condyle of tibia.** Anglo-Saxon tibia showing osteochondritis dissecans lesion in centre of lateral condyle (Fig. 11,52) (reproduced by courtesy of the late Dr Calvin Wells). Compare with radiograph of recent case (Fig. 11,53) (S.R., female, aged 11, case of Mr Lloyd-Roberts, see text).

there was a lesion of the lateral femoral condyle in the opposite knee. In a bilateral case there was a lesion at the classical site in one femoral condyle.

The circumstances in which the first case was encountered and treated are recorded.

The boy (T.J., aged 12) was first seen with giving-way incidents in the left knee, then of two years duration. A radiograph showed what was considered to be an anomaly of ossification in the lateral femoral condyle. At the same time irregularities were noted on the antero-superior aspect of the femoral condyles and in the patella which tended to confirm the probability of an anomaly of ossification. The final clinical decision made was that the symptoms were referable to his patella. His symptoms ceased within one year, but in a follow-up examination one year later he complained of pain and giving-way symptoms, this time in the right knee. When seen three years from the first examination, radiographs of both knees showed not only a lesion in the lateral femoral condyle on the left side, almost certainly the transition from anomaly of ossification to osteochondritis dissecans, but also, what had not been encountered before, a lesion in the lateral condyle of the tibia on the right side (Figs 11,54 and 11,55). He complained of pain in the right knee, the site of the tibial lesion, but had symptoms referable to the lesion in the lateral femoral condyle on the left side.

Both lesions were subjected to the 'drilling' operation as described approaching from a non-articular site at the side. Both joints were radiologically normal within a year.

### Treatment

Experience of treatment is limited to three knees, the patient described above and one bilateral case, all at an early stage and 'drilled' from the side. No operative experience of an advanced lesion has been accumulated. The author is indebted therefore to Mr G. C. Lloyd-Roberts of London for the record which follows:

The patient (S.R., female, aged 11) when referred had already undergone a negative exploratory operation. The one and only complaint was of continuous pain in the left knee since a fall two years previously. Clinical examination revealed quadriceps wasting, a 10° fixed flexion deformity and slight lateral joint line tenderness. The radiographs and later tomographs revealed the presence of a 'lesion' in the lateral condyle of the tibia (Fig. 11,53). The provisional diagnosis of cystic degeneration of the lateral meniscus in unusual form was made and operation undertaken on the basis of the prolonged nature of the disability and in spite of the previous negative exploration.

At operation the lateral meniscus was normal; but on being raised from the tibia revealed an abnormal area of articular cartilage. To gain access to the site the meniscus

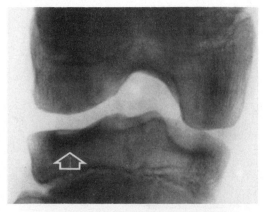

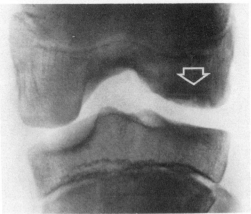

FIGS 11,54–55. **Bilateral asymmetrical osteochondritis dissecans.** Lesion of lateral femoral condyle on left side (Fig. 11,54). Lesion of lateral condyle of tibia on right side (Fig. 11,55) (see text).

was excised. The abnormal cartilage, swollen and bulging, was approximately 2·5 cm in diameter. When it was excised the underlying bone was sclerotic and the lesion in keeping with the known pathological features of osteochondritis dissecans. The histological features of the excised material, never pathognomic, were in keeping with this diagnosis.

## OSTEOCHONDRITIS DISSECANS OF PATELLA

**Incidence.** Osteochondritis dissecans of the patella is a condition of some rarity. Forty cases only have been reported including the six cases recorded by the author in 1960 (Edwards and

Bentley, 1977). Since then a further six personal cases have been encountered.

**Location.** It is an entity not to be confused with lateral marginal or with the medial tangential osteochondral fracture from single or repeated incidents of dislocation (Ch. 2). It is to be distinguished from such fractures in that the lesion tends to be located towards the inframedial aspect of the medial facet with the intact isthmus of articular cartilage on the lateral side. It does not involve the margin of the bone.

### Clinical Features

The patients, as in osteochondritis dissecans in general, are predominantly male. All the author's 12 cases were males; but examples in

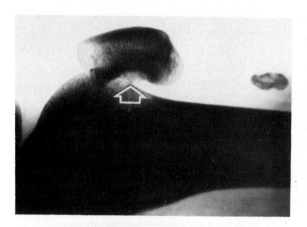

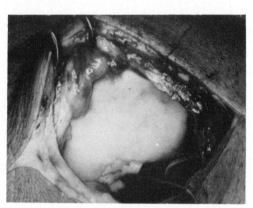

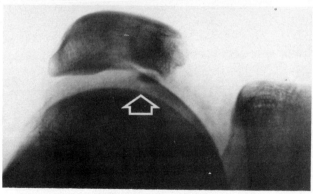

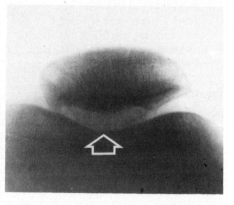

FIGS 11,56–59. **Osteochondritis dissecans of patella.** Bilateral case. Right: the fragment with large bone element has separated and is located in the suprapatellar pouch (Fig. 11,56). Left: articular surface patella from which fragment has not yet separated but clearly not amenable to restoration (Fig. 11,57) (A.D., male, aged 20). Lesion with large bone element in case treated by conservative surgery (Fig. 11,58) (G.McK., male, aged 18). Axial view to show location of lesion (Fig. 11,59) (C.E., male, aged 16).

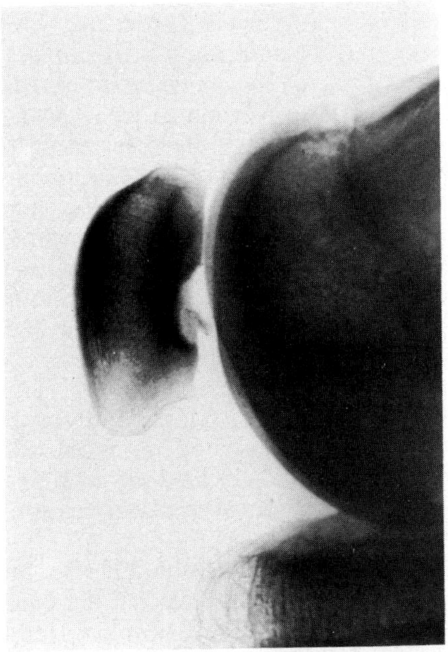

FIG. 11,60

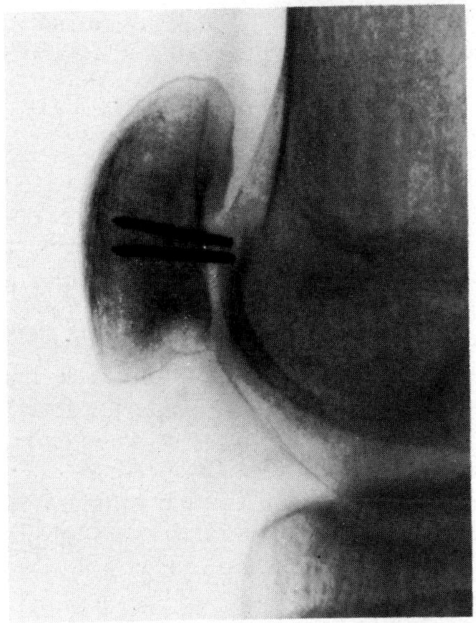

FIG. 11,61

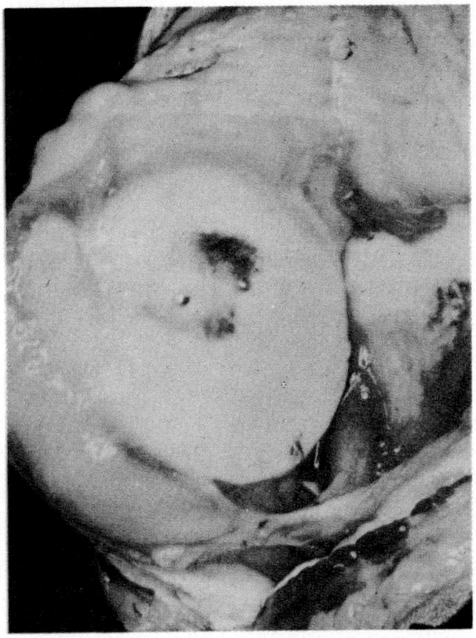

FIG. 11,62

FIGS 11,60–62. **Osteochondritis dissecans of patella: treatment.** Lesions in the patella are rare and distinguished from other lesions in that the margin of the bone is not involved (Fig. 11,60, see also Ch. 2). Circumstances arise favourable to restoration of the articular cartilage by the method described and have been successfully accomplished (Figs 11,60 and 11,61). In the radiograph taken before removal of the nails note disappearance of sclerosis in base of crater (Fig. 11,61). In the photograph taken at operation note that articular cartilage has healed and with total absence of reaction at nail heads (Fig. 11,62).

females have been reported (Edwards and Bentley, 1977). The age range is 15 to 20 with the occasional older patient with a long history. The presenting symptoms are retropatellar pain, catching and giving-way or sudden locking of the variety associated with the presence of a free loose body.

**Diagnosis.** The lateral radiograph (Figs 11,56 and 11,58) or one of the skyline views at 30°, 60° and 90° depicts the lesion (Fig. 11,59).

Arthroscopy will locate the exact site and give some indication as to whether restoration of the articular surface is possible.

The following is an example of a case:

The patient (A.D., a male aged 20) of unquestioned dysototic constitution, presented with locking of the right knee, the result of a loose body in the supra-patellar pouch (Fig. 11,56). On investigation the lesion was located in the patella and found to be bilateral and symmetrical. Both were observed at operation and, as if to make confirmation of the nature of the pathology complete, a massive lesion of the medial femoral condyle in the left knee was diagnosed radiologically and eventually repaired surgically. The patellar lesion was located midway between superior and inferior poles on the medial aspect and extended in area to the mid-line of the bone. On the right side the osteocartilaginous fragment was free as a loose body in the joint. On the left it lay in the crater anchored, as in typical osteochondritis fashion, by a remaining tag of articular cartilage. Where the fragment was free the constant motion of the bone over the femoral condyles had separated tags of articular cartilage from the periphery of the crater and these projected into the joint to be responsible for recurring mechanical incidents (Fig. 11,57).

### Treatment

The articular surface of the patella is subjected to such exceptional stresses that the condition of the cartilage element of the separating fragment is seldom such as to make restoration possible (Fig. 11,57). Nevertheless, of the 10 cases which came to operation 2, perhaps exceptionally, were capable of restoration of the articular surface by drilling and internal fixation on the lines indicated; both were successful (Figs 11,58 and 11,60 to 11,62). In the remaining cases the affected area was excised in the manner described for chondromalacia patellae (Ch. 2).

**Results of operation.** The limited experience of excision of the affected area on the lines indicated has resulted in relief of the presenting symptoms. The impression has been gained that the results are consistently better than in chondromalacia patellae and may reflect the different aetiological background.

## LOOSE BODIES

### Source of Symptoms

**1. Locking of joint.** The sudden dramatic block to movement, 'out of the blue' so to speak, in the course of normal everyday use and unrelated to athletic activity, is the classical symptom associated with the presence of a loose body in the joint. It is produced by interposition of a *small* loose body between opposing joint surfaces, usually femur and tibia but sometimes patella and femur, where the block is usually transient.

IMPLICATIONS. Incidents of locking are not innocent of implication for the welfare of the joint on a long-term basis. Articular cartilage, remarkable substance as it is, is not designed for sudden impact incidents. Split lines, as have been described in relation to meniscus lesions, are the result. Repeated incidents in particular have serious implications for the future in terms of osteoarthrosis, mono- or bi-compartmental.

**2. Interference with motion.** This symptom is associated with a loose body anchored or pedunculated and located at the margin of a femoral condyle where it interferes with movement. The presence of such a loose body is usually known to the patient.

**3. Synovial irritation.** This symptom too is associated with a loose body moveable through a small range and located at a site where mechanical irritation of synovial membrane is produced by movement.

**4. Loss of flexion or extension.** This is rarely the cause of complaint but noted in the course of examination in the presence of vague symptoms. It is caused by the presence of a *large* and gradually enlarging loose body in the intercondylar notch or in the posterior compartment.

### Indications for Operation

It will be evident from what precedes, that a small loose body, of whatever origin, producing incidents of locking in the young subject, should be removed at the earliest opportunity in the long-term interests of the joint. A loose body which is not free to move about and become interposed between the joint surfaces may be innocent of symptoms and rare instances have been cited where their presence actually conferred benefit (Ch. 3). The presence therefore of a loose body in a routine radiograph particularly in the ageing joint does not imply that symptoms are so related and is not *per se* an indication for operation.

The posterior compartment is the common site of such a loose body and the features which distinguish it from the fabella in the lateral head of gastrocnemius are described in Chapter 2.

On the other hand, and at the opposite extreme, is the grossly arthrosic joint in which the presenting clinical features are easily related to the presence of a loose body and the patient rendered symptomless by extraction through a

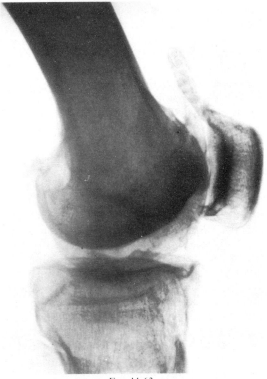

FIG. 11,63

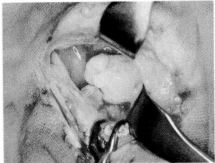

FIG. 11,64

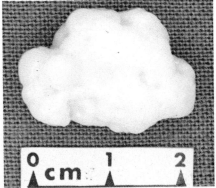

FIG. 11,65

FIGS 11,63–65. **Pan-articular osteoarthrosis based on medial torsion of the femur.** This patient had a supracondylar osteotomy in youth which healed in medial rotation. His immediate symptoms were due to the presence of a loose body in the suprapatellar pouch producing mechanical incidents in the patello-femoral joint (Figs 11,63 and 11,64). The loose body was removed (Fig. 11,65). No other action was taken. It is a gross error to deal with symptomless pathology. (G.A., male, aged 58.)

limited incision inflicting the minimal disturbance to the joint (Figs 11,63 to 11,65).

## REMOVAL OF LOOSE BODIES: PRINCIPLES OF OPERATIVE TREATMENT

### Operative Technique

It is superficially attractive to remove a loose body of known location through a 2·5 cm (1 in) incision and there are circumstances when this is the correct approach. But it has the disadvantage in the youthful subject that it precludes the possibility of repair and, more serious, it precludes inspection of the lesion on the articular surface. Patients are encountered who have suffered a second or third operation at intervals. of years for the removal of loose bodies, all of which had separated from the same situation, usually the classical site. The man whose knee locks a second time may be difficult to convince that the original loose body was, in fact, removed; and such allegations are made. In general, therefore, in the young adult, the incision used should visualise the articular lesion. This statement should not be interpreted as justification for wide destructive exposures of the joint. The incision need not be greater than that required for meniscectomy. A loose body in the suprapatellar pouch can be extracted through either incision by straightening the knee, retracting the patella from off the femoral condyles and exerting manual pressure on the pouch above.

### The Loose Body is Small

A single small loose body in the adolescent or

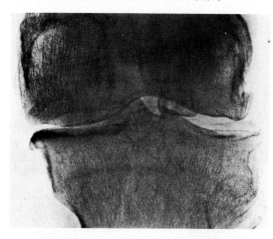

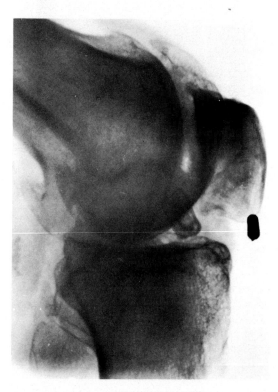

FIGS 11,66–67. **Loose body in extra-articular synovial pouch: trap for the unwary.** The radiographs suggest that this loose body is in the anterior compartment (Figs 11,66 and 11,67). When it was not seen on opening the joint a radiograph with a marker (Fig. 11,67) was taken to make certain it had not shifted. It was in fact lying free within a synovial pouch in the fat pad (G.W., male, aged 59). (See also Chapter 4.)

young adult, provided it has not arisen from a lesion of osteochondritis dissecans, can be removed without inspection of the site of origin in so far as the question of restoration of an articular defect will not arise.

**Loose body: where shall I find it?** Loose bodies, in spite of a reputation for elusiveness, are not found just anywhere. There is a pattern in human affairs, and it applies to the knee joint; and it includes exceptions.

The removal of a loose body should never be undertaken lightly; and the smaller it is the more the difficulties which may be encountered without the knowledge of where it is likely to be located. The loose body which is completely mobile, known to the patient to appear sometimes at one point and sometimes at another, is the one which at the time of operation may be anywhere. It is prudent therefore immediately prior to operation to secure radiographs after the tourniquet has been applied. The knee in such circumstances will be in extension, and, in transferring the patient to the operating table, care should be taken that it is not displaced to some completely new site. The flexed position as for meniscectomy will, in general, be the one selected if it is only for the reason that this is the position which permits inspection of the classical site for osteochondritis dissecans.

There are a number of sites at which small loose bodies are commonly located:

THE LOOSE BODY IS OUTWITH THE JOINT. It is not always appreciated that the loose body which appears in the radiograph to be within the synovial cavity may be located in a synovial pouch outwith the joint. The common sites for such pouches are the infrapatellar fat pad (Figs 11,66 and 11,67); behind the posterior capsule; the suprapatellar pouch; but, indeed, anywhere. The radiograph, which locates the anatomical site does not determine that it is within a pouch. If at this stage the radiographs confirm that it is still at the same site the fact that it is within a pouch will be evident. It can be located by palpation with the gloved finger introduced to the synovial cavity.

IT IS UNDERNEATH THE MENISCUS. It is the lateral meniscus which is most commonly affected; and with this knowledge the surgeon should be alerted as to the possibility. The type of loose body is a small one, almond-shaped,

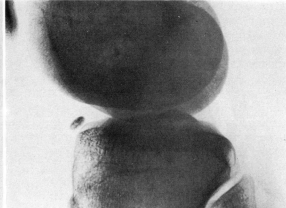

Fig. 11,68                    Fig. 11,69

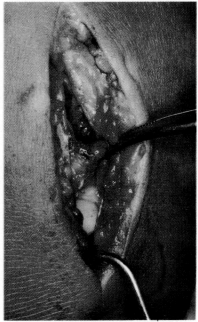

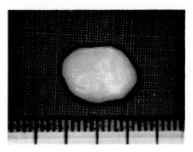

Fig. 11,71

Fig. 11,70

FIGS 11,68–71. **Loose body beneath meniscus: trap for unwary.**
This loose body was under the anterior segment of the medial meniscus (Figs 11,68 and 11,69). At operation through a short incision as for meniscectomy it is seen to lie beneath the anterior horn when the meniscus is lifted from off the tibial head (Fig. 11,70). Size and conformation of the kind of loose body which can become insinuated beneath the anterior segment (Fig. 11,71).

so that the edge is readily invaginated beneath the concave edge. It is located anteriorly rather than posteriorly because the weight-bearing bringing the meniscus into close contact with the tibial head prevents it from remaining at this site. It is therefore located anteriorly where it is not under constant compression.

The loose body located beneath the anterior segment of the lateral meniscus may be difficult

to see in a radiograph. If it is of the size and shape which can insert itself beneath the anterior segment it is unlikely to have a large bony element. Furthermore, lying within the concavity of the lateral condyle it is likely to have superimposed bone in both antero-posterior and lateral views. The hint that it is in such a position may be given at clinical examination from the fact that extension is less complete than on the opposite side. A loose body under the anterior segment of a meniscus tends to be permanently located there because weight-bearing produces an indentation in both the articular cartilage and the meniscus so that it may be trapped within two small concavities (Figs 11,68 to 11,71).

In the differential diagnosis has to be considered calcification or ossification of the meniscus. Figure 11,72 shows a situation in which confusion might arise as to the nature of the lesion. The hint as regards the pathology existed in (1) the fact that the 'loose body' is vertical. If it was under the meniscus it must be horizontal. Furthermore, there is just the suggestion of trabeculation indicating that the bone is alive. This trabeculation is more clearly shown in the radiograph of the meniscus following excision (Fig. 11,73).

*Treatment.* At operation a loose body in this situation is readily removed by making a small horizontal incision in the peripheral synovial attachment of the anterior segment. In general, however, this is an undesirable practice in so far as the resulting fibrosis may fix the meniscus anteriorly and thus be responsible for a local horizontal cleavage lesion. It may be possible by lifting the meniscus from off the tibial head with a single hook retractor to push the loose body into the concavity of the meniscus. In doing this, however, considerable care should be exercised. It is small and extremely slippery and may disappear into the posterior compartment.

THE SYNOVIAL CAVITY WHERE THE TENDON OF POPLITEUS CROSSES THE MENISCUS. The lateral side, as opposed to the medial, is a common site for the location of a small loose body. It will be found, for reasons determined by gravity and the absence of tension, in the pouch of synovial membrane immediately below the joint line or in the synovial cavity where the tendon of popliteus traverses the meniscus. It is desirable that extraction is achieved through a minimal vertical incision; and that any extensive separation of the meniscus from its peripheral synovial attachments will result in fixation by fibrosis with resulting parrot-beak tear.

In approaching the joint line it will be recalled that the inferior lateral geniculate artery is located at the periphery of the meniscus; and that it has been divided may not be appreciated under tourniquet.

### The Loose Body is Large

A large loose body other than in gross pathological processes can have arisen only from

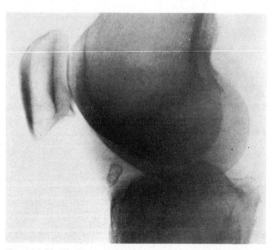

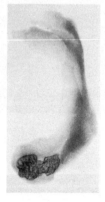

FIGS 11,72–73. **Loose body in anterior compartment: differential diagnosis. Ossification of anterior horn of meniscus.** The position is similar to that seen when the loose body is lying beneath the anterior horn of the lateral meniscus (Fig. 11,69). But it lies vertically; and this would be impossible were it beneath the meniscus. Furthermore, there is the suggestion of trabeculation indicating that it is living bone (Fig. 11,72). The radiograph shows this trabeculation in detail (Fig. 11,73). (M.McK., female, aged 55, number M8718, case of I.D.S.)

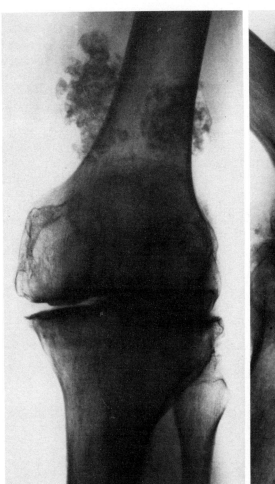

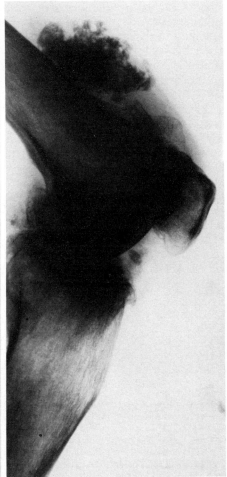

FIGS 11,74–76. **Large loose bodies in suprapatellar pouch.** The patient (C.M., male, aged 82) attributed the condition to a railway accident 50 years previously! His only symptom, limitation of flexion, was relieved when they were removed.

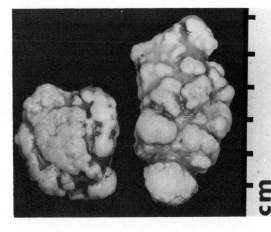

certain sites. The massive variety of osteochondritis dissecans and the tangential osteochondral fracture of the lateral femoral condyle are the outstanding examples. In other circumstances a large loose body is the result of the progressive growth of articular cartilage over the years. In the former two circumstances there is likely to be a considerable bone element but an even larger cartilagenous element so that the loose body is likely to be much larger than the radiograph depicts. It will be clear, also, that the number of sites within the joint capable of accommodating such a large loose body are small. The most likely situations are the supra-patellar pouch (Figs 11,74 to 11,76), the anterior compartment within the intercondylar notch or the posterior compartment within the intercondylar notch. A loose body of this size, and it is likely to be single, cannot move about freely and poses no problems of localisation.

In the youthful subject it is important that an attempt be made prior to operation to decide from the radiographs whether the lesion is osteo-chondritis dissecans or a tangential osteo-chondral fracture; and the site of the resulting defect in the articular surface. In either circumstance a large area of articular cartilage may be involved and the possibility of repair will arise. Both lesions are readily restored by the methods described; and it is desirable to do so if the defect is large and when the articular cartilage of the loose body is undamaged. It will be clear, however, that if the loose body has been free for any considerable length of time overgrowth of the cartilagenous margins will have occurred and tissue will require to be removed in order to attain an accurate repair of the defect. Furthermore, the bone element may require to be drilled and the crater in the condyle prepared as described under the treatment of osteochondritis dissecans.

In such circumstances the initial limited incision should be located in such a position that it exposes the lesion in the articular cartilage when a decision can be made as to the necessity for repair. In the majority of cases the loose body can be manoeuvred towards the original incision. In other circumstances a second incision may be necessary.

## REFERENCES

AHLBACK, S., BAUER, G. C. H. & BOHNE, W. H. (1968). Spontaneous osteonecrosis of the knee. *Arthritis and Rheumatism*, **11**, 705.

BAUER, G. C. H. (1968). The use of radionuclides in orthopaedics, part IV. Radionuclide scintimetry of the skeleton. *Journal of Bone and Joint Surgery*, **50A**, 1681.

BAUER, G. C. H. & SMITH, E. M. (1969). [85]Sr scintimetry in osteoarthritis of the knee. *Journal of Nuclear Medicine*, **10**, 109.

BERNSTEIN, M. A. (1925). Osteochondritis dissecans. *Journal of Bone and Joint Surgery*, **7**, 319.

CAFFEY, J., MADELL, S. H., ROYER, C. & MORALES, P. (1958). Ossification of the distal femoral epiphysis. *Journal of Bone and Joint Surgery*, **40A**, 647.

CAMERON, H. U., PILIAR, R. M. & MACNAB, I. (1974). Fixation of loose bodies in joints. *Clinical Orthopaedics and Related Research*, **100**, 308.

CHARNLEY, J. (1955). Report of a meeting of British Orthopaedic Association, London, October 1954. *Journal of Bone and Joint Surgery*, **37B**, 164.

EDWARDS, D. H. & BENTLEY, G. (1977). Osteochondritis dissecans patellae. *Journal of Bone and Joint Surgery*, **59B**, 58.

GARDINER, T. B. (1955). Osteochondritis dissecans in three members of one family. *Journal of Bone and Joint Surgery*, **37B**, 139.

GREEN, W. T. & BANKS, H. H. (1953). Osteochondritis dissecans in children. *Journal of Bone and Joint Surgery*, **35A**, 26.

HANLEY, W. B., McKUSICK, V. A. & BARRANCO, F. T. (1967). Osteochondritis dissecans with associated malformations in two brothers. *Journal of Bone and Joint Surgery*, **49A**, 925.

HELFET, A. J. (1963). *The Management of Internal Derangements of the Knee*, p. 219. London: Pitman.

HOLMBLAD, E. C. (1937). Postero-anterior X-ray view of knee in flexion. *Journal of the American Medical Association*, **109**, 1196.

JACKSON, R. W. & DANDY, D. J. (1976). *Arthroscopy of the Knee*. New York: Grune and Stratton.

LACROIX, P. (1941). L'osteochondrite dissequante. *Revue belge. Sci. méd.* **13**, 78.

LEHMANN, J. C. (1922). Die konstitutionell schwache Epiphyse und ihre Beziehungen sur Rachitis. Osteochondritis und Arthrosis deformans. *Dt. Z. Chir.*, **178**.

MAU, H. (1958). Juvenile osteochondroses—enchondral dysostosis. *Clinical Orthopaedics*, **11**, 154.

MUHEIM, G. & BOHNE, W. H. (1970). Prognosis in spontaneous osteonecrosis of the knee. *Journal of Bone and Joint Surgery*, **52B**, 605.

NOVOTNY, H. (1952). Osteochondritis dissecans in two brothers. The pre- and developed stage. *Acta radiologica (Scand.)*, **37**, 493.

PALAZZI, S., PALAZZI, C. & PALAZZI, A.-S. (1977). Osteocartilaginous autograft of the knee. *International Orthopaedics*, **1**, 48.

PICK, P. M. (1955). Familial osteochondritis dissecans. *Journal of Bone and Joint Surgery*, **37B**, 142.

RIBBING, S. (1937). Studien über hereditäre, multiple Epiphysentörungen. *Acta radiologica*, Supplementum **34.**

RIBBING, S. (1944). Zur Atiologie der Osteochondritis Dissecans. *Acta radiologica*, **25,** 732.

ROSENOER, V. M. (1961). In *Wilson's Disease: Some Current Concepts.* Edited by Walshe and Cumings. Oxford: Blackwell.

SMILLIE, I. S. (1960). *Osteochondritis Dissecans.* Edinburgh: E. & S. Livingstone.

SMITH, A. D. (1960). Osteochondritis of the knee joint. *Journal of Bone and Joint Surgery,* **42A,** 289.

STOUGAARD, J. (1961). The hereditary factor in osteochondritis dissecans. *Journal of Bone and Joint Surgery,* **43B,** 256.

STOUGAARD, J. (1964). Familial occurrence of osteochondritis dissecans. *Journal of Bone and Joint Surgery,* **46B,** 542.

TOBIN, J. (1957). Familial osteochondritis dissecans. *Journal of Bone and Joint Surgery,* **39A,** 1091.

TROELL, A. (1914). Zur Kenntnis der Entstehung von freien Körpern im Kniegelenke etc. *Archiv klinische Chirurgie,* **105,** 399.

WAGONER, C. & COHN, B. N. E. (1931). Osteochondritis dissecans. A resume of the theories of etiology and the consideration of heredity as an etiological factor. *Archives of Surgery,* **23,** 1.

WELLS, C. (1962). Joint pathology in ancient Anglo-Saxons. *Journal of Bone and Joint Surgery,* **44B,** 4, 948.

WELLS, C. (1974). Osteochondritis dissecans in ancient British skeletal material. *Medical History,* **18,** 365.

WILSON, J. N. (1967). A diagnostic sign in osteochondrites dissecans of the knee. *Journal of Bone and Joint Surgery.* **49A,** 3, 477.

# 12. Problems of Diagnosis in Women

## LESIONS REFLECTING THE BIOMECHANICAL STATUS OF THE JOINT

**Introduction.** It will be shown that many of the internal derangements and of other affections encountered in women reflect the biomechanical status of the female knee. It follows that, in contradistinction to internal derangements in the male, they are likely to present in *bilateral* form: (1) recurrent subluxation of the patella; (2) lesions of the infrapatellar fat pad in particular the premenstrual water retention syndrome; (3) transient effusion in recurvatus deformity; (4) lesions of the anterior segment of a meniscus and particularly of the lateral structure; (5) panniculitis; (6) erythrocyanosis; and (7) the congenital discoid lateral meniscus, though not of mechanical origin, are obvious examples and will be elaborated. Of the disease processes, not of mechanical origin, the most common is rheumatoid arthritis. It will be evident that these conditions, when bilateral, do not necessarily present at the same time, nor, when present, in equal degrees of intensity.

**Recurrent subluxation of patella.** If, as has been shown in Chapter 2, patella alta is the commonest single cause of recurrent subluxation, the frequency with which some degree of recurvatus, in addition to the normal valgus angulation, is encountered in the female subject, ensures that this affection is the commonest cause of serious internal derangement of the knee in a *young* woman. Testing of the stability of the patello-femoral joint is an essential feature of routine clinical examination of the young female subject. No other diagnosis should be considered until the possibility of instability has been eliminated.

**Lesions of infrapatellar fat pad.** In genu recurvatum the fat pad is subject to compression forces. Bilateral fat pad lesions of endogenous traumatic origin are essentially but not exclusively an affection of the female knee. There is a variety based on the **premenstrual water retention syndrome** and to which reference will be made later in which genu recurvatum is an additional factor in aetiology.

The influence of recurvatus deformity on the production of pain related to the fat pad is illustrated by the following case:

The patient (A.M.W., aged 26), an instructress in physical education, stated that she was capable of ski-ing all day without symptoms but on returning to the gymnasium developed, within a short time, pain in both knees. She had been examined by the college medical officer who could detect no abnormality. She had as a result been accused of malingering. The reason for the consultation was the distress caused by the accusation. 'I can assure you the pain is very real.'

Clinical examination revealed some degree of recurvatus and the typical signs of bilateral fat pad lesions. The explanation of the phenomena in the circumstances was obvious: in ski-ing the knees are flexed and the fat pad is not under compression. In the gymnasium she wore shoes without heels and the fat pads as a consequence were subjected to compression.

**Transient recurrent effusion.** Closely related to lesions of the fat pad in so far as the mechanism of production is the same is trauma inflicted on the synovial membrane, presumably that lining the fat pad, by unaccustomed exertion or long periods of standing with hyperextended knees. This syndrome has been recognised in the hyperextended knees of the heritable disorders of connective tissue but applies to any knee joint in which recurvatus is extreme.

**Lesions of the anterior segment of the meniscus.** If the fat pad can be subject to compression so also can the anterior segment of the meniscus. The lateral structure is the one most commonly affected partly from its more posterior location and partly because of the valgus angulation of the female knee. The lesion takes one of several forms. The anterior segment may be extruded, an example of which is recorded below; may be the subject of a horizontal cleavage lesion (Fig. 12,1); or may be grossly lacerated from repeated trauma. In the last instance the inferior surface may become adherent to the tibial head. When this occurs the meniscus no longer moves as a whole and as a result becomes the subject of a parrot-beak tear.

**Cystic degeneration of anterior segment of lateral meniscus.** Cystic degeneration of the anterior segment of the lateral meniscus, presenting as a large swelling extruding between patellar tendon and iliotibial band, is more common in the female subject.

If, as has been suggested in IKJ5, Chapter 5, cystic degeneration arises as a result of endogenous compressive force such abnormal compression, as applied to the anterior segment of the lateral meniscus in particular, exists in the valgus/recurvatus conformation of the female knee.

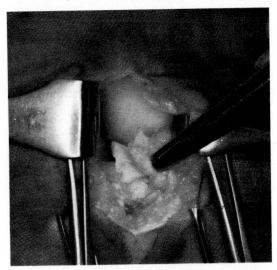

FIG. 12,1. **Internal derangements relative to the menisci.** Lesions of the anterior segments of the menisci, particularly on the lateral side, are more common in the female knee and this is explained by the frequency of recurvatus deformity in association with the normal valgus angulation. Figure 12,1 shows a horizontal cleavage lesion of the anterior segment of the lateral meniscus.

**Differential Diagnosis.**

It will be evident that difficulty will be

TABLE 12

Age and incidence of female cases
per 500 meniscectomies: 1940–74

| Years | Number of cases | Number of females | Average age |
|---|---|---|---|
| 1940–43 | 1– 500 | 1 | 22 |
| 1943–45 | 500–1000 | 2 | 23 |
| 1945–50 | 1000–1500 | 27 | 28 |
| 1950–53 | 1500–2000 | 66 | 30 |
| 1953–55 | 2000–2500 | 16 | 32 |
| 1955–57 | 2500–3000 | 44 | 35 |
| 1957–58 | 3000–3500 | 57 | 32 |
| 1958–59 | 3500–4000 | 76 | 36 |
| 1959–61 | 4000–4500 | 77 | 37 |
| 1961–62 | 4500–5000 | 60 | 37 |
| 1962–63 | 5000–5500 | 69 | 38 |
| 1963–64 | 5500–6000 | 110 | 38 |
| 1964–65 | 6000–6500 | 93 | 41 |
| 1965–66 | 6500–7000 | 82 | 42 |
| 1966–67 | 7000–7500 | 96 | 42 |
| 1967–68 | 7500–8000 | 105 | 45 |
| 1968–70 | 8000–8500 | 114 | 52 |
| 1970–71 | 8500–9000 | 131 | 48 |
| 1971–72 | 9000–9500 | 105 | 48 |
| 1972–74 | 9500–10 000 | 113 | 50 |

encountered in distinguishing a lesion of the anterior segment of the meniscus from a fat pad lesion in this variety of knee in the female subject. In the meniscus lesion the pain is situated to one or other side of the midline and tenderness which may be acute is accurately located to the joint line. In the fat pad lesion the swelling is more diffuse, located on both sides of the patellar tendon and the tenderness more generalised.

The following is an example of extrusion of the anterior segment of the medial meniscus to illustrate the difficulties of diagnosis encountered:

The patient, aged 15, grossly overweight, 13½ stones (85 kg) and showing considerable genu recurvatum on the normal side, complained that six months previously while playing table tennis she sustained a twisting injury to the knee and had suffered pain ever since.

On examination there was loss of hyperextension by comparison with the normal side and with tenderness in the anterior compartment on the medial side. In view of her age, weight and overreaction she was kept under observation. In all four examinations were carried out at fortnightly intervals. The clinical features never changed. The provisional diagnosis was that of a displaced complete longitudinal tear; but in view of the rarity of the lesion in girls of this age it could not be more than tentative. Social-domestic circumstances compelled the operation, unusual in the author's hands, of exploration. The parents were informed that the joint would be opened on the medial side but unless the expected lesion was found it would be closed without removal of the meniscus. On exposure of the meniscus, however, it was evident that the anterior segment was completely loose and could be induced to slip over the margin of the articular cartilage on to the anterior aspect of the tibia by extension of the joint. In such circumstances there was no alternative to meniscectomy. It was noted that even at this interval of time there were reactionary changes at the margin of the articular cartilage.

## ERRORS OF DIAGNOSIS IN MENISCECTOMY

In the total of 1331 women subjected to meniscectomy in the years 1940–74 (Table 12) there were 114 cases in which it was recorded that there was 'no meniscus lesion'. In addition, there were 105 in which the meniscus was recorded as normal but exhibiting a 'lax peripheral attachment'. If the latter operative finding, the explanation for which is suggested below, is not accepted as a legitimate pathological entity the aggregate of the two categories would result in a percentage of errors of diagnosis in women of 15 per cent. If 'lax peripheral attachment' is accepted this percentage is reduced to 8 per cent, still unacceptably high by comparison with the 4 per cent recorded for men (IKJ5). When the total of 219 so-called errors of diagnosis are analysed, 167 occurred on the medial side of the joint, only 52 on the lateral. An explanation of these phenomena is offered and conclusions drawn in the interests of increase in the accuracy of diagnosis.

### Ligamentous and Capsular Laxity

It will be recognised that in general the female knee exhibits, as a result of ligamentous and capsular laxity, a greater degree of mobility than that of the male subject. The ability to 'sit on the heels' is a common female accomplishment (Fig. 12,2) even in those of short stature and considerable muscular development (Figs 12,3). There are racial differences but in general the European male sits on his heels only with practice or as a result of occupation as, for example, coal mining. Furthermore, the normal valgus angulation entails laxity of medial ligament and capsule seldom encountered in the male joint.

Capsular laxity provides the explanation as to why so many errors of diagnosis occur in the female knee and why, in particular, so many normal medial menisci are removed. Reference has been made to the grosser errors such as recurrent subluxation of the patella and fat pad lesions. Both possibilities are known to experienced clinicians. In any event both are readily distinguished from meniscus lesions by clinical means. Patients from whom a normal medial meniscus, or one with 'lax peripheral attachment', has been removed, clearly had symptoms directing attention to that structure. The explanation lies in capsular laxity which permits trauma to the synovial attachments of the meniscus in the form of stretching, pinching or trapping to occur. The pain which causes the patient to complain and the tenderness to pressure cannot be other than of synovial origin. The excised meniscus in such circumstances shows no evidence of injury. The fact that the patient is cured of her symptoms following operation merely indicates that the regenerated meniscus, located in reduced joint space, is firmly fixed: the synovial attachments are no longer the subject of trauma.

Laxity of the peripheral attachment of the medial meniscus in the female subject is illustrated by the following case:

The patient (Y.T., aged 15) complained of pain on the medial aspect of the right knee; and that on certain movements she could produce a clicking sensation which she stated occurred within the joint. Examination confirmed that the patello-femoral joint was stable. No evidence of a medial meniscus tear both knees was so related. The condition settled with cessation of these particular exercises which were willingly exchanged for the non-weight-bearing quadriceps variety.

The case is quoted not only to draw attention to the general ligamentous and capsular laxity of the female knee, and that symptoms may be so related, but once again to the importance of history-taking. In this case the abnormal physical activity provided

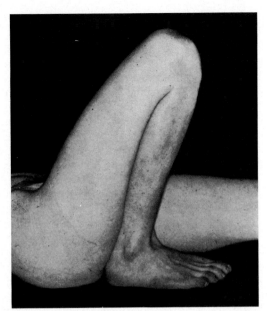

FIG. 12,2. **Mobility of the female knee joint.** In general a greater degree of mobility exists in the female than in the male knee. Few males in western countries can sit on their heels without practice or produce a situation in which the femur and tibia are almost parallel (Fig. 12,2).

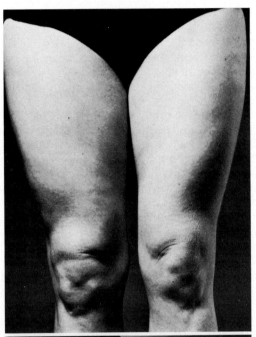

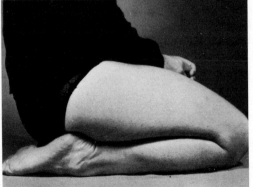

FIGS 12,3–4. **Mobility of the female knee joint.** It is unlikely that a male of this stature and quadriceps development (Fig. 12,3) could sit on his heels (Fig. 12,4).

could be elicited other than tenderness on the joint line immediately posterior to the ligament. When the situation was reviewed one month later she was, if anything, worse. Furthermore, she volunteered that similar symptoms, but in lesser degree, were taking place in the left knee. The bilaterality of the situation immediately suggested the possibility of a fat pad lesion in the form of the pre= menstrual water-retention syndrome. Examination in this regard was negative.

On leaving the room at the second examination she asked if there was any possibility that her symptoms could be related to the Yoga exercises which she had been practising recently. When she demonstrated what she was doing it was evident that she was stretching the medial side of both joints. She demonstrated also, not only sitting on her heels (Fig. 12,3) but the ability to sit on the floor between her heels. There arose thus the strong suspicion that the mobility of the medial menisci and the tenderness of the peripheral attachments on the medial side of the clue to the medial meniscus symptoms. Without this information such a patient may be subjected to meniscectomy at which the pathological finding would be no more than the only too common 'lax peripheral attachment'.

**Cosmetic defects presented as 'pain'.** Vigilance should be exercised by the clinician in the interpretation of a situation in the female subject whereby a cosmetic defect in the form of angular deformity, varus or valgus, or a torsional deformity, even in minor degree but unacceptable to the patient, is presented as 'pain in the knee'. The problem as might be expected arises in the second decade. It is assumed that the girl does not expect her complaint regarding the appearance of her legs to be taken seriously whereas a complaint of pain cannot be disregarded.

This is a situation which may be detected by the experienced clinician in that the pain is unrelated to any other symptom, is vague in distribution, affects both knees, but in any event does not fit the familiar pattern of internal derangements associated with the sex and age range. The possible bilateral diagnoses, recurrent subluxation of patella, fat pad lesions in the form of the premenstrual water retention syndrome and congenital discoid lateral meniscus are considered and eliminated. The possibility that the vague pain as described might be associated with the patella alta/genu recurvatum complex, if that is the deformity presented, is excluded. It is at this stage that the suspicions of the experienced may be aroused. It is at this stage that the inexperienced may feel obliged to make a positive diagnosis invariably involving the medial menisci; and a most unhappy train of events set in motion (see Ch. 9).

### INTERNAL DERANGEMENTS IN WOMEN RELATIVE TO THE MENISCI: PROBABILITIES IN DIAGNOSIS

#### Medial Meniscus

**Longitudinal tear.** The longitudinal tear of the medial meniscus is generally, but not exclusively an injury of youth associated with athletic activities. It is thus more likely to occur in the male than the female.

In 6500 cases (M3500 to M10 000) the percentage in men was 90, in women 10.

Errors of diagnosis in relation to lesions of the medial meniscus, in particular, are so common that before committing a patient to operation for a lesion of the medial structure the surgeon should ask himself whether the symptoms from which this patient suffers are those of a *longitudinal tear* or a *horizontal tear*. If he commits himself to a longitudinal tear he should remind himself of the rarity of such tears in women. In general, the diagnosis of a longitudinal tear should not be made in a young woman unless she has sustained an injury in some field sport such as hockey or basketball. In other circumstances, it is prudent to review the patient on a number of occasions, at, say, monthly or more intervals, rather than come to a precipitate conclusion which terminates in the excision of a normal meniscus (Fig. 12,5). Experience has shown that a proportion of cases, with patience and quadriceps exercises, eventually become symptomless.

*Horizontal tears.* If, on the other hand, the pathology is considered to be a horizontal cleavage lesion of the posterior segment and the patient is middle-aged or elderly the same degree of caution is unnecessary: the diagnosis is likely to be correct.

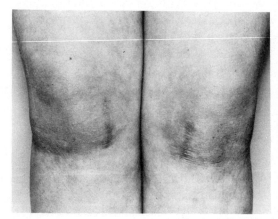

FIG. 12,5. **Error of diagnosis in the female knee joint.** This unfortunate young woman suffered the removal of two normal medial menisci without relief of symptoms. Why the second meniscus was removed when the first was shown to be normal is unexplained. The diagnosis established is the commonest in this age group in the female subject: recurrent subluxation of the patella.

This lesion is the commonest cause of internal derangement relative to the menisci in the female knee and provides the explanation of the high average age of women subjected to meniscectomy (Table 12). If there is a danger of error it is that symptoms related to the medial joint line posteriorly in the middle-aged or elderly woman are erroneously labelled osteoarthrosis when dramatic relief is afforded by simple meniscectomy.

## Lateral Meniscus

**Congenital disc.** This anomaly, for reasons not yet understood, is much more common in women than in men. In the total of 1444 women there were 156 (11 per cent) as opposed to 318 in 8556 men (4 per cent). Thus one woman in nine undergoing meniscectomy had a congenital discoid meniscus on the lateral side.

**Cystic degeneration.** The lateral meniscus is the structure most commonly affected; and the association with the congenital disc and with the parrot-beak tear in the meniscus of normal conformation is established (IKJ5).

## Diagnosis

If in general lesions of the lateral meniscus are less common and the symptoms less precise than on the medial side, statistics show that fewer errors of diagnosis occur. The reasons have been outlined above. If, therefore, the diagnosis is of an internal derangement related to the lateral meniscus, as opposed to the medial, the chances are that it will be correct.

# LESIONS OF THE FAT PAD: PREMENSTRUAL WATER-RETENTION SYNDROME

If bilateral fat pad lesions of endogenous mechanical origin are more common in the female and for reasons which have been indicated there is a variety based on the pre-menstrual water-retention which is exclusive to the female subject. Experience shows that it is a common, possibly the commonest, source of *bilateral* symptoms in the female; and that it is a

source of misdiagnosis, misunderstanding and sometimes of injustice.

**Pathological anatomy.** In the interval immediately preceding menstruation the swollen fat pad is subject to compression in extension and particularly in circumstances of hyper-extensibility such as is common in the female. If as is supposed the fat pad has a considerable nerve plexus system the result is the induction of tension pain. The synovial membrane lining the fat pad is subject to compression and with repetition of the trauma at monthly intervals secondary changes such as have been described (Ch. 4) occur. The situation therefore can rapidly become irreversible and thus the symptoms, unilateral or bilateral, continue even after hormonal adjustment has occurred.

## Clinical Features

It is not intended to repeat the clinical features of lesions of the fat pad which have been listed in some detail in Chapter 4.

Two varieties of patient are encountered: (1) the adolescent girl or young women with a relatively short history; (2) the adult with a history of many years. There are instances when (1) merges into (2). In the classical situation the complaint is of pain in both knees. It is seldom, however, that the pain is of equal intensity: one is usually worse than the other. In older patients with symptoms of some duration one knee only may be involved; but they say that at one time the other knee was affected. The condition is a clear-cut clinical entity to the initiated. In other hands it is a source of error and injustice and with possible serious implications in the long term as in the example quoted below. The teenage girl may not have her regularly repeated complaint of pain in both knees taken seriously (Fig. 12,6) and particularly when she says the pain is relieved by the use of high heels!

**Progestogens.** There is some evidence that the current use of progestogens may have increased the incidence of the condition. It is known to make it worse. In this regard and in the pursuit of confirmation in a difficult diagnosis there are circumstances in which some delicacy of approach may be necessary. The single girl may not be prepared to volunteer the information that she is on progesterone; and certainly not in the presence of her mother.

## Differential Diagnosis

The differential diagnosis of fat pad lesions has been described in Chapter 4. In the premenstrual water-retention syndrome the symptoms are bilateral and of a somewhat indefinite nature. It is prudent in such circumstances to apply the simple screening test of the ESR to eliminate the possibility that the symptoms are the earliest stage of rheumatoid arthritis.

The following case is quoted as an extreme example of the long history, consequences in terms of undesirable operations and the serious psychological effect on a young woman of the failure to diagnose fat pad lesions possibly based on the premenstrual water-retention syndrome; but in any event to the problems which can arise in the teenage female knee.

The letter of referral stated: 'I originally saw her (J.L., aged 15) three years ago. She had struck her left knee on a door, and the following day when playing tennis, noted a

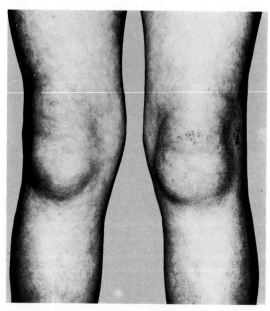

FIG. 12.6. **Bilateral fat pad lesions: premenstrual water retention syndrome.** A young woman complaining of both knees may not have her symptoms taken seriously.

click within the joint. Shortly afterwards she said she was unable to play because of pain in the knee. It remained painful on walking and she felt that she was unable to extend the knee fully. The knee gave way on two occasions. There were no symptoms in the right knee at that time.

Examination showed that she was just able to extend the knee fully; although apparently with some pain. There was no effusion. Wasting of the quadriceps was slight. There was tenderness on the medial joint line. Flexion was full. The joint was stable. There was no pain or crepitus of patello-femoral movements. Radiographs revealed no abnormality.

I thought at that time that she had sustained a minor strain. I therefore arranged for her to attend a physiotherapy department.

A month later the knee appeared to be very much better. She had few symptoms but did complain of some discomfort at the front of the knee if she used it a lot. She was advised to begin games and ballet dancing and gradually resume full activities.

On subsequent visits she complained that her symptoms were steadily increasing. She developed marked tenderness along the medial joint line. The pain appeared to become localised antero-medially. The knee continued to give way; and she complained that something became caught in the joint when the knee gave way.

It was at this stage that I therefore performed a left medial meniscectomy. There was no abnormality. The posterior horn could not be mobilised and a posterior incision was required to free it and complete the operation.

She made average progress during the immediate convalescence and thereafter attended the physiotherapy department as an out-patient. About a fortnight after the operation she was walking normally around the shops. At the end of the outing, however, the knee was aching and weak. She therefore started to use crutches, partially weight-bearing.

One month after the meniscectomy she complained that the knee had become very painful and was tending to swell. She was wakened at night by pain. At that time there was a small effusion present and general tenderness, particularly over the medial aspect. The quadriceps redevelopment was poor. I advised her to continue with physiotherapy; and to use some support when walking. One week later I had a letter from her mother stating that she was in constant pain, spent all night crying and refused to walk without crutches. When I re-examined her she was reluctant to do anything with the knee. There was, however, no finding abnormal for an interval one month from operation. In such circumstances I arranged for her to be admitted to hospital in order to mobilise the knee and to persuade her to abandon her crutches. Simple analgesic tablets relieved the pain completely within a few hours of her admission to hospital and immediately thereafter she was walking without any crutches. The next day she was able to extend the knee. She was therefore discharged to her home and shortly afterwards returned to school. It was immediately thereafter that her mother informed me that she spent most of each day in the school sick-bay doing nothing; and that she lay around in the evenings. I therefore arranged for her to attend a medical rehabilitation centre.

She continued to complain of increasing pain over the lateral aspect of the joint; and the knee was tending to swell once more. On examination at that time there was a slight effusion. There was equal tenderness medially and laterally. Flexion was restricted to 45°. She walked very slowly keeping the knee quite stiff and straight. I felt certain that her symptoms were functional and had, in fact, come to that opinion previously when she was re-admitted to hospital.

One month later she was still complaining that the knee repeatedly gave way, was very painful and felt insecure without a bandage. She stated that she had fallen on several occasions when the knee gave way. She said she was frightened to bend it in case it collapsed or locked. On questioning she stated that it had locked on three occasions. On one of these she had noted a click antero-laterally.

Subsequent to this examination she spent a fortnight at another rehabilitation centre.

Then she had further physiotherapy in the form of exercises. It was my impression still that the condition was functional in origin. The girl and the parents, the mother in particular, were agitating strongly for a further operation to remove the lateral meniscus. They felt that all her symptoms were associated with the lateral side of the knee joint.

I was extremely reluctant to consider operating on her again. The mother did not wish to take her to another consultant for a second opinion. She agreed finally to allow me to take the. child to the orthopaedic conference at a teaching hospital as a problem case. To my dismay, everybody there advised further surgery, including a patellar tendon transplant and even a patellectomy!

My hand was therefore forced and as a result I performed a left lateral arthrotomy, using a long incision. The undersurface of the patella showed no evidence of chondromalacia. I did a left lateral meniscectomy. The meniscus was intact but appeared to have a lax peripheral attachment.

She made very slow progress in the post-operative period but the knee got very slowly stronger until it eventually became completely symptomless. At this time, however, she developed symptoms in the right knee similar to those which she has had in the left.

Mother and daughter have been very anxious that I should remove both menisci from the right knee. This I have refused to do, fortunately obtaining some support for my opinion from the father.

I have just examined her again. The left knee, she says, is very much better and causes hardly any symptoms at all. She is now determined that the right knee is stopping her from playing games and indeed stopping her from doing anything at all in the way of exercise. She states that it has locked straight five times and in flexion once. She thought that the patella moved laterally when the knee locked straight.

Examination showed no effusion in the joint. The quadriceps appeared equal to the left. There was retro-patellar tenderness along the medial side of the patella. She had some patello-femoral pain on movement, but the patella-femoral joint seems stable.

U

I am under increasing pressure to carry out meniscectomies on the right side. I believe the operation to be unnecessary and undesirable.'

On examination the left·knee appeared normal other than the presence of three incisions which unfortunately had healed with somewhat broad scars. The quadriceps muscle was of excellent tone. No abnormality could be detected. There was a minimal pain-less click in the patello-femoral joint to which the patient drew attention.

On the right side the quadriceps was wasted by comparison with the left. The only abnormality was swelling of the fat pad and tenderness to pressure in the midline and on either side of the patellar tendon. There was no swelling on the joint line. The patello-femoral joint was stable and no reaction was produced by forcible attempts to displace the patella laterally. It was at this stage that the patient offered the information that she had noticed that the ache in the knee, which was of a degree which prevented her from concentrating in school, was made worse by the use of low heels. At the time of examina-tion she was wearing a heel of moderate height. There was a bilateral recurvatus deformity of moderate degree.

It appeared that here was an example of bilateral fat pad lesions possibly based on the premenstrual water-retention syndrome. The condition had been cured on the left side by reduction of the size of the fat pad in the course of two meniscectomies which undoubtedly removed normal menisci. In other words the patient had been cured on the left side by the wrong operation performed for the wrong reason.

The patient was accompanied by her father. She was highly emotional. Her father recognised her abnormal mental state and related dangers. He explained that it had been aggravated by a long period off school and the necessity to work excessively hard to maintain her position with her contemporaries. The father recognised that in the various rehabilita-tion centres and physiotherapy departments she had had many diagnoses offered to her as an explanation of her pain and why the original meniscectomy had not proved effective. She had become obsessed with the

diagnosis 'chondromalacia of the patella' which sounded serious but which neither he nor she understood.

When the diagnosis of a fat pad lesion was explained to the girl in carefully chosen words which stressed the simplicity of the pathology, it was hoped that she might accept the ache and discomfort with the reassurance that they had no serious pathological basis. She declared, however, that she had suffered the condition too long; and that as she had been cured by operation on the left side why could she not now have an operation on the right side which would cure her. The father readily accepted the explanation for the pain and, realising the psychological situation which had been created, was anxious to avoid further surgery. It was evident, however, that in this particular case reassurance would not be accepted. There seemed little alternative to advising reduction of the volume of the fat pad by operation in the manner described. The outcome is unknown.

## Treatment

**Reassurance.** Patients fear pain for which no rational explanation has been offered and are resentful that an organic basis should be questioned by a doctor. Experience has shown that a proportion of cases, and particularly those with bilateral symptoms based on the premenstrual water-retention syndrome, when offered the reason for the pain, and the explanation as to why it is relieved by the use of high-heeled shoes, etc., learn to live with the disability; and particularly when told that if they fail to do so the condition can be relieved by a relatively minor operative procedure.

**Operation.** If symptoms persist and are of a degree which demands operative action it is possible to offer near certainty of relief by the simple measure described under 'Lesions of the Fat Pad', Chapter 4. If operative action is demanded in the teenage girl kept under observation for many months, it is the author's practice to tell the mother that the side of the greater symptoms will be opened first and unless the expected lesion is found the second joint will not be entered. Such is the precision with which the pathology can be identified.

RECURRENCE. In one case only to date has a recurrence taken place:

The patient (L.K.) was operated on at the age of 16 and the lesions such as described confirmed in both knees. There was immediate relief of symptoms and she remained symptomless for two years. At the end of that time, however, there was a gradual return of the same symptoms as previously. She tolerated the situation for a further year but eventually the pain was so severe that she again sought help. On examination the fat pads were enlarged and tender to pressure and, as on the previous occasion, the symptoms were worse on the left side than on the right. She denied any relationship to menstruation. The only way she knew of obtaining relief was the use of high-heeled shoes. The symptoms were so severe that she accepted without hesitation the only apparent solution: a second operation.

At operation the salient feature of the fat pads was not only the bulk of tissue present but the amount of fibrous infiltration of the fat. When the joint was entered the surface of the synovial membrane was granular and of a dusky red appearance. There was no ligamentum mucosum present. Unfortunately, no note had been made at the previous operation as to whether a ligamentum mucosum was present and if it was, whether it had been divided. The reason for the recurrence of symptoms remains unknown. It may have been that the pre-existing mechanical defect of minimal genu recurvatum continued to subject the fat pads to constant microtrauma; and that this was the reason for the fibrosis.

All that was done was to reduce the bulk of the fat pads by a wedge resection of the extrasynovial fibro-fatty tissue in the manner described in Chapter 4. She is known to have remained symptomless two years later.

## PANNICULITIS: THE FIBRO-FATTY SYNDROME

**Definition.** An ill-defined fatty fibrous mass situated over the antero-medial aspect of the medial condyle of the tibia is a common bilateral finding in the female subject in the post-menopausal age range. The swellings, however, may be seen at any age; and since the author's interest in the subject was aroused, have been noted as young as 13.

The condition has been classified as a form of 'non-articular rheumatism', whatever that term may mean; and such a classification is an indication of the ignorance which surrounds its aetiology and pathology.

**Aetiology.** What little is known about this common condition is couched in the vaguest terms. It is presumed to be of endocrine origin; and in this regard it may not be without significance that a recent example encountered at the age of 16 was under investigation for fat pad lesions based on the premenstrual water-retention syndrome.

**Pathological anatomy.** It can be demonstrated that the upper margin of the swelling corresponds to the medial joint line. The reason for the limitation is not clear except in so far as if the fatty fibrous tissue crossed the joint line it would affect motion. The symptomatology is concerned with pain; not with interference with movement.

A characteristic feature of the condition is that when the fatty mass is picked up between finger and thumb there is a peau d'orange effect. This presumably means that there are strands of fibrous tissue attached to the skin rather than to the deeper tissue. It is when the mass of fatty fibrous tissue is picked up that the patient complains of pain. There must, therefore, be neurological features not seen in normal fat. If, in the same patient, skin and fat is picked up in an adjacent area, there is no complaint of pain.

### Clinical Features

The patient is often, but by no means always, obese. There are usually no symptoms and the condition no more than incidental finding in a post-menopausal patient with symptoms related to degenerative pathology within the joint. In the majority of cases the patient is unaware of the presence of moderately sized masses or considers them to be part of her 'overweight'. At the other extreme is the complaint of local pain, before the menopause worst prior to the menstrual period, and/or of the appearance of the masses which in some instances reach grotesque proportions (Fig. 12,7).

The only physical signs, other than the presence of a variety of degrees of swelling, are tenderness to pressure and pain and the characteristic peau d'orange effect produced by picking up the skin and subcutaneous tissues between finger and thumb (Fig. 12,8).

**Differential diagnosis.** The only source of a painful localised swelling over the antero-medial aspect of the tibial condyle is a pes anserinus bursitis. This unusual condition must be rare in the age range affected by panniculitis; and in any event should be readily distinguishable.

It should be remembered that the complaint of pain on the medial aspect of the joint with the presence of a fibro-fatty mass as described does not rule out the possible co-existence of a horizontal cleavage lesion of the posterior segment of the meniscus. In this regard the precise location of tenderness to the postero-medial joint line in addition to generalised soft tissue tenderness is of importance.

## Treatment

It has been the author's practice to offer no treatment other than explanation on the basis of a hormonal background.

In the absence of other considerations large

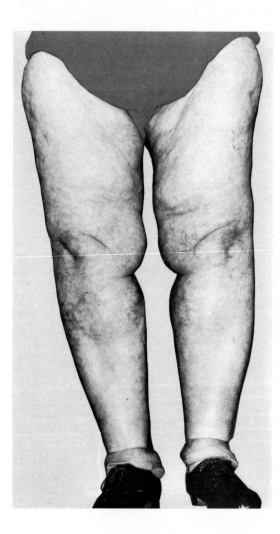
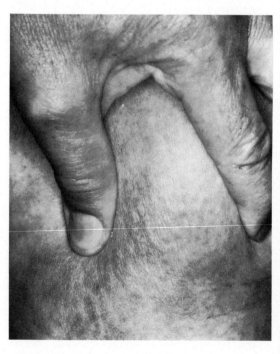

FIGS 12,7–8. **Panniculitis.** In this gross example of panniculitis the large fibro-fatty mass is located at the antero-medial aspect of the leg immediately below the knee. Note the upper limit of mass coincides with medial joint line and thus the fibro-fatty tissue does not interfere with movement (Fig. 12,7).

The peau d'orange effect when the fibro-fatty tissue is pinched between finger and thumb. In some examples with related symptoms this action is painful (Fig. 12,8).

fatty fibrous masses in the thigh and below the knee need not necessarily be a contraindication to operation. It has been recorded above that at the joint line and about the patella there may be little more than the normal thickness of subcutaneous fat. Access to the joint for the purpose of meniscectomy or debridement can be accomplished without the necessity to traverse the fatty mass. There are, however, circumstances when the existence of the condition can be of embarrassment to the surgeon faced with the problem of a meniscectomy operation for, in this age range, a horizontal cleavage lesion of the posterior segment of the medial meniscus. It may be suggested that if meniscectomy is necessary would it not be possible, at the same time, to excise the fibro-fatty mass? It has to be explained in such circumstances that the condition is bilateral and that excision of fat from one side will create a cosmetic situation whereby an essentially plastic operation is required on the 'normal' leg. Whether plastic procedures are justified in patients of this physical type and age range has yet to be determined. Patients with this condition in extreme form and who seek surgery are just as extremely obese elsewhere and with resultant disability. Care should be exercised in embarking on surgical manoeuvres in this negative background. Such patients lack motivation and are subject to every complication so related.

## ACROCYANOSUS: ERYTHROCYANOSIS: ERYTHROMELALGIA

These uncommon conditions in the peripheral vascular field affect women in the feet and lower thirds of the legs but can occur, it is said, in any part of the body surface. Minor degrees are a not uncommon finding in the female knee whereby the skin overlying the patella becomes blanched on flexion. Major degrees are uncommon but when present can produce disabling symptoms in the form of pain, local swelling, exquisite tenderness to pressure and limitation of flexion from tension within the soft tissues with consequent inability to kneel. The joint and entire cyanotic area may be cold by comparison with the opposite side and with the

skin above and below the cyanotic area even on a warm day. The appearance is similar to the blue cold sympathetic disturbance associated with paralysis below the knee in poliomyelitis, except, of course, that unlike polio the disturbance is local. Neither the cyanosis nor the associated pain may be influenced by transfer to a warm climate.

There is a relationship in the basic pathology to panniculitis in so far as some patients exhibit large fatty pads over the front of the knee with the same peau d'orange effect as panniculitis and complain of pain only when they kneel on the fatty tissue which is not only tender but produces a feeling of instability. On the other hand sensitivity of the skin over the front of the knee is such as to suggest an ischaemic neuritis of the patellar plexus. It is characteristic that the red and bluish patches change in appearance even in the course of examination.

The condition like panniculitis is extracapsular. It is distinguished from lesions of the fat pad which produce swelling on either side of the patellar tendon rather than in the midline and by the fact that it does not change in shape or consistency on straight-leg-raising.

The following is the record of an extreme example:

The patient (Mrs A.G., aged 48) was referred by an orthopaedic surgeon colleague with the history of pain in the front of the left knee which might have arisen in a minor injury three months previously. The outstanding clinical feature, he said, was swelling which involved the fat pad on both sides of the patellar tendon; but also of significance as it transpired, the soft tissues in front of the patellar tendon. One of the features of the case had been that only a small range of flexion was possible and any attempt to increase this range induced pain; and he quoted as an example that her symptoms had been exacerbated for several days when an attempt was made to secure axial views of the patella. No treatment was prescribed other than restriction of activities. It was significant, again as it transpired, that she found ice-packs helpful in reducing pain. It was mentioned also in the course of his letter of introduction that she had seen another orthopaedic surgeon who had demanded in the course of examination that she kneel; and the pain induced had produced an emotional outburst which had ended dramatically their professional relationship.

When examined there was little doubt that she had symptoms in her knee joint of a severe nature; and that in no circumstances was the situation of a hysterical nature. There was swelling of the fat pad on both sides of the patellar tendon; but there was also, as the referring orthopaedic surgeon had noted, some soft tissue swelling in front of the tendon. The nature of the pain was such that it appeared to arise in the fat pad. It was advised that this be explored.

On the night before operation examination showed a marked increase in the swelling, both of the fat pad and of the overlying soft tissues; and was, exceptionally for a fat pad lesion, superficially tender to touch. The next morning, after a night's rest, the swelling was much reduced in size. At operation, performed as described in Chapter 4, the fat pad was enlarged and oedematous. One tag only showed evidence of compression; and indeed it had to be confessed that rather less was found than had been anticipated. The operation was completed by division of the ligamentum mucosum and the stitching of the tag referred to above into the incision as described in Chapter 4.

The immediate result of the operation was good. The patient declared that the pain, which incidentally had never been marked while at rest in bed, had disappeared. The convalescence was normal. It was hoped that she had been cured. This, however, was not to be.

She returned one month later stating that while her symptoms had been altered in nature and much reduced, they had not been eliminated. She was told that no explanation could be offered. No treatment was suggested other than gentle quadriceps exercises. In a further month's time the situation had not materially changed.

On review four months later it was noted that both knees, as opposed to the legs lower down, were somewhat blue and cold; and in weather conditions when this should not have been so. The left knee, the one complained of,

showed these phenomena in more marked degree than the right (Fig. 12,10). It was noted also that when the knee was flexed to a right angle, which was as far as the patient would tolerate, the skin over the patella became blanched. There was some soft tissue swelling; and this could be shown to be anterior to the patellar tendon. There was extreme sensitivity of the skin of the region of the swelling. There was an area of apparent numbness on the lateral side of the joint. This area was remote from and could not have been caused by division of the infrapatellar branch of the saphenous nerve at the exploratory operation.

The appearance of the knees was that of the mysterious condition erythromelalgia and its curious relationship with erythrocyanosis.

She remains, having had the situation explained to her, under observation.

**Treatment.** The author is unaware of any treatment which can be proved to be effective.

## HYSTERICAL KNEE

**Introduction.** The only excuse for including hysteria in this section are certain quotations from the works of Sir Benjamin Brodie (1837):

'The liability to hysteria is, in fact, among females, one of the severest penalties of high civilisation. It is among those who enjoy what are supposed to be the advantages of affluence and an easy life that we are to look for cases of this description, not among those who, fulfilling the edict of the Deity, "eat their bread in the sweat of their face". I do not hesitate to declare that among the higher classes of society, at least four fifths of the female patients, who are commonly supposed to labour under diseases of the joints, labour under hysteria, and nothing else.'

If the statement was true in 1837 it is not true today. If Brodie was an able clinician he cannot be blamed for failing to anticipate the social changes of the 1970s and the effect of the Welfare State.

**Definition.** This is not the occasion for categorical statements regarding the background of conversion hysteria even if such were possible. In brief, when the patient develops a physical ail-

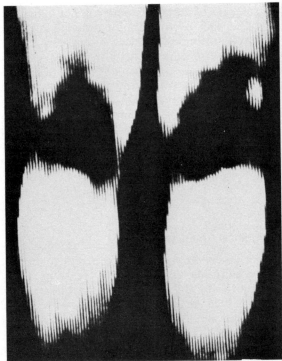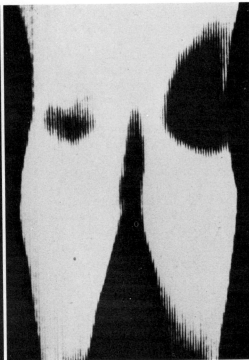

FIGS 12,9–10. **Erythrocyanosis.** Thermoscans of patients with local erythrocyanosis, bilateral (Fig. 12,9) and uni-lateral (Fig. 12,10) referred to in the text. In both cases posterior aspects of the joints were normal. (Thermoscans by courtesy of Mr W. F. Walker, Dundee, Scotland.)

ment that resolves her psychological conflict she becomes less anxious or depressed. But the symptoms are brought about by unconscious means; and this is very different from malingering.

## Manifestations in Knee Joint

Sir Benjamin continues:

'When the symptoms are referred to the knee, they bear a near resemblance to those which have been just described. There is great tenderness of the joint; but the patient suffers more from pinching the skin than from pressure, and the morbid sensibility extends for some distance up the thigh, and down the leg, perhaps as low as the foot and ankle. She suffers less from an examination when the attention is fixed on other matters than when it is directed to the affected parts; and she does not usually complain when pressure is made on the heel, so as to press the articulating surface of the tibia against that of the femur, provided that care be taken at the same time to produce no motion of the joint. *In most instances the leg is kept extended on the thigh, whereas, in cases of real disease in the knee joint, it is usually a little bent.* [Author's italics.] The symptoms may continue in this case, also, without any material alteration, for an indefinite time; for weeks, or months, even for years, the joint retaining its natural size and figure: *but occasionally a slight degree of tumefaction is observable especially on the anterior part, over, and on each side of, the ligament of the patella.* [Author's italics.] This tumefaction is not to be confounded with a general enlargement of the joint, by which surgeons are frequently perplexed and misled, the result not of the disease, but of the remedies employed. I refer to cases which have been misunderstood, and mismanaged by the application of blisters, issues, and a succession of various counter-irritants' (Fig. 12,11).

The first italicised statement is of great importance and just as true today as it was in 1837. In hysterical affections or malingering, the knee is frequently held in complete extension. The position of a slight flexion which is the natural position of a diseased or injured joint, is difficult to simulate. It is a matter of complete extension or very considerable, say right-angled, flexion; but nothing in between.

The second italicised section would cast some suspicion that the unfortunate hysterical young woman was perhaps not so hysterical as possibly suffering from the premenstrual water retention syndrome.

The greatest circumspection must be observed in the application of the label 'hysteria'. If failure to distinguish the functional from the physical has dire consequences it is important to recognise that organic disease can co-exist with hysteria. Neither condition proves the absence of the other. There are few orthopaedic

surgeons of experience who will not admit that faced with overreaction to examination of a physically impossible degree, they were eventually confronted with the physical explanation. The diagnosis should at all times be a positive one and not arrived at by a process of elimination of the physical diagnoses within the limited knowledge of the examining physician.

How many young women with pain in both knee joints with fat pad lesions based on the premenstrual water retention syndrome have been labelled 'hysteria'; and still are? Perhaps even Sir Benjamin Brodie made that mistake.

## Clinical Manifestations

**Incidence.** In what will be accepted to be a considerable experience of 'problem knees' referred by colleagues the hysterical situations have been uncommon. No record has been kept but considering the matter over the past decade not more than one proved example has been encountered each year. In the Second World War it was a different matter. Numerous cases presented in a variety of forms and frequently posed considerable problems in diagnosis.

**Features.** The importance of the condition is the diagnostic trap for the unwary and the potential for permanent physical disability. The condition usually takes the form of 'locking' or of a flexion contracture. But the clinical pattern is abnormal. The knee is held rigidly in extension, as observed by Brodie, or in 45° or more of flexion. There is no positive block to further flexion or extension. All muscles are visibly contracted to maintain the position.

If a contracture or other manifestation of hysteria has existed for any considerable length of time physical changes take place. Such changes greatly increase the difficulty of diagnosis and can mask the aetiology on a permanent basis. This is particularly true where physical measures have been applied. Examples from the author's experience include a knee placed in a plaster cast under anaesthesia to overcome a flexion contracture; a knee from which a normal medial meniscus was excised on the basis that the joint was locked despite the fact that complete extension occurred under anaesthesia; and a knee extended under

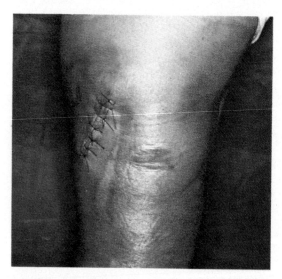

FIG. 12,11. **Fat pad lesion.** If misdiagnosis and 'mismanagement by the application of blisters, issues and a succession of various counter-irritants' was common in 1837 it continues to this day. The counter-irritant in this case took the form of a hot charcoal placed over the patellar tendon by an Arab witch doctor; and the resultant scar (Fig. 12,11). The persistent symptoms were relieved by the simple operative procedure described in Chapter 4.

anaesthesia and placed in a plaster cast with the clinical diagnosis of tuberculosis.

**Tenderness to pressure.** Overreaction to examination is an almost constant feature of hysteria but is not *per se* of diagnostic significance. In this regard the author recalls a case presented to him for opinion by an orthopaedic surgeon in Athens, Greece, with the opening remark, 'This is a very tender lady!'

It is important to remember that it is seldom that acute tenderness to palpation is present in the absence of local soft tissue swelling. An exception is meralgia hyperaesthetica, a condition encountered in a variety of forms about the knee.

**Limp.** The purpose of a limp is an attempt to reduce the weight carried by a painful joint. The patient with a painful knee walks with obvious caution in a manner readily recognised. The patient with a functional disability, or who is consciously malingering, walks often with a grotesque gait which could not other than place more weight on the joint in question than would be borne in normal walking. An 'abnormal' limp, which often puts more weight on the affected knee, rather than less, will be noticed immediately by the experienced clinician. But its very exaggeration may have the desired dramatic effect on the inexperienced audience (see case quoted below).

**Synovial effusion.** Reference is made in Chapter 2 to the means by which effusion can be induced.

EXAMINATION UNDER ANAESTHESIA. It has been indicated (Ch. 1) that circumstances may exist where examination under anaesthesia may be necessary to distinguish the functional from the physical with particular reference to the 'locked joint' or flexion contracture. This is a situation most likely to occur in the inexperienced. When such action is contemplated the possible effect on the underlying cause should be considered. In any event it seems unwise and ineffectual (see case quoted below) to place the now extended leg in a plaster cast to prevent recurrence.

### 'Hysterical Internal Derangement of the Knee'

The military conscript, but sometimes the recruit, with the complaint of internal derangement of the knee consisting of pain, giving way, locking, clicking or popping, but in which the clinical features are entirely subjective, should be well known to orthopaedic surgeons. A case reported (IKJ1, 1946) of a soldier who spent a considerable part of the Second World War in hospital while he parted with four normal menisci. Whether this was a hysterical manifestation or true malingering was not recorded. In more recent times the 'ruined knee syndrome' (IKJ5) ought to be a warning to Armed Services orthopaedic surgeons. Reference has been made in this volume (Ch. 2) to the unnecessary loss of a patella with a diagnosis of 'chondromalacia'. The background to such situations may be a variety of 'conversion hysteria'. This diagnosis, as stated previously, should be a positive one and not arrived at by a process of elimination of the physical explanations within the limiting knowledge and experience of the examining physician.

The following are three recent examples encountered of hysterical manifestations in the knee:

1. The patient (K.W., aged 15) complained that a year previously she was involved in an alarming accident: when sitting on a high stool outside the family home her sister had backed a car into the stool throwing her to the ground. There was a peculiar addition in that the dog's chain had become wrapped round the leg in question in the fall. There had been trouble with the knee ever since this accident. There was a long history of pain, instability and locking.

She was accompanied by case sheets with a large number of entries and with a variety of opinions as to the diagnosis. In brief, there had been a number of falls at school. There was a significant entry in which the knee had allegedly locked as she was ordered to turn off a television set. The locking was at a right angle. The orthopaedic surgeon who saw her suspected a functional background. Under anaesthesia the knee extended spontaneously. A padded plaster back-slab was applied to maintain extension. When the splint was removed she developed the curious quivering of the quadriceps which she alleged was paralysed. One month after the locking incident she developed total anaesthesia of the leg extending from the waist to the foot. In spite of the recognised nature of the anaesthesia, physiotherapy was continued on a once-weekly basis. There was a record of the development of the to-and-fro movement at the joint on weight-bearing referred to below.

It was at this time that her general practitioner under pressure from the mother sought a second opinion. She was accompanied by her mother and father. The mother adopted the dominant role. She was examined in the absence of the parents. She entered the room using two canes. When the leg in question was placed on the floor it vibrated in an antero-posterior movement through 15° or so for 10 seconds. It then became rigid and the good leg took a step forward, the affected leg followed and the vibrating process repeated. It was a dramatic and almost incredible performance of what she considered to be a demonstration of paralysis. When seated she was asked, in a casual manner, of her school situation. It appeared she was scheduled to attain an almost impossibly high level of examination results with the prospect of becoming, of all things, a medical student. The matter was not pursued further.

In brief it was evident that apart from any other consideration the girl was under intolerable academic and social pressures.

In view of the circumstances of the consultation and the only too obvious hysterical performance, it was felt necessary to explain in simple terms that the condition was unlikely to be resolved by physical means. The mother's lack of insight was illustrated by the fact that she sneeringly suggested that this was quite impossible as the girl was much the brightest and most intelligent member of the family! The interview continued on a more receptive level when it was explained that such affections did not occur in the dull and backward.

At the time the diagnosis was made the condition had existed for a year. There was thus, as always, the danger, possibly less important in the total scene, that what began as a functional condition was soon to develop into a physical one; and the issue confused still more.

It was recommended to her general practitioner that psychiatric help be sought. The outcome is not known.

It has been indicated that organic disease can co-exist with hysteria. The following is an example to illustrate the difficulties which can arise in distinguishing the functional from the physical:

2. The letter of referral stated: 'The patient (C.H., aged 21) was first seen at my clinic three years ago with a complaint of pain in her left knee of two years duration. Examination at this time showed quadriceps wasting and a 5° extension block. It was thought she had a torn medial meniscus and exploration of the knee was advised. She left the district at that time and no treatment was given.

She returned one year later with the continuing complaint of pain on the medial side of the knee and of a feeling of insecurity. There was a fixed flexion contracture of 30° and a small synovial effusion. The radiograph was negative.

She was admitted for meniscectomy. At operation she was found to have marked hypertrophy of the synovial membrane with numerous papillomatous swellings. The appearance was that of synovial osteochondromatosis. The meniscus was removed and considered to have an indefinite lesion of the posterior segment. The portion of synovial membrane taken for biopsy was reported to show early synovial chondromatosis. She developed a post-operative haemarthrosis and 50 cc of blood was aspirated. Following this she made good progress. On removal of stitches she had full extension and three weeks after operation had regained 90° flexion. She was discharged to her home at the time and arrangements made for her to receive physiotherapy as an outpatient.

She did not keep her physiotherapy appointments. When I next saw her she had developed a 30° flexion contracture and had only 20° active flexion. I admitted her to hospital for intensive physiotherapy. She was seen by several of my colleagues at that time who considered that an attempt should be made to straighten the knee by serial casting.

PROBLEMS OF DIAGNOSIS IN WOMEN 447

In spite of intensive treatment she has never regained full extension. The physiotherapists reported consistently that she failed to co-operate with her exercises, presumably due to pain.

She had not made any progress at the end of six months. I therefore asked a colleague with a special interest in knee surgery to see her. He considered that while there was definite underlying organic disability in the knee there was no justification for synovectomy. He considered that there was a considerable functional element to the disability. He advised me to examine the knee under anaesthesia. I was able to obtain a full flexion of the knee without any difficulty. There was a slight block to full extension. In spite of further intensive physiotherapy she never regained the range of flexion obtained under anaesthesia.

I continued to see her from time to time. A radiograph on one occasion showed ossification, presumably of one of the chondromatus tags, at the upper outer aspect of the patella. I thought this might be contributing to the loss of extension. I removed it operatively. I was not convinced that extension was increased.

I had interviewed her parents on several occasions. In discussing her management with the family doctor I was told for the first time that she had a 'nervous breakdown' and had been under the care of a psychiatrist.

The girl seems to suffer no pain. She is however walking with a flexed knee. Her life seems to revolve round horse riding. In view of the related difficulties her mother asked that a further opinion be sought.'

On examination there was loss of the last 5° of extension. Flexion was limited to 45°. There seemed to be a mechanical block to extension. There was strong muscular resistance to any attempt to increase flexion.

It was clear that if, as she stated, she was on horseback all day the type of riding she was doing would be virtually impossible with a 45° flexion deformity.

Arrangements were made to have her observed. When she swung into the saddle the knee in question flexed beyond a right angle. It therefore became necessary to pursue the reason for her hysterical deformity. It transpired eventually that she had been engaged for the purpose of 'breaking' horses. She explained that this she found to be a highly dangerous occupation; and that she had been involved in a most unpleasant accident so related.

It appeared, therefore, that what she was doing was to produce a situation of disability which allowed her to ride and to teach, but which would not permit her to undertake the dangerous task of horse-breaking.

One year later enquiries were made as to her progress. She had changed her job, worked in a different riding school and was no longer required to break horses. She had regained full flexion. There was, however, still a 5° loss of extension.

The case illustrates the point that a physical condition, in this example osteochondromatosis, can have superimposed a hysterical flexion contracture. It is a clinical situation with considerable diagnostic difficulties for the inexperienced.

3. **Self-inflicted wound.** This case was seen, in consultation with a colleague, as a problem of diagnosis and management. The patient, a dancer aged 22, gave a history that a year previously she had suffered a fall in the course of her dancing activities and injured her left knee. As a result of this injury she suffered a medial meniscectomy at the hands of an orthopaedic surgeon in her country of origin. It is not known whether the meniscus was torn. The first unusual feature of the case was that three months after the meniscectomy the scar had been excised. It was not clear in the content of language difficulties and the circumstances in which she was presented exactly why; but it was stated, and the second unusual feature, that it was because 'the wound had failed to heal'. Since this episode she had come to England with the purpose, she said, of improving her technique and professional status.

The reason for the consultation was the serious situation which had arisen in the latter regard in that she was no longer able to dance because the meniscectomy scar had broken down once again. She entered the room using one elbow crutch. The knee was held in

30° of flexion and was encased in an elastic bandage. There was a dried, but recent, blood-stain 2·5 cm square at the site where a medial meniscectomy incision is usually located.

There is a pattern in human affairs, even in those of the knee joint. This was not a familiar one. What possible reason could there be for a meniscectomy incision breaking down after a year? It could be an unrelated hair follicle infection or a retained suture. The latter possibility seemed unlikely in view of the history of excision of the scar by a plastic surgeon. When the bandage was removed no swelling of the joint was evident; nor was there local swelling at the site of the scar. There was, however, some dried blood of recent origin. When this had been removed with detergent there appeared, parallel to the meniscectomy scar, a linear scratch some 4 cm in length. It was of recent origin and without adjacent reaction. Examination with a magnifying glass confirmed the nature of the lesion. It was a self-inflicted wound!

Regrettably the outcome of this case is unknown. She was seen but once; and for the purpose only of establishing the cause of the breakdown of the scar. A superficial assessment of the situation suggested that what little brains she had were located in her feet. She had discovered, like many others, that London standards of show business were far beyond her reach. She required an excuse for failure.

**Treatment.** Limited experience would suggest that orthopaedic surgeons, confronted with parental or patient pressure to take some positive action, send such cases to a physiotherapy department to treat by physical means a condition without physical basis; even worse, a plaster cast is applied. Experience has shown that this aggravates rather than alleviates the condition in the long term. There may be exceptions. It is the author's practice to refer such cases to a sympathetic psychiatrist for advice.

REFERENCES

BRODIE, SIR BENJAMIN C. (1837). *Lectures Illustrative of Certain Local Nervous Affections, Lecture II*. London: Longman, Rees, Orme, Brown, Green & Longman.

JONES, SIR ROBERT & LOVETT, R. W. (1921). *Orthopaedic Surgery*. London: Oxford University Press.

SMILLIE, I. S. (1963). Lesions of the infrapatellar fat pad and synovial fringes: Hoffa's disease. *Acta orthopaedica Scandinavica*, **33**, 4.

SMILLIE, I. S. (1968). Internal derangements of the knee joint in women. *Proceedings of the Royal Society of Medicine*, **61**, 10.

# 13. Tumours and Tumour-like Conditions: Soft Tissue

## SIMPLE

### Cystic Degeneration of a Meniscus

The most common limited soft tissue swelling about the knee, with the possible exception of prepatellar bursitis, is located on the lateral joint line in the form of cystic degeneration of the meniscus.

The presenting symptom is pain in the form of a deep boring ache produced by a tension situation when the cysts are confined by the capsule and subject to irritation by physical activity (Fig. 13,1). This symptom complex does not apply to the medial side where the cyst, having penetrated the capsule, has unlimited space for expansion and the pain-producing tension situation does not obtain: the complaint is of the presence of a swelling (Figs 13,2 and 13,3).

The characteristic feature of the swelling on the lateral side is that it is most prominent in 45° of flexion (Fig. 13,1). It is reduced in size in extension and even more so in full flexion.

Cystic degeneration of the menisci has been considered in some detail from the viewpoint of aetiology, pathology, clinical features and treatment in IKJ5 and these aspects of what is a common and important clinical entity will not be repeated.

### Differential Diagnosis

'Ganglion' of the knee. This is a diagnosis to be made with caution if it is only for the reason that it is readily confused with a variety of other conditions and, in particular, with cystic degeneration of a meniscus on the lateral side of the joint.

In the recent past when cystic degeneration was less well recognised it was not uncommon to be presented with a knee with two or more scars resulting from removal of a so-called ganglion which had recurred. The patient was cured only when the source of the swelling was recognised and the affected meniscus removed. Nevertheless, 'ganglions' do exist and can occur anywhere in relation to ligamentous, capsular or other tissue (Figs 13,5 to 13,7). In recent examples the ganglion arose in the posterior capsule (Fig. 13,4) and in an anterior example, at the attachment of vastus lateralis. In another, it was located within the patellar tendon close to the attachment to the patella.

A common source of a ganglion-like swelling is the superior tibiofibular joint; and the possible effect on the lateral popliteal nerve will be described. Such swellings are liable to be confused with cystic degeneration of the lateral meniscus and particularly when it is recognised that cysts of the meniscus can be located at considerable distance from the site of origin.

In this regard ganglia also may be located at a situation far removed from the site of origin but connected to that site by a pedicle. In the knee joint cysts of the meniscus which have passed through the capsule are swept backwards by the action of flexion to be located in a posterior situation; and an example is cited in which a cyst which had passed through the capsule between patellar tendon and iliotibial band anteriorly when next seen was located on the joint line posteriorly. At operation the pedicle was traced forward to the point of emergence. It is possible, in the circumstances of such a case, that the swelling is in fact a ganglion; and that the meniscus need not be excised provided it is shown that a pedicle exists and is extirpated at the point of exit.

Cysts within the joint. It is not uncommon to find small cystic swellings within the joint in the course of exploration for some other condition. These may be found within the fat pad, at the anterior extremity of a meniscus or at the attachment of the anterior cruciate ligament. In such sites it cannot be determined whether they arise in the capsule, fat pad, meniscus, ligament or synovial membrane. These cysts are small and, it is repeated, usually an incidental finding. There is no record of one having recurred to the

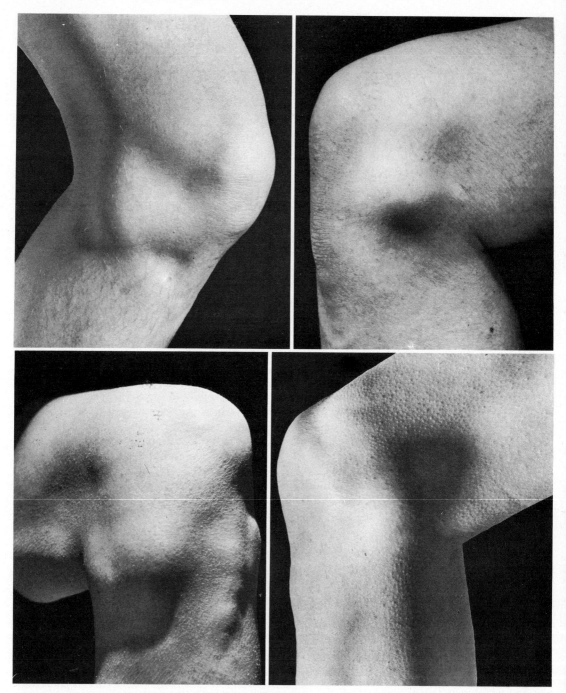

**FIGS 13,1–4. Cystic swellings on the joint line.** The commonest source of a local swelling on the lateral aspect of the knee is cystic degeneration of the meniscus. This swelling is characteristically located on the joint line and is most prominent in 45° of flexion tending to disappear in full flexion (Fig. 13,1). On the medial side cysts of the meniscus, having passed through the capsule, have room for expansion. They tend, therefore, to be larger than on the lateral side (Figs 13,2 and 13,3). Not all swellings, lateral or medial, arise in the menisci but may be ganglions or, on the medial side, bursae. This swelling was a ganglion arising in the posterior capsule (Fig 13,4).

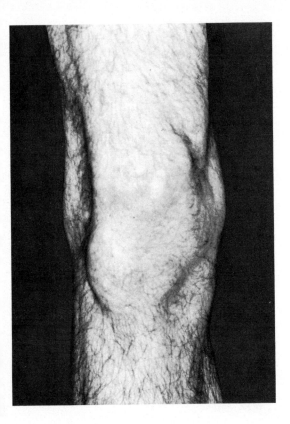

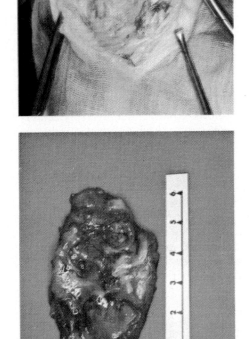

FIGS 13,5–7. **Cystic swellings about the knee.** A space-occupying lesion arising in the anterior compartment whether cystic degeneration of the anterior segment of a meniscus, 'ganglion' or other mass, presents through the weak area in the capsule between iliotibial band and patellar tendon (Fig. 13,5). The multilocular cyst which protruded on division of the capsule (Fig. 13,6). The tissue of origin of the cystic mass (Fig. 13,7) was not determined. It did not appear to arise in the anterior segment of the meniscus and the meniscus was not excised (R.D., male, aged 33).

extent that it was the source of symptoms demanding re-exploration.

**Ganglion of the superior tibio-fibular joint.** The swelling is not on the joint line as is a cyst of the meniscus. It tends from its origin to be at a lower level and located further posteriorly. It is usually larger, possibly localised but more vague in dimensions than cystic degeneration in so far as cysts produce pain and eventual internal derangement whereas ganglions produce symp-

toms on account of size and of pressure on related structures and, in particular, nerves (see below).

## Treatment

If cystic degeneration of a meniscus is not necessarily progressive in terms of size of the swelling or of related symptoms it is not therefore innocent in terms of the future of the joint.

Cystic degeneration of the lateral meniscus is associated in a large proportion of cases with a parrot-beak tear as a result of loss of local mobility from fixation of the periphery by the degenerative pathology. It has been indicated (IKJ5) that the lateral compartment of the joint is 'silent'. If it is silent in terms of symptoms it is this silence which is responsible for degeneration of the articular cartilage and eventual mono-compartmental osteoarthrosis. Cystic degeneration therefore should not be ignored. If it is the resultant meniscus lesion will produce degeneration of articular cartilage considerably in excess of what would have occurred if the meniscus had been excised. It should not be assumed, however, that every extra-articular capsular cystic swelling, particularly on the medial side, is cystic degeneration to be treated by excision of the opposing relative meniscus.

It should be recorded that intracapsular multi-locular cysts do not necessarily require to be isolated, dissected out and removed. Excision of the meniscus from which they have arisen results in resolution of the mass. Conversely, as has been indicated, excision of the mass, without the structure from which it has arisen, results in recurrence.

## LIPOMA

In theory a lipoma can arise wherever there is fatty tissue; and that is almost anywhere.

Superficial lipomata are unusual about the knee. The majority encountered have been located, not unexpectedly, in the fat pad, and in the layer of fat deep to the suprapatellar pouch; and these, significantly, are the sites implicated by Jaffe (1958).

### Clinical Features

The possibility will be considered in a small soft localised swelling in an unusual situation. In no instance in this series was the diagnosis established with certainty prior to exploration.

A lipoma within the fat pad produces a swelling of indeterminate origin. The fact that it is a local space-occupying lesion rather than some general affection of the synovial membrane is shown by the fact that there is no swelling of the suprapatellar pouch nor on the medial or

lateral joint lines; and that it protrudes in extension through the weak area in the capsule between the patellar tendon and the iliotibial band or to the medial side of the tendon.

Lipomas located within normal fat, as in the fat pad, are characterised by a thin delicate capsule which may be difficult to delineate in the course of excision:

On one occasion, well recalled (Mrs J. T., aged 56), an exploration of the anterior compartment for an expected cyst of the meniscus revealed an encapsulated lipoma which was enucleated, as it appeared at the time, *in toto*. Nine months later she presented with a swelling similar to the original; and in some degree of alarm. A second operation was advised. That recurrence took place raised the question of liposarcoma and in such circumstances wide excision was practised. The pathologist reported the apparent recurrence to be simple. Two years later, there has been no further swelling. It is assumed that at the original operation a lobule of tumour remained *in situ* to grow rapidly into the space provided.

## LOCALISED NODULAR SYNOVITIS: GIANT CELL TUMOUR OF TENDON SHEATH

**Definition.** Localised nodular synovitis refers to a form of pigmented villonodular synovitis in which a limited area only of the synovium is affected.

**Joint incidence.** The joint involved is nearly always the knee (Jaffe, 1958).

The following is the record of a case to illustrate the problems which may be encountered in the diagnosis and treatment of soft tissue tumour-like conditions about the knee joint:

The patient (Miss S.S.S., aged 22, medical student) reported that nine months ago for no obvious reason her right knee had locked; and several similar episodes of locking, temporary in nature, had occurred since then. Three days ago the joint had suddenly, and without any incident of trauma, become swollen and painful.

On examination the knee was swollen as a

result of synovial effusion. There was a localised tender swelling on the medial side immediately above the joint line. A provisional diagnosis of a loose body was made. Radiographs showed the mass to be radiotranslucent.

At operation, through a limited incision centered over the swelling, a purplish-coloured, pedunculated tumour about the size of a cherry presented on dividing the synovial membrane. The pedicle appeared to be attached to synovial membrane.

The pathological report stated the specimen to consist of a firm, oval-shaped, smooth-surfaced mass measuring $3 \times 2 \times 0.5$ cm in size. Microscopy showed the appearance of a giant cell tumour of the type associated with tendon sheaths. It was of relatively high cellularity and contained many areas of infarction of varying age as well as numerous well-formed vessels. The nodule, until very recently, must have had a vascular pedicle. The sections showed no evidence of malignancy. It was thought appropriate to remark that a growth of this kind is liable to local recurrence.

Convalescence was uneventful.

Approximately one year later she reported that during the past two months there had been a return of pain in the knee, but this time on the lateral side. The pain was increased by exercise. Examination showed a small firm swelling on the joint line and the provisional diagnosis of cystic degeneration of the lateral meniscus made. At operation, and in view of the previous history, instead of ignoring the cyst as would have been the normal practice, it was exposed for the purpose of identification. A skin incision as for lateral meniscectomy was employed. An oblique incision was made in the iliotibial tract and the mass exposed and freed from the surrounding soft tissues. The appearance was that of multilocular cystic degeneration. The joint was then entered anteriorly between iliotibial band and patellar tendon and the meniscus the subject of a parrot-beak tear together with the attached cystic mass excised.

The pathological report stated: the appearances are not those of any form of neoplasm but suggest degeneration with cystic change.

Recovery was unremarkable.

It was concluded that the cystic degeneration of the lateral meniscus was no more than coincidental and with no relationship to the giant cell tumour of a year previously.

Eighteen years have elapsed since the first operation. There has been no recurrence of the giant cell tumour and, indeed, no further trouble with the joint.

## AFFECTIONS OF NERVES

The affections of the nerves about the knee do not merit a separate chapter. The common conditions are not primary lesions, although such occur (see below), but are the result of pressure from some external source. The chapter concerned with tumours of soft tissue including as it does ganglion of the superior tibio-fibular joint, would appear appropriate.

The lesions encountered in the sensory field concern the patellar plexus and are the result of exogenous trauma, accidental or operative, endogenous trauma or of ischaemia. In the motor field the lesions encountered in the lateral and medial popliteal nerves and their branches result from the pressure of reactionary oedema and of exogenous forces incurred in the course of treatment; and, as will be recorded, from tumours.

### PATELLAR PLEXUS

**Anatomy.** The patellar plexus is characterised by the wide variation in the origin and anatomical situation of the constituent nerves (Fig. 13,8). The infrapatellar branch of the saphenous nerve, the largest involved, received the major attention and is the subject of the widest variations some of which may be of clinical significance (see below). The origin, as the description suggests, is most commonly the saphenous nerve; but it may arise from the femoral nerve and indeed elsewhere. It is the routes of distribution which may have clinical implications. It may branch from the saphenous nerve proximal to the adductor canal, in the canal or distal to the canal. It may pass through, under or over the sartorius muscle or tendon.

**Clinical implications.** The importance of the patellar plexus as a source of symptoms has not been explained except in so far as time expended by the human race in kneeling is rated in terms of activity rather than repose. That normal sensitivity is important is shown by the fact that those who work on their knees, at the extreme, coal miners, but in less arduous occupations, slaters, tile and carpet layers, and a host of other occupations, often complain of loss of local sensation after meniscectomy. Experience of a considerable number of meniscectomies would suggest that such complaint is temporary and that normal sensation is eventually restored. There are exceptions.

### NEURITIS OF PATELLAR PLEXUS: MERALGIA HYPERAESTHETICA

This condition is characterised by the complaint of momentary excruciating pain in the form of an 'electric shock' when a small well-defined area of skin overlying the patella, or the immediately adjacent regions, is subjected to the lightest touch, the patient stating that even contact with the material of the trouser leg causes him to pause abruptly in whatever he is doing.

The author is credited with the original description (IKJ1, 1946) (Wartenberg, 1954). At that time it was assumed to be the result of minor direct, but unremembered, injury. But the fact that cases are encountered in which the affection is bilateral is against such a mechanism. It seems probable that some accident of anatomy in the position of the infrapatellar branch of the saphenous, or other nerve taking part in the patellar plexus may render it vulnerable to mechanical trauma or ischaemia in movement (Fig. 13,8). If meralgia hyperaesthetica is of mechanical origin it is not surprising that it should be encountered about the knee joint. There must be few areas of the body where so much soft tissue movement occurs between full flexion and full extension as the anterior aspect of the knee. Simple flexion or extension is seldom responsible. But flexion together with some rotatory action, as in getting into bed, may induce the pain tending to confirm the sugges-

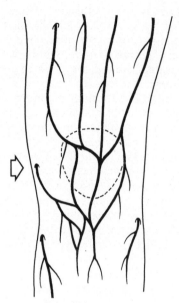

Fig. 13,8 **Patellar plexus and sensory nerves on anterior aspect of knee.** The arrow indicates the site of the infrapatellar branch of the saphenous nerve.

tion that trauma occurs where a nerve pierces the fascia. But some unknown sensitising agent must operate. The similarity of the conditions described as 'traumatic prepatellar neuralgia' (Gordon 1952) and 'gonyalgia paresthetica' (Wartenberg, 1954) is such as to suggest that they are variations of the original.

On examination the 'trigger area' can usually be found, adjacent to which is an area of hyperaesthesia in the region of the patellar plexus. On the lateral side the trauma may be produced by the ilio-tibial band. The zone of acute hyperaesthesia covers a wide area and when the attack has passed a reduced area of diminished sensation is situated in front of the head of the fibula. The patient often excuses himself for having complained of such a trivial matter, but has become apprehensive about the unexpected suddenness of the shocks and the nature of the condition. He may be reassured that although the condition may remain for a few weeks, it is self-limiting and will disappear as suddenly as it came; but that recurrence is common.

It is important that the condition be recognised as innocent and not confused with some internal derangement meriting interference.

There is another form of patellar plexus neuritis of importance if only that its existence should be recognised. In the mysterious condition erythrocyanosis in the peripheral vascular field, the extreme sensitivity of the skin in the prepatellar region and the consequent reluctance to kneel is probably due to a neuritis of the patellar plexus of ischaemic origin (see Ch. 12).

**Herpes zoster of infrapatellar branch of saphenous nerve.** It appears that the nerve can be affected by a herpetic lesion producing pain and extreme sensitivity to pressure over a wide area of the plexus accompanied by a skin lesion of spontaneous origin. It is clear that the importance of the lesion is recognition. In a recent example, the case, a young woman, was presented for diagnosis on account of severe and persistent pain on the medial side of the joint out of proportion to the severity of the original direct injury some weeks previously. There was evidence of vesiculation and general soft tissue atropy on the medial side of the knee. It is of interest that trauma to the affected part has been suggested as a common cause of reactivation of the latent virus (Juel-Jensen, 1970).

## Neuroma of Infrapatellar Branch of Saphenous Nerve

Reference has been made, IKJ5, to the vulnerability of the patellar plexus to injury, exogenous in operative incision, and endogenous, as above, from mechanical trauma at the exits from the deep fascia resulting in meralgia hyperaesthetica.

It will be evident that almost any incision about the knee divides sensory nerves concerned in the plexus; and, in general, there are no serious consequences. The most common operation is meniscectomy; and the meniscus most commonly involved that on the medial side. It appears that of the nerves concerned the infrapatellar branch of the saphenous nerve is the largest and most important. The nerve is located at some 2·5 cm distal to the superior margin of the medial tibial condyle. The inferior limit of the incision recommended on the medial side is one finger's breadth below the superior margin of the condyle; and thus, in ordinary circumstances, should avoid contact with the nerve.

It apears that injury to the nerve in the form of partial division is more likely to be productive of symptoms than the total division which must be of common occurrence. Where weak tincture of iodine (5 per cent) has been used for the immediate pre-operative skin preparation, division of the nerve will be indicated at the time of removal of the sutures by an area of skin in which desquamation has not occurred; and this corresponds to the area of anaesthesia. The presence of a neuroma will be indicated by a complaint of pain and of exquisite local tenderness and of disturbance of sensation in the area of skin involved. In experienced hands this situation is readily recognised. In other circumstances the persistent complaint of pain and giving-way incidents in the absence of effusion, local swelling or the other sign of internal derangement in the course of delayed recovery has been known to have been a source of misinterpretation and of injustice.

If doubt exists, an injection of local anaesthetic at the point of maximum tenderness confirms the diagnosis by the elimination of subjective phenomena.

**Treatment.** Excision of the scar and identification of the nerve for the purpose of confirming the existence of a neuroma followed by the excision of the segment of the nerve involved has been the treatment adopted. No example of further complaint can be recalled.

**Entrapment neuropathy of infrapatellar nerve.** Four cases have been described (House and Ahmed, 1977), which, because of the persistence of symptoms and signs similar to those described under 'neuritis' above, eventually came to exploratory operation. In two it was found that the nerve passed deep to the sartorius and was thought to be compressed against the posterior margin of the medial condyles as well as sharply angulated in its distal course. In the others the nerve passed through a musculotendinous hiatus in the sartorius and showed narrowing or kinking at this site. The symptoms were relieved in all four patients by neurolysis and translocation of the nerve from the site of entrapment.

It will be evident that the condition as described differs only in degree from 'neuritis' as above. The author has not encountered an example in which symptoms persisted.

## LATERAL POPLITEAL NERVE

This nerve in its close relationship to the knee joint is probably the most vulnerable of the sensory and motor nerves to exogenous and endogenous forces. 'Drop-foot', temporary or permanent, is a common complication of a variety of conditions, traumatic, degenerative and neoplastic in origin.

**Exogenous trauma.** The nerve in its proximity to the biceps tendon and head of the fibula (Fig. 13,9) is sensitive in the extreme to direct pressure from flexed-knee splints, cotton wool pads used to maintain flexion, plaster casts and indeed any source of direct pressure the most common of which is the compression bandage.

No instance of lateral popliteal paralysis can be recalled which could be attributed directly to the use of a tourniquet, Samway or pneumatic. Occasionally paresis occurs some days later; and at that stage it is impossible to determine whether it resulted from oedema and/or pressure from the compression bandage. The situation may be multifactorial: oedema or other source of swelling such as effusion increases the pressure exerted by the bandage and accounts for the late onset of the phenomena (see case recorded below).

**Endogenous trauma.** In this context should be considered pressure from Steinmann pins, direct or indirect in the form of local soft tissue swelling. Insertion of a pin, or pins, in the region of the flare of the tibia should take place from the lateral side, and, no matter how accurately executed, is not without risk to the lateral popliteal nerve in terms of reactionary oedema aggravated by the adverse mechanical influences created by the reduction of angular deformity by opening-wedge, or even closing-wedge, osteotomy.

No matter how much care is exercised paralysis can occur for which no obvious explanation is evident. The following is an example:

The patient (R.M., male, aged 69) underwent a medial closing-wedge osteotomy of the tibial head for mono-compartmental osteoarthrosis with valgus angulation of some 25°. No technical difficulties were encountered at operation. Stability was achieved with two staples. A compression bandage incorporating plaster slabs was used for immobilisation. He was nursed in a half-ring Thomas bed-knee splint. In pursuance of the regime recommended he commenced dorsiflexion exercises as soon as he had recovered from his anaesthetic and the following day demonstrated dorsiflexion of the foot of normal power. Six days later the physiotherapist who was supervising his exercises reported a complete drop-foot. The compression bandage was therefore removed in the expectation that a fold of blood-soaked cotton wool in the innermost layer of the bandage had dried and was exerting pressure although there had never at any time been a complaint of local pain. There was, however, no ridge of wool and no evidence of external pressure of any kind nor of soft-tissue swelling on the lateral aspect of the joint. There was thus no explanation of the phenomenon. When the stitches were removed on the tenth day a cuff-type weight-bearing plaster cast was applied. The situation permits a simple spring to be used for the control of dorsiflexion in so far as the circumferential strap below the knee

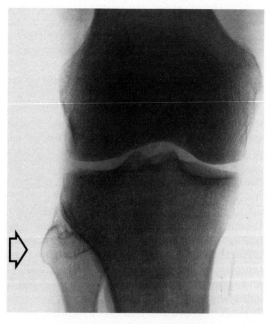

FIG. 13,9. **Lateral poplital nerve: endogenous trauma.** A prominent head of fibula as in this example can be responsible for irritation of the lateral popliteal nerve.

is outside the plaster cast and cannot therefore exert pressure on the nerve. At the end of four weeks there was evidence of return of function. At the end of four months he had regained right-angle flexion in the knee. Dorsiflexion of the foot was slowly improving but had not reached a stage at which apparatus could be discarded. The final outcome is unknown.

(For compression of lateral popliteal nerve by fabella in lateral head of gastrocnemius, see Chapter 2.)

### Ganglion of Superior Tibio-fibular Joint: Intraneural Ganglion of Lateral Popliteal Nerve

**Definition.** Invasion of the lateral popliteal nerve by a ganglion arising in the superior tibio-fibular joint is a recognised clinical syndrome presenting in the form of pain on the lateral aspect of the joint accompanied by paralysis, partial or complete, of the muscles of the anterior compartment of the leg. There is palpable swelling of the lateral popliteal nerve.

**Pathological anatomy.** The invading tumour is generally accepted to arise in the superior tibio-fibular joint from whence it tracks along the sheath of the recurrent articular branch of the lateral popliteal nerve to the sheath of the main nerve where it enlarges and expands usually in a proximal direction. The fact that the recurrent articular branch arises from that part of the trunk which is about to become the anterior branch probably accounts for the muscles of the anterior compartment being more severely affected than those of the lateral compartment (Parkes, 1961).

### Clinical Features

PAIN. The presenting symptom is pain initially situated in the region of the head of the fibula. Later it may be located in the cutaneous distribution of the lateral popliteal nerve.

PARALYSIS. There is weakness, partial or complete, of the muscles of the anterior compartment.

SENSATION. There may be blunting of sensation in the direction of the lateral popliteal nerve.

SWELLING. There is swelling of the lateral popliteal nerve posterior to the head of the fibula; and it may extend upwards into the popliteal space.

**Differential diagnosis.** It will be evident that a condition presenting as pain, paralysis of the muscles of the anterior compartment of the leg coupled with sensory disturbance is capable of a wide range of interpretations and particularly in the similarity to the common lumbar-disc syndrome. Where pain is aggravated by exercise, possible confusion with intermittent claudication, or the anterior compartment or peroneal compartment syndromes, will arise. In circumstances where the presence of the swelling is known to the patient, or deliberately sought, the problem will be reduced at least to one of local pressure. In the presence of palpable swelling in the course of the nerve the differential diagnosis will raise the possibility of a primary tumour in the form of Schwannoma. The origin of the swelling may be resolved only at exploration.

### Treatment

**Operation.** Exploration without delay is the treatment of choice. An essential feature of operation is the location and extirpation of the pedicle which connects the ganglion with the superior tibio-fibular joint. The multilocular cyst is decompressed. No attempt is made to remove the walls from within the nerve sheath. It is considered to be unnecessary and liable to damage of nerve fibres resulting in incomplete recovery of muscle power (Parkes, 1961).

**Results.** Treatment on the lines indicated results in recovery of muscle power complete or virtually complete. Recurrence is not uncommon (three out of eight cases: Muckart, 1976).

## MALIGNANT TUMOURS: PRINCIPLES OF TREATMENT

In a soft tissue tumour liable to local recurrence, as, for example, a desmoid, necessitating wide excision of tissue including muscle and skin, it is necessary to look into the future and to the possibility that amputation may be required. If excision of muscle is such that the function of the knee is virtually destroyed, excision of skin should be such that the formation of flaps for the amputation stump of the future is not, if possible, prejudiced.

The desmoid tumour, the one quoted, is of course rare, and the situation has arisen once only in the experience of the author. Recurrences up to six times, however, have been recorded (Ackeman, 1964). The same author states that only rarely does local aggression necessitate amputation.

## FIBROSARCOMA

**Incidence.** Fibrosarcoma is the most common of the malignant soft tissue tumours.

### Clinical Features

It presents in the form of a soft tissue mass which may be adherent to skin and to the deep tissues. It is not usually painful except in an advanced stage involving invasion of bone. It tends to grow slowly and may be present even for years before a sudden increase in size leads the patient to seek advice.

### Treatment

Whether the tumour is well or poorly differentiated, recurrence is almost certain unless it is subject to radical excision. Metastases do not occur in the early stages and thus if the initial intervention is radical the prognosis is not unduly unfavourable. In general, and understandably in the absence of precise diagnosis, the initial intervention is usually inadequate. More than 60 per cent of poorly differentiated tumours recur and more than 40 per cent succumb to metastases (Jaffe, 1958).

Amputation should thus be considered once the diagnosis is established with certainty.

The clinical features are reproduced in the case to be reported:

> The patient (M.F., female, aged 75) reported that for the past eight months she had been aware of a swelling on the lateral aspect of the left knee. It had never been painful but recently it appeared to be growing rapidly; and this was the reason she had sought the advice of her general practitioner. On examination an exceptionally large mass was present which was solid to touch and was

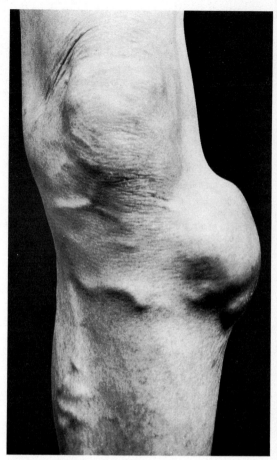

FIG. 13,10. **Fibrosarcoma.** The patient presented with a swelling on the lateral aspect of the joint with a history of recent rapid increase in size. The tumour was of rubber-like consistency and measured $8 \times 7 \times 4$ cm (M.F., female, aged 75, see text).

adherent to skin and to the deep soft tissues at the joint line (Fig. 13,10). Radiographs were taken but showed no involvement of the underlying bone. No precise diagnosis was made but the adherence to skin raised the question of possible malignancy. At operation, the mass, including an ellipse of skin to which it adhered, was removed. It had appeared to be adherent to the capsule. It could not be said with certainty that the excision was wide of the tumour. The pathologist reported the mass to be a cellular sarcoma probably arising in fibrous tissue. Three weeks later as a result of this report she received radiotherapy. She was reviewed at two monthly intervals and appeared to be progressing favourably.

: Sixteen months later her general practitioner referred her back in so far as two nodules, the larger of which was 3 cm in diameter, had appeared in the scar. Neither was adherent to the deep structures. The question of her further treatment arose. Amputation was considered to be the measure of necessity. The patient, however, would not countenance the possibility. The matter, in view of her age, was not pressed. Instead a radical excision was carried out. This consisted of encircling the area of skin involved. The upper nodule was cleared by some 6 cm and the lower nodule by about 4 cm. The dissection was carried into the popliteal fossa. It was evident that sacrifice of the lateral popliteal nerve would be necessary. Finally, the entire tumour area with attached skin, the superior 5 cm of the fibula and a considerable amount of muscle from the anterior compartment, was excised. The anterior tibial vessels were preserved. The resultant defect was skin grafted. The wound healed well and she was discharged from hospital six weeks later wearing a below-knee brace to control the drop-foot which had resulted from division of the lateral popliteal nerve.

Nine months later there was no evidence of local recurrence and the patient was apparently well. Four months later, however, her general practitioner wrote to say that she had died in an emaciated state, he believed the result of metastic deposits in the lungs.

In retrospect, it is probable that the correct treatment in this particular case, and which might have saved her life, was amputation, just as soon as the diagnosis was established with certainty. Such treatment was understandably unacceptable in a patient of her age and was not pressed.

## Neuro-fibrosarcoma

Tumours of nerves may occur anywhere. There is no predilection for the region of the knee joint.

The following is an example of a malignant tumour encountered in the course of compilation of this work and a summary recorded for the purpose illustrating the mode of presentation and the problems of treatment, social and surgical which were encountered:

The patient (Mrs M.W., aged 36, case of J.H.) was referred with the history that she had suffered pain behind the left knee and down the leg for the past two years. The condition had become worse in the last six months and progressing in the past week. The referring practitioner had noticed tenderness in the sciatic distribution above the knee and absence of the ankle jerk: the possible diagnosis of the lumbar disc syndrome was offered.

The salient feature of examination was apparent extreme tenderness in the popliteal region; but her apprehension was such that a suspected swelling could be palpated but not with certainty. The absence of the ankle jerk was confirmed. A routine radiograph of the joint revealed the presence of a calcified mass in the line of the lateral popliteal nerve which explained, at least, the neurological finding (Fig. 13,11). Exploration was advised. At operation an ovoid swelling was found within the lateral popliteal division of the sciatic nerve (Fig. 13,12). This swelling was excised but not without difficulty. The pathological report reflected problems of identification of the tissue but concluded with the diagnosis of a neuro-fibrosarcoma. It was recommended that the segment of the nerve should be resected. It was at this stage that considerable delay occurred. A visit from a social worker, after failure to keep appointments offered for the purpose of discussing further treatment, revealed social-domestic problems of some magnitude. It was not until six months from the original exploration that the nerve was resected and apparatus fitted to control the drop-foot which resulted. She was last reviewed two years from the date of resection. She was fit, well and without evidence of recurrence.

## Synovioma: Synovial Sarcoma

**Definition.** The term synovioma is reserved for the rare but highly malignant synovial sarcoma which is encountered in the vicinity of a large joint of the lower limb. The term 'benign

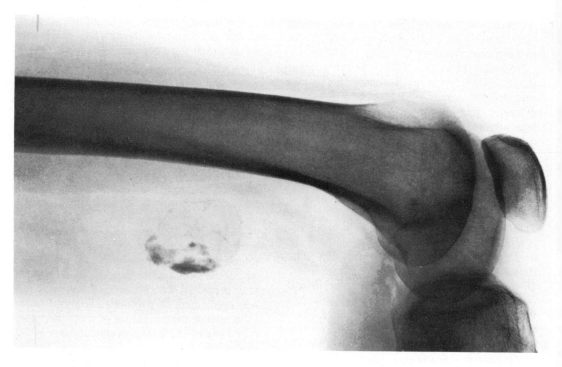

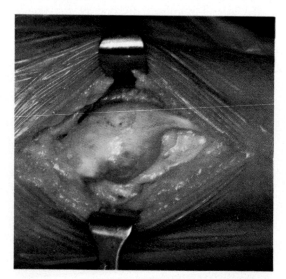

FIGS 13,11–12. **Neuro-fibrosarcoma of lateral popliteal nerve.** The patient complained of pain behind the knee referred down the leg. A tender palpable mass was present. The radiograph showed that the mass was calcified (Fig. 13,11). The mass was removed initially without section of the nerve (Fig. 13,12) but when the nature of the tumour was established the segment involved was excised (M.W., female, aged 36).

synovioma' refers to lesions such as pigmented villonodular synovitis and should be avoided in any connection (Jaffe, 1958).

**Incidence.** The knee is the joint most commonly affected.

**Gross pathology.** The name implies that the tumour originates in the synovial lining of the capsule but, according to Jaffe, this occurs only infrequently. He states that the tumour usually starts in the para-articular soft tissues just beyond the confines of the capsule although it may eventually penetrate the latter structure and invade the synovial membrane. It is assumed that occurring where there is no synovial tissue it must arise as a result of differentiation of non-specific connective tissue.

**Age range.** The majority of the subjects are young adults. The remainder are adolescents or middle-aged. A few only are young children or elderly.

## Clinical Features

The diagnosis is virtually never established prior to operation. In the limited experience of

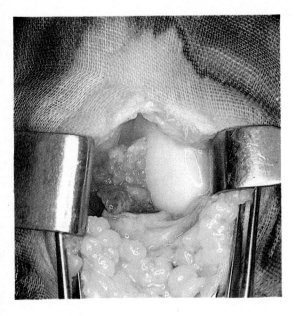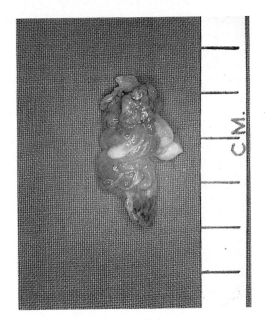

FIGS 13,13–14. **Synovioma.** This intra-articular tumour was reported to be a synovioma. The final outcome is unknown.

a few examples the tumour was encountered unexpectedly in the course of an operation for a 'firm swelling'; and the fact that growth is characteristically slow adds to the difficulty. The commonest firm swelling about the knee is cystic degeneration of a meniscus; and this has been the pre-operative diagnosis in the majority of cases. The duration of the complaints therefore vary between a few months and two or three years. The complaint, apart from the possible knowledge of the existence of the lump, is the usual one of pain increased by exercise. On examination there is a palpable mass tender to touch with possible increase of local temperature if the tumour has attained any considerable size.

There are no radiological findings.

The course of events at operation has been as follows: the mass, thought to be a cyst, was usually large enough to demand local exploration and at exposure it was evident that the swelling was a solid doubtfully unencapsulated tumour. It was appreciated that such a mass might be a synovioma and wide excision undertaken.

### Treatment

If suspicion is aroused in the course of operation as to the nature of the swelling as wide an excision as is practical is performed. The tumour is not radiosensitive and amputation in the circumstances probably offers the best chance of survival.

**Prognosis.** The diagnosis of synovioma is associated with a prognosis of the utmost gravity. Recurrence after excision is as characteristic as is the slow growth. In a recent series of 39 cases (Cameron and Kostuik, 1974) 25 per cent of which affected the knee, the average rate of 5-year survival was 45 per cent; of 10-year survival, 30 per cent and of survival for more than 10 years, 10 per cent. This series confirms that primary amputation is the treatment of choice.

X

## REFERENCES

ACKEMAN, L. V. (1964). *Surgical Pathology*, p. 965, 3rd edn. London: Henry Kimpton.

CAMERON, H. U. & KOSTUIK, J. P. (1974). A long-term follow-up of synovial sarcome. *Journal of Bone and Joint Surgery*, **56B,** 613.

GORDON, G. C. (1952). Traumatic prepatellar neuralgia. *Journal of Bone and Joint Surgery*, **34B,** 41.

HOUSE, J. H. & AHMED, K. (1977). Entrapment neuropathy of the infrapatellar branch of the saphenous nerve. *American Journal of Sports Medicine*, **5,** 217.

JAFFE, H. L. (1958). *Tumors and Tumorous Conditions*, p. 576. London: Henry Kimpton.

JUEL-JENSEN, B. E. (1970). The natural history of shingles. Events associated with reactivation of *Varicella-zoster* virus. *Journal of the College of General Practitioners*, **20,** 323.

MUCKART, R. D. (1976). Compression of the common peroneal nerve by intramuscular ganglion from the superior tibio-fibular joint. *Journal of Bone and Joint Surgery*, **58B,** 241.

PARKES, A. (1961). Intraneural ganglion of the lateral popliteal nerve. *Journal of Bone and Joint Surgery*, **43B,** 4, 784.

SMILLIE, I. S. (1946). *Injuries of the Knee Joint*, 1st Edition. Edinburgh: E. & S. Livingstone.

WARTENBERG, R. (1954). Digitalia paresthetica and gonyalgia paresthetica. *Neurology*, **4,** 106.

# 14. Tumours and Tumour-like Conditions: Bone

## SIMPLE

### SOLITARY AND MULTIPLE OSTEOCARTILAGINOUS EXOSTOSES

The most common simple tumour arising in the bones about the knee is a solitary exostosis and the most common location is the medial aspect of the medial condyle of the tibia.

**Definition.** Osteocartilaginous exostoses take two forms: (1) **solitary** and (2) **multiple.** In the solitary variety one site only in the skeleton is affected.

The forms differ in so far as multiple exostoses is a hereditary disorder with implications for modification of the architecture and mechanics of the joint. The solitary exostosis is apparently not of hereditary origin:

In this regard it is of interest that in the course of compilation of this work twin girls were encountered (A. and S.Z., aged 11, cases of I.D.S.), one with a single exostosis of left femur, the other with a single exostosis of left tibia, both of a size interfering with function and demanding resection.

The implications for alteration of joint mechanics are minimal in the solitary variety. It is important as the more likely to be the source of diagnostic error.

**Joint incidence.** The knee is the joint most commonly implicated in either variety.

### SOLITARY EXOSTOSIS

**Aetiology.** It is presumed that a fragment of the growth plate becomes displaced and gives rise to a cartilage-capped bony exostosis. It is presumed also that displacement of the fragment is related to muscular activity. It will not have escaped unnoticed and cannot be without significance that a solitary exostosis is encountered most commonly on the medial, as opposed to the lateral, aspect of the tibial head (Figs 14,1 to 14,4). On the medial side is located the insertion of the sartorius, gracilis and semitendinosus—

the pes anserinus. It seems likely that the insertion of these tendons is implicated; and to the extent that the avulsion of tissue with growth potential is the explanation. Although Jaffe (1958) states that there is no significant sex difference in the incidence, it is the impression (which cannot however be substantiated) that males predominate in the cases treated; and this would be related to greater physical activity. It is unlikely to be coincidental that the case illustrated in Figure 14,3 had, in addition, a traction epiphysitis (Osgood-Schlatter's disease) on the same side.

**Pathological Anatomy.**

Osteocartilaginous exostoses take one of two forms: **sessile** or **pedunculated.**

**Sessile.** The contour of a sessile lesion may be smooth (Fig. 14,3) or, in other instances, irregular. This is the variety of solitary exostosis most likely to produce some alteration in the architecture of the tibial head (Fig. 14,3). Symptoms other than the knowledge of the presence of a lump are rare (Figs 14,5 to 14,7).

**Pedunculated.** This is the common variety. The stem varies in length and may or may not be capped by cartilage. Whether in the tibia or femur it points in the direction of the shaft of the bone and is usually bent towards the bone in the form of a hook (Fig. 14,9). It is commonly mushroom-shaped. It is this feature combined with the bending towards the shaft which is responsible in the tibia for the semitendinosis becoming locked beneath the hook.

The exostosis is covered by periosteum which is continuous with that covering the adjacent cortex. It grows by endochondral ossification on the inner surface of the cartilaginous cap after the manner of growth of an epiphyseal cartilage plate. As a rule growth ceases at the time of closure of the main epiphyseal plate; occasionally before maturity is achieved. The remnants of the quiescent cartilage cap can exist into adult life.

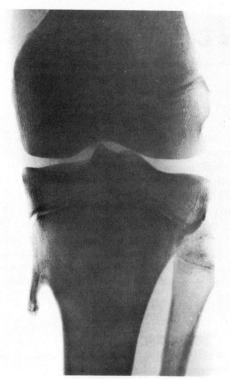

Fig. 14,1

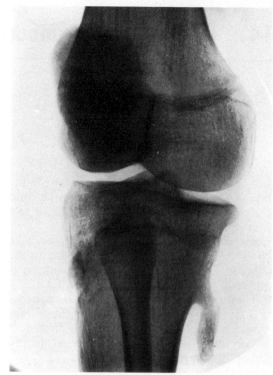

Fig. 14,2

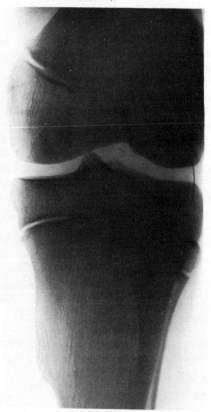

Fig. 14,3

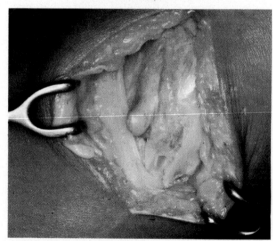

Fig. 14,4

Figs 14,1–4. **Solitary exostosis.** In the tibia the single exostosis occurs on the medial aspect of the medial condyle (Fig. 14,1). An exostosis of this length (Fig. 14,2) is liable to fracture as has occurred in this example. The sessile variety (Fig. 14,3). Note effect on contour of tibial head (see Fig. 14,9). It is of interest in relation to aetiology that this patient (G.W., male, aged 13) had a traction epiphysitis of the tibial tubercle on the same side.

A common cause of symptoms is interference with pes anserinus and particularly with the tendon of semitendinosus. The cartilage-capped exostosis exposed within the tendons (Fig. 14,4).

Note in all examples that the growth plates at the time of presentation were open.

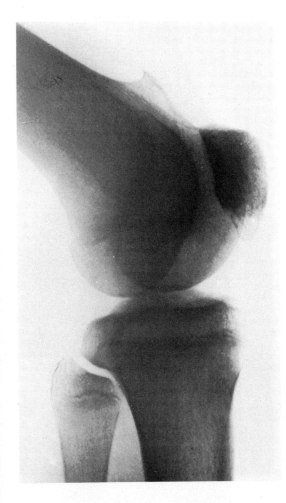

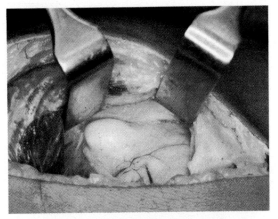

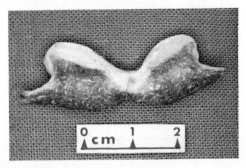

FIGS 14,5–7. **Solitary sessile exostosis.** This exostosis lay beneath the vastus medialis and interfered with movement (Fig. 14,5). Exostosis *in situ* with vastus medialis retracted upwards and laterally (Fig. 14,6). Exostosis split to show thickness of the cartilaginous cap (Fig. 14,7). (R.D., male, aged 16.)

## DIAPHYSEAL (METAPHYSEAL) ACLASIS (HEREDITARY MULTIPLE EXOSTOSES)

Diaphyseal aclasis is a common aberration of skeletal development. In those severely affected there is retardation of growth but otherwise it has surprisingly little effect on function. Complications are infrequent, but varied, the most serious of which is sarcomatous degeneration. In so far as the knee joint is concerned alterations in growth produce angular deformity which results in osteoarthrosis. Local phenomena include pressure on nerves and vessels and interference with action of muscles and tendons (Figs 14,12 to 14,14).

**Sex incidence.** This condition shows a definite predilection for males who account for 70 per cent of cases. It has been pointed out, however, that a proportion of unaffected females in families showing the disorder are able to transmit the disease. It is the fact that these latent cases show no clinical abnormality that is mainly responsible for the relatively low incidence in females (Jaffe, 1958).

### Aetiology

The condition has for long been considered to be inherited. Recent work has established the genetic background. Increased mucopolysaccharide excretion has been demonstrated

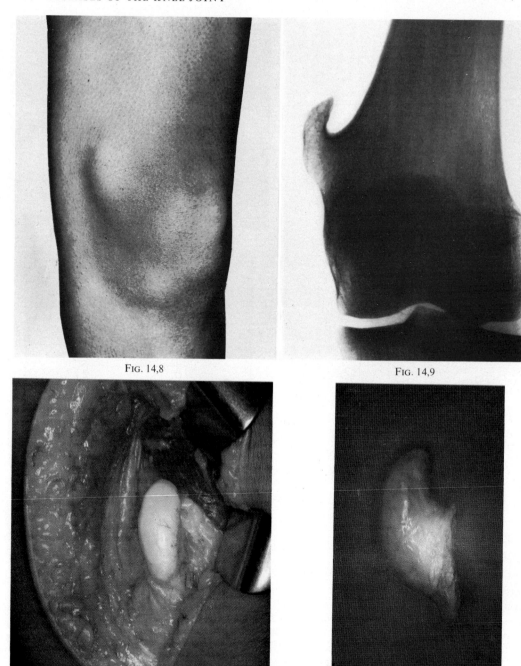

FIG. 14,8

FIG. 14,9

FIG. 14,10

FIG. 14,11

FIGS 14,8–11. **Solitary exostosis:** This example on the medial aspect of the lower end of femur produced a visible and palpable mass interfering with action of vastus medialis. Note effect of even single exostosis on conformation of related bone (Figs 14,8 and 14,9). Exostosis exposed at operation to show cartilaginous cap (Fig. 14,10) and to show shape in profile (Fig. 14,11) (M.L., female, aged 17).

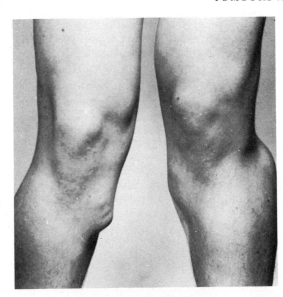

FIGS 14,12–14. **Metaphyseal aclasia: hereditary multiple exostoses.** The exostosis on the tibia on the right side was interfering with the action of gracilis, semimembranosis and semitendinosus. The exostosis arising in the head of the fibula on the left side was exerting pressure on the lateral popliteal nerve.

It appears that interference with the action of tendons about the knee does not occur until about adolescence and probably coincides with rapid skeletal growth. Note development of angular deformity on the left side. (J.A., male, aged 13.)

FIG. 14,12

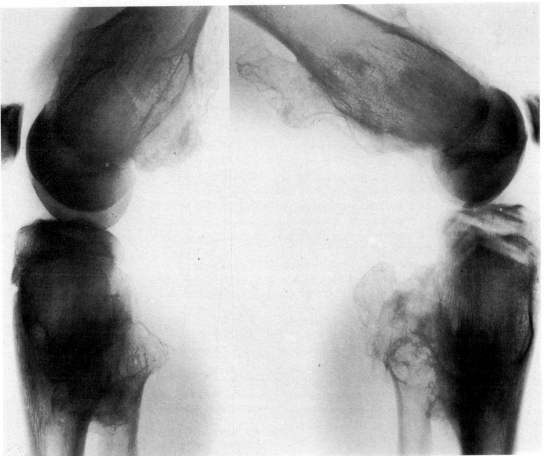

FIG. 14,13                                    FIG. 14,14

suggesting an underlying metabolic disturbance (Rigal, 1969). The experimental work of this observer has shown that the presence of the exostosis influences in the course of growth the shape of the entire bone in addition to the effect on local trabecular pattern. In the tibia bone is resorbed laterally and forms on the medial side between the growth plate and the exostosis. This has the apparent effect of bulging of the exostosis area medially producing a curved bone even in solitary examples (Fig. 14,15). The effect of the exostosis is three-fold: (1) it alters the local architectural pattern as well as producing a bony swelling: (2) it produces stunting of growth by acting in competition with the growth plate: (3) it deforms the outline of the tibia.

### Exostoses: Clinical Features

The patient with a solitary exostosis is usually in the age range 10 to 15, presumably as the result of rapid growth at that time. The commonest site is the medial tibial condyle. There may be no symptoms other than the presence of a lump. But symptoms can arise in a number of ways:

**'Snapping knee'.** The slipping of tendon, usually that of semitendinosus, over an exostosis can produce a well-marked 'snap' and has been known to be confused with that produced by a torn meniscus. On the lateral side of the joint confusion with the symptoms produced by a congenital discoid meniscus has occurred.

**'Pseudo-locking'.** A sharp-pointed exostosis may button-hole the pes anserinus or a tendon, usually that of semitendinosus, may become immobilised on the inferior surface of an exostosis producing fixation of the joint in some degree of flexion. Both these complications are known to have been responsible for errors of diagnosis resulting in the excision of a normal meniscus, the 'locking' being erroneously attributed to a displaced longitudinal tear.

**Fracture.** A long pedunculated exostosis is liable to fracture near its base from exogenous trauma, or endogenous, in the form of local muscle action. If the existence of the exostosis is known the diagnosis will not present difficulty. If the patient is unaware of its presence, the sudden appearance of a large tender mass may occasion alarm (Fig. 14,2).

**Bursitis.** An adventitious bursa may develop in relation to an exostosis in contact with moving soft parts. The bursa, like bursae elsewhere, may be the subject of effusion or haemorrhage from trauma; or from infection.

**Popliteal aneurysm.** Nine cases of popliteal aneurysm caused by an osteocartilaginous exostosis of the femur in single or multiple form have been reported (Schoene, Berthelsen and Ahn, 1973). In most of the cases there was no cartilaginous cap on the exostosis: the protruding tip consisted of sharp cancellous bone. In the ninth case reported by Schoene *et al.*, there was a cartilaginous cap (Stevenson and Zuska, 1957). It was thought that the wall of the artery tethered at the adduction canal had been worn away as it pulsated against the osteochondroma.

In six of the nine cases recorded there was a history of superimposed trauma.

CLINICAL FEATURES. In all the cases described the existence of a mass in the popliteal space was known to the patient; and pain in the

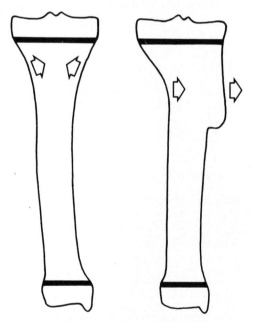

FIG. 14,15. **Exostosis: effect on conformation of tibia.** Diagram to show how the presence of an exostosis dictates bone accretion on the medial side of the metaphysis while normal bone resorption continues on the lateral side. As a result, the tibia becomes convex to the medial side (after Rigal). See also Figures 14,3 and 14,9.

region of the mass the outstanding complaint. The fact that the mass pulsated or a bruit was detected was noted in five of the examples quoted.

TREATMENT. Operative excision of the offending exostosis combined with operative repair of the defect in the arterial wall is the treatment of choice.

**Chondrosarcoma.** It appears that chondrosarcoma may evolve from the cartilaginous cap of an exostosis or out of the residium of the cap. It is said that the complication occurs in no more than 1 per cent of solitary exostosis but in more than 10 per cent of the hereditary multiple variety. The exact figure is not yet known. The area of the hip joint is more often implicated than the knee (Jaffe, 1958).

CLINICAL FEATURES. A sudden increase in size of a known bone mass should be regarded with suspicion.

TREATMENT. A chondrosarcoma in the region of the knee joint is readily accessible and does not offer the gloomy prognosis of osteogenic sarcoma. In general, as has been referred to elsewhere, the surgical decision should avoid conservatism; and in particular a joint not otherwise normal. The amputation should be performed well above the site of the lesion.

## Treatment: General, Single or Multiple

The known existence of a solitary exostosis which is not interfering with function is not necessarily an indication for surgery. The patient, however, aware of an abnormal bony swelling, may desire its removal on cosmetic or other grounds; and this should not be refused.

In other circumstances of interference with the action of tendons, vessels or nerves, the exostosis should be excised through a limited incision. In theory the local periosteal covering should be excised together with a proportion of the cortex from which it arises. If there is any question of a sudden increase in size a wide resection should be practised.

The presence of multiple exostoses is not a reason for surgical intervention. The indications for surgery are: (1) pain from pressure on moving structures or mechanical interference with the action of tendons or muscles or local pressure on nerves or vessels; (2) cosmetic

reasons: the osteocartilaginous out-growths are particularly noticeable about the knee joint and removal is justified on cosmetic grounds; (3) liability to recurrent injury; (4) the intervention of a complication.

TECHNIQUE. In theory the excision of the offending area should include the overlying periosteum.

### OSTEOCHONDROMA

A variety of osteochondromata varying in cartilaginous and bone content are encountered at the lower end of the femur calling attention to their presence in the patello-femoral joint by interfering with movement or producing a positive block to the completion of extension (Figs 14,16 to 14,19). At other adjacent sites the patient is conscious of the presence of a 'lump' which may or may not interfere with muscle action. With the exception of the last circumstance, in which some variety of bone tumour is anticipated, the diagnosis conforms to the pattern of bone tumour diagnosis in occurring as an unexpected radiological finding.

TREATMENT. In the example located in the suprapatellar pouch the tumour is approached through a limited lateral incision. When the extent has been defined the area from which it has arisen is excised with a margin of, say, 1 cm on all sides.

In tumours located within the confines of the quadriceps, new bone formation with related adherence of muscle, may pose problems of loss of flexion.

The following is an example of such a case. It is recorded with the purpose of indicating how persistent adhesion of muscle with resultant loss of flexion can be overcome:

The patient (G.H., male, aged 14, case of L.C.) first complained of loss of extension in the right knee coupled with the known existence of a swelling on the anterior aspect of the thigh immediately above the patella. On examination a bony tumour large mass could be palpated, and the radiograph (Fig. 14,20) identified the mass as an osteochondroma. At operation it was excised with an area of surrounding bone. The result, however, 18 months later was totally

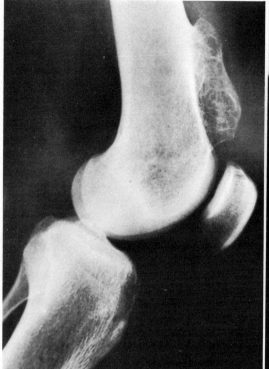

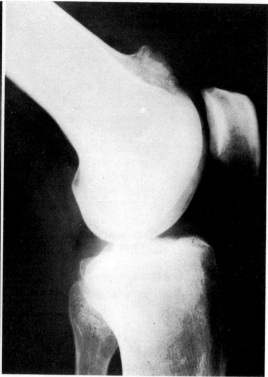

FIGS 14,16–17

FIG. 14,18

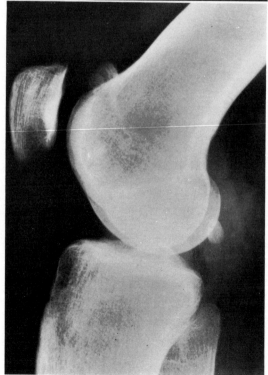

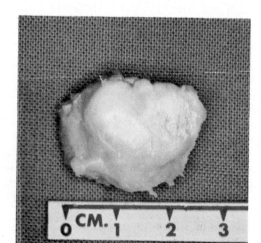

FIG. 14,19

FIGS 14,16–19. **Osteochondroma patello-femoral joint.**
Massive tumour producing block to extension (Fig. 14,16).
Smaller lobulated mass obstructing extension (Fig. 14,17).
Small solitary tumour interfering with action of patella
(Figs 14,18 and 14,19). (E.G., female, nurse, aged 23.)

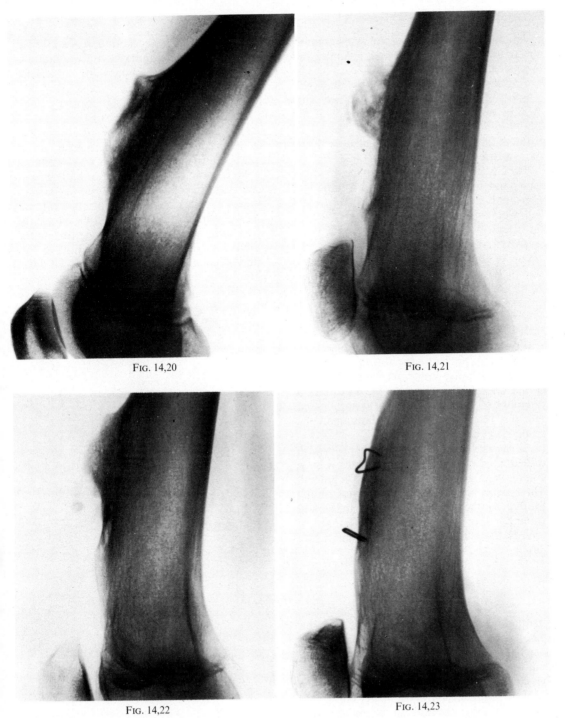

FIG. 14,20

FIG. 14,21

FIG. 14,22

FIG. 14,23

FIGS 14,20–23. **Osteochondroma.** This simple tumour on the anterior aspect of the lower end of femoral shaft produced a large mass in the quadriceps (Fig. 14,20). Two months after excision there was evidence of new bone formation (Fig. 14,21). The result 18 months later. The new bone limited flexion to 30° (Fig. 14,22). The appearance three months later following re-excision of the mass and the application of a Teflon sheet to the operation site. The staples secured the Teflon sheet in position. At the time of this radiograph the patient had regained a full range of flexion (Fig. 14,23). (G.H., male, aged 14.)

unsatisfactory from the patient's viewpoint in so far as that whereas he had regained full extension, flexion was limited to 30°. The radiograph (Fig. 14,22) showed that there was a mass of new bone at the operation site. It was presumed that as a result of the stimulus of early movement new bone had formed. There was no radiological evidence of a recurrence of the tumour.

The situation, amounting from the practical viewpoint to myositis ossificans traumatica, indicated that excision was likely to be followed by further production of new bone. At operation the mass of heterotopic bone was excised, but on this occasion a sheet of teflon of a size about 12 cm by 9 cm and completely covering the raw area was applied to the femoral surface and stapled in position in a similar manner to that described in synovectomy (Ch. 6). It was hoped that the interposition membrane would stop the formation of new bone; but in addition, and in any event, prevent adhesion of the vastus intermedius to the femur. At the termination of the operation it was possible to obtain a full range of passive flexion. It was anticipated that if a return of flexion was obtained the teflon sheet could be removed.

At the end of three months there was no evidence of reformation of bone and a complete range of flexion had been regained. The patient was at that time playing rugby football for the school XV with the teflon and staples *in situ* (Fig. 14,23). It is proposed to remove the teflon and staples at some future date.

## SOLITARY BONE CYST

**Definition.** The solitary bone cyst is not a tumour in the strict sense of this description but is covered by the description of 'tumour-like' conditions of bone.

**Bone incidence.** The common site is the proximal half of the humeral shaft. The lower end of the femur, as in the example to be recorded, is unusual.

**Aetiology.** The origin of the cyst is unknown. The theory that it is of traumatic origin, the result of an intramedullary haemorrhage, seems

unlikely in so far as the common situation is the upper end of the humeral shaft, a site less liable to trauma than the bones about the knee joint (Jaffe, 1958).
Report of a case:

The only example encountered occurred as an unexpected radiological finding as is the usual pattern in tumours of bone. The patient (T.McC., male, aged 43, football coach) reported with persistent symptoms in the knee which he located to the patello-femoral joint. Clinical examination confirmed the site of the symptoms; and there was pain on pressing the patella against the femur. A tentative but unconvincing diagnosis of an area of local chondromalacia was made. The routine radiographs revealed the unexpected presence of the cyst (Fig. 14,24).

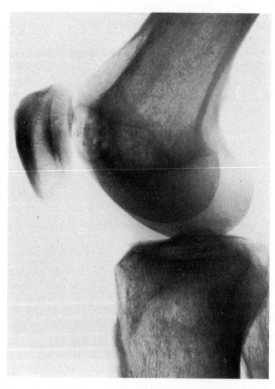

FIG. 14,24. **Simple subchondral cyst.** This solitary cyst gave rise to symptoms in the patello-femoral joint: a tentative diagnosis of chondromalacia was made. The routine radiographs revealed the unexpected presence of the cyst (see text).

The cyst was located in the lateral condyle and thus it was considered that a simple lateral approach would gain access and have the advantage of being non-destructive. An incision about the length of the patella was made on the lateral side and the patella retracted medially. A flat area was seen on the articular cartilage of the lateral condyle and a large hypertrophied tag of synovial membrane seen to be projecting backwards into the joint at the extreme limit of the infralateral margin of the patella where it joins the fat pad. This tag was thickened and injected and was large enough to have been of itself the cause of symptoms. The surface of the patella was smooth. It was decided that it would be possible to approach the cyst from the lateral aspect of the lateral condyle and thus avoid disturbance to the articular surface. The flat soft area in the articular cartilage was not of a degree of irregularity to be the cause of serious mechanical upset. A small gouge was entered on the lateral aspect of the lateral condyle behind the junction of the articular margin. The cyst was entered at the first attempt and the jelly-like content evacuated. The sclerotic margins of the wall were broken down with a hand gouge and the cyst thoroughly curetted. The cavity was then packed with bone chips taken from the ilium. The small incision in the synovial membrane was then closed over the gouge entrance and the wound closed in layers.

Recovery was unremarkable. When last seen one year later he had returned to football coaching and regarded his knee as normal.

## OSTEOID OSTEOMA

**Definition.** Osteoid osteoma (Jaffe, 1935) is a benign neoplasm the characteristic feature of which is severe but poorly localised pain.
**Bone incidence.** The lower extremities more frequently involved than the upper.
**Sex.** Males more frequently affected than females.
**Age.** The peak incidence is the second decade. Cases are seldom encountered over the age of 30 suggesting that the condition may be self-limiting.

**Relevance.** Unusual cause of pain in the knee particularly liable to misdiagnosis in that the severity of the pain, worst at night, is out of proportion to the physical and radiological findings.
**Radiological examination.** The essential radiographic feature is a zone of bone sclerosis surrounding a small area of translucency in the centre of which is seen a dense nidus of irregular calcification. In a recently reported case (Micheli and Jupiter, 1978) the lesion was located in the medial condylar epiphysis of the femur.
**Differential diagnosis.** The radiological features are not dissimilar from those of chronic bone infection in the form of a Brodie's abscess. Diagnosis depends eventually on the histological examination of the excised tissue.
**Treatment.** Accurate localisation of the lesion by tomography followed by excision of a block of bone containing the lesion is the treatment of choice.
**Histological findings.** In the excised material there is in general a circumscribed mass of irregular osteoid tissue within a vascular stroma of connective tissue containing osteoblastic cells. The demonstration of the presence of the nidus is essential to the diagnosis.

## TUMOURS OF PATELLA

Primary tumours of the patella are rare. Benign growths, exostoses and chondromata are even less common than malignant ones. Giant-cell tumour appears to be the most frequent neoplasm at this site.

Goodwin (1961) reporting a case of osteosarcoma states that this malignant tumour is rare in the patella. Christensen (1925), reviewing 1000 cases of bone tumours collected from the Codman Registry and from the literature, found only one case. Hambly (1959) put the number of acceptable cases in the literature at 13.
**Single exostosis.** This simple tumour may be less rare than is generally accepted in so far as, because of the unusual natural history, it may pass unrecognised as such. On clinical examination, and in radiographs, it may appear to be a sessile excrescence of periosteal new bone the result of trauma. In a true exostosis there may

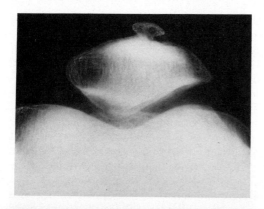

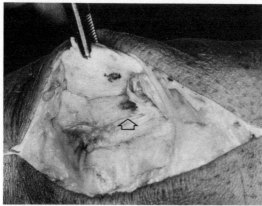

FIGS 14,25–26. **Patella: single exostosis.** This pedunculated simple tumour was readily seen in the skyline view (Fig. 14,25). At operation the mass of the exostosis, held between forceps, was lying parallel to the anterior surface with a bony pedicle, marked with an arrow, at the upper end (Fig. 14,26).

be a pedicle at the upper end; but the exostosis, instead of protruding outwards as is the usual pattern, is subject to the influence of knee flexion by the overlying skin and is thus flattened against the anterior surface (Fig. 14,26).

**Clinical features.** Pain due to irritation of the patellar plexus or a prepatellar adventitious bursa are presenting symptoms. The patient may, or may not, be aware of the bony swelling the nature of which may not be recognised unless lateral and skyline radiographs (Fig. 14,25) are obtained.

**Treatment.** The mass is excised through a limited lateral parapatellar incision. When the overlying fascia has been excised the existence of a bony pedicle may be revealed (Fig. 14,26).

## MALIGNANT AND POTENTIALLY MALIGNANT

The knee joint region is a common site for tumours of bone, simple or malignant. Fortunately malignant tumours are uncommon, almost rare, by comparison with the conditions with which this volume is principally concerned.

This is not the occasion for a review of the diagnosis and treatment of malignant tumours of bone. The principles involved are determined by the site in so far as it is accessible and with the possibility for a radical approach to treatment which may not obtain elsewhere. In such circumstances it is proposed to outline a practical approach to the problem, present the clinical features of certain classical examples and finally to quote a selection of cases to illustrate the problems encountered in a variety of tumours located at or about the knee joint.

### Clinical Features: General

There is no pattern. A diagnosis from clinical examination is possible only when the patient is presented at an advanced stage when pain, particularly night pain, associated with bony swelling accompanied by increase of local temperature, may make the diagnosis obvious. In other circumstances it is a radiological diagnosis in the course of a routine investigation often in the absence of any clear-cut pattern of symptoms or of positive clinical diagnosis.

**Diagnosis.** It has been indicated that in general tumours are an incidental, usually unexpected, radiological finding. Initially, therefore, the diagnosis depends on the opinion of a radiologist probably unconcerned with the ultimate decision regarding treatment. The value of the contribution of the orthopaedic surgeon depends on his experience, but particularly on his interest, in such matters. The experience of any individual surgeon must be limited. In such circumstances no effort should be spared to obtain the most expert opinion, radiological and pathological, and with reference to a Bone Tumour Registry where such exists, before undertaking treatment, local in the form of resection or radical in the form of amputation. In the latter circumstance, inquiry should be made as to the form it should take.

## Principles of Treatment

In the course of revising personal cases, those of colleagues referred to in the Preface, and of the considerable literature, it became evident that a radical aggressive attitude to tumours should be adopted. Orthopaedic surgeons are naturally conservative in outlook and are opposed to destructive procedures. They do not readily sacrifice a joint or ablate a limb. This outlook should not be applied to malignant tumours in the region of the knee. In the limited experience of the individual surgeon in such matters, and approaching the subject in retrospect, it is evident that the multiple operations necessitated by recurrence, the long periods of hospitalisation and of invalidism were due, in considerable degree, to the failure of the surgeon to adopt a sufficiently aggressive attitude in the first instance.

Radical measures to be considered are:

**Block resection.** Many tumours have a predilection for the metaphyseal region; and this is an ideal site for block resection of the entire tumour without destroying the continuity of the bone (Fig. 14,27). The defect can be bridged by a graft either sliding from above or elsewhere and the cavity obliterated with autogenous or homologenous cancellous bone (Fig. 14,28).

**Block excision/arthrodesis.** The decision to sacrifice a knee joint in favour of arthrodesis, or, even the entire limb in favour of amputation, are radical decisions, to be faced in circumstances which involve multiple operations, repeated hospitalisation, long-term invalidism, domestic and economic consequences, and indeed, risk to life.

**Amputation.** In highly malignant or aggressive tumours in the region of the joint treatment may require to be radical in the extreme. There are circumstances, however, when without the knowledge of the ultimate prognosis, a decision must be made whether a mutilating operation is advisable in the short-term view in favour of no treatment at all (see osteosarcoma).

### Indications

**Block excision/arthrodesis.** In any neoplastic bone growth, with the exception of such highly malignant tumours classified as osteogenic,

Ewing's and reticulum-cell sarcoma, the initial definitive operative procedure should offer the reasonable likelihood of cure. If the tumour is of a size, type and location, or has invaded the joint, so that local resection with preservation of the articulation is impossible, segmental resection of femur or tibia with sacrifice of the joint may be indicated if the limb is to be preserved (Fig. 14,29). The reconstruction of the site entails autogenous bone grafting with massive grafts of tibia or femur or both supplemented with autogenous bone chips taken from the ilium, with internal fixation by intermedullary nail, with screws and possibly circumferential wires (Wilson and Lance, 1965). The manner in which this may be accomplished is illustrated in Figure 14,30.

Block excision of tumour-bearing bone is indicated in the following circumstances (Parrish, 1966):

1. Recurrence of the tumour one or more times;
2. Tumour invading the joint;
3. Thinning or expansion, or both, of the entire cortical circumference;
4. Unclassified tumours with questionable malignant potential;

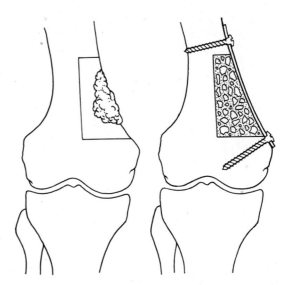

FIGS 14,27–28. **Malignant or potentially malignant tumours: treatment: block resection.** Tumours in the metaphyseal region (Fig. 14,27) are ideal for block resection and repair by sliding or autogenous graft supplemented by autogenous cancellous chips (Fig. 14,28). In young patients injury to the epiphyseal plate must be avoided (after Parrish).

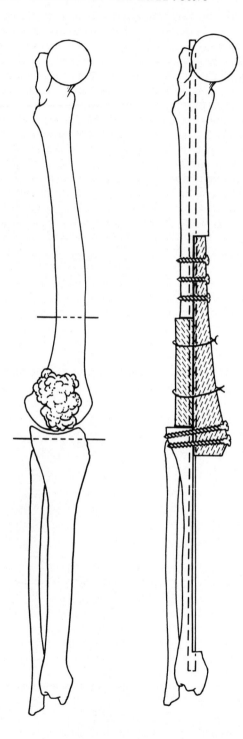

5. Tumours invading wide areas of subchondral bone such as multilocular lesions; and

6. Tumours with a natural history characterised by recurrence or tendency to become malignant with eventual metastasis after a period of years such as central chondroma in adults, giant-cell tumours of bone and parosteal osteoma.

## Operation

The principles and requirements for the resection-reconstruction operation as applied to the knee joint based on the recommendations of Wilson and Lance are as follows:

### Pre-operative Treatment

1. The diagnosis must be established with certainty, preferably by open biopsy.

2. The plan of resection and reconstruction must be prepared including measurements of the limits of resection, the size of the graft and the means of internal fixation likely to be required.

3. A 48-hour skin preparation of the operative and donor sites is advisable.

4. Prophylactic antibiotic therapy should be started 48 hours prior to operation.

5. Blood loss may be considerable particularly if a tourniquet cannot be used and the necessity for replacement should be anticipated.

### Operative Technique

**Resection.** (1) En bloc excision of the tumour-bearing bone with an envelope of soft tissue, including the biopsy wound, should be performed. (2) Adequate margins of normal tissue at the limits of resection should be confirmed by frozen section if possible.

### Reconstruction by Arthrodesis

1. Sound internal fixation is important. An intermedullary nail is the method of choice.

FIGS 14,29–30. **Malignant or potentially malignant tumours: treatment: block excision/arthrodesis.** If the tumour is of a size, type and location, or has invaded the joint, segmental section of the femur (or tibia) with sacrifice of the joint may be indicated (Fig. 14,29). Reconstruction of the site entails massive autogenous grafts and internal fixation by inter-medullary nail supplemented with screws and circumferential wires as indicated (Fig. 14,30) (after Wilson and Lance).

2. The defect should be bridged with massive sliding autogenous bone grafts supplemented with autogenous cancellous chips and with appropriate local internal fixation.

3. Suction drainage is advisable.

4. The overlying soft tissues should be closed in layers and the skin sutured without tension.

**After-treatment.** At the termination of operation a massive compression bandage is applied supplemented by plaster slabs in the outer layers for additional splinting and the patient nursed in a half-ring Thomas bed-knee splint. Antibiotic therapy is continued until the stitches are removed on the fourteenth day and the skin noted to be healed. It is at this time that a skin-tight plaster cast is applied. It will be recognised that the revascularisation of such massive grafts is a slow process and external support in the form of plaster cast, and later, corset-caliper, may be required for at least a year from the date of operation if the risk of fracture is to be avoided.

**Results.** In reporting the experience of a series of 20 cases treated by such methods over a period of 17 years (Enneking and Shirley, 1977), all of which united, there was one example only of local recurrence of the tumour. The 16 cases which survived (there were 4 deaths from metastases) were all ambulatory and active within the limits of arthrodesis.

## CHONDROMYXOID FIBROMA

**Definition.** The tumour, chondromyxoid fibroma, which is benign, received the name by which it is known from Jaffe and Lichtenstein (1948). It is important in that the histological appearances suggest chondrosarcoma. It is probable that until it was described and defined patients suffering from it had been subjected to unnecessary radical measures. Local recurrence, however, has been recorded; and this is what occurred in the case to be described.

**Joint incidence.** The areas most commonly

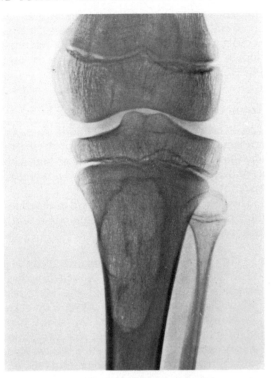

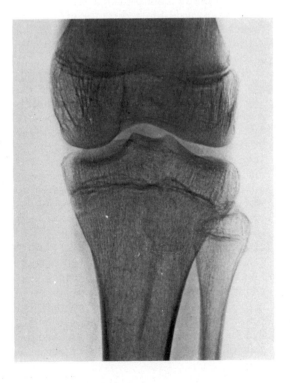

FIGS 14,31–32. **Chondromyxoid fibroma.** The tumour as originally presented (Fig. 14,31) and treated by currettage and packing with autogenous bone chips. The result six years later reflects the favourable prognosis in this tumour. Note virtually normal trabeculation of the bone (Fig. 14,32) (M.B., female, aged 9).

affected are the lower end of the femur and the upper end of the tibia. The lesion arises usually, as did the case to be described, in close relationship to the epiphyseal plate (Figs 14,31 and 14,32).

### Treatment

This is another example of a tumour classified academically as simple but with problems of identification. In such circumstances, and with a predilection for the metaphysical region, block resection is indicated.

The case record which follows demonstrates the practical difficulties encountered in both diagnosis and treatment:

The patient (D.McI., female, aged 11) (Hutchison and Park, 1960) presented with a swelling at the upper end of the left tibia which she had noticed several weeks previously. She complained of slight discomfort in the area but not of pain except on injury to the site. On examination the swelling was diffuse, firm to touch, and painful only on pressure or percussion. It extended from the joint line on the antero-medial aspect of the knee downwards for a distance of 8 centimetres (Fig. 14,33). General examination revealed no other abnormality and routine investigations were negative.

RADIOLOGICAL EXAMINATION. Radiographs showed an area of rarefaction in the antero-medial part of the metaphysis and with a multilocular appearance. There was a marked defect in the tibial cortex at the lower limit of which was subperiosteal new bone (Figs 14,34 and 14,35). A precise radiological diagnosis was not achieved. The provisional pre-operative diagnosis was that the cortex was eroded, and with the extension of the process into the soft tissues, raised a suspicion of malignancy. It was decided, therefore, to explore the swelling for the purpose of biopsy.

At operation a poorly encapsulated, lobulated tumour was revealed which had extruded through a defect in the tibial cortex and extended upwards as far as the joint line beneath the deep fascia. The cavity in the tibia had septa dividing it into compartments, the walls of which appeared to consist of relatively compact bone. When an attempt was made to curette out the cavity it was found that the upper limit was the epiphyseal plate. In view of the unfamiliar consistency of the cavity content the question of malignancy arose. It was for this reason that the cavity was not packed initially with bone chips.

The patient was kept under observation and radiographs taken at six-monthly intervals. The impression made was that the cavity was undergoing a slow obliteration. Two and a half years after the original operation, however, radiographs revealed that small cystic areas which had appeared in the lower part of the lesion were increasing in size. In the interval, bone growth had occurred and resulted in the lesion becoming apparently more remote from the epiphyseal plate. In such circumstances it was decided that a more radical operation could be undertaken without the risk of subsequent deformity.

At the second operation, some three years after the original, two cysts were located and found, as on the previous occasion, to have penetrated the cortex. The cysts and a zone of surrounding healthy bone was excised. The defect which resulted was filled with cancellous banked bone (Fig. 14,36).

The patient was last seen three years after the second operation and at that time there was no evidence, clinically or radiologically, of recurrence.

## ANEURYSMAL BONE CYST

**Definition.** This benign bone lesion received its name from Jaffe. In explanation he states that 'aneurysmal' relates to the distortion of part of the contour of the affected area of bone which produces the striking radiological appearance often presented by the lesion. The term 'bone cyst' relates to the fact that when the cyst is entered it is found to contain blood as was the experience in the example to be quoted.

Report of a case:

The patient (F.O., male, aged 23, case of J.H.) illustrates (1) the incidental finding of a tumour; (2) the difficulties of precise diagnosis

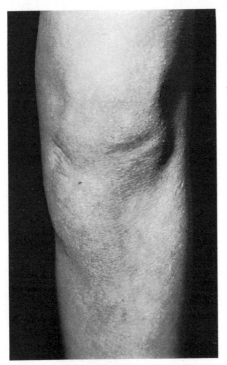

FIG. 14,33

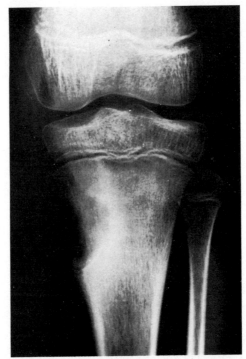

FIG. 14,34

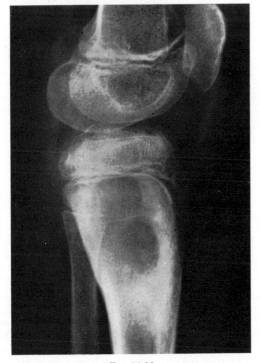

FIG. 14,35

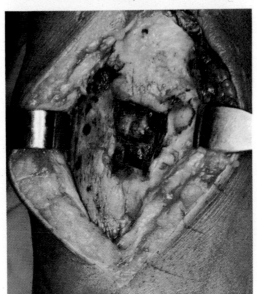

FIG. 14,36

FIGS 14,33–36. **Chondromyxoid fibroma.** This patient
(D.McI., female, aged 11) presented with a swelling at the
upper end of the left tibia (Fig. 14,33). The radiographs
showed an area of rarefaction of multilocular appearance
shown by biopsy to be a chondromyxoid fibroma (Figs
14,34 and 14,35). The window in the cortex showing the
tumour material and through which the cavity was eventually
curretted and packed with cancellous chips (Fig. 14,36) (see
text).

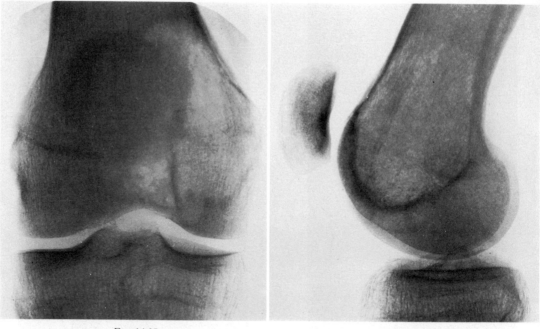

FIG. 14,37

FIG. 14,38

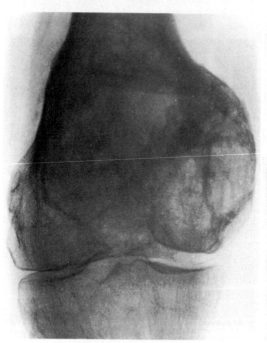

FIG. 14,39

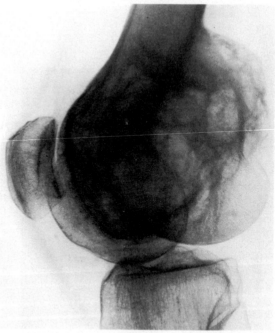

FIG. 14,40

FIGS 14,37–40. **Aneurysmal bone cyst.** The osteolytic lesion in the medial condyle was demonstrated by biopsy to be an aneurysmal bone cyst. Note pathological fracture with overlying periosteal reaction on the medial side. (Figs 14,37 and 14,38). It was treated initially by currettage and packing with bone chips; and later, when it was evident that the tumour was advancing, by irradiation. The radiographs (Figs 14,39 and 14,40) 18 months from the date of irradiation suggested that the destructive process had been arrested (F.O., male, aged 23; see text).

which can occur and (3) the problems which such lack of precision entail.

He gave a history that five weeks previously he received a hyperflexion injury not of great severity but which caused marked swelling of the joint. It had been treated by the application of heat.

On examination there was some wasting of his quadriceps, but no swelling nor tenderness of the joint. The only positive finding was pain on forced flexion. All the possibilities of internal derangement were considered, but no positive clinical diagnosis made other than of 'sprain'. The radiographs, however, showed a large osteolytic lesion involving the medial condyle of the femur with a pathological fracture through the cortex on the medial side (Figs 14,37 and 14,38). The latter finding explained what had happened in the hyperflexion injury: the swelling was the result of the haemorrhage from the fracture site. When the radiological lesion was discovered the patient was questioned further regarding his symptoms. He stated, in retrospect, that he had suffered a dull ache in his knee for some three months. All further investigations proved negative. The sedimentation rate was 4. It was decided therefore that a biopsy was indicated. At operation through an 8 cm skin incision over the medial aspect of the femoral condyle the cyst was found to be devoid of contents other than blood. A portion of the wall was taken for examination. It was reported to be an aneurysmal bone cyst.

It was decided in view of the extreme proximity to the articular surface and the implications for the future function of the joint, to pursue the matter of the pathology further before embarking on treatment. The report received was that the condition was one of a giant-cell tumour. Thus once again the well-known difficulty in defining this lesion arose and to which reference has been made by Jaffe. In such circumstances consideration was given to the possibility of block resection of the site as has been referred to elsewhere in this section. It will be evident, however, from study of the radiographs, that such a measure was impossible without destruction of the joint. It was decided therefore to employ curettage and packing with autogenous bone

chips. Unfortunately, seven months later it became evident that the tumour had not been eliminated, rather the reverse, and indeed it had broken through the cortex into the soft tissues. There was swelling palpable both anteriorly and posteriorly. Lateral radiographs confirmed that the tumour had broken out posteriorly.

The radiologist who reviewed the films suggested that a rescrutiny of the histology should be undertaken. The decision made, in consultation with the radiotherapist, was that the tumour should be irradiated; and this was carried out. Four months later radiographs suggested that further extension of the tumour had occurred. A surgeon consulted at that time was of the opinion that amputation should not be deferred. This decision was not acceptable to the patient. He was kept under observation at monthly intervals. At four months from the time of irradiation there was no longer any pain. The radiotherapist held the view that there was evidence that the lesion was attempting to heal. The attitude of the patient towards the lesion, in so far as there is no longer any pain, was further resistance to radical measures. In such circumstances there was no alternative but to continue to keep him under observation.

Reviews took place at two monthly intervals. Progress was better than had been anticipated. The last radiographs which are available (Figs 14,39 and 14,40) were taken at an interval of two years from the date of operation and approximately 18 months from the date of irradiation. They showed consolidation; and that the destructive process had been arrested. The patient was satisfied subjectively in so far as there was no pain. He had retained a range of 90° of flexion. Extension of the joint was complete.

## GIANT-CELL TUMOUR OF BONE

**Background note.** Giant-cell tumours of bone are rare and individual experience limited. In the most important recent review (Goldenberg, Campbell and Bonfiglio, 1970) an analysis of 218 cases from a multiplicity of sources was made using the strictest diagnostic criteria. It is largely upon the findings of this review, in so far as it concerns tumours in the region of the knee joint, that this section is based.

**Joint incidence.** The ends of the long bones which comprise the knee joint are the most common site of the tumour. In the series referred to there were 96 tumours so located out of a total of 222 lesions in 218 patients.

**Age and sex.** In the 57 patients with tumours of the distal end of the femur the age range was 16 to 58 with an average of 30. In the 39 patients with tumours at the proximal end of the tibia the age range was 13 to 62 with an average of 33. Skeletal maturity, as shown by closure of the epiphysis, was present in all cases; and this may explain the predominance of females in patients less than 20 years of age.

If the epiphyses are open doubt should be cast on the provisional diagnosis and the histological sections obtained at biopsy reviewed accordingly.

## Clinical Features

It has been indicated that there are no distinctive symptoms or signs related to tumours; and this applies to the giant-cell tumours. The most common complaint is of pain; and to possibly a progressively enlarging swelling. Local tenderness is a consistent finding if a tumour mass is present and is related to the degree of expansion of the tumour and the existence of cortical fractures. The presence of limp and quadriceps wasting is not specific but is indicative of proximity to the joint.

**Radiological features.** There are no characteristic appearances. The tumour appears as an expanded radiotranslucent lesion located in the epiphyseal end of a long bone in a skeletally mature patient in the age range 15 to 40 years. The related cortex is thinned, perforated or even fractured. The articular cartilage may be destroyed and invasion of the joint evident. The

FIGS 14,41–42. **Giant-cell tumour of bone.** It is unlikely that the tumour could be eliminated other than by block excision/arthrodesis.

When these radiographs were obtained the patient (C.S., female, aged 47) was under treatment for her knee symptoms by walking caliper! The outcome is unknown. Note that patient is skeletally mature; and the absence of osteogenic features.

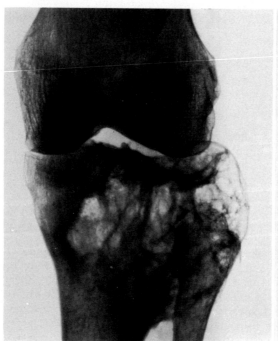
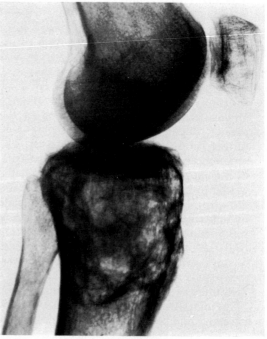

radiotranslucency is the result of destruction of cancellous and cortical bone. There is no stippling or calcification of the tumour mass. A giant-cell tumour is without osteogenic features except in the common complication of fracture (Figs 14,41 and 14,42).

### Diagnosis

**Biopsy.** The ultimate diagnosis is dependent on the result of histological examination of a specimen obtained at biopsy. In planning the biopsy it is necessary to anticipate the necessity for future definite surgery. The incision should be so placed that it is not re-entered but excised en bloc with the tumour mass.

### Treatment

**Resection with total replacement of the knee.** When block resection entails sacrifice of the joint consideration should be given to the possibility of replacement by a prosthesis. The Stanmore hinged total knee replacement (Ch. 6) is based on an original endoprosthesis designed to replace the lower third of the femur and upper end of the tibia. In all, 13 knee replacements have been specially made for the inpatients with tumours and tumour-like conditions (Wilson, Lettin and Scales, 1974). Initially fixation of the prosthesis to the bones was effected by plates and bolts. In recent years the plates have been replaced by medullary stems. The latest design (Ch. 6) is readily adapted for use in patients with destructive lesions about the knee. The standard prosthesis is altered by cementing an extension piece of the required length on to the medullary stem. The extension consists of a titanium type 160 tube into one end of which is bolted a titanium type 318 alloy stem (Fig. 14,43).

**Resection and bone grafting.** In view of the well known tendency for local recurrence following curettage and packing with cancellous bone

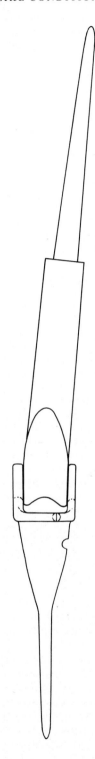

FIG. 14,43. **Tumours lower end femur: treatment.** Where sacrifice of the joint is necessary the possibilities of replacement should be considered. The Stanmore hinged total knee replacement can be adapted by extending the intermedullary stem with a titanium tube of the length demanded by the resection.

chips (85 per cent: Goldenberg, Campbell and Bonfiglio, 1970) and indeed as occurred in the example quoted, it is probably best to attempt block resection extending into normal cancellous bone on either side of the tumour, combined with bone grafting in the first instance. Occasionally block resection means that the joint as such must be sacrificed. In such circumstances arthrodesis is performed using a sliding graft from adjacent healthy tibia.

**Amputation.** In cases which appear to be malignant or have perforated the cortex and soft tissues or which demand such radical resection that joint function cannot be preserved, primary amputation is the operation of choice. In other circumstances amputation may be preferred to the prolonged convalescence necessitated by bone grafting or arthrodesis.

RADIOTHERAPY. Giant-cell tumours of bone are not notably radiosensitive; and the use of such therapy involves the risk of fractures (one case in four: Coley, 1949) and danger of post-irradiation sarcoma. It is to be employed only in cases which cannot be treated by surgical means. Experience has shown that the combination of radiotherapy and surgery is not to be recommended (Goldenberg *et al.*, 1970).

The following is an example of a case finally successfully treated by block resection and bone grafting after a recurrence following curretage and packing with bone chips:

The patient (J.McC., female, aged 27, case of G.M.) complained of pain in the right knee of 10 months duration. Following the birth of her fourth child 13 weeks previously the pain became suddenly worse. It was of a constant dull ache made worse by any physical activity. At the time the pain became worse she noticed a swelling on the lateral aspect of the leg below the knee. On examination there was a firm tender swelling of the lateral condyle of the tibia. Movements of the joint were full and free. There were no inguinal glands. Radiographs revealed an osteolytic lesion in the lateral aspect of the upper end of the tibia with an ill-defined margin on the medial side. The cortex appeared to be eroded and possibly penetrated on the medial side. The appearance is that of a giant-cell tumour. The biopsy was reported provisionally to have the appearance of a giant-cell tumour. Two weeks later the scar of the biopsy was excised, the tumour curetted leaving a thin and apparently uninvolved layer of the roof of the condyle. The joint was not involved and was not entered. The resulting cavity was packed with cancellous chips taken from the iliac crests. The immediate post-operative phase was unremarkable and she returned home in two weeks wearing a protective plaster cast. She was reviewed at intervals of three months. At the end of six months the bone chips appeared to have been incorporated in the main mass of the bone. She had no symptoms and a complete range of movement. At the end of 15 months it was thought possible to discharge her from review. Arrangements were made for follow-up radiographs in one year's time.

The initial success however was not maintained. Before the year had elapsed, and indeed approximately two years from the original referral, her general practitioner requested an urgent review of the situation in so far as she reported a return of pain of a deep nagging nature but which was not of a degree of intensity to disturb her sleep. He noted tenderness in the lower part of the operation scar and could induce pain in the previous tumour site by forceful hyperextension of the knee. Radiographs taken at this time revealed recurrence of activity in the lower part of the zone of reconstituted bone (Fig. 14,44). A further operation was recommended. On this occasion block resection was practised. The block, excised with reciprocating saw, measured $8 \times 2 \cdot 5 \times 2.5$ cm. It was confirmed that the limits of the defect so produced was radiologically normal bone and that the entire tumour had been excised (Figs 14,45 and 14,46). The cavity was packed

FIGS 14,44–47. **Giant-cell tumour of bone: treatment.** Appearance after recurrence of tumour one year after original curettage and packing with bone chips (Fig. 14,44). Radiographs taken at time of block resection (Figs 14,45 and 14,46). Radiograph two years later to show bone blocks used to obliterate the cavity. Note that some compression of the weight-bearing surface of the condyle has occurred (Fig. 14,47). The patient (J.McC., female, age 27) is known to be fit and well and with no recurrence four years from the date of block resection.

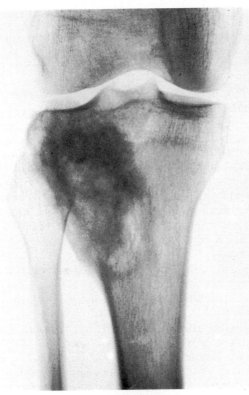

FIG. 14,44

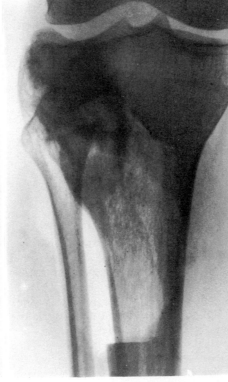

FIG. 14,45

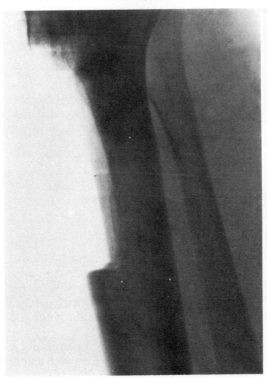

FIG. 14,46

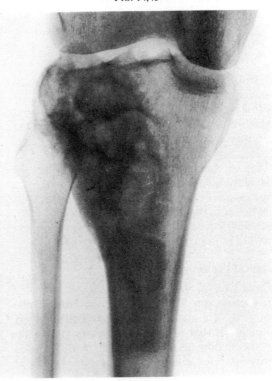

FIG. 14,47

with blocks of Kiel bone. Post-operative treatment was uneventful. She returned home three weeks later ambulant in a cuff-type plaster cast and with the use of crutches. In view of the implications of recurrence sections of the tumour were submitted for opinion to two authorities on bone tumours. It appears that the histological appearance was not without abnormal features. The concensus of opinion favoured a giant-cell tumour. 'All giant-cell tumours are, of course, potentially malignant and can recur or even metastasise without showing atypical histological features.'

Her further progress was entirely favourable. The plaster cast was discarded after four months had elapsed. Crutches were used for a total of six months to limit compressive forces on the grafted area. She was last examined two years from the date of resection. She walked without limp and had a full range of movements in the knee. Her ESR was 8. Radiographs showed no signs of activity. The bone blocks used to obliterate the cavity could still be outlined (Fig. 14,47). Two years later, that is to say four years from the date of block resection, she is known to be fit and well.

## OSTEOSARCOMA

**Definition.** A malignant tumour the cells of which form bone.
**Site distribution.** The ends of the long bones which comprise the knee joint are the most common sites (63 per cent: Jeffree and Price, 1976).
**Varieties. Central and parosteal.** The latter has the more favourable prognosis.
**Age range.** Two-thirds of the cases encountered are under the age of 25 (Jeffree and Price, 1976).
**Sex distribution.** There is a marked preponderance of males.

### Clinical Features

There are, as has been indicated, no early distinctive symptoms or signs indicating the presence of a malignant tumour. The common situation is that of a child complaining of pain in the region of the joint and possibly of a progressively enlarging swelling. Seen in advanced form the tumour is suspected. In other circumstances it is revealed by the radiograph.

### Radiological Features: Differential Diagnosis

**Subperiosteal ossification.** The anterior aspect of the femur immediately above the knee is vulnerable to direct injury most commonly a kick in a football game. Subperiosteal ossification may follow the haemorrhage produced by such trauma. A similar situation may occur in the bleeding diseases of haemophilia and scurvy. The importance of the appearance is the radiological simulation of osteogenic sarcoma particularly when there is no obvious predisposing cause.
**Myositis ossificans.** This condition in its various forms has certain similarities to osteosarcoma. The differential diagnosis has been described in Chapter 2.
**Pelligrini Stieda's disease.** This condition, the result of a sprain or partial avulsion of the upper femoral attachment of the medial ligament, is characterised by new bone formation, producing radiological appearances which vary from a thin elongated shadow in the **stable** type indicating raising of the periosteum, to massive new bone formation in the **evolutive** variety. These appearances can be alarming to a physician unfamiliar with the syndrome and particularly when the precipitating injury may be trivial amounting to no more than a twist. It is well-known as a source of misdiagnosis and of injustice in the industrial accident field. The location of the shadow is characteristic. A selection of the radiological varieties encountered are illustrated in IKJ5.
**Stress fracture.** The wide-ended bones which comprise the knee joint are not a common site for stress fractures. It is for this reason that the case recorded below gave rise to anxiety.

The patient (J.L., male, aged 17) was referred complaining of pain and swelling on the antero-medial aspect of the tibia below the left knee joint. The only possible related injury was a twist of the joint when he jumped down from a height. He thought nothing of the injury at the time.

On examination there was a bony enlargement of the upper end of the tibia with tender-

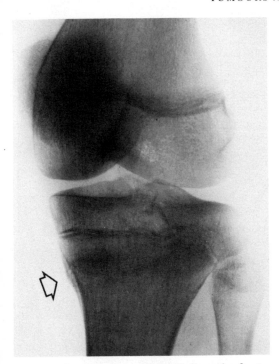

FIG. 14,48. **Stress fracture: differential diagnosis of osteosarcoma.** The clinical features of pain, bony swelling and tenderness together with periosteal reaction immediately below the epiphyseal plate on the medial side raised the possibility of osteosarcoma. The line of sclerosis running from the periphery obliquely across the tibia to the epiphyseal plate provided the clue that the appearance was that of a stress fracture (J.L., male, aged 17).

ness to pressure over the medial side where the swelling was most marked. No explanation was forthcoming as to the cause of the bony swelling. At the age at which the patient presented the possibility of a tumour arose. When the radiographs became available there was a marked periosteal reaction immediately below the epiphyseal line. There was, however, a line of sclerosis running from the periphery, where the periosteal reaction was present, into the epiphyseal plate (Fig. 14,48). The appearances were those of a stress fracture. No stress fracture had been encountered at this site previously; and thus the suspicion remained. His ESR, however, was normal and all other investigations relating to the possibility of tumour also proved negative. He was kept under close observation. Later radiographs, which were not of

a quality to warrant reproduction, confirmed with certainty that the condition had been a stress fracture despite the unusual site. The lesion healed rapidly and without residual disability.

**Infection.** A common cause of the raising of periosteum is infection; and the situation is complicated by the current indiscriminate use of antibiotics. On a number of occasions in the past, four of which spring to memory, cases considered clinically to be a osteogenic sarcoma were reported, after biopsy, to be osteomyelitis. The clinical assessment was the more accurate: all died of secondary deposits. Microscopical examination is a matter of opinion and no more an exact science than clinical opinion; it can be the less.

In the field of infection should be mentioned the chronic variety encountered in the form of Brodie's abscess. In common with osteosarcoma is the symptom of intense deep boring ache at night. An example of an osteosarcoma in which chronic osteomyelitis of this type was the provisional diagnosis will be quoted.

PALM THORN GRANULOMA: THORN INDUCED 'TUMOURS' OF BONE. In countries where palm trees abound but, indeed, anywhere where thorn-bearing bushes are common, there exists a problem of diagnosis related to the penetration of the knee joint by such thorns.

*Clinical features.* A child while playing falls on a palm leaf and a thorn (or thorns) penetrates the skin about the knee and breaks off (Fig. 14,53). A parent, examining the wound, may not see the thorn if it has broken beneath the surface, or may withdraw one that is visible and leave another that is concealed. A few days later he may complain of pain and develop a limp. There may be swelling at the site of penetration. A general practitioner presented with the case may find no evidence of trauma for by that time the entrance wound will have healed. There may be some synovial effusion and limitation of movement so related. There is no systemic reaction; no leucocytosis. The ESR is not raised. Aspirated fluid may reveal an increased number of leucocytes but is sterile. Radiological examination at this early stage reveals no abnormality (Cozen and Fonda, 1953). It is at a later date between the fourth and sixteenth week

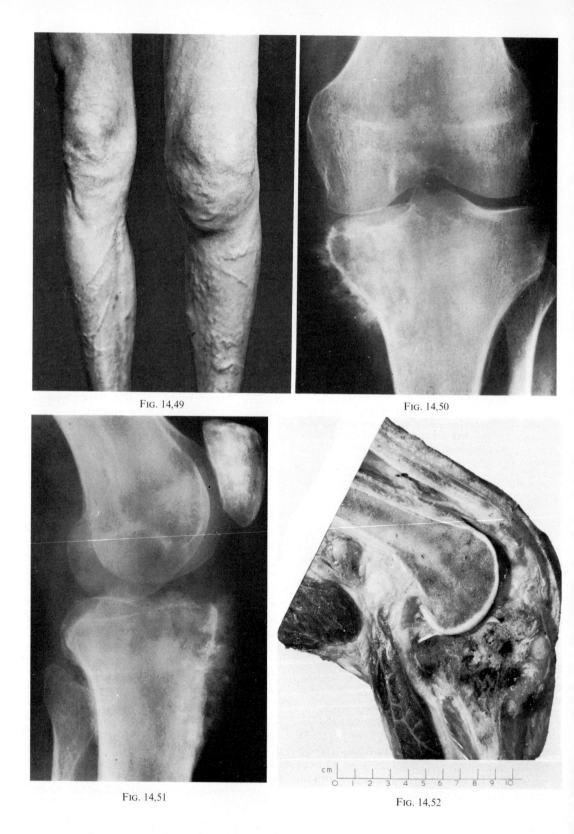

Fig. 14,49

Fig. 14,50

Fig. 14,51

Fig. 14,52

that even greater problems of diagnosis arise. There persists a painful swelling without reaction, local or general, and without leucocytosis or enlargement of related lymph glands. Moreover the radiographs at this time reveal an osteolytic lesion and/or periosteal reaction with appearances not unlike a malignant tumour (Maylahn, 1952). The situation in a child becomes particularly alarming when as a result of the length of the quiescent period before the secondary manifestations develop the causative accident has been forgotten.

*Diagnosis.* This diagnosis will be achieved only in circumstances of (1) a clear-cut history of the injury; (2) familiarity with the condition and (3) a high index of clinical suspicion.

*Treatment.* Exploration of the site and removal of the thorn results in rapid recovery.

The following is an example of a case reproduced by courtesy of Dr J. Harold La Briola, Los Angeles, California, who first drew my attention to the condition in the differential diagnosis of malignant bone tumours about the knee in children:

The patient, a boy aged 11, incurred a puncture wound of the left knee with a palm thorn. The thorn was removed by his family doctor on the day of injury. The wound healed without complications. One month later, when playing, his left knee became painful and swelling was noted that evening.

At examination two days later there was a minimal elevation of temperature of 99·8°F. There was a moderate synovial effusion. The joint was tender to palpation over the anterior surface. There was loss of complete extension. Flexion was limited to a right angle. There was increase in local temperature, but there was no erythema. The regional lymph glands were not enlarged.

Radiographs of both knees in AP and lateral planes were negative.

FIGS 14,49–52. **Fibrosarcoma.** This patient was referred with the complaint of 'recurrent swelling of the left knee' (Fig. 14,49). The radiographs (Figs 14,50 and 14,51) revealed an evident malignant tumour established by biopsy to be a fibrosarcoma. In spite of hind quarter amputation from which the specimen (Fig. 14,52) was obtained he died 8 months later reflecting the grave prognosis in this tumour in the past (W.C., male, aged 59).

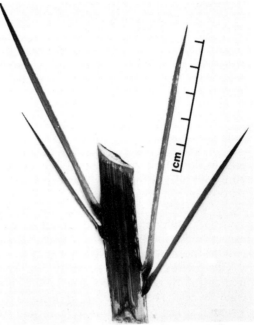

FIG. 14,53. **Palm thorn granuloma: differential diagnosis of sarcoma.** Section of leaf of Senegal date palm to show the lethal thorns which are 6 to 10 cm in length (by courtesy of Dr Harold la Briola, Los Angeles).

Aspiration of the left knee produced 20 cc of cloudy, serosanguinous fluid. Microscopic examination disclosed 'many' WBC's but no organisms. Cultures were negative in 48 hours. Blood examination revealed:

| | |
|---|---|
| Hgb: | 13·6 gm |
| WBC: | 12,000 |
| Segs: | 61 |
| Stabs: | 2 |
| Lymphs: | 35 |
| Monos: | 2 |
| ESR: | 30 mm/hr. |

Diagnoses considered were: (1) palm thorn granuloma; (2) pyogenic arthritis; (3) acute traumatic arthritis.

The patient was started on aureomycin 250 mg q. 6 hours prior to receiving the above reports. The limb was immobilised and bedrest prescribed. He continued to run an elevated temperature. The swelling and pain did not subside. On the third day the joint was again aspirated. The cloudy fluid again revealed many WBC's. Culture revealed anaerobic streptocci, Group A, Lancefield. A guinea pig was inoculated with the synovial fluid for acid-fast bacilli (this was reported negative two months later). On the sixth day 2 000 000 units of penicillin were injected intra-articularly and was followed by a moderate decrease in effusion and pain.

At this time synovial swelling was still present but there was no local heat, and pain only on motion.

Two weeks from the start of the illness and due to failure of the condition to subside an exploratory arthrotomy was carried out. At operation a granulomatous area containing a palm thorn was located within the synovial membrane in the antero-medial aspect of the joint. The pathological tissue, and the thorn, were excised.

The patient's post-operative course was uneventful. He returned to full activity within eight weeks. There was no recurrence of symptoms. The radiographs were normal six months later.

Cultures of the palm thorn were negative.

**Biopsy.** The ultimate diagnosis is dependent on the result of histological examination of a specimen obtained at biopsy. There is no evidence that this essential diagnostic measure is harmful.

## Treatment

**Chemotherapy.** The advent of powerful chemotherapeutic agents has changed dramatically the dismal prognosis associated with this tumour in the past. In the current, but changing, scene methotrexate alone or in combination with adriamycin are the drugs most favoured. Their use dictates the nature and timing of operative action in so far as resection with the use of an endoprosthesis (see later) may be undertaken rather than amputation. But if amputation is considered desirable, in so far as chemotherapy is most effective in minimal disease, the timing of operation is determined by the retarding influence of the drugs on soft tissue healing (Jaffe and Watts, 1976). The relationship of chemotherapy to radiotherapy is in the course of investigation. A definite synergism, as regards eradication of tumours, is said to exist between irradiation and high-dose methotrexate (Satow

*et al.*, 1976). If these potent drugs signal the arrival of a new era in the treatment of osteosarcoma it should be recognised that they exhibit an exceptionally high level of toxicity and with a mortality rate which varies from institution to institution but with an average of approximately 6 per cent (Jaffe and Watts, 1976). In these circumstances such chemotherapy should be undertaken only in centres staffed by experts in this narrow but highly specialised field.

**Metastases.** Recent statistics suggest that chemotherapy administered by various regimes will prevent metastases in about 60 per cent of cases. Many of the remaining 40 per cent are ultimately rendered disease-free as a result of an aggressive attack on their metastases by chemotherapy, thoracotomy and radiation therapy. Even if metastases appear, chemotherapy seems to decrease their number and thus render them more amenable to resection (Jaffe and Watts, 1976).

**Traditional methods.** If chemotherapy has revolutionised the treatment of osteosarcoma it is important that the principles underlining traditional methods be remembered. The tumour is located in an accessible extremity and thus there is a strong temptation to recommend immediate primary amputation. In recent years doubt has been cast on the wisdom of such a mutilating operation particularly in a child. In brief, the following sequence of events, based on the recommendations of Cade (1947) and confirmed (Sweetnam, Knowelden and Seddon, 1971), should be observed:

1. The diagnosis is established, with the degree of certainty which human error will permit, by biopsy.
2. The course of radiotherapy indicated is given.
3. The next step depends on the reaction to radiotherapy. If the local and radiological response is unsatisfactory there is an indication for amputation. Those cases which react favourably should be reviewed four to five months later at which time 75 per cent of those who will die have already developed pulmonary metastases. If there are no metastases there is a good chance of survival. It is this last group of patients for whom amputation is indicated.

The following are examples of cases so-treated.

**1. Femur.** The patient (K.R., male, aged 24, case of J.H.) was referred to hospital complaining of a painful swelling of the right knee which developed shortly after he started a new job as a tile-layer. Initially his general practitioner considered that his symptoms were related to this change of occupation, regarded the swelling as a possible bursitis and prescribed a crêpe bandage. The pain continued and in some degree of intensity. It was decided that radiological investigation was indicated. This revealed a lesion in the lower end of the femur. On first inspection it was considered to be a Brodie's abscess; and this diagnosis thought to be consistent with the night pain which was preventing him from sleeping. It was decided that the abscess should be decompressed. At exploration a week after his initial referral instead of the expected abscess a cavity containing a mass of soft tissue was found. The material was such as to cause suspicion that it might be neoplastic in origin. Histological examination showed that it was an osteosarcoma. He was treated by radiotherapy; and this resulted in a considerable reduction of pain. In addition, the tumour ceased to advance both clinically and radiologically. He was kept under observation and permitted partial weight-bearing using crutches.

Six months later the radiographs of the tumour remained unchanged. A skeletal survey and radiographs of the lung fields showed no metastases. It was at this stage, and observing the rules outlined above, that amputation was advised. The patient, who no longer had pain and in his own opinion greatly improved, was astonished that such a radical measure should be suggested. He refused operation. About this time, however, he developed pain in the knee due, it was thought, to increased activity and in an attempt to prove that amputation was unnecessary. The return of pain enabled some pressure to be exerted. Nevertheless, a month had passed, and further investigation demanded. No evidence of local spread (Figs 14,54 and 14,55) nor of pulmonary metastases was forthcoming. He agreed on mature consideration to amputation.

The final outcome is unknown.

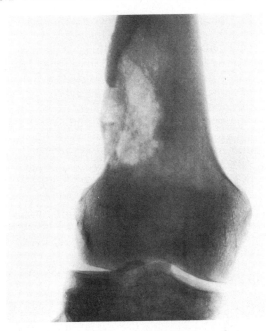

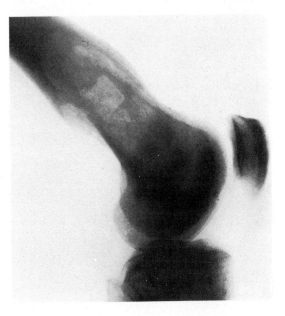

FIGS 14,54–55. **Osteogenic sarcoma.** Osteolytic lesion at lower end of femur is an osteogenic sarcoma. Radiographs following radiotherapy and immediately before amputation was performed (Figs 14,54 and 14,55) (K.R., male, aged 24, case of J.H., see text).

The window in the cortex is that of the original biopsy.

**2. Tibia.** The patient (G.P., male, aged 37, case of I.D.S.) first reported in February 1963 with a history of an aching pain of increasing severity just below the right knee for the past 6 to 8 weeks. Examination showed a diffuse soft tissue swelling over the lateral condyle of the tibia accompanied by increase of local temperature and tenderness to pressure. The antero-posterior radiograph showed increase of density in the lateral condyle of the tibia with a break in the cortex accompanied by new bone formation suggesting the presence of an osteogenic sarcoma (Fig. 14,56). Further investigations showed his chest to be clear of metastases. His blood picture and ESR were normal. He was informed of the seriousness of the lesion. He stated that he was prepared to accept whatever advice was offered.

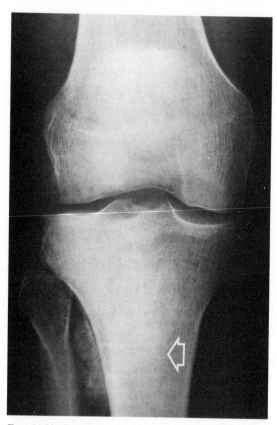

FIG. 14,56. **Osteogenic sarcoma.** Lesion at upper end of tibia is an osteogenic sarcoma treated by radiotherapy followed by amputation and known to be fit and well 12 years later (G.P., male, aged 37, case of I.D.S., see text).

A biopsy was performed which confirmed the diagnosis to be an osteogenic sarcoma. Intensive radiotherapy resulted in reduction of pain. It was at this point, some three months since first reporting, that he returned to his work which was that of a postal clerk.

He was reviewed at monthly intervals when routine local and chest radiographs were obtained. In October, eight months since beginning treatment and in the absence of metastases in the lungs, an above-knee amputation was performed. He was last seen in October 1975, 12 years from the date of amputation. His reason for reporting at that time was the development of pain in his left knee. He was worried lest the cause was the same as occurred on the right side. The symptoms were those of a horizontal cleavage lesion of the medial meniscus. When reassured as to the nature of the lesion he declined operation. At that time he was otherwise fit and well. His artificial limb was satisfactory. He was able to play golf.

## FIBROSARCOMA OF BONE

**Definition.** Fibrosarcoma of bone is a rare and distinct malignant primary neoplasm believed to arise from the connective tissue of the skeleton either centrally (medullary) or peripherally (parosteal).

**Incidence.** It is about one-third as common as osteosarcoma.

**Site distribution.** The ends of the long bones which comprise the knee joint are the most common sites (50 per cent: Larsson, Lorentzon and Boquist, 1976; Jeffree and Price, 1976).

**Age range.** The age distribution differs from osteosarcoma only in the absence of the juvenile-adolescent peak of osteosarcoma.

### Clinical Features

The most common presenting symptom is pain. There may be local swelling and limitation of movement in the knee. The tumour is osteolytic in nature. A pathological fracture is the presenting feature in about one-third of cases which is a much higher percentage than obtains in osteosarcoma.

The ESR is usually markedly raised.

**Radiographs.** The appearance is that of an expanded osteolytic lesion in the metaphyseal region on which is superimposed a spontaneous fracture in one-third of cases.

For differential diagnoses see 'Osteosarcoma'.

**Biopsy.** The ultimate diagnosis is dependent on the result of histological examination of a specimen obtained at biopsy.

## Treatment

Radical surgery in the form of amputation, supplemented by chemotherapy, immunotherapy and radiotherapy as may be indicated, offers the best hope of cure. See also 'Osteosarcoma'.

## DISEASES OF BONE

It is not intended to compile a catalogue of diseases of bone and their effect on the mechanics of the knee joint. There is, in any event, no pattern to be defined. It is evident that conditions such as osteomyelitis, poliomyelitis and general bone conditions with dystrophic effect influence the size and shape of the opposing condyles; and the earlier in youth the condition is manifest the greater is likely to be the resultant architectural abnormality. The effect of exostoses, single and multiple, on the shape of the bone and the conformation of the adjacent joint has been described. Nevertheless, reasonable function, particularly in terms of motion, is consistent with gross anatomical changes. Experienced clinicians continue to be surprised at the level of function experienced by patients carrying such deformities into middle life. It may not be until this stage is reached with progressive increase in weight and the superimposed related stresses that serious symptoms ensue. At the opposite extreme is the phenomenon whereby the deformed and paralytic knee joints of poliomyelitis have an apparent advantage over normal joints in that they do not develop osteoarthrosis; and the reason has been explained in Chapter 10. It is one more example of the maxim repeated throughout this text that clinical decisions relate to function and only exceptionally depend on radiological appearances. These observations do not apply to angular deformities acquired as a result of a disease process late in life when adaptive changes occur less easily. Even then, as has been shown, deformity in the form of varus angulation acquired slowly over the years is consistent with acceptable function. (See 'Paget's Disease', below.)

It is proposed to cite examples only of the effect of diseases of bone on the function of the knee joint, at one end of the spectrum a common condition Paget's disease, at the other, a rare condition Pyle's disease.

## PAGET'S DISEASE OF BONE: OSTEITIS DEFORMANS

### Gross Pathology

The condition as it effects the components of the joint is peculiar in that it effects femur and not tibia; tibia and not femur; tibia and patella and not femur; femur and patella and not tibia (Fig. 14,57). But if this is the accepted pattern there are exceptions. A case was encountered in the course of writing this monograph in which both tibia and femur were involved, the tibia in major degree, the femur in lesser degree but nonetheless definite (Figs 14,58 to 14,61).

Paget's disease entails an increase of blood supply in subchondral bone and therefore destruction of articular cartilage. It is thus a cause of osteoarthritis apart from the mechanical effect of angular deformity produced by the gross manifestations readily recognised on clinical examination. It appears however that gross osteoarthritis such as is encountered in the hip is not common in the knee; and this may be explained by the phenomena that the disease frequently crosses the hip joint but seldom crosses the joint of the knee.

In other circumstances the disease is encountered by surprise in routine radiographs taken in the course of investigation of a pain situation for which clinical examination did not provide an explanation.

Reference has been made to Paget's disease as a cause of increase of local temperature encountered in the course of clinical examination (Ch. 1).

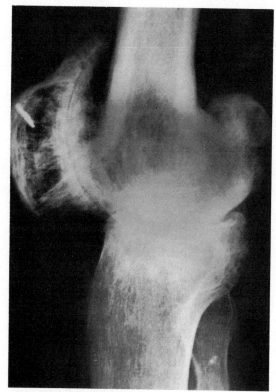

Fig. 14.57. **Paget's disease.** In this example the disease affected femur and patella. The tibia is not apparently involved. The destruction of articular cartilage of patello-femoral joint and to a lesser extent of tibio-femoral joint as indicated by the loss of joint space is due to the increase of blood supply in the underlying bone. The presence of a wire suture in the patella suggests that it has been the subject of a previous fracture. Note, however, that extension is complete. There was no angular deformity. The function of this knee as a result was reasonably good in spite of the gross radiological features.

### Clinical Features

The deformity encountered is varus angulation (Fig. 14,58); not, apparently, the reverse. The angulation reflects presumably the effect of the forces involved during the active stage of the disease when the tibia, less likely the femur, are plastic.

It is the common observation that even in severe varus angulation the complaint of pain is unexpectedly unusual; and this is said to be the result of the insidious development of the deformity and the gradual mechanical adjust-ments which take place in the process. Never-theless, there are exceptions when there is complaint of severe pain in the joint, loss of function from angular deformity and related stress fractures.

### TREATMENT

The basic pathology in Paget's disease, for reasons unknown, is the high ratio of bone formation and resorption. In recent years it has been shown that calcitonin lowers plasma-alkaline-phosphatase and urinary hydroxy-proline levels (Haddad, Birge and Aviolo, 1970; Neer *et al.*, 1970) and thus is effective in Paget's disease (Bijvoet *et al.*, 1970). It is not, however, the only available drug. It has been shown that the diphosphonates, which can inhibit crystal-lisation, crystal growth or crystal dissolution, all of which are concerned at some stage in bone mineralisation and bone resorption, can inhibit bone turnover which in Paget's disease is said to be as high as 50 times the normal rate (*Lancet*, Editorial, 1971). It has been demonstrated that the diphosphonates can produce a fall in plasma-alkaline-phosphate and plasma and urinary hydroxyproline levels far beyond the spon-taneous variations normally encountered in Paget's disease (Smith, Russell and Bishop, 1971). Furthermore, mithramycin, an inhibitor of RNA synthesis (Yarbro, Kennedy and Barnum, 1966), has been found to induce hypo-calcaemia by an inhibitory effect on osteoclasts (Parsons, Baum and Self, 1967). It is rapid in action. It is most effective in combination with calcilonin (Hadjipavlou *et al.*, 1977).

These are matters which remain in the experi-mental stage. There is already, however, evi-dence that this common, painful and often severely disabling disease can be controlled. There is even evidence of improvement in the radiological picture (Woodhouse *et al.*, 1972; Palmieri *et al.*, 1972).

**Indications.** In the current scene the indications for treatment are persistent, intractable pain unrelieved by simple analgesics; in repeated pathological fractures (Evans and Slee, 1977); and immobilisation hypercalcaemia. In such circumstances relief can be anticipated within a few weeks. Response should be measured bio-chemically as well as clinically. The most con-

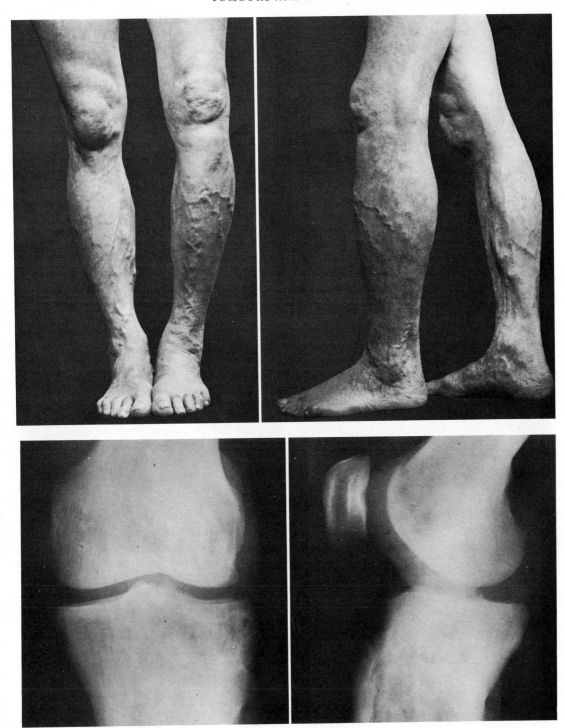

Figs 14,58–61. **Paget's disease.** If it is unusual for the disease to cross the tibio-femoral joint, there are exceptions. This patient had major involvement of the tibia and minor involvement of the femur (G.M., male, aged 60).

venient assessment measures the serum alkaline phosphatase concentration and the urinary hydroxyproline excretion which reflect osteoblastic and osteoclastic activity respectively. It is useless, and expensive, to continue calcitonin injections without evidence of continuing suppression of bone overactivity (Smith, 1977).

**Source of pain.** It is at all times necessary to distinguish 'Paget pain' from that of the osteoarthrosis which is the outcome of destruction of articular cartilage the result of hyperaemic disease process in the underlying bone. Calcitonin cannot be expected to influence pain of the latter origin. In this regard it is suggested that injection of local anaesthetic into the joint is a simple method of identification of source and saves the cost and time of a two-month course of calcitonin (Stevens, 1976). An alternative method is the effect of a two-day course of mithramycin (Heath, 1976).

A case treated with calcitonin while still in the experimental phase, but which resulted in dramatic reduction of pain, is recorded later.

### Complications

**Vascular.** Vascular disease is thought to occur prematurely and with increased incidence in patients with Paget's disease. Calcification of the popliteal artery is a common finding. This vascular disease is thought to be independent of 'high output' heart failure.

It is important that the possibility of vascular complications be recognised in a patient in whom operation is necessary. In such circumstances the number of bones involved should be estimated. The greater the number, the greater the increased vascularity which may represent a significant, and at times intolerable, burden on the heart similar to that of arteriovenous fistulae leading to high output failure.

The vascularity of bone may constitute a problem of haemostasis.

**Pathological fractures.** A characteristic feature of long bones affected by Paget's disease is the presence of incomplete, and often parallel, fissure fractures on the convex aspect of the cortex, in so far as the knee joint is concerned, in the upper half of the tibia (Fig. 14,62). In most instances they are symptomless but may be associated with pain and increased local temperature. They present the constant threat that a complete fracture may occur at any time.

The most common cause of admission to hospital is a pathological fracture. They are not as a rule close to the knee joint but such can occur (Fig. 14,63). The patella, however, when affected, is readily fractured (Fig. 14,64); and it is possibly not without significance that an earlier radiograph (Fig. 14,57) showing involvement of the patella indicates that at some time the bone has been the site of a fracture requiring internal fixation.

Union of fractures of the tibia, which are characteristically transverse, occurs rapidly and without the necessity for operation or internal fixation. Fractures of the patella may require internal fixation by the means described in IKJ5. Re-fracture, however, is common. A case has been encountered in which fracture without trauma occurred on three separate occasions at three different sites. In the circumstances of a second fracture consideration would require to be given to excision of the bone.

**Preparation for operation.** If operative procedures such as described below are required in patients with widespread disease the inherent hazards so-related are such as to demand preparation for operation. Since radiological improvement takes a year or more to become apparent a two-year course of treatment is necessary before surgery is contemplated.

**Osteomy.** Reference has been made to the necessity to distinguish between pain of vascular origin and that of osteoarthrosis of biomechanical origin the result of deformity. If calcetonin can be expected to relieve the former in a matter of two months there remains a residue of patients with varus and bowing of the tibia (Fig. 14,58) who continue to have pain in the knee or ankle or both. Such patients may be candidates for corrective osteotomy in the knowledge that calcitonin cover by decreasing vascularity of the bone and adjacent soft tissue reduces the hazards of operation.

**Technique of operation.** The technique advised is that of a V osteotomy apex upwards performed through drill holes and located at or about the apex of the deformity. If medial torsion is such as to demand correction a transverse linear osteotomy, performed also through multiple drill holes, is required (Meyers and Singer, 1978).

**After-treatment.** The original padded post-operative plaster cast is changed in favour of an above-knee skin-tight walking cast at the end of two weeks. This cast is retained for 8 to 12 weeks or until such time as clinical and radiological union can be demonstrated.

**Arthrodesis.** The considerable experience of arthrodesis reflected in Table 8 (Ch. 6) contains

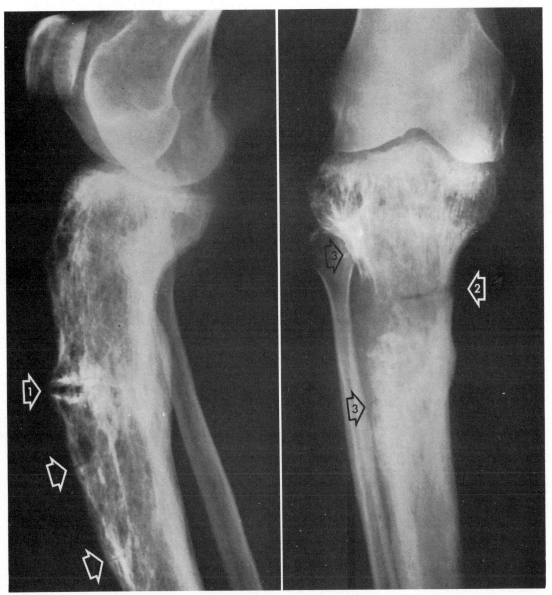

FIGS 14,62–63. **Paget's disease of tibia.** Example to illustrate the principal complications. Pathological fractures incomplete (1) (Fig. 14,62). Radiograph of the same patient four years later to show a complete fracture (2) and an osteolytic lesion in the form of a sarcoma (3) (Fig. 14,63) (H.L., male, aged 60: see text). The complete fracture has been superimposed on the sarcoma.

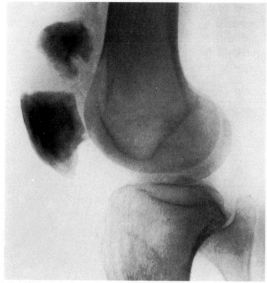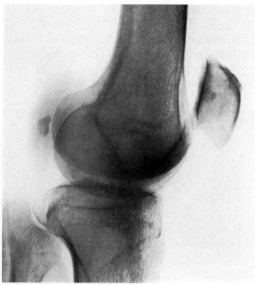

FIGS 14,64–65. **Paget's disease.** Spontaneous fracture of left patella sustained in the course of normal activity and without intervening trauma. The adjacent femur and tibia were not affected (Fig. 14,64); nor the opposing knee (Fig. 14,65). Note size of affected patella in comparison with the normal side.

A skeletal survey confirmed Paget's disease of the fifth lumbar vertebra and of the ilium, head and neck of the femur on the right side.

no example of Paget's disease. Whether this indicates the absence of clinical indications or whether it indicates unwillingness to accept the implications of the operation cannot be determined by reflection. The necessity and successful accomplishment of the procedure using the method of compression has been recorded (Barry, 1969). If the operation has not been undertaken personally, the immediate result of a successful fusion, using the compression technique, has been observed in the form of a stress fracture of the femoral shaft in the subtrochanteric region; but whether the fracture, sustained in a fall, was the direct result of the arthrodesis, known to be responsible for falls, or whether it occurred in the natural course of Paget's disease was impossible to determine.

It is, of course, a mistake to operate on symptomless deformities no matter how gross; and the most extreme examples are encountered. If, for mechanical reasons, operation is necessary, care should be exercised to remember the possibility, if many bones are involved, of high output heart failure; and, of course, the necessity for calcitonin cover.

It does not appear to have been recorded whether the disease, previously confined to one bone, crosses the joint after fusion.

## Sarcoma

**Incidence.** 'The tendency towards sarcomatous transformation sets off Paget's disease sharply from all other metabolic bone disease' (Jaffe, 1958). The exact incidence is unknown. Opinion varies between 2 per cent where there is minimal skeletal involvement and 10 per cent where skeletal involvement is widespread.

**Clinical features.** Pain is an early and striking feature of the complication. A complaint of increasing pain at a site known to be involved should be regarded with suspicion. Concurrently with the change in the pattern of symptoms is the appearance of a tumorous mass which grows rapidly.

**Radiological features.** An irregular subchondral osteolytic lesion appearing in a femur or tibia shown to be involved in Paget's disease should be regarded with suspicion [Fig. 14,63(3)].

**Treatment.** Radiotherapy is in common use as a

palliative measure in the hope of reduction of pain. Surgical treatment as applied to the complication in the region of the knee joint is synonymous with amputation which may be required for intractable pain but which in any event provides a chance of survival.

The following is an example of such a case:

The patient (H.L., male, aged 60, case of W.W.), on admission for investigation gave a history of pain and of deformity in the right tibia for the past 18 years. He had suffered numerous spontaneous fractures from minimal trauma. His main complaint was of gradually increasing but intermittent boring pain in the right lower limb below the knee, made worse by prolonged standing. He had noticed, in answer to the direct question, an increase in the size of hats he wears.

A year ago pain was such that he required large amounts of analgesics. He had been required to resort to crutches. He had no other complaints other than frequent nocturnal cramps and occasional episodes of palpitations which he treats with quinidine.

Ten years ago he had radiotherapy on several occasions to bones involved by Paget's disease and for the purpose of alleviation of pain.

On examination he was somewhat overweight. B.P. 140/85. Pulse rate 80/minute. Auscultation of the heart and chest were normal. There was no evidence of cardiomegaly or cardiac failure. The fundi were normal.

Examination of the right tibia revealed anterior bowing with increase in local temperature. On the left side there was lateral bowing of the femur.

Radiographs revealed Paget's disease of the right tibia with incomplete fractures in upper third (Fig. 14,62). The left half of pelvis, upper half of the left femur and the left humerus were involved also.

**Routine investigations.** Full blood count— serial Hb varied between 13·8 and 14·1 g per cent with normal PCV and MCHC. The ESR lay between 2 and 6 mm/hr. Platelets were present in normal numbers. The white cells count lay between 2·8 and 6·1 with a normal differential. Blood film was normal. Pro-

thrombin time ranged between 1 and 1·7 to 1 BCR.

On admission—calcium 9·1; magnesium 1·8; phosphate 2·85 mg per cent. Serum creatinine—0·95 mg per cent.

ECG was within normal limits.

Thyroid radioiodine tests showed an uptake of 16·4 per cent at 4 hours.

Serum PBI 3·8 and 4·2 micrograms per cent.

Alk. phosphatase lay between 221 and 328 iu/l.

Serum enzymes—LDH 173 iu/l. SGOT 12 and 15 iu/l.

Thymol turbidity—1.

CCFT negative.

Serum bilirubin—0·6 mg per cent.

Total protein—7·6 g per cent, albumin 59·6 per cent, alpha 1 globulin 4·1 per cent, alpha 2 globulin 8·4 per cent, beta globulin 13·0 per cent, gamma globulin 14·9 per cent.

Serum uric acid 4·8 mg per cent.

Serum cholesterol—195 mg per cent.

Acid phosphatase—5·1 iu/l with a prostatic fraction of 0·5 iu.

MSU sterile.

Radiograph of chest showed the heart to be enlarged, the CTR being 170/320.

**Treatment and progress.** Metabolic balance tests for calcium, phosphate, magnesium and creatinin with the use of faecal chromium markers, i.e. strontium administered for periodic strontium scans of the tibiae were undertaken. Treatment with calcitonin was coincident with remission of symptoms; he had no further recourse to analgesics. Coincidently a reduction in local temperature of the tibia occurred.

On return home he continued with calcitonin therapy. Alkaline phosphatase estimations were carried out at weekly intervals and remained during treatment in the region of 25 KA units. The reduction in pain was maintained; and the feeling of heat experienced in the tibia. There were side effects. These were negligible in relation to the benefit obtained.

Approximately one year after discharge

from hospital he reported that he had twisted his right knee. Examination revealed tenderness over the medial condyle of the tibia. It was thought clinically that the symptoms related to a further stress fracture. When radiographs were taken to confirm this suggestion it was noted that no new fracture had occurred. In comparison with old films, however, an osteolytic area was present which had not been noted previously [Fig. 14,58(3)]. The question of sarcoma was raised and biopsy performed. The decalcified section confirmed the bone to show the changes typical of Paget's disease on which was superimposed sarcomatous infiltration. A through-knee amputation was performed.

He survived for 18 months, thus reflecting the grave prognosis. Amputation was indicated primarily for pain. It has minimum effect on survival.

# PYLE'S DISEASE: CRANIOMETAPHYSEAL DYSPLASIA TARDA

**Definition.** This rare bone dysplasia is of interest in that it illustrates bone growth unmodified by the natural resorptive processes. During normal growth as bone is laid down in the metaphyses the calibre of the shaft is gradually reduced by internal and external resorption or modelling. As a result of failure of absorption of the secondary spongiosa normal modelling and funnelisation of the metaphyses fails to take place. The metaphyses in the tarda variety therefore appear splayed or widened as all the bone formed as a result of endochondral bone formation persists; but this becomes evident only after considerable growth has occurred (Rubin, 1964). Thus in craniometaphyseal dysplasia tarda, in contrast with the congenital form, the

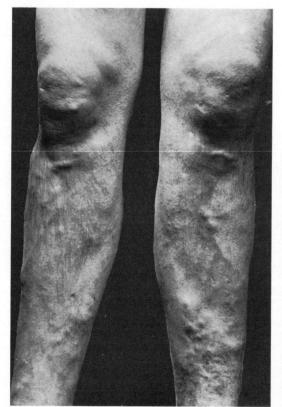

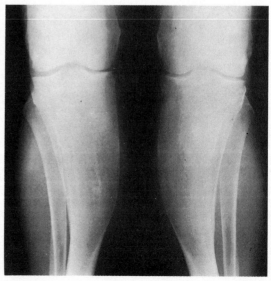

FIGS 14,66–67. **Pyle's disease (craniometaphyseal dysplasia tarda).** The clinical appearance, not grossly abnormal, suggestive of Paget's disease except that the deformity is symmetrical (Fig. 14,66). The radiographs to show Erlenmyer flask deformities of femora and the S-shaped deformities of the tibiae (Fig. 14,67).

predominant feature is splaying or widening of the metaphyseal regions of the long bones, well demonstrated in the distal femora which exhibit 'Erlenmeyer flask' deformities. The mid-diaphyseal portions of the long bones are not sclerotic in appearance and the cortices are only slightly thickened.

The diagnosis is based solely on the radiological findings which include changes elsewhere. In the cranium there are varying degrees of diffuse symmetrical hyperostosis of the vault and the base associated hypertelorism, prognathism and retarded or absent pneumatisation of the paranasal sinuses and mastoids. These changes are very similar to those found in 'leontiasis ossea' (Girdwood, Gibson and Mackintosh, 1969).

That such a bone dysplasia can have manifestations in the joint is illustrated by the following case:

The patient (W.J.M., male, aged 58), a slater, was involved in an accident when he fell from scaffolding injuring his left knee. The precise diagnosis remained in doubt for some time but, five months later, it was decided that the lateral meniscus was implicated and it was excised. It is not known whether the meniscus was the subject of pathological changes. The point at issue, and the reason for the author's involvement, was assessment of his residual disability for a Social Security Department: he had never attained more than right-angle flexion since the operation.

The salient feature of examination, apart from limitation of active and passive flexion to a right angle, was deformity at the upper end of the tibia particularly affecting the medial side. The immediate reaction was to consider the possibility of Paget's disease. The deformity however, was noted to be bilateral and symmetrical (Fig. 14,66). On questioning, the patient stated that the condition had always been present but had not troubled him previously. The appearance of the radiograph (Fig. 14,67) was that of the condition craniometaphyseal dysplasia tarda, so-called Pyle's disease.

The radiological appearance of the joint surfaces, as opposed to the flask-shaped expansion of the opposing bones, did not show a positive bony block to flexion. The exact reason for the loss of flexion remained in doubt, with the strong possibility that loss of flexion had existed unrecognised until the accident occurred. In such circumstances the acceptance of permanent loss of flexion was advised.

## REFERENCES

BARRY, H. C. (1969). *Paget's Disease of Bone*. Edinburgh & London: E. & S. Livingstone, Ltd.

BIJVOET, O. L. M., VAN DER SLUYS VEER, J., WILDIERS, J. & SMEENK, D. (1970). Proceedings of the Second International Symposium, 531, London.

CADE, S. (1947). *British Journal of Radiology*, **20,** 10.

CHRISTENSEN, F. C. (1925). Bone tumours. *Annals of Surgery*, **81,** 1074.

CLARK, P. M. & KEOKARN, T. (1965). Popliteal aneurysm complicating benign osteocartilaginous exostosis. *Journal of Bone and Joint Surgery*, **47A,** 7, 1386.

COLEY, B. L. (1949). *Neoplasms of Bone and Related Conditions. Their Etiology, Pathogenesis, Diagnosis and Treatment*. New York: Paul B. Hoeber, Inc.

COZEN, L. & FONDA, M. (1953). Palm thorn injuries. *California Medicine*, **79,** 40.

EDITORIAL (1971). Treatment of Paget's disease. *Lancet*, **i,** 955.

ENNEKING, W. F. & SHIRLEY, P. D. (1977). Resection—arthrodesis for malignant and potentially malignant lesions about the knee using an intramedullary rod and local bone grafts. *Journal of Bone and Joint Surgery*, **59A,** 233.

EVANS, G. A. & SLEE, G. C. (1977). Calcitonin for multiple fractures in Paget's disease. *British Medical Journal*, **i,** 357.

GIRDWOOD, T. G., GIBSON, W. J. A. & MACKINTOSH, T. F. (1969). Craniometaphyseal dysplasia congenita—Pyle's disease in a young child. *British Journal of Radiology*, **42,** 299.

GOLDENBERG, R. R., CAMPBELL, C. J. & BONFIGLIO, M. (1970). Giant-cell tumour of bone. *Journal of Bone and Joint Surgery*, **52A,** 4, 619.

GOODWIN, M. A. (1961). Primary osteosarcoma of the patella. *Journal of Bone and Joint Surgery*, **43B,** 2, 338.

HADDAD, J. G., JR., BIRGE, S. J. & AVIOLO, L. V. (1970). *New England Journal of Medicine*, **283,** 549.

HADJIPAVLOU, A. G., TSOUKAS, G. M., SILLER, T. N., DANAIS, S. & GREENWOOD, F. (1977). Combination drug therapy in treatment of Paget's disease of bone. *Journal of Bone and Joint Surgery,* **59A,** 8, 1045.

HAMBLY, E. (1959). Primary tumour of the patella. *Proceedings of the Royal Society of Medicine,* **52,** 576.

HEATH, D. A. (1976). *Bone Disease and Calcitonin.* Symposium Proceedings, p. 69, Armour Pharmaceutical Company, Ltd.

HUTCHISON, J. & PARK, W. W. (1960). Chondromyxoid fibroma of bone. *Journal of Bone and Joint Surgery,* **42B,** 3, 524–548.

JAFFE, H. L. (1935). Osteoid osteoma. *Archives of Surgery,* **31,** 709.

JAFFE, H. L. (1958). *Tumours and Tumourous Conditions.* London: Henry Kimpton.

JAFFE, H. L. & LICHENSTEIN, L. (1948). Chondromyxoid fibroma of bone: a distinctive benign tumour likely to be mistaken especially for chondrosarcoma. *Archives of Pathology,* **45,** 541.

JAFFE, N. & WATTS, H. G. (1976). Multidrug chemotherapy in primary treatment of osteosarcoma. *Journal of Bone and Joint Surgery,* **58A,** 634.

JEFFREE, G. M. & PRICE, C. H. G. (1976). Metastatic spread of fibrosarcoma of bone. *Journal of Bone and Joint Surgery,* **58B,** 418.

LARSSON, S. E., LORENTZON, R. & BOQUIST, L. (1976). Fibrosarcoma of bone. *Journal of Bone and Joint Surgery,* **58B,** 412.

MCGRATH, P. J. (1972). Giant-cell tumour of bone. *Journal of Bone and Joint Surgery,* **54B,** 2, 216.

MAYLAHN, D. J. (1952). Thorn-induced 'tumours' of bone. *Journal of Bone and Joint Surgery,* **34A,** 386.

MICHELI, L. J. & JUPITER, J. (1978). Osteoid osteoma as a cause of knee pain in the young athlete. *American Journal of Sports Medicine,* **6,** No. 4, 199.

MYERS, M. H. & SINGER, F. R. (1978). Osteotomy for tibia vara in Paget's disease under cover of calcetonin. *Journal of Bone and Joint Surgery,* **60A,** 810.

NEER, R. M., PARSONS, J. A., KRANE, S. M. & POTTS, J. T. JR. (1970). *Journal of Clinical Investigation,* **49,** 89a.

PALMIERI, G. M. A., EATON, B., BEAHM, D. E., JOEL, W., GROZEA, P. & HAWRYLKO, J. (1972). Effect of calcitonin and vitamin D on radiological changes in Paget's disease. *Lancet,* **ii,** 1250.

PARRISH, F. F. (1966). Treatment of bone tumours by total excision and replacement with massive autologous and homologous grafts. *Journal of Bone and Joint Surgery,* **48A,** 968.

PARSONS, V., BAUM, M. & SELF, M. (1967). Effect of mithramycin on calcium and hydroxyproline metabolism in patients with malignant disease. *British Medical Journal,* **i,** 474.

RIGAL, W. M. (1969). *The Growth Plate and its Disorders.* Edinburgh: E. & S. Livingstone Ltd.

RUBIN, P. (1964). *Dynamic Classification of Bone Dysplasias,* 1st edn. Chicago: Year Book Medical Publishers Inc.

SATOW, W. W., GEHAN, E. A., VIETTI, T. J., FRIAS, A. E. & DYMENT, P. G. (1976). Multidrug chemotherapy in primary treatment of osteosarcoma. *Journal of Bone and Joint Surgery,* **58A,** 629.

SCHOENE, H. R., BERTHELSEN, S. & AHN, C. (1973). Aneurysm of femoral artery secondary to osteochondroma. *Journal of Bone and Joint Surgery,* **55A,** 847.

SMITH, R. (1977). Paget's disease of bone, osteogenesis imperfecta, and fibrous dysplasia. *British Medical Journal,* **i,** 365.

SMITH, R., RUSSELL, R. G. G. & BISHOP, M. (1971). Diphosphonates and Paget's disease of bone. *Lancet,* **i,** 945.

STEVENS, J. (1976). *Bone Disease and Calcitonin.* Symposium Proceedings, p. 69, Armour Pharmaceutical Company, Ltd.

STEVENSON, C. A. & ZUSKA, J. J. (1957). Aneurysm of the popliteal artery from perforation by a solitary exostosis of the femur. A case report. *Journal of Bone and Joint Surgery,* **39A,** 431.

SWEETNAM, R., KNOWELDEN, J. & SEDDON, SIR HERBERT (1971). Bone sarcoma: treatment by irradiation, amputation, or a combination of the two. *British Medical Journal,* **ii,** 363.

WILSON, P. D. & LANCE, E. M. (1965). Surgical reconstruction of the skeleton following segmental resection for bone tumours. *Journal of Bone and Joint Surgery,* **47A,** 1629.

WILSON, J. N., LETTIN, A. W. F. & SCALES, J. T. (1974). Twenty years evolution of the Stanmore hinged total knee replacement. *Conference on Total Knee Replacement,* The Institution of Mechanical Engineers, London.

WOODHOUSE, N. J. Y., JOPLIN, G. F., MACINTYRE, I. & DOYLE, F. H. (1972). Radiological regression in Paget's disease treated by human calcitonin. *Lancet,* **ii,** 922.

YARBRO, J. W., KENNEDY, B. J. & BARNUM, C. P. (1966). Mithramycin inhibition of ribonucleic acid synthesis. *Cancer Research,* **26,** 36.

# Index